Nervous System and Neuroplasticity

Nervous System and Neuroplasticity

Edited by Ryder Dixon

hayle medical

New York

Hayle Medical,
750 Third Avenue, 9th Floor,
New York, NY 10017, USA

Visit us on the World Wide Web at:
www.haylemedical.com

ISBN: 978-1-63241-680-3

Printed in China.

Cataloging-in-Publication Data

Nervous system and neuroplasticity / edited by Ryder Dixon.
p. cm.
Includes bibliographical references and index.
ISBN 978-1-63241-680-3
1. Nervous system. 2. Neuroplasticity. 3. Neurosciences. 4. Nervous system--Diseases.
I. Dixon, Ryder.
RC346 .N47 2019
616.8--dc23

Table of Contents

Preface

Every book is initially just a concept; it takes months of research and hard work to give it the final shape in which the readers receive it. In its early stages, this book also went through rigorous reviewing. The notable contributions made by experts from across the globe were first molded into patterned chapters and then arranged in a sensibly sequential manner to bring out the best results.

The nervous system is the organ system concerned with the transmission of signals from one cell to the other, or between one body part to another. With the help of neurons and neural networks, the nervous system provides a point-to-point signal transmission and thus offers a high degree of specificity and speed. An incredible aspect of the nervous system is its ability to change with time. The adult brain does not have fixed neuronal circuits. Cortical and subcortical rewiring of these circuits and neurogenesis can persist up to old age. Synapses may weaken or strengthen over time, the proportion of grey matter may change, cortical remapping may also arise as a response to injury, etc. Neuroplasticity plays a crucial role in advancing functional outcomes with respect to post-stroke physical therapy. This book aims to shed light on some of the unexplored aspects of the nervous system and neuroplasticity, and the recent researches in this field. The various advancements in these fields are glanced at and their implications as well as ramifications looked in detail. This book, with its detailed analyses and data, will prove immensely beneficial to professionals and students involved in these areas at various levels.

It has been my immense pleasure to be a part of this project and to contribute my years of learning in such a meaningful form. I would like to take this opportunity to thank all the people who have been associated with the completion of this book at any step.

Editor

Mu Suppression Is Sensitive to Observational Practice but Results in Different Patterns of Activation in Comparison with Physical Practice

Najah Alhajri,[1] Nicola J. Hodges,[2] Jill G. Zwicker,[3,4] and Naznin Virji-Babul[5,6]

[1]*Graduate Program in Rehabilitation Sciences, University of British Columbia, Vancouver, BC, Canada*
[2]*School of Kinesiology, Faculty of Education, University of British Columbia, Vancouver, BC, Canada*
[3]*Department of Occupational Science & Occupational Therapy, University of British Columbia, Vancouver, BC, Canada*
[4]*BC Children's Hospital Research Institute, Vancouver, BC, Canada*
[5]*Department of Physical Therapy, University of British Columbia, Vancouver, BC, Canada*
[6]*Djavad Mowafaghian Centre for Brain Health, University of British Columbia, Vancouver, BC, Canada*

Correspondence should be addressed to Nicola J. Hodges; nicola.hodges@ubc.ca

Academic Editor: Thierry Pozzo

Research has shown the effectiveness of observational practice for motor learning, but there continues to be debate about the mechanisms underlying effectiveness. Although cortical processes can be moderated during observation, after both physical and observational practice, how these processes change with respect to behavioural measures of learning has not been studied. Here we compared short-term physical and observational practice during the acquisition and retention of a novel motor task to evaluate how each type of practice modulates EEG mu rhythm (8–13 Hz). Thirty healthy individuals were randomly assigned to one of three groups: (1) physical practice (PP), (2) observational practice (OP), and (3) no practice (NP) control. There were four testing stages: baseline EEG, practice, postpractice observation, and delayed retention. There was significant bilateral suppression of mu rhythm during PP but only left lateralized mu suppression during OP. In the postpractice observation phase, mu suppression was bilateral and larger after PP compared to that after OP. NP control showed no evidence of suppression and was significantly different to both the OP and PP groups. When comparing the three groups in retention, the groups did not differ with respect to tracing times, but the PP group showed fewer errors, especially in comparison to the NP group. Therefore, although the neurophysiological measures index changes in the OP group, which are similar but moderated in comparison to PP, changes in these processes are not manifest in observational practice outcomes when assessed in a delayed retention test.

1. Introduction

A common instructional method in the teaching of motor skills has been to watch repeated demonstrations with the intention of later reproduction, so termed observational practice or observational learning (for recent reviews regarding its relative efficacy, see [1–6]). Many individuals, perhaps as a result of injury, neurological impairment, or fatigue, cannot engage in physical practice, at least all of the time, such that learning through observation serves as an alternative practice method for motor gains [7]. Despite the potential efficacy of this approach, at least in comparison to no-practice conditions, the mechanisms underpinning its efficacy are still debated, as well as its relative benefits in comparison to actual physical practice. In this paper, we evaluate the similarities and differences between observation and physical practice, in terms of both behavioural performance and learning outcomes as well as neurophysiological processes assessed through EEG and mu rhythm suppression.

We now know that watching others perform skills that are part of their existing motor repertoire engenders similar cortical neural processes to those apparent during actual action execution. There is a considerable body of research pointing towards a motor simulation circuit or mirror-neuron system in the human brain that responds in a similar way to observed and executed movements, supporting the idea of a shared neural representation between action observation and action execution (for reviews, see [8–11]). There are a wide range of brain areas that are activated during both observation and execution of actions, with the primary regions including the ventral and dorsal premotor cortex (PMC) [12–16], the intraparietal cortex [13, 17] and the superior and inferior parietal lobule [14, 15, 18]. For a recent review of these areas, see a meta-analysis by Caspers et al. [19].

One index of mirror neuron activity that has been extensively studied in humans is mu (8–13 Hz) suppression. At rest, neurons in the sensorimotor area fire synchronously, resulting in large-amplitude EEG and MEG oscillations in the mu frequency band. When participants perform an action, imagine movement, or observe movements, these neurons fire asynchronously, decreasing the power of the mu band [20–25]. This suppression is known as alpha-band or mu-rhythm suppression (also related to event-related desynchronization (ERD)). It has been hypothesized that the mu rhythms reflect downstream modulation of primary sensorimotor areas by mirror neuron activity, representing a critical information processing function translating perception into action [26]. When comparisons have been made across execution and observation conditions, suppression is typically stronger in execution conditions [23]. For very simple movements (e.g., repetitive finger pointing [20]), as well as more functional movements (e.g., reaching and grasping a coffee cup [24]), bilateral suppression, particularly in central electrode sites, has been noted. Importantly, Virji-Babul et al. [27] showed that although both conditions activate similar brain areas, there were distinct differences in the timing and pattern of the activation. During movement execution, the earliest activation was observed in the left premotor and somatosensory regions, followed closely by left primary motor and superior temporal gyrus (STG) at the time of movement onset. In contrast, during observation, there was a shift in the timing of activation with the earliest activity occurring in the right temporal region followed by activity in the left motor areas, suggesting that there are important differences underlying the neural processes of action execution and action observation.

While there is now a significant body of literature linking perception and action in well-learned actions, studies looking at processes underpinning observation practice of new actions are still rather scarce. With respect to behavioural work, generally it has been shown that observation and physical practice can lead to similar behavioural (though weaker in observation) motor outcomes [4, 28, 29] (for a meta-analysis see Ashford et al. [30]). However, notable differences have also been reported. For example, although people learn from watching others perform novel visuomotor adaptation tasks, where people learn to move to radially aligned targets that are rotated from their veridical spatial position, observers do not show after-effects that are nearly always seen in physical practice participants [5, 31]. The absence of after-effects after observational practice has led to conclusions that the two modes of learning implicate distinct brain networks, with an absence or reduction in motor-system (implicit) adaptation following only observation practice.

There is also evidence supporting the idea that observation and physical practice involve similar "motor-related" mechanisms and networks. For example, in studies of sequence learning, observation learning effectiveness was specific to the observed hand [29, 32], suggesting effector-specific modulation of the motor system during observation. In studies where observers watched a learner adapt to a dynamic perturbation controlled by a robot arm, at least some of the observation learning effects appeared to be mediated by the observer's motor system (e.g., [33, 34]). This was shown through dual-task interference effects associated with performing a motor task during the observation practice phase as well as interference from a postobservation practice period of repetitive TMS (transcranial magnetic stimulation) to the primary motor cortex (M1).

There have been two general hypotheses concerning the transfer of information during observation learning [35]. The first is that information is primarily cognitively mediated (also termed late mediation), such that the motor system does not play a role in learning until the later physical enactment stage. The second is a primarily motor-mediated learning (also known as early mediation), whereby observation is thought to automatically activate the motor representations of the observed action in the observer's brain. This motor resonance or simulation is thought to allow for action understanding, and hence learning, to occur [35, 36]. Behavioural studies provide support for both proposals, suggesting that information transfer during observational practice could be a result of either or both processes. There have been no studies to date where measurement of both the neurophysiological and behavioural processes of observation and physical practice of the same task has been determined concurrently during both types of practice.

In relation to observational practice, Nakano et al. [37] recorded EEG signals during the observation, preparation, and execution of five trials of a two-ball-rotation task. Across all three conditions, mu suppression in the fifth trial was significantly greater than that in the first trial. However, no comparisons were made between a pure observation practice-only group and a physical practice group (i.e., after the first trial, the second observation phase was a combination of both observation and execution) and no efforts were made to assess learning, as based on a retention or transfer test [38, 39].

Neurophysiological responses have been probed during action observation under conditions where motor/physical practice experiences have already been attained. For example, EEG was recorded in professional dancers and nondancers while they watched video clips of dance movements and everyday movements. Expert dancers exhibited significantly more mu suppression compared to nondancers, with no difference between the two groups during the observation of everyday movements [40] (see also [41, 42]). However, Babiloni et al. [43] reported that long-term experience was associated with less mu rhythm suppression in action-observation-related areas during the observation of familiar actions.

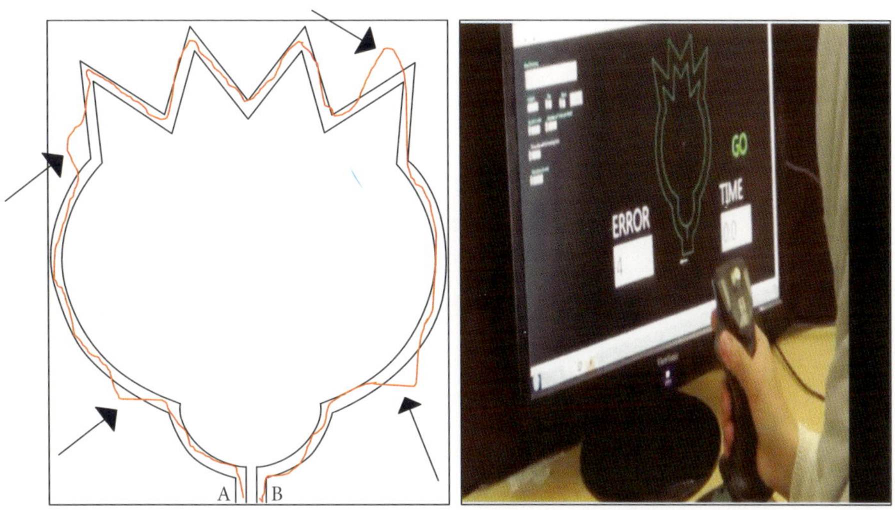

Figure 1: The flower-tracing task. Each arrow represents an error. The total tracing time starts at A and ends at B.

Despite evidence that physical experience modulates a subsequent observation phase with respect to EEG activity, to date, no researchers have studied how visual or physical/motor experiences with a novel motor task modulate EEG activity (specifically mu rhythm) during actual practice. Moreover, there have been no attempts to determine whether cortical activity changes noted in practice are evidenced in behavioural measures of motor learning, as assessed on a retention test. Therefore, in the present study, we compared short-term physical and observation practice during the acquisition and retention of a novel motor tracing task and evaluated how EEG mu rhythm is moderated during each type of practice. Our primary research question related to whether observational practice brings about change in EEG mu rhythm, comparable to that seen during physical practice, during "practice" of a novel motor task, and during a subsequent postpractice observation phase for both groups. To answer this question, EEG measurements were collected during either physical or observational practice across 45 trials of a flower-tracing task performed using a joystick. We also compared these two practice groups to a third, no-practice control group in a postpractice observation-only session. Relative to resting baseline, we hypothesized that mu rhythm would be suppressed at all the central interpolated channels for both the physical practice and the observation practice groups in comparison to the no-practice group, with greater suppression during physical practice.

Our second research question pertained to whether observational practice brings about behavioural evidence of motor learning, based on comparisons of the three groups in a delayed retention test. This delayed testing under the same conditions is regarded as a critical way of assessing motor learning, such that long-term effects of practice can be ascertained, uninfluenced by temporary factors associated with fatigue, motivation, or the conditions of practice [38, 39]. This delayed retention test was conducted without EEG, but all three groups were compared. We predicted that behavioural performance following physical practice would be improved when measured in a retention test compared to observation practice and no practice. However, if there are benefits to be gained from observation practice, we predicted that this group would perform faster and more accurately than the control group would. We expected that any differences in mu rhythm noted during practice and in the postpractice observation session would be evidenced in behavioural measures of motor learning as assessed on the delayed retention test.

2. Materials and Methods

2.1. Participants. Thirty healthy individuals between the ages of 19 and 40 years were recruited from the community. Participants were pseudo-randomly assigned to one of three groups with the constraint of $n = 10$/group and equal distributions of males and females (males = 3/group): physical practice (PP) ($M_{age} = 26.60$ yr, SD = 7.18), observation practice (OP) ($M_{age} = 24.4$ yr, SD = 3.37), and no practice (NP) control group ($M_{age} = 27.70$ yr, SD = 6.0). All participants were right-handed as confirmed by the Edinburgh Handedness Inventory [44]. They reported normal or corrected-to-normal vision, no motor problems, and no known neurological disorders. The experiment was conducted over two days, and informed consent was obtained from all participants according to the ethical guidelines of the University of British Columbia.

2.2. Motor Task. We used a computerized version of the flower-tracing task used in the Movement Assessment Battery for Children (MABC [45]). The flower figure was displayed on a computer screen using custom LabVIEW 7.1 software (National Instruments Co., Austin, TX). Participants were instructed to trace the figure between the two solid lines of the flower figure (Figure 1) as quickly and accurately as possible in a clockwise direction using a joystick. An error was registered each time the participant crossed beyond the two solid lines of the flower. The number of errors and

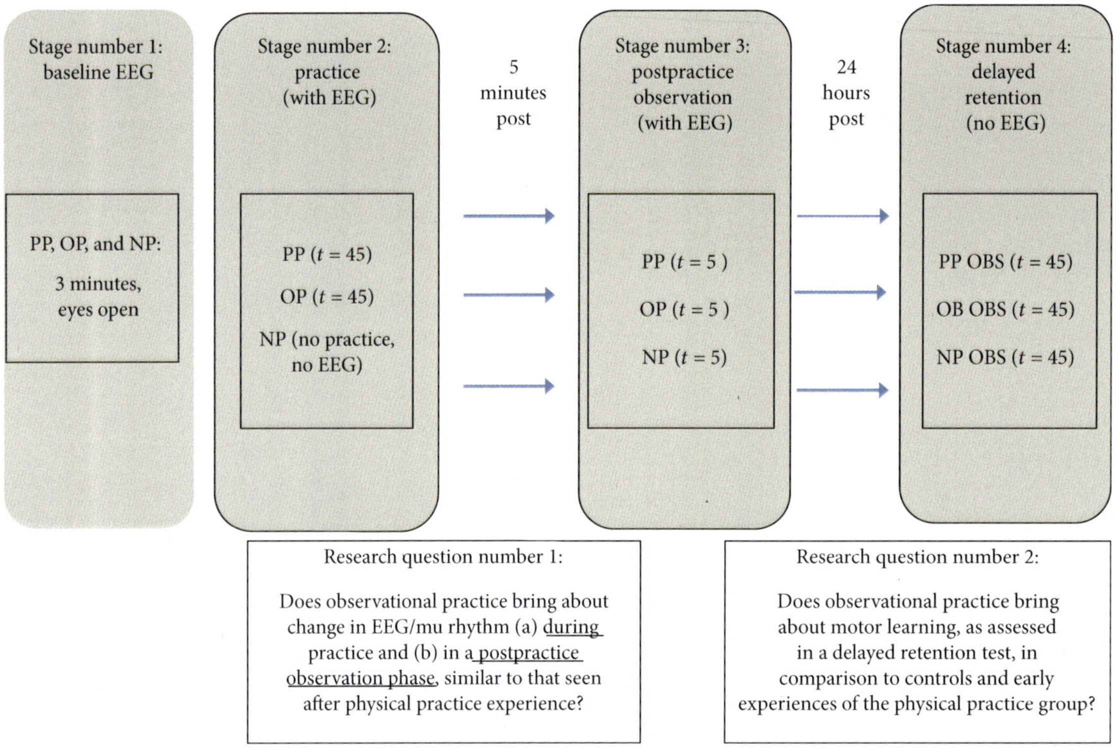

FIGURE 2: Research design and research questions.

the time it took the participant to complete the trial were displayed on the screen following each trial.

2.3. EEG Recording. EEG was recorded using a 64-channel HydroCel Geodesic Sensor Net with a Net Amps 300 amplifier at a sampling rate of 250 Hz via EGI software (Net Station, Electrical Geodesics Inc., Eugene, OR). At the start of the acquisition, impedance values for all EEG channels were less than 50 kΩ. The collected signals were referenced to the vertex (CZ).

2.4. Procedure. The experiment was divided into four sessions: (1) baseline EEG, (2) practice, (3) postpractice observation, and (4) delayed retention. Figure 2 shows the design of the experiment as well as the primary and secondary research questions related to the design.

2.4.1. Baseline EEG. Baseline EEG data were first collected on all participants for 3 minutes while they were viewing a blank screen. They were asked to keep their eyes open and to sit still without moving their limbs or eyes.

2.4.2. Practice Sessions

(1) Physical Practice (PP) Group. Participants were familiarized with the joystick by tracing a cross on the computer screen for 60 seconds. Once familiar with the movement of the joystick, they performed three blocks of the flower-tracing task for a total of 45 trials. Participants were instructed to trace the flower figure between the two solid lines using the joystick as quickly and accurately as possible. A 2-minute rest was provided between each block of 15 trials. EEG was recorded during all trials.

(2) Observation Practice (OP) Group. Participants in this group observed video clips of a model performing the flower-tracing task. The model in the video clips was right-handed and was a novice to the task. She was selected over several performers as she showed the least trial-to-trial variability in performance, yielding the most typical learning curve.

Each video clip represented one trial, with a total of 45 trials. Similar to the PP group, a 2-minute break was provided between each block of 15 trials. The video clips used in the observation trials were recorded at a resolution of 1280 × 720 pixels and a frame rate of 60 Hz. Additionally, the recording was from a first-person perspective, as this results in improved learning [46] and stronger hemispheric activation [47, 48] compared to the third-person perspective. Observers were instructed to refrain from any movement, and their behaviour was monitored via a video camera. EEG was recorded during all trials.

Participants were instructed to pay attention to the model's movement and were told that they would be doing the same task the following day. To ensure that participants were paying attention to the recordings, each participant was asked to state the tracing time or/and the number of errors made by the model at the end of each trial. These questions were randomized so the observers did not identify the pattern and focus on observing one measure on the screen.

(3) No Practice (NP) Control Group. Participants in this group did not receive physical or observation training. Participants in this group just completed the baseline EEG trials and the postpractice observation stage (as below).

2.4.3. Postpractice Observation Session. Five minutes after the training session, participants in the PP and OP groups viewed a video of the same model observed by the OP group performing the last five trials of the learning experience. The NP group began the session with the postpractice observation. All participants were instructed to pay attention to the model's performance. EEG was recorded as participants observed the model's movements.

2.4.4. Delayed Retention. Twenty-four hours after the training session, participants in all groups performed 45 trials of the motor task (again with 2-minute rests every 15 trials). No EEG was recorded during the retention session.

2.5. EEG Processing and Analysis. EEG data collected from each participant were processed and analyzed using Brain Electrical Source Analysis (BESA) software (MEGIS Software GmbH). Data were first manually screened for eye blinks and eye motion. Trials where eye movement occurred at the time of the task were removed. This resulted in approximately 10% of the total trials from all groups and all conditions being removed from further analysis. Data were filtered at 4–40 Hz and a notch filter of 60 Hz was applied. Independent component analysis (ICA) was then performed on the whole data set using an extended infomax algorithm for mixed sub-Gaussian and super-Gaussian sources in BESA. Using this approach, spatial topographies of the motion artifacts were first defined manually and then the brain signal topographies were determined. The artifact signal at each electrode was reconstructed with a spatial filter taking into account the artifact as well as the brain signal subspace. The reconstructed artifact signal was then subtracted from the original EEG segment.

EEG data were then transformed to a virtual montage using BESA. Virtual montages estimate the voltage at idealized locations of the standard electrodes into 27 channels using spherical spline interpolation. We used the 10-10 virtual standard montage. The average reference was computed for each time point as the mean voltage over the interpolated amplitudes of the standard virtual scalp electrodes. For each clean segment, the power in the 8–13 Hz range was computed using fast Fourier transforms (FFT). The data were segmented into epochs of 2 seconds for each trial in each condition. FFT was performed on the epoched single trials (1024 points) and averaged for each block in each condition to obtain the experimental mu value for each condition. For the baseline mu value, FFT was performed on one minute of the epoched resting state data. Using these values, the Mu suppression index (MSI) was calculated.

2.6. Mu Suppression Index (MSI). We calculated the ratio of the mu power in the experimental condition relative to the mu power in the baseline condition. The ratio is used to control for variability in absolute mu power as a result of individual differences, such as scalp thickness and electrode impedance [49]. Because ratio data are inherently skewed, a log transform was used for the purposes of parametric analysis [49]. The MSI is a change score of absolute mu power (8–13 Hz) between the baseline and experimental conditions. It was calculated as

$$\text{MSI} = \log \frac{\text{mu power experimental}}{\text{mu power baseline}}. \tag{1}$$

A log value below zero in the area of C3, C4, and CZ indicates mu suppression or activation of premotor or sensorimotor neurons and is considered an index of mirror neuron system functioning. A value of zero indicates no suppression or no change from baseline. Values above zero indicate synchronization or deactivation of the premotor or sensorimotor neurons, perhaps indicating inhibition of these premotor regions.

The MSI was calculated for each participant (using rest as baseline) for the electrodes C3, CZ, and C4. These central electrodes record the activity of the left, middle, and right sensorimotor regions, respectively.

For statistical analysis, we first compared MSI for the PP and OP groups in acquisition (stage 2) across 3 practice blocks ($t = 15$/block) and the three electrode sites. These data were compared in a 2 group × 3 electrode site × 3 block mixed-design ANOVA with repeated measures on the second and third factors. Our primary aim with this first analysis was to assess for group differences as a function of the type of experience (observation versus physical practice) as well as to determine any changes across practice blocks. Second, we compared the MSI values to zero for each electrode site to assess whether there was evidence of suppression for each group. This allowed us to determine at the within-group level, if there was evidence of suppression (and where based on electrode site). As such, we performed single sample t-tests (comparing against zero), with Bonferroni-corrected p values based on the number of electrodes ($.05/3 = .017$).

A second analysis was performed on the postpractice observation session (stage 3) for all 3 groups. Again, we first compared across groups (PP, OP, and NP) and electrodes in a 3 group × 3 electrode RM ANOVA, with repeated measures on the second factor. We also compared MSI against zero in single sample t-tests for each group and each electrode (again based on Bonferroni-corrected t-tests).

2.7. Behavioural Measures and Analysis. Two behavioural measures were used to assess learning: (1) error, which was denoted as the number of times the participant crossed out of the flower figure's bounds, and (2) total trace time, which was described as the time it took the participant to complete each trace/trial. These two measures were analyzed in retention testing in a 3 group (PP, OP, NP) × 9 block (5 trials/block), mixed-design ANOVA, with repeated measures on the second factor. Greenhouse-Geisser corrections were applied to violations to sphericity associated with the repeated-measures factor. Significant interaction effects were followed up with Tukey HSD post hoc comparisons ($p < .05$). Due to errors in processing, we were missing data from one control group participant (NP) and from one block of a PP

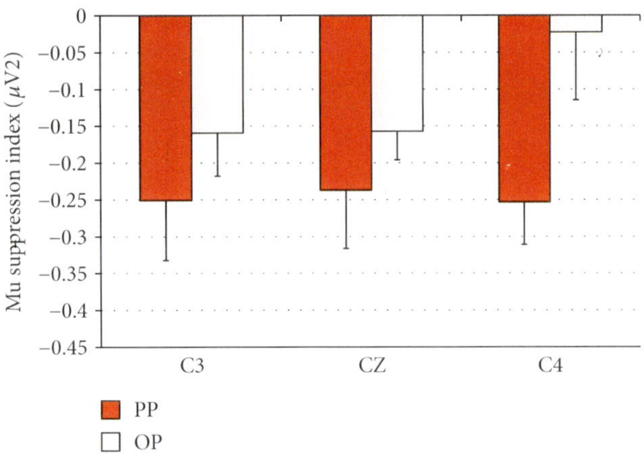

FIGURE 3: Mu suppression index during physical (PP) and observational practice (OP) (i.e., stage 2 testing) at the central interpolated electrodes C3, CZ, and C4. Values represent the mean log ratio of mu power at the frequency range of 8–13 Hz in the experimental condition compared to baseline. A ratio of negative value indicates suppression. Error bars represent standard error of the mean SE.

participant; these individuals were not included in the reported statistical analyses. As a check, we re-ran the analysis with the PP participant using estimated values (interpolating based on means for surrounding blocks), and this did not affect the behavioural results.

3. Results

3.1. Does Observational Practice Bring about Change in EEG Mu Rhythm Similar to That Seen after Physical Practice?

3.1.1. Mu Suppression during Practice for Both OP and PP Groups. In general, mu suppression across the two groups and across practice blocks and electrodes looked similar. The results of the mixed ANOVA on MSI showed neither significant main effects nor significant interactions (all $Fs < 1.37$, except the group main effect, where $F(1, 18) = 2.78$, $p = .11$, $\eta_p^2 = 0.13$). In Figure 3, we have plotted the MSI for the PP and OP groups for each of the three electrodes averaged across all trials. Based on comparisons to zero, there was evidence of bilateral mu suppression during PP, but only left lateralized mu suppression during OP. This was confirmed through single sample t-tests for both the PP and OP groups for each electrode, as displayed in Table 1. During PP, the average MSI at C3, CZ, and C4 was significantly less than zero. During OP, the average MSI at C3 and CZ was significantly less than zero, but it was not at C4.

3.1.2. Mu Suppression during the Postpractice Observation Phase. Comparison of the three groups during postpractice observation yielded a significant group main effect, $F(2, 27) = 9.68$, $p = .001$, $\eta_p^2 = 0.42$, but no electrode effect ($F < 1$). In Figure 4, we have plotted the MSI values for each electrode as a function of group. Based on Tukey HSD post hoc comparisons, the PP group showed more overall suppression than both the OP and NP groups and the OP group showed more suppression than the NP control group did. The interaction between group and electrode approached conventional levels of significance, $F(4, 54) = 2.52$, $p = .051$, $\eta_p^2 = 0.26$. As can be seen in Figure 4 and based on Tukey post hoc comparisons, the PP group displayed significantly greater MSI compared to the NP group at all electrodes (i.e., strong bilateral activation across both hemispheres). However, MSI values of the PP group were only significantly higher than were those of the OP group at C4, in the right hemisphere. An additional analysis was run on the baseline mu results for each electrode to test for pre-existing group differences, in a 3 group × 3 electrode RM ANOVA. There were no group differences in baseline mu all group $Fs < 1$. Group mean values varied from 6.7 to 12.2.

To test for evidence of suppression, single sample t-tests comparing the MSI value to zero for each group and electrode showed that for the PP group, MSI at all three electrodes (C3, CZ, and C4) was significantly less than zero ($p < .006$). For the OP group, only the middle, central electrode, CZ, had a significantly lower MSI value ($p = .004$). For the NP control group, MSI was significantly higher than the baseline at CZ ($p = .003$).

3.2. Does Observational Practice Bring about Motor Learning? In Figure 5(a), we have plotted the average number of errors for the three groups during the nine blocks of testing for the delayed retention test. For illustrative comparison, we have also plotted the acquisition data for the PP group. There does not appear to be any savings associated with previous observational practice for the OP group, when comparing their performance to the PP and NP groups. The PP group had the fewest number of errors in retention, particularly across the first few retention blocks, but across groups, number of errors decreased across blocks. With respect to statistical confirmation of the descriptive data, although the main effect of group was not significant, $F(2, 25) = 2.88$, $p = .075$, $\eta_p^2 = 0.19$, there was a significant block, $F(5.05, 126.23) = 24.04$, $p < .001 \eta_p^2 = 0.49$, and a significant group × block interaction, $F(10.10, 126.23) = 2.21$, $p = .021$, $\eta_p^2 = 0.15$. The block effect comprised significant linear and quadratic trend components ($p < .001$). Tukey's post hoc analysis of the interaction showed significant differences between the PP and NP group for blocks 1, 2, and 3, with the PP group showing fewer errors than the NP group. The PP and OP groups were only significantly different on block 1. However, there was no significant difference between the OP and NP groups for any practice block.

We have also plotted data for the first 10 trials of physical practice for all groups in order to better describe group effects and illustrate how differences in performance were not apparent on these first 10 trials, but rather emerged with practice. These data are shown in Figure 6 (i.e., first 10 trials of retention for all groups in addition to the first 10 trials of acquisition for the PP group). A group × trial ANOVA comparing the PP group during acquisition and the NP and OP groups during retention confirmed the absence of any group effect, $F(2, 26) = 1.30$, $p = .29$, $\eta_p^2 = 0.09$, nor a group × trial interaction ($F < 1$).

TABLE 1: Single sample t-test results (and Cohen's d), comparing MSI to zero for each electrode site for PP and OP groups during the stage 2 practice session.

	PP				OP			
	df	t_{obs}	d	p	df	t_{obs}	d	p
Electrode								
C3	9	−3.06	0.97	.007*	9	−2.71	0.86	.012*
CZ	9	−3.01	0.95	.008*	9	−4.08	1.2	.002*
C4	9	−4.39	1.3	.001*	9	−0.25	0.08	.405

*Statistical significance based on Bonferroni-corrected alpha values (.05/3 = .017).

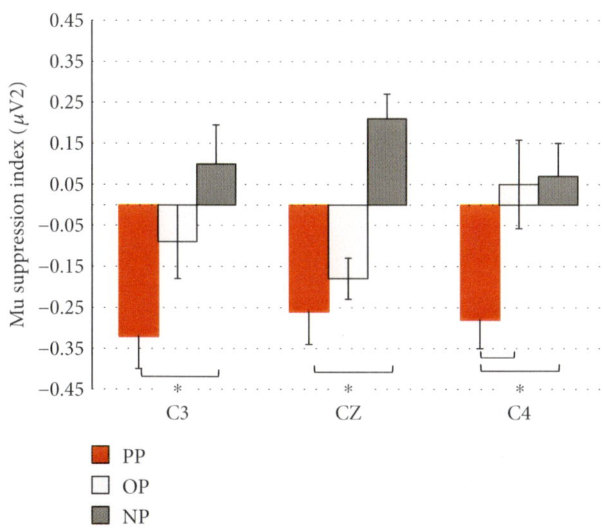

FIGURE 4: Mu suppression index for the PP, OP, and NP groups during postpractice observation (stage 3 testing). Error bars represent standard error of the mean (SE). Asterisks indicate significant between group differences ($p < .05$).

For tracing time, the data are illustrated in Figure 5(b), again with the PP group's acquisition data illustrated for comparison purposes. Although there was still a main effect of block, $F(3.08, 77.01) = 12.25$, $p < .001$, $\eta_p^2 = 0.33$, which comprised a significant linear trend component ($p < .001$) due to decreasing times as retention testing continued, there was no group or group × block interaction (both $Fs < 1$).

4. Discussion

This study is the first to investigate how mu suppression changes as a function of both observation and physical practice and what this means in terms of behavioural indices of motor learning. As predicted, the behavioural results showed that during the retention phase, the PP group made the least number of errors compared to the OP and NP control groups. However, the groups did not differ in average tracing time during retention. This suggests that benefits from physical practice were mostly a result of spatial accuracy improvements, rather than speed. Although both the PP and OP groups showed evidence of mu suppression, in both practice and postpractice observation (especially when compared to the control group), the patterns and degree of suppression differed across the groups. Therefore, although there was evidence of suppression in the OP group, suggestive of changes in cortical processing due to observational practice experience, these patterns of activation did not appear to manifest in improved motor learning, when the OP group was compared to the NP control and PP groups on a delayed retention test.

With respect to the behavioural data, there was no evidence of motor learning in the OP group. For tracing times, there were no significant group-related differences. There was no evidence that prior physical practice resulted in tracing time benefits. Rather, there was a trend for the PP group to be slower than the NP and OP groups. However, there was also no evidence that prior observation aided performance times, when comparing the NP and OP groups. The behavioural effects related to prior physical experience were evidenced in tracing errors. The PP group showed fewer errors in retention during the first five trials, when compared to both the NP and OP groups and across the first 15 trials when compared to the NP group. However, the OP group did not differ statistically from the NP group. Because accuracy could be compromised as a function of speed, it may be that the slower tracing times for the PP group (at least descriptively) were compensated for by fewer errors. We do not have a good reason why the PP group might have weighted accuracy more highly than tracing time. We would have expected the NP group in retention to have looked like the PP group in acquisition, but as can be seen from Figures 5(a) and 5(b), the PP group showed fewer errors and longer tracing times right from the start.

The lack of differences between the NP group and the PP and OP groups for the behavioural measures of motor learning might be due to the five 30–40 s observation trials shown during the postpractice observation testing session. It is possible that learners did not need to observe all 45 visual trials to show gains in subsequent execution and that these five trials of "good" performance may have been adequate to bring about performance benefits in retention, at least with respect to tracing time. If so, this suggests that covert practice benefits were likely more strategically mediated, associated with familiarity with the flower shape, rather than a motor-mediated strategy based on action simulation. This does not mean that there was no action simulation, as appeared to be evidenced by the EEG mu suppression data, but that this suppression or simulation was not associated with behavioural indices of motor learning.

The neurophysiological results showed that, compared to baseline, mu rhythm was significantly suppressed over both hemispheres during PP and only over the left hemisphere during OP. However, the magnitude of this suppression did not change, as a function of practice. This result is not consistent with studies that reported changes in the magnitude of MNS activity during practice. Nakano et al. [37], for example, reported a significant difference in suppression between the first and last of 5 trials of observation of a ball rotation task. Although the authors associated this decrease in suppression

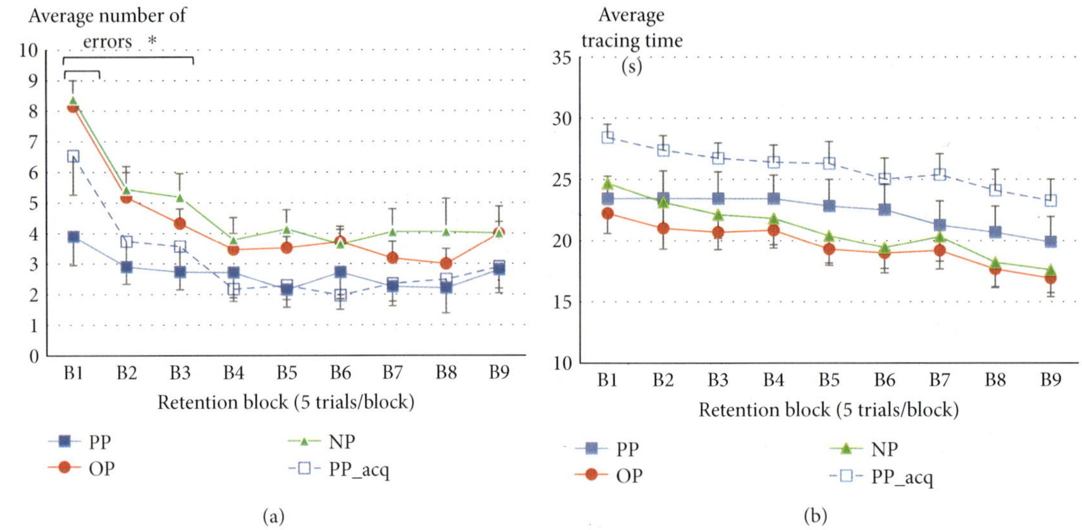

FIGURE 5: (a) Average number of errors across 9 blocks of retention testing ($t = 9$/blk) for the physical practice (PP), observational practice (OP), and no practice (NP) groups and first-day acquisition trials for the PP group (PP_acq). Error bars represent standard error (SE). *PP group significantly different to NP group B1–B3. PP group significantly different to OP group (B1). (b) Average tracing time across 9 blocks of retention testing ($t = 9$/blk) for the physical practice (PP), observational practice (OP), and no practice (NP) groups and first-day acquisition trials for the PP group (PP_acq). Error bars represent standard error (SE). There was no interaction.

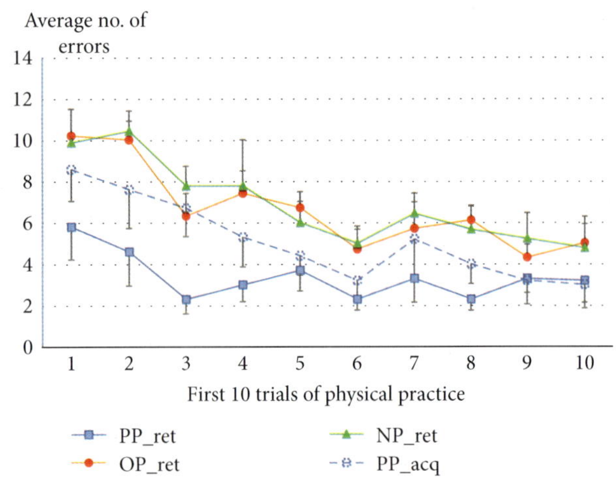

FIGURE 6: Average number of errors across the first 10 trials of physical practice in retention for the physical practice (PP), observational practice (OP), and no practice (NP) groups as well as during first-day acquisition for the PP group (PP_acq). Error bars represent standard error (SE). There were no group differences comparing PP_acq to the OP_ret and NP_ret.

with motor learning, it is difficult to draw a conclusion about motor learning based on so few trials (in our study, there were 45 trials of practice). The unchanged magnitude of mu suppression is also not in line with the neural efficiency hypothesis, which associates improved learning with less cortical activation [50]. Several lines of evidence show that experts exhibit less suppression during the execution and observation of motor skills, suggesting that more experience eventually leads to a more efficient neural processing [43]. However, contrary to our study, which focused on short-term practice, these studies tested individuals with years of experience and researchers have identified different brain networks, with different activation patterns, involved in short-term and long-term motor practice [51].

As expected, mu suppression during physical practice was bilateral, showing that both hemispheres were active during movement performance. Contrary to our hypothesis, however, mu suppression during observational practice was higher in magnitude in the left hemisphere compared to the right hemisphere and hence did not show a similar bilateral suppression as noted for physical practice. Given that both the model and the study participants were right-handed and that the observers watched the movement from a first-person perspective, bilateral suppression of mu rhythm would be expected based on previous work [52].

Despite this research above, which was primarily based on observation of already experienced actions, there is evidence that action observation can lead to a more lateralized activation pattern. For example, Perry and Bentin [53] showed that when they examined right-handed participants while observing movements of both right and left hands from a first-person perspective, mu suppression was evidenced at the frequency range of 8–13 Hz. This suppression was stronger in the hemisphere contralateral to the hand being observed compared to the hemisphere ipsilateral to the observed hand (similar to our data). Similarly, when Quandt et al. [54, 55] presented video clips of a right-handed model from a first-person perspective, action observation was associated with greater suppression at the alpha frequency range in the left hemisphere compared with the right hemisphere. In a different study, when a third-person, action-observation paradigm was employed, suppression was greater over the right hemisphere compared with the left hemisphere [55]. The left-lateralized activation reported in this study is also consistent with fMRI studies. These studies have revealed that watching right-hand reaching-and-grasping movements from a first-person, egocentric perspective elicited larger BOLD responses in the left anterior intraparietal cortex of right-handed observers [17]. This contralateral effect, however, was replaced by an ipsilateral response (i.e., the right hemisphere) in the anterior superior parietal lobule when the right-handed observers viewed the right-handed movements from an allocentric perspective (i.e., facing the model) [56].

Complementing the EEG differences in practice between OP and PP, the postpractice observation testing session also yielded differences between groups based on experience. Although for the OP group, these postobservation trials had already been viewed, whereas these were novel videos for the PP and NP groups, there was no suggestion that the patterns of activation were affected by novelty. There was no significant block effect in acquisition, such that the patterns of activation shown in the first block of practice were maintained throughout practice. Moreover, patterns of activation seen for the PP group while acting were also maintained for this group while observing. Again, this suggests that prior experience, rather than novelty or familiarity, was responsible for these effects.

For the PP group, postpractice observation was characterized by bilateral suppression. For the OP group, observing the same stimuli as the PP group, action observation was characterized by left-lateralized suppression. It appears that observation without any physical practice activates only a subset of brain regions, which also explains the lateralized effect during observation practice. The absence of suppression for the NP group, however, suggests that more than 5 trials of observation are needed for this suppression to be evidenced or that a learning model who shows improvement across trials is necessary for suppression. The model shown in the postpractice observation session only was of near perfect performance (i.e., the last five trials from practice). Behavioural studies that have compared expert and learning models have provided evidence that watching learning models engages the observer in a problem-solving mode in which he/she considers all the relations between the movement patterns and their outcomes to optimize performance [57]. Given the association between the left hemisphere and relational reasoning [58], the left-lateralized suppression during visual training could be moderated by model type, which continues to influence patterns of activation during near-perfect performance. In light of this explanation, it is possible that the bilateral effect during observation reported in other studies in this area was because the observers viewed error-free hand movements, with no learning component.

What is important from the postpractice observation data is the fact that differences existed between the groups based on the types of experience, despite the fact that all three groups were watching the same action stimuli and that we only collected data from 5 trials in practice (each trial lasting ~60 s). Differences in activation between the OP and PP groups might simply be a carryover effect from practice, such that whatever areas of the brain were activated during initial exposure continued to be activated during a subsequent observation phase. Because the observe-only group never physically practiced and did not show bilateral suppression, there was no reason to think that this would be observed postpractice as nothing had changed. For the PP group, it appears that it was able to resonate and engage in action simulation, based on previous physical experience with the task, such that the patterns of activations resembled these early learning physical practice experiences. In comparing the size of suppression and making conclusions about motor-mediated learning in observation conditions, the PP group exhibited the strongest suppression compared to the OP and NP control groups. This suggests that for observation to induce significant suppression, it has to be preceded by active motor experience with the motor skill of interest. This result corroborates with EEG studies that have stressed the role of prior active motor experience (long- or short-term) in modulating mu responses during observation [59].

Although previous PP in this study involved both hemispheres and led to the strongest suppression, comparable suppression between OP and PP groups was shown at the medial central site (i.e., CZ), especially in comparison to the NP control group. Interestingly, although the NP control was not that different to the PP and OP group with respect to their behavioural performance in retention, at least with respect to tracing times, the five trials of EEG collected during the observation-testing session revealed significant differences between these groups. No suppression was observed at all three central sites (in fact, there was significant synchronization in comparison to baseline). Even though the participants in the control group were observing a motor task, their preceding lack of experience with this task either covertly or overtly moderated any motor system suppression at this central location. Therefore, action-observation does not always induce suppression, supporting the suggestion that the MNS and mu suppression more specifically is sensitive to previous experiences with the task, both visual and physical (see also [60]). Prior physical and observation practice experiences caused mu suppression in our study, but to different degrees and in qualitatively different ways.

This study has some limitations that deserve mention. One of these concerns potential accuracy-speed trade-offs. Any improvement in one measure could be attributed to a decrease in the other. Although not reported, correlations between these two measures in retention were all small ($rs < 0.25$) and nonsignificant. However, in future work, fixing one measure of the task to examine the changes in the other would rule out any possible trade-off influences and narrow down alternative explanations for the observed effects (e.g., requiring zero-error performance).

Monitoring the observers' motion only via a video camera, without a stringent control for muscle activation, introduced another limitation. Although the activation during PP was different from that during OP, there is still a possibility that any mu suppression could be due to muscle activation. To avoid such confounding effects, electromyography (EMG) should be used to accurately detect any possible movement.

The lack of change in the magnitude of mu suppression throughout both types of practice could be a result of the number of training trials (i.e., 45 trials). This number was used because in pilot testing, it was shown that behavioural measures of performance leveled out (i.e., plateaued) around the 45th trial. Increasing the number of trials could also cause participants possible discomfort with the EEG net, which in turn could negatively impact performance. Nevertheless, in future work it would be important to increase the amount of practice, especially as behavioural plateaus do not indicate the absence of learning [61]. Moreover, it may be that for observational learning benefits to be realized in this task, observational practice trials should be increased. Although behaviourally, the OP group did not look different to the NP group, which might suggest that five observation trials were enough to bring about some performance gains, watching 45 trials of practice from a learning model did lead to differences in cortical activation. In future work, it will be important to test motor performance of a no-practice control group in the absence of any observational practice trials to better appreciate the short-term effects of watching and the volume of practice which is needed to bring about observational-related changes.

Finally, although mu rhythm is mainly described as EEG oscillations at the frequency range of 8–13 Hz, some authors limited mu rhythm to the frequency band of 8–10 Hz (e.g., [26]). EEG researchers have identified two frequency ranges within the alpha range (8–13 Hz): the lower alpha (8–10) Hz and the upper alpha (10–13) Hz. The lower alpha emanates from the somatosensory cortex and is modulated by motor activity, showing a more anterior and asymmetrical hemispheric effect. The upper band, in contrast, consists of posterior bilateral waves, which cluster mainly around the parietooccipital cortices and is primarily modulated by visual stimulation [62]. Given that the observed suppression in this study could be a result of visual stimulation or motor activation or both, examining each component separately would shed more light on both the hemispheric activation and the source of stimulation. It may also be of interest in future work to conduct time frequency analysis on the EEG, to help provide more information about the complex network dynamics underlying observational practice [63].

In conclusion, we have demonstrated that observation practice induces neurophysiological changes as indexed by mu suppression at central sites, which provides evidence for motor-based processes during observational practice. However, there was no evidence that these motor-related processes were related to motor learning and behavioural measures of learning in retention. The lateralized suppression during observation practice suggests that cortical processes involved in this covert type of practice might not be entirely motor-based and that the lateralized activation during OP and the bilateral activation during PP at the central sites suggest that OP does not trigger all brain areas activated during PP. Therefore, observation practice cannot replace physical practice, even though in some instances there may be benefits to be gained behaviourally from this type of practice (at least in comparison to not practicing). Because of EEG differences between OP and NP control conditions during a postpractice observation phase, there is evidence that OP is leading to neurophysiological changes, although we did not have evidence that this suppression was linked to motor learning outcomes.

Importantly, we confirm the vital role of previous motor experience in modulating mu responses during observation, suggesting that employing movements that are within the observer's motor repertoire (i.e., prior physical exposure) is more likely to result in optimal activation during a subsequent practice phase. To a lesser extent, observers without this experience could benefit from watching movements where they have only had previous visual experience. Although both physical and observational practice might share some similarities, the underlying mechanisms by which each of them operates appears to be different both qualitatively and quantitatively. To better understand the relationship between mu responses and motor learning during observational practice, researchers should address other factors that could influence this relationship, such as handedness, observation perspective, the amount of visual familiarity, model's expertise, and the type of motor task. Further study of the relation between these types of practice and their neurophysiology would help to elucidate on the dominant mechanisms underpinning observation practice and the conditions which maximize motor-mediated learning under these conditions. It has yet to be shown that an increase in motor-related areas during observation practice is responsible for better learning. One possible future method to help determine how cortical activation in motor-related areas of the brain relates to learning is to use methods to stimulate the brain either during or before a period of observational practice, potentially through transcranial direct current stimulation (tDCS).

Disclosure

The manuscript is based on the Masters' thesis of the first author, Najah Alhajri (June 2017), comparing motor learning and mu suppression under short-term physical and observational practice in adults (University of British Columbia).

Conflicts of Interest

The authors declare that they have no conflicts of interest.

References

[1] N. J. Hodges and D. Ste-Marie, "Observation as an instructional method," in *Developing Sport Expertise: Researchers and Coaches put Theory into Practice*, D. Farrow, J. Baker, and C. MacMahon, Eds., pp. 115–128, Routledge, Abingdon, UK, 2nd edition, 2013.

[2] N. J. Hodges, "Observations on action-observation research: an autobiographical retrospective across the past two decades," *Kinesiology Review*, vol. 6, no. 3, pp. 240–260, 2017.

[3] N. J. Hodges, A. M. Williams, S. J. Hayes, and G. Breslin, "What is modelled during observational learning?," *Journal of Sports Sciences*, vol. 25, no. 5, pp. 531–545, 2007.

[4] D. Maslovat, S. J. Hayes, R. Horn, and N. J. Hodges, "Motor learning through observation," in *Vision and Goal-Directed Movement: Neurobehavioral Perspectives*, D. Elliott and M.

Khan, Eds., pp. 315–340, Human Kinetics, Champaign, IL, USA, 2010.

[5] N. T. Ong and N. J. Hodges, "Mixing it up a little: how to schedule observational practice," in *Skill Acquisition in Sport: Research, Theory and practice*, N. J. Hodges and A. M. Williams, Eds., pp. 48–65, Routledge, London, UK, 2nd edition, 2012.

[6] D. M. Ste-Marie, B. Law, A. M. Rymal, O. Jenny, C. Hall, and P. McCullagh, "Observation interventions for motor skill learning and performance: an applied model for the use of observation," *International Review of Sport and Exercise Psychology*, vol. 5, no. 2, pp. 145–176, 2012.

[7] M. Bassolino, G. Sandini, and T. Pozzo, "Activating the motor system through action observation: is this an efficient approach in adults and children?," *Developmental Medicine and Child Neurology*, vol. 57, Supplement 2, pp. 42–45, 2015.

[8] P. Molenberghs, R. Cunnington, and J. B. Mattingley, "Is the mirror neuron system involved in imitation? A short review and meta-analysis," *Neuroscience and Biobehavioral Reviews*, vol. 33, no. 7, pp. 975–980, 2009.

[9] L. Cattaneo and G. Rizzolatti, "The mirror neuron system," *Archives of Neurology*, vol. 66, no. 5, pp. 557–560, 2009.

[10] G. Rizzolatti and L. Craighero, "The mirror-neuron system," *Annual Review of Neuroscience*, vol. 27, no. 1, pp. 169–192, 2004.

[11] K. Zentgraf, J. Munzert, M. Bischoff, and R. D. Newman-Norlund, "Simulation during observation of human actions–theories, empirical studies, applications," *Vision Research*, vol. 51, no. 8, pp. 827–835, 2011.

[12] G. Buccino, S. Vogt, A. Ritzl et al., "Neural circuits underlying imitation learning of hand actions: an event-related fMRI study," *Neuron*, vol. 42, no. 2, pp. 323–334, 2004.

[13] I. Dinstein, U. Hasson, N. Rubin, and D. J. Heeger, "Brain areas selective for both observed and executed movements," *Journal of Neurophysiology*, vol. 98, no. 3, pp. 1415–1427, 2007.

[14] F. Filimon, C. A. Rieth, M. I. Sereno, and G. W. Cottrell, "Observed, executed, and imagined action representations can be decoded from ventral and dorsal areas," *Cerebral Cortex*, vol. 25, no. 9, pp. 3144–3158, 2015.

[15] V. Gazzola and C. Keysers, "The observation and execution of actions share motor and somatosensory voxels in all tested subjects: single-subject analyses of unsmoothed fMRI data," *Cerebral Cortex*, vol. 19, no. 6, pp. 1239–1255, 2009.

[16] M. Iacoboni, I. Molnar-Szakacs, V. Gallese, G. Buccino, J. C. Mazziotta, and G. Rizzolatti, "Grasping the intentions of others with one's own mirror neuron system," *PLoS Biology*, vol. 3, no. 3, article e79, 2005.

[17] L. Shmuelof and E. Zohary, "Dissociation between ventral and dorsal fMRI activation during object and action recognition," *Neuron*, vol. 47, no. 3, pp. 457–470, 2005.

[18] T. T.-J. Chong, R. Cunnington, M. A. Williams, N. Kanwisher, and J. B. Mattingley, "fMRI adaptation reveals mirror neurons in human inferior parietal cortex," *Current Biology*, vol. 18, no. 20, pp. 1576–1580, 2008.

[19] S. Caspers, K. Zilles, A. R. Laird, and S. B. Eickhoff, "ALE meta-analysis of action observation and imitation in the human brain," *NeuroImage*, vol. 50, no. 3, pp. 1148–1167, 2010.

[20] C. Babiloni, F. Babiloni, F. Carducci et al., "Human cortical electroencephalography (EEG) rhythms during the observation of simple aimless movements: a high-resolution EEG study," *NeuroImage*, vol. 17, no. 2, pp. 559–572, 2002.

[21] S. Cochin, C. Barthelemy, B. Lejeune, S. Roux, and J. Martineau, "Perception of motion and qEEG activity in human adults," *Electroencephalography and Clinical Neurophysiology*, vol. 107, no. 4, pp. 287–295, 1998.

[22] S. D. Muthukumaraswamy, B. W. Johnson, and N. A. McNair, "Mu rhythm modulation during observation of an object-directed grasp," *Cognitive Brain Research*, vol. 19, no. 2, pp. 195–201, 2004.

[23] J. A. Pineda, B. Z. Allison, and A. Vankov, "The effects of self-movement, observation, and imagination on mu rhythms and readiness potentials (RP's): toward a brain-computer interface (BCI)," *IEEE Transactions on Rehabilitation Engineering*, vol. 8, no. 2, pp. 219–222, 2000.

[24] N. Virji-Babul, A. Moiseev, T. Cheung, D. Weeks, D. Cheyne, and U. Ribary, "Changes in mu rhythm during action observation and execution in adults with Down syndrome: implications for action representation," *Neuroscience Letters*, vol. 436, no. 2, pp. 177–180, 2008.

[25] C. C. Woodruff and S. Maaske, "Action execution engages human mirror neuron system more than action observation," *Neuroreport*, vol. 21, no. 6, pp. 432–435, 2010.

[26] J. A. Pineda, "The functional significance of mu rhythms: translating "seeing" and "hearing" into "doing"," *Brain Research Reviews*, vol. 50, no. 1, pp. 57–68, 2005.

[27] N. Virji-Babul, A. Moiseev, T. Cheung, D. Weeks, D. Cheyne, and U. Ribary, "Spatial-temporal dynamics of cortical activity underlying reaching and grasping," *Human Brain Mapping*, vol. 31, no. 1, pp. 160–171, 2010.

[28] R. Gatti, A. Tettamanti, P. M. Gough, E. Riboldi, L. Marinoni, and G. Buccino, "Action observation versus motor imagery in learning a complex motor task: a short review of literature and a kinematics study," *Neuroscience Letters*, vol. 540, pp. 37–42, 2013.

[29] C. M. Heyes and C. L. Foster, "Motor learning by observation: evidence from a serial reaction time task," *The Quarterly Journal of Experimental Psychology*, vol. 55, no. 2, pp. 593–607, 2002.

[30] D. Ashford, S. J. Bennett, and K. Davids, "Observational modeling effects for movement dynamics and movement outcome measures across differing task constraints: a meta-analysis," *Journal of Motor Behavior*, vol. 38, no. 3, pp. 185–205, 2006.

[31] N. T. Ong and N. J. Hodges, "Absence of after-effects for observers after watching a visuomotor adaptation," *Experimental Brain Research*, vol. 205, no. 3, pp. 325–334, 2010.

[32] G. Bird and C. Heyes, "Effector-dependent learning by observation of a finger movement sequence," *Journal of Experimental Psychology: Human Perception and Performance*, vol. 31, no. 2, pp. 262–275, 2005.

[33] L. E. Brown, E. T. Wilson, and P. L. Gribble, "Repetitive transcranial magnetic stimulation to the primary motor cortex interferes with motor learning by observing," *Journal of Cognitive Neuroscience*, vol. 21, no. 5, pp. 1013–1022, 2009.

[34] A. A. G. Mattar and P. L. Gribble, "Motor learning by observing," *Neuron*, vol. 46, no. 1, pp. 153–160, 2005.

[35] S. Vogt and R. Thomaschke, "From visuo-motor interactions to imitation learning: behavioural and brain imaging studies," *Journal of Sports Sciences*, vol. 25, no. 5, pp. 497–517, 2007.

[36] S. Vogt, "Visuomotor couplings in object-oriented and imitative actions," in *The Imitative Mind: Development, Evolution,*

and Brain Bases, A. N. Meltzoff and W. Prinz, Eds., pp. 206–220, CUP, Cambridge UK, 2002.

[37] H. Nakano, M. Osumi, K. Ueta, T. Kodama, and S. Morioka, "Changes in electroencephalographic activity during observation, preparation, and execution of a motor learning task," *The International Journal of Neuroscience*, vol. 123, no. 12, pp. 866–875, 2013.

[38] S. S. Kantak and C. J. Winstein, "Learning-performance distinction and memory processes for motor skills: a focused review and perspective," *Behavioural Brain Research*, vol. 228, no. 1, pp. 219–231, 2012.

[39] R. A. Schmidt and T. D. Lee, *Motor Control and Learning: a Behavioral Emphasis*, Human Kinetics, Champaign, IL, USA, 2005.

[40] G. Orgs, J. H. Dombrowski, M. Heil, and P. Jansen-Osmann, "Expertise in dance modulates alpha/beta event-related desynchronization during action observation," *The European Journal of Neuroscience*, vol. 27, no. 12, pp. 3380–3384, 2008.

[41] L. P. Behmer Jr and K. J. Jantzen, "Reading sheet music facilitates sensorimotor mu-desynchronization in musicians," *Clinical Neurophysiology*, vol. 122, no. 7, pp. 1342–1347, 2011.

[42] E. S. Cross, D. J. M. Kraemer, A. F. . C. Hamilton, W. M. Kelley, and S. T. Grafton, "Sensitivity of the action observation network to physical and observational learning," *Cerebral Cortex*, vol. 19, no. 2, pp. 315–326, 2009.

[43] C. Babiloni, C. del Percio, P. M. Rossini et al., "Judgment of actions in experts: a high-resolution EEG study in elite athletes," *NeuroImage*, vol. 45, no. 2, pp. 512–521, 2009.

[44] R. C. Oldfield, "The assessment and analysis of handedness: the Edinburgh inventory," *Neuropsychologia*, vol. 9, no. 1, pp. 97–113, 1971.

[45] S. E. Henderson, D. A. Sugden, and A. L. Barnett, *Movement Assessment Battery for Children*, Psychological Corporation, London, UK, 1992.

[46] T. Ishikura and K. Inomata, "Effects of angle of model-demonstration on learning of motor skill," *Perceptual and Motor Skills*, vol. 80, no. 2, pp. 651–658, 1995.

[47] P. L. Jackson, A. N. Meltzoff, and J. Decety, "Neural circuits involved in imitation and perspective-taking," *NeuroImage*, vol. 31, no. 1, pp. 429–439, 2006.

[48] S. Pilgramm, B. Lorey, R. Stark, J. Munzert, D. Vaitl, and K. Zentgraf, "Differential activation of the lateral premotor cortex during action observation," *BMC Neuroscience*, vol. 11, no. 1, p. 89, 2010.

[49] A. Perry, N. F. Troje, and S. Bentin, "Exploring motor system contributions to the perception of social information: evidence from EEG activity in the mu/alpha frequency range," *Social Neuroscience*, vol. 5, no. 3, pp. 272–284, 2010.

[50] R. J. Haier, B. V. Siegel Jr, K. H. Nuechterlein et al., "Cortical glucose metabolic rate correlates of abstract reasoning and attention studied with positron emission tomography," *Intelligence*, vol. 12, no. 2, pp. 199–217, 1988.

[51] A. Floyer-Lea and P. M. Matthews, "Distinguishable brain activation networks for short- and long-term motor skill learning," *Journal of Neurophysiology*, vol. 94, no. 1, pp. 512–518, 2005.

[52] A. Streltsova, C. Berchio, V. Gallese, and M. A. Umilta', "Time course and specificity of sensory-motor alpha modulation during the observation of hand motor acts and gestures: a high density EEG study," *Experimental Brain Research*, vol. 205, no. 3, pp. 363–373, 2010.

[53] A. Perry and S. Bentin, "Mirror activity in the human brain while observing hand movements: a comparison between EEG desynchronization in the μ-range and previous fMRI results," *Brain Research*, vol. 1282, pp. 126–132, 2009.

[54] L. C. Quandt, P. J. Marshall, C. A. Bouquet, and T. F. Shipley, "Somatosensory experiences with action modulate alpha and beta power during subsequent action observation," *Brain Research*, vol. 1534, pp. 55–65, 2013.

[55] L. C. Quandt, P. J. Marshall, T. F. Shipley, S. L. Beilock, and S. Goldin-Meadow, "Sensitivity of alpha and beta oscillations to sensorimotor characteristics of action: an EEG study of action production and gesture observation," *Neuropsychologia*, vol. 50, no. 12, pp. 2745–2751, 2012.

[56] L. Shmuelof and E. Zohary, "Mirror-image representation of action in the anterior parietal cortex," *Nature Neuroscience*, vol. 11, no. 11, pp. 1267–1269, 2008.

[57] C. B. Black and D. L. Wright, "Can observational practice facilitate error recognition and movement production?," *Research Quarterly for Exercise and Sport*, vol. 71, no. 4, pp. 331–339, 2000.

[58] S. A. Bunge, E. H. Helskog, and C. Wendelken, "Left, but not right, rostrolateral prefrontal cortex meets a stringent test of the relational integration hypothesis," *NeuroImage*, vol. 46, no. 1, pp. 338–342, 2009.

[59] L. C. Quandt, P. J. Marshall, C. A. Bouquet, T. Young, and T. F. Shipley, "Experience with novel actions modulates frontal alpha EEG desynchronization," *Neuroscience Letters*, vol. 499, no. 1, pp. 37–41, 2011.

[60] N. N. Rüther, E. C. Brown, A. Klepp, and C. Bellebaum, "Observed manipulation of novel tools leads to mu rhythm suppression over sensory-motor cortices," *Behavioural Brain Research*, vol. 261, pp. 328–335, 2014.

[61] J. A. Adams, "Historical review and appraisal of research on the learning, retention, and transfer of human motor skills," *Psychological Bulletin*, vol. 101, no. 1, pp. 41–74, 1987.

[62] G. Pfurtscheller and C. Neuper, "Motor imagery activates primary sensorimotor area in humans," *Neuroscience Letters*, vol. 239, no. 2-3, pp. 65–68, 1997.

[63] A. M. Cebolla, E. Palmero-Soler, A. Leroy, and G. Cheron, "EEG spectral generators involved in motor imagery: a swLORETA Study," *Frontiers in Psychology*, vol. 8, p. 2133, 2017.

2

Aberrances of Cortex Excitability and Connectivity Underlying Motor Deficit in Acute Stroke

Juan Du,[1] Jianping Hu,[2] Jingze Hu,[1] Qiang Xu,[2] Qirui Zhang,[2] Ling Liu,[1] Minmin Ma,[1] Gelin Xu,[1] Yong Zhang,[3] Xinfeng Liu,[1] Guangming Lu,[2,4] Zhiqiang Zhang,[2,4] and Fang Yang[1]

[1]*Department of Neurology, Jinling Hospital, Nanjing University School of Medicine, Nanjing 210002, China*
[2]*Department of Medical Imaging, Jinling Hospital, Nanjing University School of Medicine, Nanjing 210002, China*
[3]*MR Research, GE Healthcare, Shanghai 201203, China*
[4]*State Key Laboratory of Analytical Chemistry for Life Science, Nanjing University, Nanjing 210002, China*

Correspondence should be addressed to Zhiqiang Zhang; zhangzq2001@126.com and Fang Yang; yangfang021011@163.com

Academic Editor: Malgorzata Kossut

Purpose. This study was aimed at evaluating the motor cortical excitability and connectivity underlying the neural mechanism of motor deficit in acute stroke by the combination of functional magnetic resonance imaging (fMRI) and electrophysiological measures. *Methods.* Twenty-five patients with motor deficit after acute ischemic stroke were involved. General linear model and dynamic causal model analyses were applied to fMRI data for detecting motor-related activation and effective connectivity of the motor cortices. Motor cortical excitability was determined as a resting motor threshold (RMT) of motor evoked potential detected by transcranial magnetic stimulation (TMS). fMRI results were correlated with cortical excitability and upper extremity Fugl-Meyer assessment scores, respectively. *Results.* Greater fMRI activation likelihood and motor cortical excitability in the ipsilesional primary motor area (M1) region were associated with better motor performance. During hand movements, the inhibitory connectivity from the contralesional to the ipsilesional M1 was correlated with the degree of motor impairment. Furthermore, ipsilesional motor cortex excitability was correlated with an enhancement of promoting connectivity in ipsilesional M1 or a reduction of interhemispheric inhibition in contralesional M1. *Conclusions.* The study suggested that a dysfunction of the ipsilesional M1 and abnormal interhemispheric interactions might underlie the motor disability in acute ischemic stroke. Modifying the excitability of the motor cortex and correcting the abnormal motor network connectivity associated with the motor deficit might be the therapeutic target in early neurorehabilitation for stroke patients.

1. Introduction

Stroke is a leading cause of long-term disability worldwide [1]; approximately 80% of acute stroke survivors suffer from persistent different degrees of motor impairment [2]. Research on the neural mechanism of stroke-induced motor impairment is essential for the rehabilitation of the disease. Currently, two related hypotheses have been offered to explain motor impairment of stroke patients. In the first theory, dysfunction of ipsilesional motor areas underlies deficits in motor control after stroke [3, 4], and another posits that transcallosal inhibition (e.g., the contralesional hemisphere exerts a pathologically enhanced inhibitory influences on the ipsilesional hemisphere) thereby contributes to the reduced motor performance of stroke patients [5–7]. In the acute phase of stroke, changes in the brain at different levels from the molecular level to the network level are especially active and accelerate the brain's self-repair processes [8, 9]. Earlier rehabilitation in stroke is more critical for motor functional recovery and has been considered to be associated with better outcomes [10]. Therefore, it is more significant to investigate the neural mechanisms underlying motor deficits in the early stage of stroke, which may provide important theoretical evidence for early neurorehabilitation of ischemic stroke.

Over recent years, multimodality imaging techniques, represented by functional magnetic resource imaging (fMRI), have been widely used for investigating the neural mechanism of the motor deficits in ischemic stroke. By using sophisticated analysis approaches, fMRI has revealed the abnormalities of local activation and connectivity associated with motor deficits after stroke [11]. Dynamic causal modeling (DCM) analysis based on fMRI is a promising approach to capture effective connectivity among key regions of the cortical motor system [12]. As a complementary approach, electrophysiological assessment such as the assessment of the motor evoked potentials (MEPs) by transcranial magnetic stimulation (TMS) provides information about the excitability of the corticomotor system in stroke patients [13]. Nonetheless, these numerous studies used electrophysiological or fMRI measures in isolation. Moreover, most available evidence was primarily limited to the chronic stage after stroke, in which the mechanisms underlying neural reorganization may have returned to being stable [14]. There is little specific information on the characteristics of the motor cortical network in the acute stage following stroke.

Therefore, in the present study, we combined functional MRI and electrophysiological assessments, as well as analyses of effective connectivity to investigate the neural mechanisms underlying motor deficits in acute stroke. We first hypothesized that the early movement-related cortical activation patterns were paralleled by the motor cortical excitability measured by TMS and both relates to the degree of motor impairment after stroke. Then, combining DCM with electrophysiological assessment, we further hypothesized that pathological transcallosal inhibition originating from contralesional M1 to ipsilesional M1 could also occur in the acute stage of stroke and relate to the degree of motor impairment and motor cortical excitability.

2. Materials and Methods

2.1. Patients. Twenty-five patients (8 females and 17 males; age: 53 ± 10 years) with a first ever ischemic stroke participated in this study. The detailed inclusive criteria included the following: (1) patients being in the acute stage of stroke and having a time from stroke of less than two weeks, (2) single lesion located within the middle cerebral artery territory, as shown by structural MRI, (3) symptoms of motor deficit in the unilateral upper extremity, and (4) absence of aphasia, neglect, apraxia, or epilepsy, which were evaluated according to the patients' clinical symptoms and signs. This study was approved by the Internal Review Board of Jinling Hospital, and written informed consent was obtained from each participant.

2.2. Clinical Assessments. The clinical deficit and stroke severity were assessed using the National Institutes of Health Stroke Scale (NIHSS) [15] and the modified Rankin Scale (mRS) [16]. The following motor tests were used to assess the affected upper limb: (1) Fugl-Meyer assessment (FMA) [17] and (2) Medical Research Council (MRC) scale [18] for wrist extension of the affected hand. The FMA is a reliable and standardized motor impairment scale, which ranges from 0 (hemiplegia) to a maximum of 100 points (normal motor performance). It is divided into 66 points for the upper limb (FMA-UL) and 34 points for the lower limb (FMA-LL), scored on a 3-point ordinal scale (0 = cannot perform, 1 = performs partially, and 2 = performs fully). MRC is also used to assess the muscle strength of the hemiplegic side (ranging from 0 to 5; 5 = normal power and 0 = no movement).

2.3. Determination of Motor Cortex Excitability. Motor cortex excitability in each hemisphere was measured using single-pulse TMS [19, 20]. TMS was performed using a MagproX100 stimulator (MagVenture Company, Farum, Denmark) with a figure-of-eight coil (outer diameter of one wing 9 cm). Electromyography (EMG) recordings from the bilateral abductor pollicis brevis (APB) were detected using two pairs of silver-silver chloride surface electrodes (Alpine Biomed ApS, Skovlunde, Denmark). The RMT was defined as the minimal stimulus intensity, which could produce a MEP with a peak-to-peak amplitude of at least 50 μV in at least 5 of 10 subsequent trials. The amplitude of MEP to cortical stimulation was measured according to the peak-to-peak voltage (mV) of the EMG response. The latency of MEP was determined as the interval between the onset of the stimulation and the onset of the EMG response (ms). The presence of a TMS-elicited MEP was categorized as present or absent.

2.4. fMRI Paradigm. A block-designed motor task, for which the thumb and the forefinger of the affected and unaffected hand had to be tapped together at a rate of 1 Hz, was used as an fMRI activation paradigm. The MRI session consists of five trainings, lasting 5 minutes in total. Each training contained three blocks: a 20-second block of movement of the affected hand, a 20-second block of movement of the unaffected hand, and a 20-second rest block. Two motor task blocks were pseudorandomized and separated by a rest block. Every block was repeated 5 times in total. An investigator carried out the passive movement in the scanner room and ensured the consistency of the motor tasks. All patients underwent motor task training before MRI scanning and performed the passive movements during task-evoked fMRI scanning.

2.5. fMRI Data Acquisition. Whole-brain fMRI scans were performed using a GE MR750 3.0 Tesla Scanner (General Electric, USA). We used a gradient echo planar imaging (EPI) sequence with the following imaging parameters: TR = 2000 ms; TE = 30 ms; flip angle = 80°; FOV = 240 mm × 240 mm; matrix = 64 × 64; slice thickness = 3.2 mm, no gap; and slice number = 43 and 160 volumes. The slices covered the whole brain extending from the frontoparietal cortex to lower parts of the cerebellum. We also used 3D-BRAVO sequence to generate high-resolution 3D T1-weighted structural images, with these parameters: TR = 8.2 ms, TE = 3.2 ms, flip angle = 12°, FOV = 220 mm × 20 mm, matrix = 256 × 256, and slice thickness = 1 mm.

2.6. MRI Data Preprocess. Considering the effect of stroke lesion on the spatial normalization, a cost function modification was used to remove the presence of a lesion [21]. First, the lesion masks were manually traced on the individual structural 3D T1-weighted images independently by 2

Table 1: Individual fMRI activation maxima used as ROIs for DCM.

	M1_L			M1_R			SMA_L			SAM_R			PMC_L			PMC_R		
Subj1	−39	−24	45	42	−21	54	−12	−18	51	6	−3	57	−51	−3	33	54	−3	21
Subj2	−39	−24	63	33	−27	57	−3	0	72	9	−9	72	−54	−3	42	60	−6	36
Subj3	−39	−21	66	36	−27	69	−6	−3	63	3	−6	69	−51	−3	42	51	−9	33
Subj4	−45	−12	54	36	−21	57	−12	0	66	6	−3	69	−48	0	33	57	−6	42
Subj5	−39	−36	63	39	−21	57	−9	−6	66	12	−9	75	−57	−3	33	60	−9	42
Subj6	−39	−24	66	48	−15	60	−12	3	69	6	−6	66	−42	6	48	60	6	39
Subj7	−36	−30	63	39	−30	63	−6	−6	69	6	−21	69	−54	0	45	51	−3	45
Subj8	−48	−15	54	42	−21	66	−9	9	72	9	−6	72	−54	−3	36	57	0	39
Subj9	−45	−15	48	51	−15	45	−9	6	63	9	6	66	−48	−3	42	60	3	36
Subj10	−48	−15	45	39	−21	57	−9	12	69	6	−6	69	−57	0	30	57	0	42
Subj11	−45	−15	51	45	−15	57	−6	−6	69	9	−12	60	−51	−3	33	60	3	33
Subj12	−39	−21	60	39	−24	54	−6	−12	69	9	6	69	−51	−6	36	51	−3	33
Subj13	−39	−15	57	42	−15	57	−3	9	69	9	6	54	−45	−9	36	57	−6	33
Subj14	−33	−27	54	36	−24	54	−6	−3	69	9	−3	69	−57	0	30	54	0	45
Subj15	−36	−27	66	36	−27	63	−3	−3	69	6	0	66	−54	0	36	60	3	33
Subj16	−39	−21	57	39	−21	57	−6	0	57	9	6	60	−60	3	33	51	−3	39
Subj17	−39	−21	63	48	−15	57	−9	−12	69	6	−6	72	−51	−3	39	51	0	42
Subj18	−39	−24	60	36	−21	54	−3	−9	69	9	6	54	−48	−6	36	60	−3	36
Subj19	−48	−15	54	42	−24	66	−6	−3	69	9	−3	69	−60	0	24	57	0	33
Subj20	−48	−18	51	42	−24	57	−9	−12	66	9	−9	69	−54	−6	36	54	−6	36
Subj21	−36	−27	51	42	−18	57	−6	6	63	6	−3	60	−48	−6	33	57	−9	36
Subj22	−48	−18	45	39	−33	66	−6	3	66	9	−12	72	−54	0	30	51	−3	39
Subj23	−36	−24	51	36	−27	60	−9	−12	69	9	−9	66	−45	−3	45	54	−6	36
Subj24	−39	−18	60	39	−24	57	−6	21	63	9	18	66	−42	−3	45	54	−3	39
Subj25	−45	−15	48	42	−18	60	−6	6	51	6	−12	63	−42	−3	36	51	−9	42

Note: six motor regions of interest (ROIs) from the fMRI motor task activation were selected for the DCM analysis: the primary motor area (M1), the premotor cortex (PMC), and the supplementary motor area (SMA) from both hemispheres of each subject.

radiologists (Hu JP and Zeng FY), with the guide of the DWI image. Second, a group-sample-specific brain template was generated. For each subject, the lesion-removed whole-brain mask was used as the cost function, to normalize the 3D T1-weighted image into the standard brain template of the Montreal Neurological Institute (MNI) by using a 12-parameter affine transformation with nonlinear adjustments with 78×7 basis functions. All individual-normalized 3D T1-weighted anatomical images and all lesion-removed masks were averaged to yield sample-specific brain templates. Third, the averaged 3D T1-weighted anatomical image was segmented using unified segment function of SPM8, with the averaged lesion-removed mask as the cost function. Fourth, the individual space 3D T1-weighted images were segmented using unified segment function. The segment issues of the third step process were used as the templates of the current segment process, and the individual lesion-removed brain mask was used as the cost function. The segment parameters contained the affine transition matrix, which would be used in the functional MRI image normalization [21, 22].

For the functional MRI data, the process was done by DPARSF (http://rfmri.org/DPARSF) and SPM8 (http://www.fil.ion.ucl.ac.uk). Prior to data analysis, images from patients with right-sided lesions were flipped to the left side at the midsagittal plane, so that the affected hemisphere corresponded to the left hemisphere in all patients. First, slice timing and realignment were performed. Translation or rotation parameters in any given data set did not exceed 1.5 mm or 1.5 degree. Second, the functional images were coregistered to the individual 3D T1-weighted images. Third, the segment parameters were applied to the coregistered functional images for the normalization of functional images, with resample of $3 \times 3 \times 3\,\text{mm}^3$ voxel size. Fourth, spatial smoothing (FWHM = 8 mm) was performed to the normalized functional images [21, 22].

2.7. fMRI Data Analysis

2.7.1. Motor Activation Detection. For each subject, the experimental conditions were modeled in the framework of the general linear model (GLM). The block designs were convolved with a canonical hemodynamic response function applied in SPM8, and the first-order temporal derivatives were also generated. The design matrix also contained the head motion parameters to remove the effects. The contrast maps of the affected and unaffected hand movement were regrouped to calculate the second-level group effect by using SPM8.

Table 2: Demographical, imaging, and clinical data of stroke patients.

Patient	Age, y	Sex	Hand dominance	AH	Stroke location	Infarct volume, mL	Lesion age, d	MEP of AH	NIHSS	mRS	BI	FMA	MRC
1	66	F	R	R	CR, BG	3.1	1	Present	7	4	45	33	3
2	68	M	R	R	Temporal parietal region, BG, CR	21.8	2	Present	12	4	25	19	2
3	61	M	R	R	CR	0.5	8	Absent	5	3	65	44	3
4	68	M	R	R	Parietal occipital region	3.7	6	Present	3	2	90	33	2
5	67	F	R	L	Frontoparietal region	8.1	3	Absent	13	4	25	2	1
6	50	F	R	L	BG	4.7	14	Absent	14	4	20	3	1
7	44	M	R	L	CR	0.8	1	Present	6	2	80	53	4
8	40	M	R	L	BG	0.4	2	Present	8	3	70	38	4
9	59	F	R	L	Frontotemporal region	72	2	Present	13	4	30	36	3
10	60	F	R	R	CR	1.2	8	Present	7	4	50	38	2
11	44	M	R	L	BG	2.8	3	Present	7	4	35	46	3
12	56	M	R	R	BG	0.4	6	Present	13	4	25	2	1
13	50	M	R	R	BG, CR	6.3	1	Present	7	4	50	33	3
14	45	F	R	L	BG	6.1	3	present	5	3	60	59	4
15	50	M	R	R	BG	1.8	7	Present	4	2	65	56	4
16	49	M	R	L	BG, CR	2.3	8	Present	11	4	45	46	3
17	36	M	R	L	BG, CR	2.1	13	Present	6	4	50	26	2
18	58	M	R	L	Parietal occipital region, CR	0.5	7	Present	5	3	80	44	3
19	38	M	R	R	BG	2.6	5	Present	5	4	65	27	2
20	47	F	R	R	Frontotemporal region	9.9	6	Present	9	4	40	33	3
21	52	F	R	L	Frontotemporal region	13.5	3	Absent	12	4	35	21	2
22	43	M	R	L	BG	1.2	3	Present	6	3	75	48	4
23	61	M	R	L	BG	4.6	6	Present	9	4	35	40	3
24	39	M	R	L	BG	1.5	3	Absent	7	4	60	38	3
25	66	M	R	R	BG, CR	6.6	2	Present	9	4	45	32	2

M = male; F = female; R = right; L = left; AH = affected hemisphere; UH = unaffected hemisphere; IC = internal capsule; CR = corona radiata; BG = basal ganglia; MEPs = motor evoked potentials; NIHSS = National Institutes of Health Stroke Scale; mRS = modified Rankin Scale; BI = Barthel index; FMA = Fugl-Meyer assessment of upper extremity; MRC = Medical Research Council scale for hand muscles.

2.7.2. Dynamic Causal Modeling. Dynamic causal modeling [23] was used to assess effective connectivity within bilateral cortical motor areas activated by the fMRI motor task. Connectivity parameters represent the connectivity strength from one brain region to another. According to the previous studies [5, 12], six motor regions of interest (ROIs) from the fMRI motor task activation were selected for the DCM analysis: the primary motor area (M1), the premotor cortex (PMC), and the supplementary motor area (SMA) from both hemispheres of each subject (Table 1). A 4 mm radius sphere was applied to the ROI extraction. Principal component analysis was used to extract the ROI that represents signals. Based on previous studies on anatomical and functional connectivity in animals and human beings [4, 5, 12, 24], we supposed the intrinsic connection of these motor areas: connections between SMA and ipsilateral and contralateral M1, between SMA and ipsilateral PMC, and between PMC and ipsilateral M1 and transcallosal connections between M1-M1 and SMA-SMA. Bayes factors were computed for the "winning" model providing the best fit between accuracy and generalizability.

2.8. Statistical Analysis. Statistical analyses were performed on SPSS for Windows version 22 (IBM Corp., Armonk, NY). The comparison of neurophysiological measures in the bilateral hemisphere was analyzed by a two-tailed paired t-test, with a statistical significance set at $p < 0.05$. The estimated connectivity parameters of the "winning" model in patients were tested for statistical significance by means of one-sample t-tests ($p < 0.05$). Pearson correlation analyses were used to test the relationships between fMRI results (neural activity and connectivity parameters) and motor performance, as well as cortical excitability measures. The level of significance was set at $p < 0.05$.

3. Results

Table 2 shows the demographic, imaging, and clinical characteristics of these patients.

3.1. Cortical Excitability. In this study, MEPs could not be elicited in five of the 25 patients that were excluded from neurophysiological data analysis. We found a significant

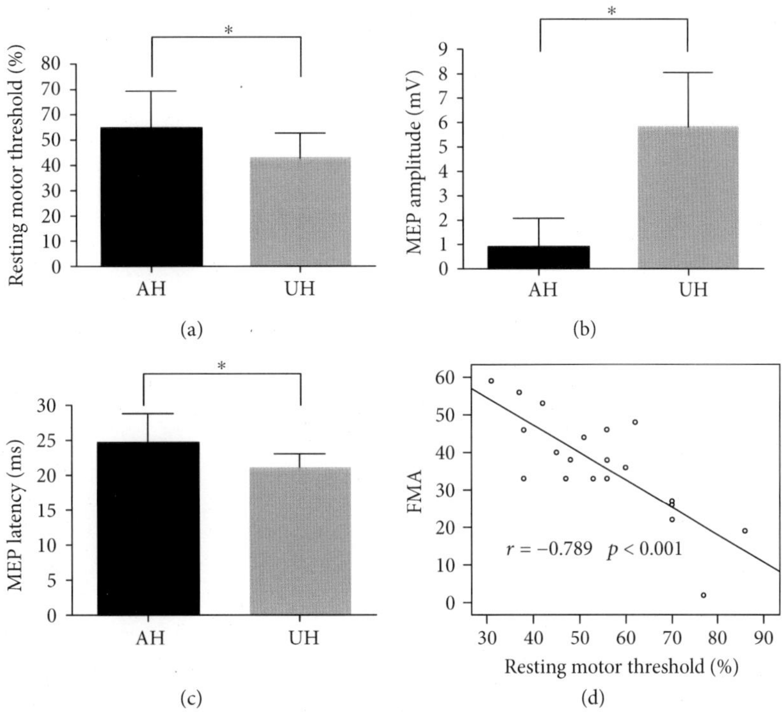

FIGURE 1: Cortical excitability as a resting motor threshold (a), MEP amplitude (b), and MEP latency (c) of the ipsilesional and contralesional hemisphere in patients. Significantly decreased cortical excitability in the ipsilesional hemisphere compared to the contralesional hemisphere ($p < 0.05$, pair t-test). (d) A significant negative correlation was evident between the resting motor threshold of the ipsilesional hemisphere and the FMA score, with reduced cortical excitability in the ipsilesional hemisphere featuring stronger motor impairment. FMA: Fugl-Meyer assessment. *Significant P value < 0.05.

decreased cortical excitability in the ipsilesional hemisphere (increased RMT, reduced MEP amplitude, and prolonged MEP latency) compared to the contralesional hemisphere ($p < 0.001$, $p < 0.001$, and $p = 0.001$, resp., paired t-test) (Figures 1(a)–1(c)). The RMT of the ipsilesional hemisphere significantly correlated with FMA scores of the affected limb ($r = -0.789$, $p < 0.001$) (Figure 1(d)), suggesting that better motor performance and less intensity were needed to evoke an MEP in ipsilesional M1. However, no significant correlation was evident between the RMT of the contralesional hemisphere and FMA scores of the affected limb ($r = -0.229$, $p = 0.331$).

3.2. fMRI Motor Activation. We first examined the task-related activation during hand movements. Movements of the unaffected hand were associated with significant BOLD activity in the contralateral M1, SMA, bilateral PMC, and the contralateral somatosensory cortex, consistent with previous studies in healthy subjects [25]. In contrast, although movements of the affected hand revealed BOLD activity in areas homologous to those just mentioned, neural activity decreased in both hemispheres, especially within M1 of the ipsilesional hemisphere (Figure 2(a)).

We next tested for correlations between brain activation early after stroke and motor impairment as well as motor cortical excitability. In the analysis of the relationship between brain activation and motor performance, we ruled out three outliers that were the patients with FMA 2-3 (patients 5, 6, and 12). A significant positive correlation was evident between the levels of BOLD activation within ipsilesional M1 and FMA ($r = 0.543$, $p = 0.009$), with better motor performance in patients featuring higher levels of BOLD activation in ipsilesional M1 during movement of the affected hand (Figure 2(b)). In 20 patients with the presence of MEP, we also found a significant correlation between cortical excitability of ipsilesional M1 and the BOLD activation in the ipsilesional sensorimotor area for movement of the affected hand ($r = 0.743$, $p < 0.001$) (Figure 2(c)). In contrast, the level of the BOLD signal in the contralesional hemisphere did not correlate with motor function as well as with cortical excitability of either hemisphere.

3.3. DCM. Figure 3(a) shows the winning model for endogenous neural coupling. We first analyzed the hand-movement-associated effective connectivity among bilateral motor networks (Figure 3(b)). The interhemispheric connections between ipsilesional and contralesional M1 showed negative connectivity parameters, indicating a mutual suppression of M1-M1 interactions during movement of the affected or unaffected hand ($p < 0.05$, corrected). Furthermore, we also found an additional inhibitory connectivity from contralesional SMA to M1 during movement of the affected hand, as has been described in the previous study [26].

In the next step, we performed correlation analysis of the connectivity parameters and motor function of the affected upper limb. We found that the FMA correlated negatively with inhibitory connectivity from contralesional

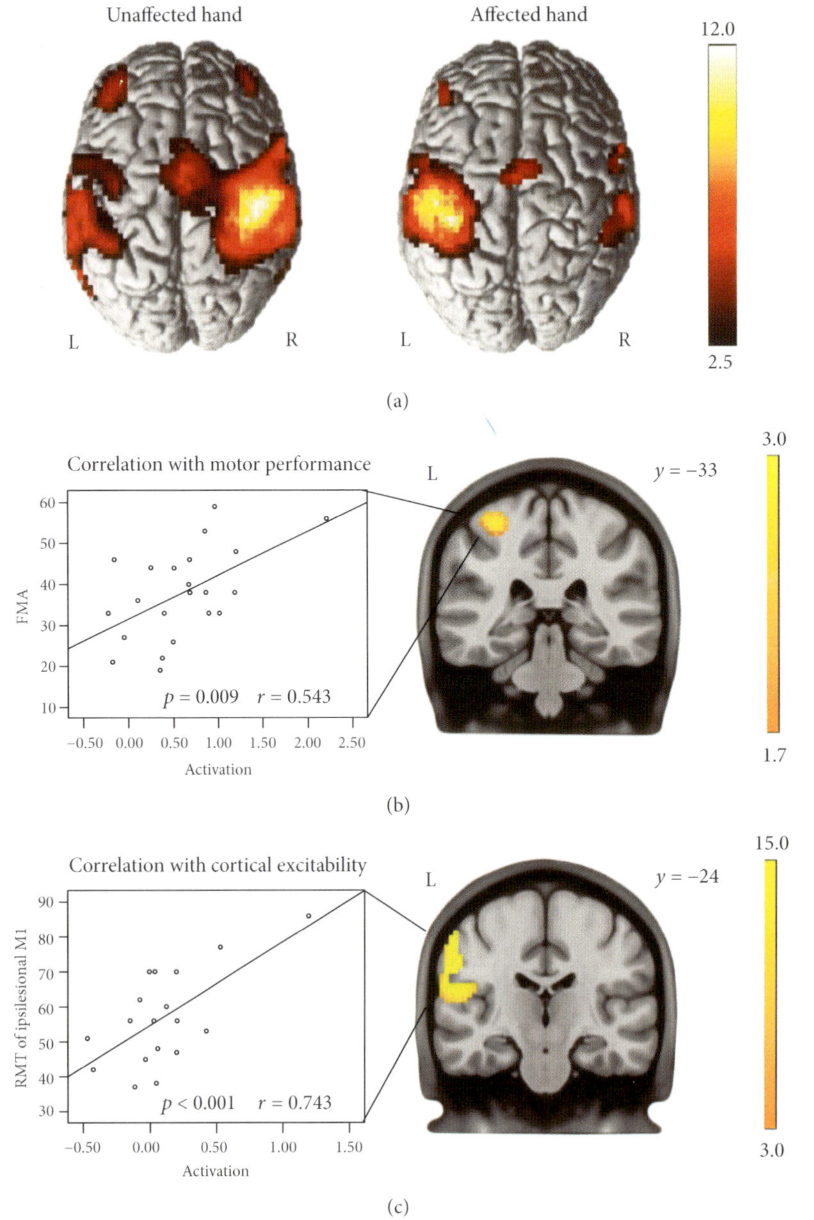

FIGURE 2: (a) Neural activity during movements of the unaffected and affected hands ($p < 0.01$, FDR corrected). (b) Significant correlation of BOLD activity with FMA of the upper extremity in ipsilesional M1 ($p < 0.05$, uncorrected) for movements of the affected hand. (c) Significant correlation of BOLD activity with the RMT of the ipsilesional hemisphere in the ipsilesional sensorimotor area ($p < 0.05$, uncorrected). L: left; R: right.

M1 to ipsilesional M1 ($p = 0.047$, $r = -0.461$) and positively with inhibitory connectivity from contralesional SMA to M1 ($p = 0.041$, $r = 0.533$) during movements of the affected hand. For movements of the unaffected hand, the FMA correlated with promoting connectivity from contralesional SMA to ipsilesional M1 ($r = 0.472$, $p = 0.036$) as well as with the M1-M1 inhibition (reduced inhibition of ipsilesional M1) ($r = -0.486$, $p = 0.022$, resp.) (Figure 4(a)). These findings were consistent with our fMRI result showing that BOLD activity within the ipsilesional M1 correlated with better motor performance (Figure 2(b)).

Finally, when correlating DCM connectivity parameters with cortical excitability, we found that the stronger the promoting connectivity from ipsilesional PMC to M1 during movement of the affected hand was, the more active the motor cortex excitability was present in the ipsilesional hemisphere ($r = -0.457$, $p = 0.043$; Figure 4(b)). In addition, we also found a statistically significant correlation between the M1-M1 inhibition and RMT of the ipsilesional hemisphere during movement of the unaffected hand (ipsilesional M1-contralesional M1, $r = -0.472$, $p = 0.036$; contralesional M1-ipsilesional M1, $r = 0.542$, $p = 0.02$) (Figure 4(b)). Hence, lower motor cortex excitability (higher intensities are needed to evoke MEP) in the ipsilesional hemisphere featured more intra- or interhemispheric inhibition of ipsilesional M1 and a relative disinhibition of contralesional M1.

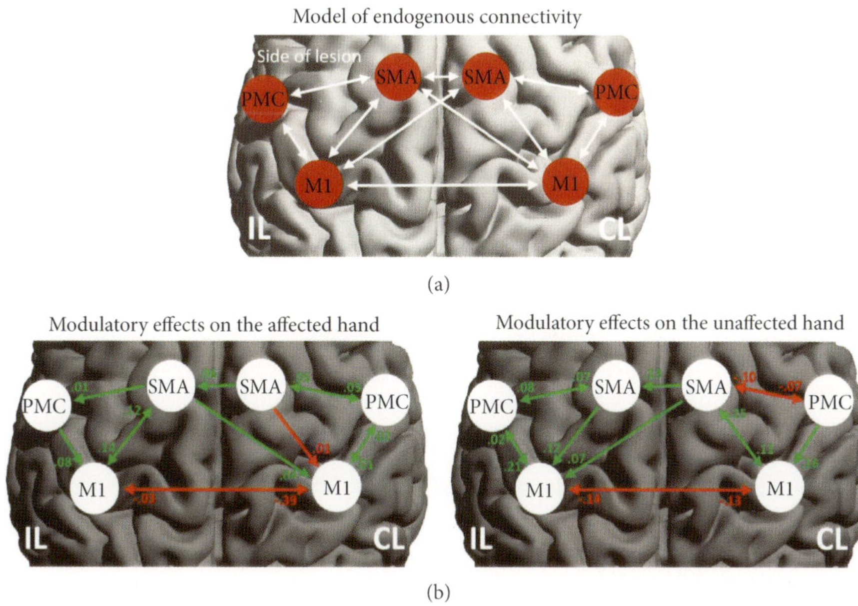

FIGURE 3: (a) Regions of interest (ROI) and connectivity model used for estimating interregional connectivity. Scans from patients with right-sided lesions were flipped, so that all patients were assumed to have left hemispheric lesions. (b) Task-dependent modulations of connectivity during movements of the affected and unaffected hands. Positive (green) values refer to the promotion of neural activity. Negative (red) values mean the inhibitory influence on neuronal activity. IL: ipsilesional hemisphere; CL: contralesional hemisphere.

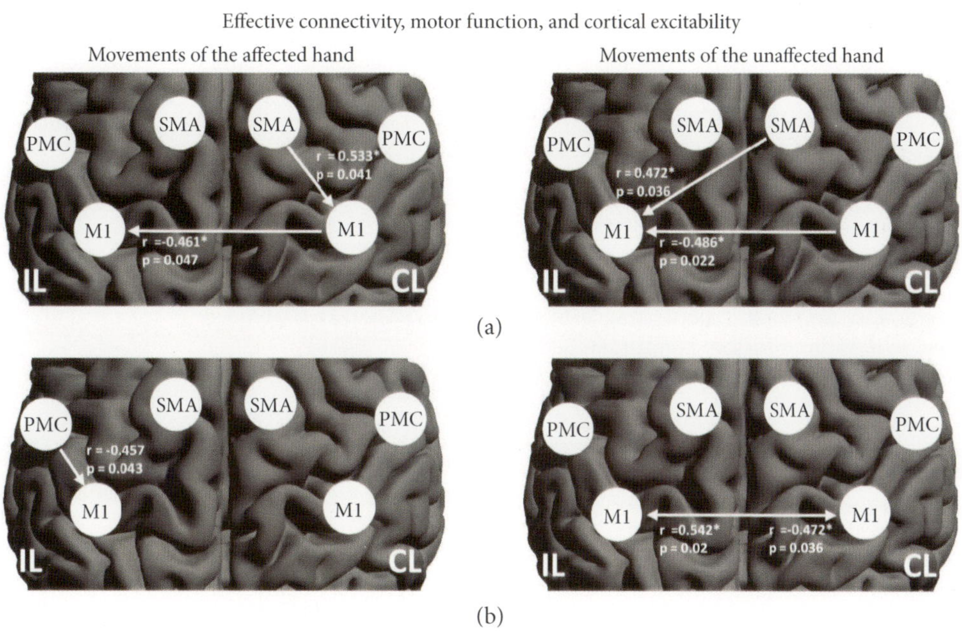

FIGURE 4: Significant Pearson correlation of DCM connectivity parameters with motor function and cortical excitability. (a) The interhemispheric connections from contralesional-ipsilesional M1 correlated with the degree of motor impairment irrespective of the affected or unaffected hand movements. The motor function also correlated with both contralesional SMA-M1 for the affected hand movement and contralesional SMA-ipsilesional M1 for the unaffected hand movement. (b) Motor excitability of the ipsilesional hemisphere significantly correlated with ipsilesional PMC-M1 during movement of the affected hand and interhemispheric M1-M1 inhibition. IL: ipsilesional hemisphere; CL: contralesional hemisphere.

4. Discussion

Combining neuroimaging and electrophysiological measures, the present study examined the relationships of effective connectivity with motor performance and motor cortical excitability in acute ischemic stroke. We first found that the brain region responding to the affected hand had weaker fMRI activation and cortical excitability relative to those of the unaffected hand. The fMRI activation and cortical excitability in the ipsilesional M1 during movement of the affected hand showed a positive correlation with motor performance. Importantly, DCM analysis revealed both enhancement of positive connectivity in the ipsilesional M1 and negative connectivity in the contralesional M1 correlated with motor performance and the ipsilesional cortical excitability.

4.1. Motor Cortical Excitability and Activity. In the present study, the assessments of neural activity and motor cortical excitability provided direct multimodal evidence that the less ipsilesional M1 recruitment signifies poor motor performance in the acute phase after stroke. Our data identified that the reduced cortical excitability and activity in the ipsilesional M1 were associated with the degree of motor impairment in stroke patients. The results were in line with a recent meta-analysis indicating activity in ipsilesional M1 characterizing favorable motor recovery after stroke [27]. Furthermore, we also found a positive correlation between the brain activity in the ipsilesional sensorimotor area and RMT of ipsilesional M1, which implied that the more recruited ipsilesional sensorimotor motor cortex, the less decreased motor cortical excitability of the ipsilesional hemisphere. The parietal lobe of the cortex is responsible for somatosensation and has been shown to be involved in sensorimotor integration for hand coordination [28]. This finding may, at least in part, be related to the fact that passive motor task influenced the neural activity in the somatosensory cortex. However, due to the variance in RMT that was considerably larger in the ipsilesional motor cortex, this observation needs further investigation.

4.2. Effective Connectivity in Motor Areas. Importantly, we combined fMRI and neurophysiological measures to investigate the effective connectivity in key motor regions in relation to cortical excitability and motor performance in the acute stage of stroke. Our findings further confirmed the former studies enrolling subacute or chronic stroke patients and demonstrated that a reduction of pathological transcallosal influences (originating from contralesional M1 to ipsilesional M1) may underlie improved motor performance [3, 26].

In the concept of interhemispheric inhibition model theory, both hemispheric M1 exhibit a mutual inhibitory influence on each other [29, 30], which is reflected in the present study data by showing a mutual suppression of M1-M1 connections. We demonstrated that patients with more enhanced inhibitory connectivity to ipsilesional M1 or less intra- and interhemispheric inhibition to contralesional M1 showed stronger motor impairment and lower ipsilesional cortical excitability. In addition, our data demonstrated that the neural coupling between contralesional SMA and contralesional M1, as well as ipsilesional M1, significantly correlated with the degree of motor impairment. More recent neuroimaging and electrophysiological data provided the evidence of the role of SMA showing that a large proportion of SMA neurons exclusively respond to contralateral hand movements only [12, 31]. These findings are compatible with our data suggesting that the SMA might represent a key region promoting or inhibiting the influence on the cortical motor network during movements of the affected or unaffected hand.

4.3. Limitation. Several limitations were noteworthy. Firstly, given the cross-sectional design of the study, we can only provide preliminary evidence of correlations across different modalities, without identifying their causative interactions. Future longitudinal studies can be performed to investigate whether the factors identified in the present study (combination of RMT, BOLD activation, and effective connectivity) have a predictive value in the acute poststroke phase for long-term recovery. Secondly, this study did not involve the healthy participants as controls.

5. Conclusions

By combining fMRI and electrophysiological measures, this study revealed the aberrances of cortex excitability and connectivity in the acute stage of stroke. The findings contributed to the understanding of the pathophysiology of motor impairment in the early phase of stroke. The inhibitory connectivity to ipsilesional M1 and a relative disinhibition of contralesional M1 may constitute an important pathophysiological aspect of motor disability in acute stroke. Moreover, the present findings might have important implication for early rehabilitative therapy in stroke patients. Aberrances of the cortical excitability and connectivity in the ipsilesional M1 might be considered the therapeutic targets in a few of novel therapeutic strategies (e.g., noninvasive brain stimulation) for the early stage of stroke [32–34].

Additional Points

Highlights. The neural mechanisms of motor deficit in acute stroke remain unclear. This multimodal study demonstrated the relationships of cortical excitability, effective connectivity, and motor impairment following stroke. Our findings provided important theoretical implication for early rehabilitative therapy in stroke patients.

Disclosure

Juan Du and Jianping Hu share the first authorship.

Conflicts of Interest

The authors declare no conflict of interest.

Authors' Contributions

Juan Du and Jianping Hu contributed equally to this work.

Acknowledgments

This work was supported by the National Natural Science Foundation of China (nos. 81530038, 81501193, 81220108008, 81701299, and 81771424), Natural Science Foundation of Jiangsu Province (no. BK20141373), the special scientific research fund of Public Welfare Profession of National Health and Family Planning Commission of the People's Republic of China (no. 201402019), the independent research project in State Key Laboratory of Analytical Chemistry for Life Science (no. 5431ZZXM1716).

References

[1] V. L. Feigin, M. H. Forouzanfar, R. Krishnamurthi et al., "Global and regional burden of stroke during 1990-2010: findings from the Global Burden of Disease Study 2010," *The Lancet*, vol. 383, no. 9913, pp. 245–255, 2014.

[2] N. E. Mayo, S. Wood-Dauphinee, S. Ahmed et al., "Disablement following stroke," *Disability and Rehabilitation*, vol. 21, no. 5-6, pp. 258–268, 1999.

[3] A. K. Rehme, S. B. Eickhoff, C. Rottschy, G. R. Fink, and C. Grefkes, "Activation likelihood estimation meta-analysis of motor-related neural activity after stroke," *NeuroImage*, vol. 59, no. 3, pp. 2771–2782, 2012.

[4] A. K. Rehme, S. B. Eickhoff, L. E. Wang, G. R. Fink, and C. Grefkes, "Dynamic causal modeling of cortical activity from the acute to the chronic stage after stroke," *NeuroImage*, vol. 55, no. 3, pp. 1147–1158, 2011.

[5] C. Grefkes, D. A. Nowak, S. B. Eickhoff et al., "Cortical connectivity after subcortical stroke assessed with functional magnetic resonance imaging," *Annals of Neurology*, vol. 63, no. 2, pp. 236–246, 2008.

[6] J. Duque, F. Hummel, P. Celnik, N. Murase, R. Mazzocchio, and L. G. Cohen, "Transcallosal inhibition in chronic subcortical stroke," *NeuroImage*, vol. 28, no. 4, pp. 940–946, 2005.

[7] N. Murase, J. Duque, R. Mazzocchio, and L. G. Cohen, "Influence of interhemispheric interactions on motor function in chronic stroke," *Annals of Neurology*, vol. 55, no. 3, pp. 400–409, 2004.

[8] S. C. Cramer and J. D. Riley, "Neuroplasticity and brain repair after stroke," *Current Opinion in Neurology*, vol. 21, no. 1, pp. 76–82, 2008.

[9] R. J. Nudo, "Mechanisms for recovery of motor function following cortical damage," *Current Opinion in Neurobiology*, vol. 16, no. 6, pp. 638–644, 2006.

[10] S. D. Horn, G. DeJong, R. J. Smout, J. Gassaway, R. James, and B. Conroy, "Stroke rehabilitation patients, practice, and outcomes: is earlier and more aggressive therapy better?," *Archives of Physical Medicine and Rehabilitation*, vol. 86, no. 12, pp. 101–114, 2005.

[11] C. Grefkes and G. R. Fink, "Reorganization of cerebral networks after stroke: new insights from neuroimaging with connectivity approaches," *Brain*, vol. 134, no. 5, pp. 1264–1276, 2011.

[12] C. Grefkes, S. B. Eickhoff, D. A. Nowak, M. Dafotakis, and G. R. Fink, "Dynamic intra- and interhemispheric interactions during unilateral and bilateral hand movements assessed with fMRI and DCM," *NeuroImage*, vol. 41, no. 4, pp. 1382–1394, 2008.

[13] M. C. Smith and C. M. Stinear, "Transcranial magnetic stimulation (TMS) in stroke: ready for clinical practice?," *Journal of Clinical Neuroscience*, vol. 31, pp. 10–14, 2016.

[14] C. Grefkes and G. R. Fink, "Disruption of motor network connectivity post-stroke and its noninvasive neuromodulation," *Current Opinion in Neurology*, vol. 25, no. 6, pp. 670–675, 2012.

[15] T. Brott, H. J. Adams, C. P. Olinger et al., "Measurements of acute cerebral infarction: a clinical examination scale," *Stroke*, vol. 20, no. 7, pp. 864–870, 1989.

[16] J. T. Wilson, A. Hareendran, M. Grant et al., "Improving the assessment of outcomes in stroke: use of a structured interview to assign grades on the modified Rankin scale," *Stroke*, vol. 33, no. 9, pp. 2243–2246, 2002.

[17] D. J. Gladstone, C. J. Danells, and S. E. Black, "The Fugl-Meyer assessment of motor recovery after stroke: a critical review of its measurement properties," *Neurorehabilitation and Neural Repair*, vol. 16, no. 3, pp. 232–240, 2002.

[18] A. Compston, "Aids to the investigation of peripheral nerve injuries. Medical Research Council: Nerve Injuries Research Committee. His Majesty's Stationery Office: 1942; pp. 48 (iii) and 74 figures and 7 diagrams; *with* aids to the examination of the peripheral nervous system. By Michael O'Brien for the Guarantors of Brain. Saunders Elsevier: 2010; pp. [8] 64 and 94 figures," *Brain*, vol. 133, no. 10, pp. 2838–2844, 2010.

[19] P. M. Rossini, D. Burke, R. Chen et al., "Non-invasive electrical and magnetic stimulation of the brain, spinal cord, roots and peripheral nerves: basic principles and procedures for routine clinical and research application. An updated report from an I.F.C.N. Committee," *Clinical Neurophysiology*, vol. 126, no. 6, pp. 1071–1107, 2015.

[20] S. Groppa, A. Oliviero, A. Eisen et al., "A practical guide to diagnostic transcranial magnetic stimulation: report of an IFCN committee," *Clinical Neurophysiology*, vol. 123, no. 5, pp. 858–882, 2012.

[21] G. T. Stebbins, D. L. Nyenhuis, C. Wang et al., "Gray matter atrophy in patients with ischemic stroke with cognitive impairment," *Stroke*, vol. 39, no. 3, pp. 785–793, 2008.

[22] W. Wei, Z. Zhang, Q. Xu, F. Yang, K. Sun, and G. Lu, "More severe extratemporal damages in mesial temporal lobe epilepsy with hippocampal sclerosis than that with other lesions: a multimodality MRI study," *Medicine*, vol. 95, no. 10, article e3020, 2016.

[23] K. J. Friston, L. Harrison, and W. Penny, "Dynamic causal modelling," *NeuroImage*, vol. 19, no. 4, pp. 1273–1302, 2003.

[24] C. Grefkes, D. A. Nowak, L. E. Wang, M. Dafotakis, S. B. Eickhoff, and G. R. Fink, "Modulating cortical connectivity in stroke patients by rTMS assessed with fMRI and dynamic causal modeling," *NeuroImage*, vol. 50, no. 1, pp. 233–242, 2010.

[25] S. M. Rao, J. R. Binder, P. A. Bandettini et al., "Functional magnetic resonance imaging of complex human movements," *Neurology*, vol. 43, no. 11, pp. 2311–2318, 1993.

[26] L. J. Volz, A. S. Sarfeld, S. Diekhoff et al., "Motor cortex excitability and connectivity in chronic stroke: a multimodal model of functional reorganization," *Brain Structure & Function*, vol. 220, no. 2, pp. 1093–1107, 2015.

[27] I. Favre, T. A. Zeffiro, O. Detante, A. Krainik, M. Hommel, and A. Jaillard, "Upper limb recovery after stroke is associated with ipsilesional primary motor cortical activity: a meta-analysis," *Stroke*, vol. 45, no. 4, pp. 1077–1083, 2014.

[28] Y. E. Cohen and R. A. Andersen, "A common reference frame for movement plans in the posterior parietal cortex," *Nature Reviews. Neuroscience*, vol. 3, no. 7, pp. 553–562, 2002.

[29] A. Ferbert, A. Priori, J. C. Rothwell, B. L. Day, J. G. Colebatch, and C. D. Marsden, "Interhemispheric inhibition of the human motor cortex," *The Journal of Physiology*, vol. 453, no. 1, pp. 525–546, 1992.

[30] E. M. Wassermann, P. Fuhr, L. G. Cohen, and M. Hallett, "Effects of transcranial magnetic stimulation on ipsilateral muscles," *Neurology*, vol. 41, no. 11, pp. 1795–1799, 1991.

[31] O. Kazennikov, B. Hyland, M. Corboz, A. Babalian, E. M. Rouiller, and M. Wiesendanger, "Neural activity of supplementary and primary motor areas in monkeys and its relation to bimanual and unimanual movement sequences," *Neuroscience*, vol. 89, no. 3, pp. 661–674, 1999.

[32] Y. H. Kim, S. H. You, M. H. Ko et al., "Repetitive transcranial magnetic stimulation-induced corticomotor excitability and associated motor skill acquisition in chronic stroke," *Stroke*, vol. 37, no. 6, pp. 1471–1476, 2006.

[33] W. H. Sung, C. P. Wang, C. L. Chou, Y. C. Chen, Y. C. Chang, and P. Y. Tsai, "Efficacy of coupling inhibitory and facilitatory repetitive transcranial magnetic stimulation to enhance motor recovery in hemiplegic stroke patients," *Stroke*, vol. 44, no. 5, pp. 1375–1382, 2013.

[34] C. M. Stinear, M. A. Petoe, and W. D. Byblow, "Primary motor cortex excitability during recovery after stroke: implications for neuromodulation," *Brain Stimulation*, vol. 8, no. 6, pp. 1183–1190, 2015.

3

The Role of Autoimmunity in the Pathogenesis of Sudden Sensorineural Hearing Loss

Guangfei Li,[1] Dan You,[1] Jiaoyao Ma,[1] Wen Li,[1] Huawei Li,[1,2] and Shan Sun[1]

[1]*Key Laboratory of Hearing Medicine of NHFPC, ENT Institute and Otorhinolaryngology Department, Shanghai Engineering Research Centre of Cochlear Implant, Affiliated Eye and ENT Hospital, State Key Laboratory of Medical Neurobiology, Fudan University, Shanghai 200031, China*
[2]*Institutes of Biomedical Sciences and The Institutes of Brain Science and the Collaborative Innovation Center for Brain Science, Fudan University, Shanghai 200032, China*

Correspondence should be addressed to Huawei Li; hwli@shmu.edu.cn and Shan Sun; shansun@fudan.edu.cn

Academic Editor: Hai Huang

Sudden sensorineural hearing loss (SSHL) is a clinically common acute symptom in otolaryngology. Although the incidence of SSHL has increased around the world in recent years, the etiology of the disease is still unclear. It has been reported that infections, ototoxic drugs, membrane labyrinth rupture, carcinomas, circulatory system diseases, autoimmune diseases, brain lesions, mental diseases, congenital or inherited diseases, and so on, are all risk factors for SSHL. Here, we discuss the autoimmune mechanisms behind SSHL, which might be induced by type II–IV allergic reactions. We also introduce the main immunosuppressive medications that have been used to treat SSHL, which will help us to identify potential targets for immune therapy.

1. Introduction

Sudden sensorineural hearing loss (SSHL) or "idiopathic sudden sensorineural hearing loss" refers to the sudden, unexplained hearing loss of more than 30 dB across all frequencies. The main clinical symptom is hearing loss, sometimes accompanied by tinnitus, ear blockage, dizziness, nausea, and/or vomiting. The pathogenesis of SSHL involves complex systemic or regional symptoms, and there are as yet no effective treatments. Here, we review our current understanding of SSHL and inner ear structures and cells as the fundamental platform for immune surveillance and responsiveness in hearing loss, and we present a summary of SSHL that results from immune system dysfunction. We think that immune-modulating medications support the clinical findings and suggest some potential targets for therapy in clinics.

2. The Evidence for Autoimmunity in SSHL

The inner ear and brain are traditionally viewed as being immune privileged because there is a blood-labyrinthine barrier that acts in a similar manner as the blood-brain barrier, and only a few macrophages are present in these organs [1]. However, a large number of experimental and clinical cases of SSHL have been identified in which SSHL is a symptom associated with other autoimmune diseases or is the primary symptom of spontaneous systemic autoimmune diseases such as autoimmune hepatitis [2], sympathetic neural hyperalgesia edema syndrome [3], Cogan's syndrome [4, 5], systemic lupus erythematosus [6, 7], multiple sclerosis [8–10], rheumatoid arthritis [11], nodular polyarteritis [12], Crohn's disease [13], and so on. Increasing experimental evidence suggesting an autoimmune component in the pathology of SSHL has emerged since 1979 when McCabe first identified 18 patients with autoimmune-associated SSHL who were effectively medicated with glucocorticoid and vincristine [14]. The presence of antibodies against the inner ear 68 kDa antigen and the recovery of hearing after immunosuppressive therapy have further confirmed the immune-mediated mechanism of hearing loss [15–18]. Immunohistochemistry and other techniques have been used to show that immune cells, including lymphocytes,

TABLE 1: The main autoimmune target antigens in the inner ear.

Inner ear antigen	Distribution	References
Collagen type II	In the subepithelial layer of the endolymphatic duct and spiral ligament.	[26, 64–68]
HSP-70	Hair cells and supporting cells.	[16, 17, 69–73]
β-Tubulin	Hair cells, supporting cells, the spiral ligament of the stria vascularis, and the spiral ganglion.	[54, 74–78]
Cochlin	In the regions of the fibrocytes of the spiral limbus and the spiral ligament and in the cochlear and vestibular labyrinth.	[52, 53, 79–82]
Beta-tectorin	Hair cells in the basal region of the hair bundle lying over the apical surface of the auditory epithelium, in the basilar papilla, in the clear cells and the cuboidal cells, and in the striolar region of the lagena macula.	[52, 53, 77, 83, 84]
Kresge Hearing Research Institute-3 (KHRI-3)	This is a protein specific to the inner ear and is expressed in the saccular wall cells and transitional epithelial cells in the utricle and ampules, by cells in the endolymphatic sac, and by supporting cells.	[85, 86]

leukocytes, and macrophages, are present in the inner ear as well as to analyze the interactions between these immune cells [19–22]. The following inner ear antigens (see Table 1) are considered to be the main targets of harmful antibodies: 68 kDa protein [23, 24], 30 kDa protein (also called myelin protein zero (P0)) [25], collagen type II [26, 27], tubulin [28], cochlin [29, 30], and inner ear supporting cell antigen [23]. Moscicki et al. have confirmed the clinical relationship between idiopathic SSHL and anti-68 kDa protein antibodies in patient serum [22, 31]. Furthermore, Billings et al. [24] and Bloch et al. [16, 17] have confirmed that the 68 kDa protein is heat shock protein 70 (HSP-70). These studies have provided a basis for the diagnosis and treatment of autoimmune-related SSHL.

3. The Immune Response in the Inner Ear

The immune system plays an important role in protecting the inner ear from damage caused by bacteria, viruses, and other pathogenic microorganisms. However, in the pathogenesis of autoimmune hearing loss, the immune system itself damages the inner ear. Although the exact mechanism of its pathogenesis is not yet fully understood, studies in patients with SSHL and in experimental animal models have identified a number of factors that are involved in autoimmune SSHL. The immune response in the inner ear relies on cytokines, especially IL-1β [32, 33], IL-2, and TNF-α [34], that play important roles in regulating the immune response of the inner ear. Some inflammatory cells in the inner ear are also involved, including macrophages (or microglia-like cells), T lymphocytes, and leukocytes. Our previous work has demonstrated that the ototoxicity of neomycin (an aminoglycoside antibiotic) is mediated through the activation of microglia-like cells that release proinflammatory cytokines that cause damage to the hair cells of the inner ear [35, 36].

3.1. The Physiological Immune Defense in the Inner Ear. The inner ear is fully capable of initiating an immune response to the invasion of external antigens. Previous studies have shown that the lymphatic sac contains several of the immunological components of the immune response and is the primary site of the immune response [37, 38]. The antigens in the inner ear are often used as targets for such immune responses. Recognition of these antigens by the inner ear's innate immune cells (neutrophils, macrophages, dendritic cells, etc.; see Table 2 and Figure 1) stimulates the release of IL-1β, which in turn triggers a series of adaptive immune responses. The cytokines that are released as part of these responses then recruit lymphocytes from the circulatory system into the inner ear where they cause irreversible tissue damage [39].

3.2. Pathological Immunity in the Inner Ear. No lymphocytes are present in the normal endolymphatic sac, and there is no evidence that the lymphocytes present in the cochlea during the immune response are derived from the endolymphatic sac; thus, they must originate mainly from the peripheral circulatory system [40]. Lymphocytes in the circulatory system are predominantly migrating from the spiral vessels and their branches [41]. When they reach the other organs of the body, they initiate the process of antigen absorption, presentation, and degradation. IL-1 plays an important role in regulating the innate immune response, and it acts as an agonist of resting helper T cells and B cells. The helper T cells, once activated by IL-1, will produce IL-2. The secretion of IL-2 results in pluripotent stem cells differentiating into helper T cells, cytotoxic T cells, and suppressor T cells. IL-2 also assists helper T cells in activating B lymphocytes and might play an important role in regulating the immune response in the inner ear [42].

IL-1β and TNF-α are involved in the initiation and amplification of immune responses. IL-1β is mainly expressed in the fibroblasts of the spiral ligament in the case of nonspecific trauma such as surgery or acoustic neuroma, while TNF-α is mainly expressed in infiltrating circulating inflammatory cells or innate immune cells in the endolymphatic sac under the stimulation of external antigens. The release of TNF-α in animal models is a part of the adaptive immune response. When an antigen is injected into the mouse inner ear, both IL-1β and TNF-α are secreted and a normal immune response occurs. However, when the antigen flows from the cerebrospinal fluid to the inner ear and the inner ear is not traumatized, only TNF-α is secreted and only a very weak immune response is initiated. It is

Table 2: The innate immune cells and adaptive immune cells in the inner ear.

Immune cells			Function	Distribution	References
Innate immune cells	Macrophages		Promote the proliferation of T cells and B cells; Process and present antigens and participate in the regulation of adaptive immune responses; Phagocytosis and digestion of pathogenic microorganisms; Mediate and promote inflammatory responses	Endolymphatic sac and subepithelial and endoluminal space and the scala tympani and scala vestibuli.	[37, 38, 87, 88]
	Granulocytes		Anti-inflammatory, release of some inflammatory factors.	In the scala tympani, in the scala vestibuli from the basal turn to the apex, and in the modiolus.	[88–90]
Adaptive immune cells	B cells		Antigen identification and presentation. Activated B cells differentiate into plasma cells that secrete antibodies.	Peripheral circulation system, infiltrating into the endolymph and perilymph of the scala tympani and the scala vestibule and the endolymphatic sac.	[38, 91]
	Helper T cells	Th1 cells	Mediate cellular immunity; Secrete some cytokines, such as IFN-γ.	From the peripheral circulation system, infiltrate into the scala tympani, the scala vestibuli, and the perisaccular connective tissue of the endolymphatic sac and the modiolar vessels.	[20, 21, 52, 54, 82, 87, 91, 92]
		Th2 cells	Mediate humoral immunity; Secrete cytokines IL-4, IL-5, and IL-13.		
		Th17 cells	Secrete inflammatory cytokines IL-17 and IL-22; act as inflammation-initiating cells.		
	Suppressor T cells	$CD4^+/CD25^+$ Th cells	Negative regulator of immune response; $CD4^+CD25^+$ regulatory T cells play an immunosuppressive function in the periphery;	From the circulation, infiltrate into the modiolus, the scala tympani, and the perisaccular connective tissue of the endolymphatic sac.	[55, 87, 92, 93]
		Antigen-specific regulatory T cells (inducible regulatory T cells (iTregs))	iTregs can secrete the suppressive cytokines IL-10 and TGF-β.		
	Lymphocytes		Anti-inflammatory	In the scala tympani, in all turns of the cochlea, and in smaller numbers in the scala vestibuli.	[51]

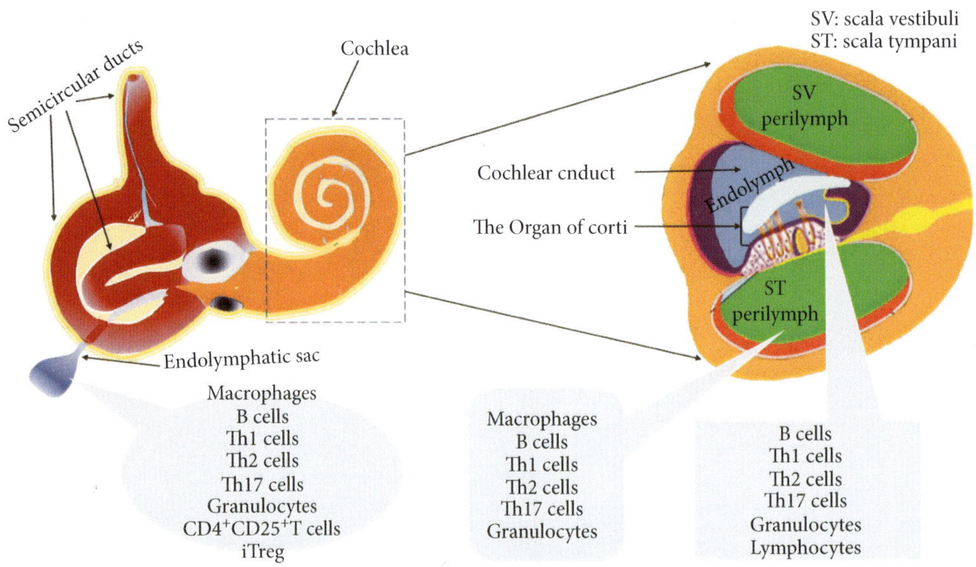

FIGURE 1: The distribution of immune cells in the inner ear when the immune response is initiated.

worth noting that damage to the cochlea alone can also lead to a slight immune response [43]. These results all show that the nonspecific and specific components of the immune response act synergistically in the inner ear so as to maximize the effect of the immune response.

Therefore, if the cochlea is damaged or antigens are injected into the cochlea (or a patient with an autoimmune disease has immune cells directly attacking the inner ear antigen), both nonspecific and specific immune responses are activated simultaneously, and these can result in simultaneous IL-1β and TNF-α production that amplifies the inflammatory effect and then leads to extensive damage to the inner ear tissue. Animal model experiments have confirmed that the innate immune response predominates in the inner ear until the regulatory immune response produces enough of an inflammatory response to cause damage to the inner ear. Therefore, when innate and specific immune responses are activated at the same time, it might be possible to avoid excessive immune responses by downregulating or inhibiting specific immune responses, particularly those that inhibit the effects of TNF-α.

4. The Immune Pathogenesis of Hearing Loss

Although it is known that immune responses in the inner ear can lead to tissue damage, the exact mechanism behind the injury process remains unclear, and thus we can use other autoimmune diseases as a reference to understand such injury processes in the inner ear. In general, immune response damage is mediated by both humoral and cellular immunity, and autoimmune damage can be classified as type I allergic reactions to type IV allergic reactions. Type I allergic reactions (immediate-type allergic reactions) are mainly caused by the interactions of an antigen with an antibody (usually IgE) on the surface of immune cells that activate the cells and causes them to release active mediators such as histamine and serotonin to induce a rapid immune response. Type II allergic reactions (cytotoxic allergies) are mediated by IgG or IgM, and when the antibody binds to the antigen on the foreign cell surface, the cells are destroyed due to the action of the complement system, phagocytes, or nature killer cells. Type III allergic reactions (immune complex allergies) are caused by the deposition of medium-sized soluble antigen-antibody complexes into capillary walls or tissues, which activates the complement system or leads to the recruitment of leukocytes. Type IV allergic reactions (delayed-type allergies) cause tissue injury that is mediated by T cells. Type I allergic reactions are not associated with autoimmune hearing loss, but types II–IV (see Figure 2) have been shown to be potential mechanisms that lead to inner ear damage in autoimmune SSHL [44], and these are described in the following sections.

4.1. Type II Allergic Reactions (Cytotoxic Allergies). Type II cytotoxic antibody-mediated damage can be confirmed from previous animal studies and clinical studies. Harris [45, 46] injected KLH protein, a metalloprotein extracted from snails, into susceptible guinea pigs. The exposure to KLH resulted in the production of anti-KLH antibodies. Subsequent injection of bovine inner ear antigen into guinea pigs resulted in hearing loss, and circulating antibodies specific to bovine inner ear antigen were found in the serum and perilymph. In patients with SSHL, analysis of antibodies in the inner ear using Western blotting revealed that there were IgG antibodies against the inner ear-specific proteins cochlin and β-tectorin and the nonspecific protein HSP-70. This study revealed that the direct antibody response to inner ear proteins can lead to SSHL and that such antibodies can be used as a marker for disease diagnosis. Using antigen-specific Western blot analysis of patient and healthy sera, it was found that anti-cochlin IgG antibodies were more prevalent in patients with idiopathic sensorineural hearing loss than anti-β-tectorin-specific IgG antibodies, whereas anti-HSP-70 IgG antibodies were more common

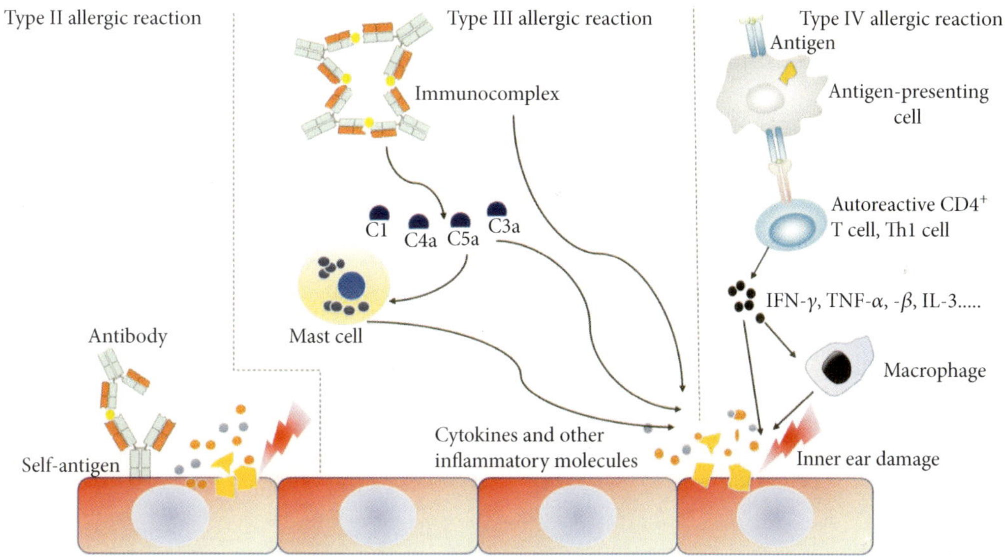

FIGURE 2: The mechanisms of inner ear damage by the type II–IV allergic reactions.

than anti-cochlin IgG antibodies and anti-β-tectorin-specific IgG antibodies in all of the patients [47]. These animal experiments and clinical studies have provided compelling evidence that in at least some patients with SSHL the pathology is due to antibody-mediated tissue damage in the inner ear.

4.2. Type III Allergic Reactions (Immune Complex Allergies). Type III immunocomplex-mediated hearing loss mechanisms have been identified in animal models of SSHL. Especially in C3H/lpr autoimmune mice with progressive hearing loss, one can find deposition of immunocomplexes in the vascular stria [48], and the deposition of IgM and IgG immunocomplexes can be seen in NZB/kl mice that have high incidences of hearing loss [49]. Trune et al. found the presence of DNA antibodies in the inner ear of MRL/lpr mice, and such anti-DNA or DNA-anti-DNA antibody immunocomplexes result in the destruction of endothelial cell integrity that affects the function of the blood-labyrinthine barrier resulting in SSHL [50]. Although the transfer of findings from animal models to patients is still speculative, the link between systemic autoimmune diseases and SSHL can provide additional evidence for the existence of such a mechanism. Many clinical cases have described hearing loss patients with associated systemic autoimmune disorders, and many of these systemic autoimmune diseases have been confirmed as type III allergic reactions with immunocomplex deposition resulting in tissue damage. For example, a 19-year-old girl with SSHL and mouth ulcers and bleeding under the nails was diagnosed with systemic lupus erythematosus. The histological sections revealed deposition of IgG, C3, C1q, and IgM immunocomplexes, obstruction of the vasculature of the inner ear by the formation of microthrombi, and damage to the organization of the inner ear. This patient's hearing recovered significantly with the use of methylprednisolone and other hormones [6]. Systemic autoimmune diseases such as multiple sclerosis, rheumatoid arthritis, and nodular arteriosclerosis are all associated with SSHL and are believed to form circulating immunocomplexes that deposit in the inner ear's vascular tissue thus causing SSHL.

4.3. Type IV Allergic Reactions (Delayed-Type Allergies): Autoreactive T Cell-Mediated Inflammatory Lesions. SSHL caused by type IV allergic reactions can be observed in animal models. Gloddek et al. used radioactive isotopes of chromium to label lymphocytes in susceptible experimental animals and demonstrated that lymphocytes migrate to the inner ear in response to antigenic stimulation and that infiltrated lymphocytes are found in the basal membrane and in the vestibule of the cochlea [51]. Hearing loss at all frequencies in the auditory brainstem response of mice was observed 5 weeks after immunization with the inner ear-specific protein cochlin 131–150 or β-tectorin in SWXJ mice. Each of the tested peptides activated Th1-like $CD4^+$ T cells with proinflammatory effects as observed by flow cytometry analysis, and after 6 weeks of selective transfer of peptide-activated $CD4^+$ T cells to unimmunized SWXJ mice, the auditory brainstem response threshold was significantly increased. This indicated that T cell-mediated tissue damage can lead to the development of autoimmune hearing loss, and immunocytochemistry analysis showed that the infiltration of leukocytes in the inner ear was associated with the observed hearing loss [52]. Billings also immunized SWXJ mice with cochlin 131–150 and confirmed that $CD45^+$ T cells infiltrate the cochlea and cause autoimmune SSHL [53]. Zhou et al. used the inner ear autoantigen β-tubulin to create a mouse model of experimental spontaneous immune hearing loss. They showed that the response to β-tubulin involves $CD4^+$ T cells producing γ-interferon, whereas T cell-mediated experimental autoimmune hearing loss is primarily caused by the induction of β-tubulin-activated $CD4^+$ T cells in neonatal BALB/c mice and increased auditory brainstem responses were seen in mice in which these cells were activated. Furthermore, a significant decrease in $CD4^+/CD25^+/$

Foxp3$^+$ regulatory T cells was observed in mice immunized with β-tubulin, which inhibited the proliferation of effector $CD4^+/CD25^-$ T cells [54]. Xia et al. used flow cytometry to analyze the clinical T cell subtypes in 17 patients with autoimmune sensorineural hearing loss, 16 patients with noise-induced hearing loss, and 100 individuals with normal hearing. There was no significant difference in the T cell subtypes among the three groups, except that the proportion of $CD4^+$ T cells in the patients with sensorineural hearing loss increased and the function of $CD4^+/CD25^+$ regulatory T cells was absent [55]. The above experimental animal models and clinical cases have confirmed that autoimmune hearing loss can be caused by cytotoxic T cell-mediated organ-specific autoimmune disorders of the inner ear.

5. Immunosuppressive Therapy for SSHL

Glucocorticoids have remained the main stay of treatment over the past four decades since McCabe [14] first treated SSHL with glucocorticoids, and the symptoms of patients were improved significantly. Owing to the systemic side effects of long-term treatment with glucocorticoids, other therapeutic methods also have been investigated. Ruckenstein et al. [56] and Trune et al. [57] used MRL/lpr mice to show that prednisolone can protect against hearing loss. In addition, Satoh et al. [58] and Wang et al. [59] used etanercept, a TNF-α antagonist, to treat SSHL and showed that it can reduce inflammation in the inner ear and prevent hearing loss. Clinically, Xenellis et al. [60] have shown that the intratympanic injection of steroids is a safe and effective method for SSHL treatment, and Haynes et al. [61] have shown that intratympanic injection of dexamethasone can also improve hearing in SSHL patients when systemic medications fail. Furthermore, Battaglia et al. [62] used a combination therapy of intratympanic dexamethasone with high-dose prednisone taper for SSHL and showed that the patients receiving the combination therapy had significant improvements in speech-discrimination score and pure-tone average and recovered their hearing quickly. More recently, azathioprine has been confirmed to maintain the hearing threshold, decrease the risk of relapse, and slow down the rate at which patients relapse [63].

The evidence to date suggests that autoimmune SSHL is mainly mediated by autoantibodies or T cells or by both. As autoimmune reactions are increasingly considered to be a cause of SSHL, animal models and clinical trials have shown that autoimmune processes cause damage to the inner ear through various mechanisms. Humoral immunity and cellular immune-mediated autoimmune damage have both been shown to play a role in the pathogenesis of autoimmune hearing loss. Although the precise diagnosis of autoimmune SSHL is still difficult, the response to immunosuppressive therapy is generally positive for these patients. Therefore, the immune mechanism of SSHL needs further study in order to identify specific antigens of the inner ear and specific diagnostic markers that can provide a more accurate and timely diagnosis and contribute to a more effective treatment plan.

Conflicts of Interest

The authors declare that there is no conflict of interest regarding the publication of this paper.

Authors' Contributions

Guangfei Li and Dan You contributed equally to this work.

Acknowledgments

Funding was provided by the National Key R&D Program of China (nos. 2017YFA0103900 and 2016YFC0905200), the National Natural Science Foundation of China (nos. 81570913 and 81620108005), and the Shanghai Pujiang Talents Plan (18PJ1401700).

References

[1] S. K. Juhn, L. P. Rybak, and S. Prado, "Nature of blood-labyrinth barrier in experimental conditions," *The Annals of Otology, Rhinology, and Laryngology*, vol. 90, no. 2, pp. 135–141, 1981.

[2] M. Düzlü, M. Çolak, İ. K. Önal, H. Tutar, R. Karamert, and Ç. Gökdoğan, "Audiological findings in autoimmune hepatitis: hearing loss at high frequencies," *Gazi Medical Journal*, vol. 28, no. 4, 2017.

[3] J. H. Check, "Sympathetic neural hyperalgesia edema syndrome as a cause of autoimmune hearing loss," *Clinical and Experimental Obstetrics & Gynecology*, vol. 44, no. 1, pp. 133-134, 2017.

[4] S. Montes, S. Rodríguez-Muguruza, V. Soria, and A. Olivé, "Atypical Cogan' syndrome associated with sudden deafness and glucocorticoid response," *Reumatología Clínica*, vol. 10, no. 4, pp. 267-268, 2014.

[5] A. Bacciu, E. Pasanisi, F. di Lella, M. Guida, S. Bacciu, and V. Vincenti, "Cochlear implantation in patients with Cogan syndrome: long-term results," *European Archives of Oto-Rhino-Laryngology*, vol. 272, no. 11, pp. 3201–3207, 2015.

[6] S. Chawki, J. Aouizerate, S. Trad, J. Prinseau, and T. Hanslik, "Bilateral sudden sensorineural hearing loss as a presenting feature of systemic lupus erythematosus: case report and brief review of other published cases," *Medicine*, vol. 95, no. 36, article e4345, 2016.

[7] C. A. Bowman, F. H. Linthicum Jr, R. A. Nelson, K. Mikami, and F. Quismorio, "Sensorineural hearing-loss associated with systemic lupus erythematosus," *Otolaryngology-Head and Neck Surgery*, vol. 94, no. 2, pp. 197–204, 1986.

[8] M. Tanaka and K. Tanaka, "Sudden hearing loss as the initial symptom in Japanese patients with multiple sclerosis and seropositive neuromyelitis optica spectrum disorders," *Journal of Neuroimmunology*, vol. 298, pp. 16–18, 2016.

[9] M. Tekin, G. O. Acar, O. H. Cam, and F. M. Hanege, "Sudden sensorineural hearing loss in a multiple sclerosis case," *Northern Clinics of Istanbul*, vol. 1, no. 2, pp. 109–113, 2014.

[10] M. A. Hellmann, I. Steiner, and R. Mosberg-Galili, "Sudden sensorineural hearing loss in multiple sclerosis: clinical course and possible pathogenesis," *Acta Neurologica Scandinavica*, vol. 124, no. 4, pp. 245–249, 2011.

[11] M. A. Melikoglu and K. Senel, "Sudden hearing loss in a patient with rheumatoid arthritis; a case report and review of

the literature," *Acta Reumatológica Portuguesa*, vol. 38, no. 2, pp. 138-139, 2013.

[12] F. Rubin, N. Tran Khai Hoan, and P. Bonfils, "Sudden bilateral hearing loss revealing polyarteritis nodosa," *European Annals of Otorhinolaryngology, Head and Neck Diseases*, vol. 131, no. 4, pp. 265-266, 2014.

[13] G. Tirelli, P. Tomietto, E. Quatela et al., "Sudden hearing loss and Crohn disease: when Cogan syndrome must be suspected," *American Journal of Otolaryngology*, vol. 36, no. 4, pp. 590–597, 2015.

[14] B. F. McCabe, "Autoimmune sensorineural hearing loss," *The Annals of Otology, Rhinology, and Laryngology*, vol. 88, no. 5, pp. 585–589, 1979.

[15] A. Sismanis, C. Wise, and G. Johnson, "Methotrexate management of immune-mediated cochleovestibular disorders," *Otolaryngology and Head and Neck Surgery*, vol. 116, no. 2, pp. 146–152, 1997.

[16] D. B. Bloch, J. A. Gutierrez, V. Guerriero Jr, S. D. Rauch, and K. J. Bloch, "Recognition of a dominant epitope in bovine heat-shock protein 70 in inner ear disease," *Laryngoscope*, vol. 109, no. 4, pp. 621–625, 1999.

[17] D. B. Bloch, J. E. San Martin, S. D. Rauch, R. A. Moscicki, and K. J. Bloch, "Serum antibodies to heat shock protein 70 in sensorineural hearing loss," *Archives of Otolaryngology–Head & Neck Surgery*, vol. 121, no. 10, pp. 1167–1171, 1995.

[18] L. Xu, C. R. Pfaltz, and W. Arnold, "Human leukocyte antigens in patients with inner ear diseases of unknown etiology," *ORL*, vol. 55, no. 3, pp. 125–134, 1993.

[19] H. Iwai, K. Tomoda, M. Inaba et al., "Evidence of cellular supplies to the endolymphatic sac from the systemic circulation," *Acta Oto-Laryngologica*, vol. 115, no. 4, pp. 509–511, 2009.

[20] H. Iwai, M. Inaba, K. Tomoda, S. Ikehara, K. Sugiura, and T. Yamashita, "T cells infiltrating from the systemic circulation proliferate in the endolymphatic sac," *The Annals of Otology, Rhinology, and Laryngology*, vol. 108, no. 12, pp. 1146–1150, 1999.

[21] B. Gloddek, J. Gloddek, and W. Arnold, "A rat T-cell line that mediates autoimmune disease of the inner ear in the Lewis rat," *ORL*, vol. 61, no. 4, pp. 181–187, 1999.

[22] R. A. Moscicki, J. E. San Martin, C. H. Quintero, S. D. Rauch, Nadol JB Jr, and K. J. Bloch, "Serum antibody to inner ear proteins in patients with progressive hearing loss. Correlation with disease activity and response to corticosteroid treatment," *JAMA*, vol. 272, no. 8, pp. 611–616, 1994.

[23] J. Dhingra and M. Mahalingam, "Antibodies to 68 kd antigen-specific for inner ear disease?," *Laryngoscope*, vol. 107, no. 3, pp. 405-406, 1997.

[24] P. B. Billings, E. M. Keithley, and J. P. Harris, "Evidence linking the 68 kilodalton antigen identified in progressive sensorineural hearing loss patient sera with heat shock protein 70," *The Annals of Otology, Rhinology, and Laryngology*, vol. 104, no. 3, pp. 181–188, 1995.

[25] G. B. Hughes, B. P. Barna, S. E. Kinney, L. H. Calabrese, and N. J. Nalepa, "Clinical diagnosis of immune inner-ear disease," *Laryngoscope*, vol. 98, no. 3, pp. 251–3, 1988.

[26] J. P. Harris, N. K. Woolf, and A. F. Ryan, "A reexamination of experimental type II collagen autoimmunity: middle and inner ear morphology and function," *The Annals of Otology, Rhinology, and Laryngology*, vol. 95, no. 2, pp. 176–180, 1986.

[27] K. C. Campbell and J. J. Klemens, "Sudden hearing loss and autoimmune inner ear disease," *Journal of the American Academy of Audiology*, vol. 11, no. 7, pp. 361–7, 2000.

[28] R. Hallworth, M. McCoy, and J. Polan-Curtain, "Tubulin expression in the developing and adult gerbil organ of Corti," *Hearing Research*, vol. 139, no. 1-2, pp. 31–41, 2000.

[29] M. Komori, Y. Yamamoto, Y. Yaguchi, T. Ikezono, and H. Kojima, "Cochlin-tomoprotein test and hearing outcomes in surgically treated true idiopathic perilymph fistula," *Acta Oto-Laryngologica*, vol. 136, no. 9, pp. 901–904, 2016.

[30] P. Baruah, "Cochlin in autoimmune inner ear disease: is the search for an inner ear autoantigen over?," *Auris Nasus Larynx*, vol. 41, no. 6, pp. 499–501, 2014.

[31] M. Gross, R. Eliashar, A. Ben-Yaakov, R. Ulmansky, and J. Elidan, "Prevalence and clinical significance of anticardiolipin, anti-β_2-glycoprotein-1, and anti-heat shock protein-70 autoantibodies in sudden sensorineural hearing loss," *Audiology & Neuro-Otology*, vol. 13, no. 4, pp. 231–238, 2008.

[32] S. Pathak, E. Goldofsky, E. X. Vivas, V. R. Bonagura, and A. Vambutas, "IL-1β is overexpressed and aberrantly regulated in corticosteroid nonresponders with autoimmune inner ear disease," *Journal of Immunology*, vol. 186, no. 3, pp. 1870–1879, 2011.

[33] S. D. Rauch, "IL-1β inhibition in autoimmune inner ear disease: can you hear me now?," *The Journal of Clinical Investigation*, vol. 124, no. 9, pp. 3685–3687, 2014.

[34] S. Pathak, C. Stern, and A. Vambutas, "*N*-Acetylcysteine attenuates tumor necrosis factor alpha levels in autoimmune inner ear disease patients," *Immunologic Research*, vol. 63, no. 1–3, pp. 236–245, 2015.

[35] S. Sun, H. Yu, H. Yu et al., "Inhibition of the activation and recruitment of microglia-like cells protects against neomycin-induced ototoxicity," *Molecular Neurobiology*, vol. 51, no. 1, pp. 252–267, 2015.

[36] Z. Wang and H. Li, "Microglia-like cells in rat organ of corti following aminoglycoside ototoxicity," *Neuroreport*, vol. 11, no. 7, pp. 1389–1393, 2000.

[37] M. Barbara, G. Attanasio, V. Petrozza, A. Modesti, and R. Filipo, "The endolymphatic sac as the immunocompetent organ of the inner ear," *Annals of the New York Academy of Sciences*, vol. 830, pp. 243–252, 1997.

[38] S. Tomiyama and J. Harris, "The role of the endolymphatic sac in inner ear immunity," *Acta Oto-Laryngologica*, vol. 103, no. 3, pp. 182–188, 1987.

[39] S. Hashimoto, P. Billings, J. P. Harris, G. S. Firestein, and E. M. Keithley, "Innate immunity contributes to cochlear adaptive immune responses," *Audiology and Neuro-Otology*, vol. 10, no. 1, pp. 35–43, 2005.

[40] J. Harris and A. Ryan, "Fundamental immune mechanisms of the brain and inner ear," *Otolaryngology-Head and Neck Surgery*, vol. 112, no. 6, pp. 639–653, 1995.

[41] J. P. Harris, S. Fukuda, and E. M. Keithley, "Spiral Modiolar vein: Its importance in inner ear inflammation," *Acta Oto-Laryngologica*, vol. 110, no. 3-4, pp. 357–364, 1990.

[42] B. Gloddek and J. P. Harris, "Role of lymphokines in the immune response of the inner ear," *Acta Oto-Laryngologica*, vol. 108, no. 1-2, pp. 68–75, 2009.

[43] H. Satoh, G. S. Firestein, P. B. Billings, J. P. Harris, and E. M. Keithley, "Proinflammatory cytokine expression in the endolymphatic sac during inner ear inflammation," *Journal of the*

Association for Research in Otolaryngology, vol. 4, no. 2, pp. 139–147, 2003.

[44] Q. Gopen, E. M. Keithley, and J. P. Harris, "Mechanisms underlying autoimmune inner ear disease," *Drug Discovery Today: Disease Mechanisms*, vol. 3, no. 1, pp. 137–142, 2006.

[45] J. P. Harris, "Immunology of the inner ear: response of the inner ear to antigen challenge," *Otolaryngology-Head and Neck Surgery*, vol. 91, no. 1, pp. 18–23, 1983.

[46] J. P. Harris, "Immunology of the inner ear: evidence of local antibody production," *Annals of Otology, Rhinology & Laryngology*, vol. 93, no. 2, pp. 157–162, 2016.

[47] A. Naumann, J. M. Hempel, and K. Schorn, "Detection of humoral immune response to inner ear proteins in patients with sensorineural hearing loss," *Laryngo- Rhino- Otologie*, vol. 80, no. 5, pp. 237–244, 2001.

[48] D. R. Trune, J. P. Craven, J. I. Morton, and C. Mitchell, "Autoimmune disease and cochlear pathology in the C3H/*lpr* strain mouse," *Hearing Research*, vol. 38, no. 1-2, pp. 57–66, 1989.

[49] H. Nariuchi, M. Sone, C. Tago, T. Kurata, and K. Saito, "Mechanisms of hearing disturbance in an autoimmune model mouse NZB/kl," *Acta Oto-Laryngologica. Supplementum*, vol. 514, pp. 127–131, 1994.

[50] D. R. Trune, J. B. Kempton, S. H. Hefeneider, and R. M. Bennett, "Inner ear DNA receptors in MRL/lpr autoimmune mice: potential 30 and 70 kDa link between autoimmune disease and hearing loss," *Hearing Research*, vol. 105, no. 1-2, pp. 57–64, 1997.

[51] B. Gloddek, A. F. Ryan, and J. P. Harris, "Homing of lymphocytes to the inner ear," *Acta Oto-Laryngologica*, vol. 111, no. 6, pp. 1051–1059, 2009.

[52] C. A. Solares, A. E. Edling, J. M. Johnson et al., "Murine autoimmune hearing loss mediated by $CD4^+$ T cells specific for inner ear peptides," *Journal of Clinical Investigation*, vol. 113, no. 8, pp. 1210–1217, 2004.

[53] P. Billings, "Experimental autoimmune hearing loss," *Journal of Clinical Investigation*, vol. 113, no. 8, pp. 1114–1117, 2004.

[54] B. Zhou, M. H. Kermany, J. Glickstein et al., "Murine autoimmune hearing loss mediated by $CD4^+$ T cells specific for β-tubulin," *Clinical Immunology*, vol. 138, no. 2, pp. 222–230, 2011.

[55] M. Xia, H. B. Zhang, F. Liu, H. Y. Yin, and A. T. Xu, "Impaired $CD4^+CD25^+$ regulatory T cell activity in the peripheral blood of patients with autoimmune sensorineural hearing loss," *European Archives of Oto-Rhino-Laryngology*, vol. 265, no. 9, pp. 1027–1033, 2008.

[56] M. J. Ruckenstein, A. Sarwar, L. Hu, H. Shami, and T. N. Marion, "Effects of immunosuppression on the development of cochlear disease in the MRL-Fas^{lpr} mouse," *Laryngoscope*, vol. 109, no. 4, pp. 626–630, 1999.

[57] D. R. Trune, R. J. Wobig, J. B. Kempton, and S. H. Hefeneider, "Steroid treatment in young MRL.MpJ-*Fas^{lpr}* autoimmune mice prevents cochlear dysfunction," *Hearing Research*, vol. 137, no. 1-2, pp. 167–173, 1999.

[58] H. Satoh, G. S. Firestein, P. B. Billings, J. P. Harris, and E. M. Keithley, "Tumor necrosis factor-α, an initiator, and etanercept, an inhibitor of cochlear inflammation," *Laryngoscope*, vol. 112, no. 9, pp. 1627–1634, 2002.

[59] X. Wang, T. Truong, P. B. Billings, J. P. Harris, and E. M. Keithley, "Blockage of immune-mediated inner ear damage by etanercept," *Otology & Neurotology*, vol. 24, no. 1, pp. 52–57, 2003.

[60] J. Xenellis, N. Papadimitriou, T. Nikolopoulos et al., "Intratympanic steroid treatment in idiopathic sudden sensorineural hearing loss: a control study," *Otolaryngology and Head and Neck Surgery*, vol. 134, no. 6, pp. 940–945, 2016.

[61] B. J. Balough, "Intratympanic dexamethasone for sudden sensorineural hearing loss after failure of systemic therapy," *Yearbook of Otolaryngology-Head and Neck Surgery*, vol. 2008, pp. 45–47, 2008.

[62] A. Battaglia, R. Burchette, and R. Cueva, "Combination therapy (intratympanic dexamethasone + high-dose prednisone taper) for the treatment of idiopathic sudden sensorineural hearing loss," *Otology & Neurotology*, vol. 29, no. 4, pp. 453–460, 2008.

[63] N. Mata-Castro, J. Gavilanes-Plasencia, R. Ramírez-Camacho, A. García-Fernández, and J. R. García-Berrocal, "Azathioprine reduces the risk of audiometric relapse in immune-mediated hearing loss," *Acta Otorrinolaringológica Española*, 2018.

[64] T. J. Yoo, M. A. Cremer, K. Tomoda, A. S. Townes, J. M. Stuart, and A. H. Kang, "Type II collagen-induced autoimmune sensorineural hearing loss and vestibular dysfunction in rats," *Annals of Otology, Rhinology & Laryngology*, vol. 92, no. 3, pp. 267–271, 1983.

[65] T. Yoo, Y. Yazawa, K. Tomoda, and R. Floyd, "Type II collagen-induced autoimmune endolymphatic hydrops in guinea-pig," *Science*, vol. 222, no. 4619, pp. 65–67, 1983.

[66] P. Berger, M. Hillman, M. Tabak, and M. Vollrath, "The lymphocyte transformation test with type II collagen as a diagnostic tool of autoimmune sensorineural hearing loss," *Laryngoscope*, vol. 101, no. 8, pp. 895–899, 1991.

[67] L. F. Bertoli, D. G. Pappas, J. C. Barton, and J. C. Barton, "Serum immunoglobulins in 28 adults with autoimmune sensorineural hearing loss: increased prevalence of subnormal immunoglobulin G1 and immunoglobulin G3," *BMC Immunology*, vol. 15, no. 1, p. 43, 2014.

[68] T. J. Yoo, K. Tomoda, and A. D. Hernandez, "Type II collagen induced autoimmune inner ear lesions in guinea pigs," *Annals of Otology, Rhinology & Laryngology*, vol. 93, Supplement 5, pp. 3–5, 1984.

[69] P. B. Billings, S. O. Shin, and J. P. Harris, "Assessing the role of anti-hsp70 in cochlear impairment," *Hearing Research*, vol. 126, no. 1-2, pp. 210–212, 1998.

[70] C. Ianuale, G. Cadoni, E. de Feo et al., "A systematic review and meta-analysis of the diagnostic accuracy of anti-heat shock protein 70 antibodies for the detection of autoimmune hearing loss," *Otology & Neurotology*, vol. 34, no. 2, pp. 214–219, 2013.

[71] K. Yeom, J. Gray, T. S. Nair et al., "Antibodies to HSP-70 in normal donors and autoimmune hearing loss patients," *Laryngoscope*, vol. 113, no. 10, pp. 1770–1776, 2003.

[72] S. Charchat, L. Lavinsky, E. Cohen, C. A. Muhlen, and C. Bonorino, "Use of HSP70 for diagnosis and treatment of patients of sensorineural autoimmune hearing loss," *Cell Stress & Chaperones*, vol. 5, no. 4, pp. 384–384, 2000.

[73] C. Bonaguri, J. G. Orsoni, L. Zavota et al., "Anti-68 kDa antibodies in autoimmune sensorineural hearing loss - are these autoantibodies really a diagnostic tool?," *Autoimmunity*, vol. 40, no. 1, pp. 73–78, 2007.

[74] T. J. Yoo, X. Ge, O. Sener et al., "Presence of autoantibodies in the sera of Meniere's disease," *Annals of Otology, Rhinology & Laryngology*, vol. 110, no. 5, pp. 425–429, 2001.

[75] T. J. Yoo, H. Tanaka, S. S. Kwon et al., "β-Tubulin as an autoantigen for autoimmune inner ear disease," *International Congress Series*, vol. 1240, pp. 1207–1210, 2003.

[76] T. J. Yoo, X. Du, and S. S. Kwon, "Molecular mechanism of autoimmune hearing loss," *Acta Oto-Laryngologica*, vol. 122, no. 5, pp. 3–9, 2002.

[77] X. Du, T. Yoo, and R. Mora, "Distribution of beta-tubulin in guinea pig inner ear," *ORL*, vol. 65, no. 1, pp. 7–16, 2003.

[78] Q. Cai, X. du, B. Zhou, C. Cai, M. H. Kermany, and T. Yoo, "Induction of tolerance by oral administration of beta-tubulin in an animal model of autoimmune inner ear disease," *ORL*, vol. 71, no. 3, pp. 135–141, 2009.

[79] N. G. Robertson, L. Lu, S. Heller et al., "Mutations in a novel cochlear gene cause DFNA9, a human nonsyndromic deafness with vestibular dysfunction," *Nature Genetics*, vol. 20, no. 3, pp. 299–303, 1998.

[80] N. G. Robertson, B. L. Resendes, J. S. Lin et al., "Inner ear localization of mRNA and protein products of COCH, mutated in the sensorineural deafness and vestibular disorder, DFNA9," *Human Molecular Genetics*, vol. 10, no. 22, pp. 2493–2500, 2001.

[81] T. Ikezono, A. Omori, S. Ichinose, R. Pawankar, A. Watanabe, and T. Yagi, "Identification of the protein product of the Coch gene (hereditary deafness gene) as the major component of bovine inner ear protein," *Biochimica et Biophysica Acta-Molecular Basis of Disease*, vol. 1535, no. 3, pp. 258–265, 2001.

[82] M. J. Baek, H. M. Park, J. M. Johnson et al., "Increased frequencies of cochlin-specific T cells in patients with autoimmune sensorineural hearing loss," *Journal of Immunology*, vol. 177, no. 6, pp. 4203–4210, 2006.

[83] R. Killick, P. K. Legan, C. Malenczak, and G. P. Richardson, "Molecular cloning of chick beta-tectorin, an extracellular matrix molecule of the inner ear," *Journal of Cell Biology*, vol. 129, no. 2, pp. 535–547, 1995.

[84] P. K. Legan, A. Rau, J. N. Keen, and G. P. Richardson, "The mouse tectorins - modular matrix proteins of the inner ear homologous to components of the sperm-egg adhesion system," *Journal of Biological Chemistry*, vol. 272, no. 13, pp. 8791–8801, 1997.

[85] T. S. Nair, D. M. Prieskorn, J. M. Miller, A. Mori, J. Gray, and T. E. Carey, "In vivo binding and hearing loss after intracochlear infusion of KHRI-3 antibody," *Hearing Research*, vol. 107, no. 1-2, pp. 93–101, 1997.

[86] M. Ptok, T. Nair, T. E. Carey, and R. A. Altschuler, "Distribution of KHRI 3 epitopes in the inner ear," *Hearing Research*, vol. 66, no. 2, pp. 245–252, 1993.

[87] M. Takahashi and J. P. Harris, "Analysis of immunocompetent cells following inner ear immunostimulation," *Laryngoscope*, vol. 98, no. 10, pp. 1133–1138, 1988.

[88] M. Takahashi and J. P. Harris, "Anatomic distribution and localization of immunocompetent cells in normal mouse endolymphatic sac," *Acta Oto-Laryngologica*, vol. 106, no. 5-6, pp. 409–416, 1988.

[89] H. F. Schuknecht, "Inner ear pathology in autoimmune disease," *Progress in Human Auditory and Vestibular Histopathology*, Kugler Publications, 1997.

[90] H. F. Schuknecht, "Ear pathology in autoimmune disease," *Advances in Oto-Rhino-Laryngology*, vol. 46, pp. 50–70, 1991.

[91] H. Kawauchi, N. Kaneda, I. Ichimiya, and G. Mogi, "Distribution of immunocompetent cells in the endolymphatic sac," *The Annals of Otology, Rhinology & Laryngology*, vol. 101, Supplement 10, pp. 39–47, 1992.

[92] H. Cantor, F. W. Shen, and E. A. Boyse, "Separation of helper T-cells from suppressor T-cells expressing different Ly components. II. Activation by antigen: after immunization, antigen-specific suppressor and helper activities are mediated by distinct T-cell subclasses," *Journal of Experimental Medicine*, vol. 143, no. 6, pp. 1391–1340, 1976.

[93] A. M. Bilate and J. J. Lafaille, "Induced $CD4^+Foxp3^+$ regulatory T cells in immune tolerance," *Annual Review of Immunology*, vol. 30, no. 1, pp. 733–758, 2012.

4

Activation State-Dependent Substrate Gating in Ca^{2+}/Calmodulin-Dependent Protein Kinase II

D. E. Johnson and A. Hudmon

Biochemistry and Molecular Biology, Stark Neuroscience Research Institute, Indiana University School of Medicine, Indianapolis, IN 46202, USA

Correspondence should be addressed to A. Hudmon; ahudmon@purdue.edu

Academic Editor: Yi Zhou

Calcium/calmodulin-dependent protein kinase II (CaMKII) is highly concentrated in the brain where its activation by the Ca^{2+} sensor CaM, multivalent structure, and complex autoregulatory features make it an ideal translator of Ca^{2+} signals created by different patterns of neuronal activity. We provide direct evidence that graded levels of kinase activity and extent of T^{287} (T^{286} α isoform) autophosphorylation drive changes in catalytic output and substrate selectivity. The catalytic domains of CaMKII phosphorylate purified PSDs much more effectively when tethered together in the holoenzyme versus individual subunits. Using multisubstrate SPOT arrays, high-affinity substrates are preferentially phosphorylated with limited subunit activity per holoenzyme, whereas multiple subunits or maximal subunit activation is required for intermediate- and low-affinity, weak substrates, respectively. Using a monomeric form of CaMKII to control T^{287} autophosphorylation, we demonstrate that increased Ca^{2+}/CaM-dependent activity for all substrates tested, with the extent of weak, low-affinity substrate phosphorylation governed by the extent of T^{287} autophosphorylation. Our data suggest T^{287} autophosphorylation regulates substrate gating, an intrinsic property of the catalytic domain, which is amplified within the multivalent architecture of the CaMKII holoenzyme.

1. Introduction

Long-term potentiation (LTP) is a long-lasting enhancement of excitatory postsynaptic currents that many believe to be a cellular correlate of learning and memory [1]. While LTP can be observed in multiple areas of the mammalian brain (as well as in lower organisms), the Schaffer collateral/CA3 synapses onto CA1 pyramidal neurons of the hippocampus are a classic example whereby brief patterns of high-frequency activity favor LTP to enhance neuronal connectivity [2]. The opposing change in synaptic plasticity, long-term depression (LTD), is produced by low firing frequencies [2]. As might be expected, activity-dependent forms of plasticity like LTP and LTD both require the second messenger calcium (Ca^{2+}). While LTP has been historically ascribed to kinase activity and LTD to dephosphorylation and phosphatase activity [3], a common effector system capable of decoding Ca^{2+} spike frequency into different functional outputs would be strategically positioned to regulate both LTP and LTD. The Ca^{2+}/calmodulin- (CaM-) dependent protein kinase II (CaMKII) is an ideal regulator of synaptic plasticity because it has complex autoregulatory features that make it ideally suited for regulating activity-dependent plasticity [4–7].

In mammals, CaMKII family is composed of four closely related isoforms (α, β, γ, and δ) where it regulates diverse substrates in cellular processes ranging from metabolism and cell cycle control to Ca^{2+} homoeostasis and excitability [8]. Thus, like other multifunctional serine/threonine protein kinases (e.g., PKA and PKC), CaMKII phosphorylates many different cellular substrates in different subcellular compartments to globally coordinate cellular function. CaM is a ubiquitous Ca^{2+} sensor that activates CaMKII by binding to a target domain that disinhibits the autoregulatory domain

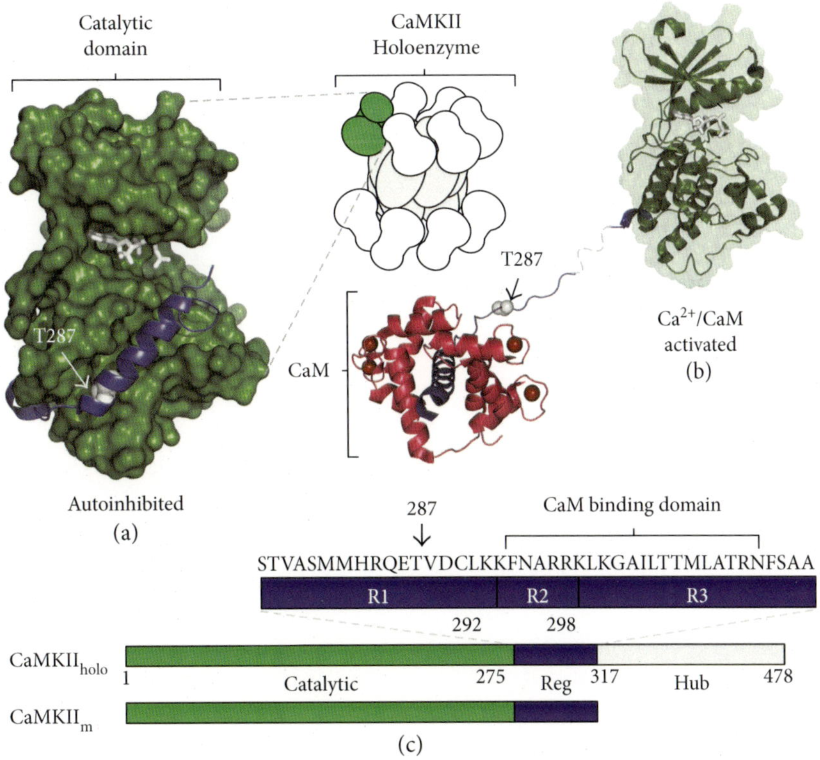

FIGURE 1: Molecular structure and schematic models for CaMKII autoregulation and activation. (a–c) Structural representations of CaMKII's catalytic domain (green), autoregulatory domain (ARD) (blue), and hub domain (gray). (a) Illustration of CaMKII holoenzyme with detailed view of the catalytic domain. Adapted X-ray crystal structure shows monomeric human CaMKIIδ_{11-309} (PDB ID: 2VN9; [11]) in the autoinhibited state with the ARD (blue) and modified to include ATP in the active site (PDB ID: 1ATP; [71]). (b) hCaMKIIδ_{11-335} activated (PDB ID: 2WEL; [11]) by Ca^{2+} (red spheres) and calmodulin (CaM) (magenta) and exposing T^{287} (white) for autophosphorylation. (c) Linear schematic of CaMKII holoenzyme (CaMKII$_{holo}$) and monomeric CaMKII (CaMKII$_m$, or CaMKII$_{1-317}$). Expanded view shows the ARD (blue) with subdivisions R1 (T^{287} containing region) and R2/R3 (CaM-binding region) [72].

(ARD) to allow substrate binding to the catalytic surface (Figures 1(a), 1(b), and 1(c)).

The unique multivalent structure of CaMKII permits complex forms of autoregulation [9, 10]. The CaMKII holoenzyme is comprised of 12–14 subunits [11–13] that permits coincident CaM binding to support an intraholoenzyme-intersubunit autophosphorylation [14, 15] (T^{286} α isoform and T^{287} β, γ, and δ isoforms) reaction (for convenience, we use T^{287} throughout the paper). While CaMKII is known to undergo autophosphorylation on multiple sites [16], many of which have unknown functions, the T^{287} autophosphorylation site within the ARD leads to enhanced CaM binding affinity in the presence of Ca^{2+} [17] and Ca^{2+}/CaM-independent activity (autonomous) in low Ca^{2+} [18, 19]. The unique structure and autoregulation make CaMKII an ideal sensor to encode Ca^{2+}-spike frequency into T^{287} autophosphorylation; a process influenced by Ca^{2+}-spike duration and amplitude [20], phosphatase activity [21], alternative spliced linker length, and CaM availability [22, 23].

While CaMKII is present throughout the body, it is highly enriched at neuronal connections. In fact, CaMKII is one of the most abundant proteins in the postsynaptic density (PSD) [24–26], a cytoskeletal organelle located just underneath the spine plasma membrane that localizes the postsynaptic signaling machinery with presynaptic release sites. While CaMKII appears to have multiple functions in synaptic plasticity, phosphorylation of GluA1 receptors to regulate their trafficking and signaling appears to be critical for LTP [7]. CaMKII's role in LTP and Ca^{2+} signaling in the postsynaptic compartment is also linked to its ability to undergo translocation to NMDA receptors and undergo autophosphorylation [5, 27, 28], processes that might serve to restrict the kinase to its targets within the PSD. However, like the second messenger Ca^{2+}, CaMKII is also implicated in LTD [29, 30]. And while the role of CaMKII in postsynaptic LTD has not been as intensively studied as its role in LTP [4], CaMKII was recently shown to differentially phosphorylate two different phosphoacceptor sites on GluA1 in LTP versus LTD [31]. Because LTP is promoted by strong stimuli versus weak for LTD, one plausible explanation is that graded levels of CaMKII activity and/or autophosphorylation promote differential substrate phosphorylation to induce the opposing forms of synaptic plasticity. However, recent studies have revealed little or no impact of autophosphorylation on the catalytic output of CaMKII [32, 33]. Using purified PSDs and immobilized peptide arrays to create a well-defined multisubstrate system, we test the hypothesis that the catalytic output and substrate selectivity of CaMKII are regulated by its activation state. Our data support a model whereby T^{287} autophosphorylation regulates substrate gating, an intrinsic property of the catalytic domain, which is amplified within the multivalent architecture of the CaMKII holoenzyme.

2. Results

CaMKII translocation and phosphorylation of PSD proteins are believed to play an important role in postsynaptic modifications supporting LTP [4–7]. We determined whether PSD phosphorylation by CaMKII induced by saturating Ca^{2+}/CaM is *equivalent* or *different* to monomeric CaMKII catalytic activity. Conceptually, one might expect that a similar number of activated T^{287} autophosphorylated subunits (T^{286} in alpha isoform) would produce similar levels of substrate phosphorylation within the PSD regardless of whether the catalytic subunits are within a holoenzyme or monomeric. While all four CaMKII isoforms exhibit a high degree of sequence identity in their catalytic and regulatory domains, we selected the human δCaMKII isoform for its enhanced stability in our kinase assays. While the association domain hub was deleted from monomeric CaMKII (1-317) (Figures 1(a), 1(b), and 1(c)), this recombinant kinase, like the native holoenzyme, retains its Ca^{2+}/CaM dependence and undergoes T^{287} autophosphorylation as an intersubunit reaction mechanism which we accomplished in a prereaction (see Materials and Methods). Postsynaptic densities were acquired from adult rats (male and female Sprague-Dawley) using differential centrifugation and detergent extraction to obtain the PSD Triton-insoluble fraction (see Materials and Methods) [34, 35]. The PSD preparation displayed a characteristic size and ultrastructure (data not shown) and SDS-PAGE separation and a Coomassie blue staining revealed the complex protein profile characteristic of PSD preparations.

Our intent was to focus on characterizing PSD phosphorylation from exogenously added CaMKII; therefore, several steps were taken to accomplish this. First, rat brains were extracted and snap frozen in liquid nitrogen as rapidly as possible (~90 secs) after animal sacrifice to reduce CaMKII translocation to the PSDs in response to decapitation [36]. Second, to minimize autonomous activity of endogenous PSD CaMKII, isolated PSDs were dephosphorylated overnight using a PP1α catalytic fragment. The 6X-His-tagged phosphatase was removed the next day using immobilized metal affinity chromatography. Third, the allosteric small molecule CaMKII inhibitor, KN93, was included in the PSD phosphorylation reaction to inhibit endogenous CaMKII from undergoing T^{287} autophosphorylation with addition of Ca^{2+}/CaM (as KN93 prevents Ca^{2+}/CaM binding/activation but does not inhibit activated T^{287} autophosphorylated CaMKII). Fourth, phosphatase and protease inhibitor cocktails were used in the PSD phosphorylation reactions to disrupt dephosphorylation and proteolysis reactions. Finally, exogenous CaMKII was preautophosphorylated at T^{287} with thiol-ATP (ATPγS) to limit potential dephosphorylation and to minimize subsequent incorporation of ^{32}P in exogenous CaMKII autophosphorylation sites.

Postsynaptic densities were phosphorylated (plus [γ-^{32}P-] ATP) with T^{287} autophosphorylated holoenzyme ($CaMKII_{holo}^{+P}$) or monomer ($CaMKII_m^{+P}$) in the presence of Ca^{2+}/CaM. Similar levels of catalytic activity were applied for both forms of the autophosphorylated CaMKII (see Materials and Methods). To control for endogenous Ca^{2+}/CaM-dependent or Ca^{2+}/CaM-independent kinase activity, PSDs were also phosphorylated in the presence of Ca^{2+}/CaM or EGTA, respectively. As described in detail in Materials and Methods, PSD phosphorylation was quantified by phosphorimaging of the ^{32}P incorporation following SDS-PAGE separation of the proteins (Figures 2(a) and 2(b)). The corresponding phosphorylation data (autoradiography of ^{32}P incorporated bands) (Figures 2(c) and 2(d)) was scaled to the total PSD protein in a given sample based on the area under the curve (AUC) as described in Materials and Methods. Under these conditions, the addition of Ca^{2+}/CaM alone produced less than a 2-fold increase in the total phosphorylation compared to other Ca^{2+}/CaM-independent kinases (the EGTA condition; Figure 2(d)). The inclusion of exogenous $CaMKII_m^{+P}$ produced ~2-fold increase in the phosphorylation compared to Ca^{2+}/CaM-activated PSDs alone, suggesting that PSD substrates were available to exogenously added kinase (Figure 2(d)). The $CaMKII_{holo}^{+P}$ produced a 6.4-fold increase in phosphorylation compared to Ca^{2+}/CaM-activated PSDs (Figure 2(d)). More importantly, compared to the T^{287} autophosphorylated monomer, there was a 4.4-fold increase in total phosphorylation when corrected for endogenous Ca^{2+}/CaM-stimulated phosphorylation (Figure 2(d)) even though the holoenzyme might be expected to have less accessibility to substrates in the PSD compared to the monomer because of their size difference (~750 kDa versus 35 kDa, resp.).

The amount of CaMKII enzymatic activity (both Ca^{2+}/CaM stimulated and autonomous) added to the PSD phosphorylation reaction was determined both before and after the experiment via a soluble kinase assay using the CaMKII-specific peptide AC-2 (see Materials and Methods). While the catalytic activity of the monomeric kinase was greater than the holoenzyme at the initiation of the PSD phosphorylation reaction, the level of activity at the end of the PSD phosphorylation was similar between monomeric and multimeric CaMKII (Figure 2(e)). While it is unclear why a loss of monomeric activity is observed at the end of the PSD reaction, no loss of enzymatic activity is observed for either $CaMKII_{holo}^{+P}$ or $CaMKII_m^{+P}$ in the absence of PSD protein (data not shown). Thus, while the enzymatic activity of monomeric CaMKII is favored or equal (start or end of the reaction) to that of the holoenzyme CaMKII, substrate phosphorylation is higher for CaMKII when multiple subunits are activated within the holoenzyme for a diffusion-restricted environment like the PSD.

Specificity for the switch-like behavior in CaMKII critical for LTP [3] may arise from this enzyme's ability to translate Ca^{2+}-spike frequency produced by brief patterns of high-frequency stimulation into graded levels of activity and T^{287} autophosphorylation [20]. Thus, we tested whether regulating the extent of activation within the CaMKII holoenzyme regulates substrate selectivity. However, endogenous effectors,

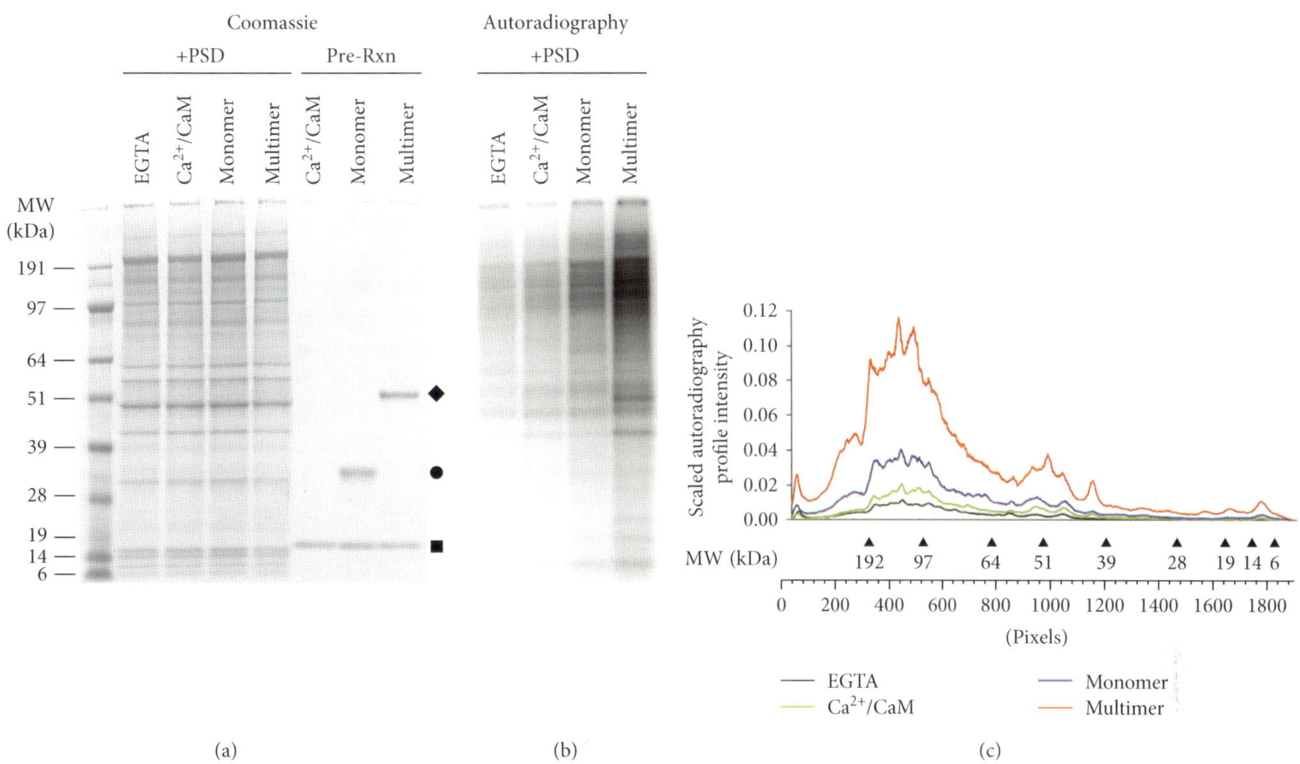

	PSD + EGTA	PSD + Ca^{2+}/CaM	PSD + monomer	PSD + monomer
AUC (arbitrary units)	0.16	0.27	0.59	1.72
Corrected AUC (for endogenous CaM-activated kinase)	N/A	0	0.33	1.46

(d)

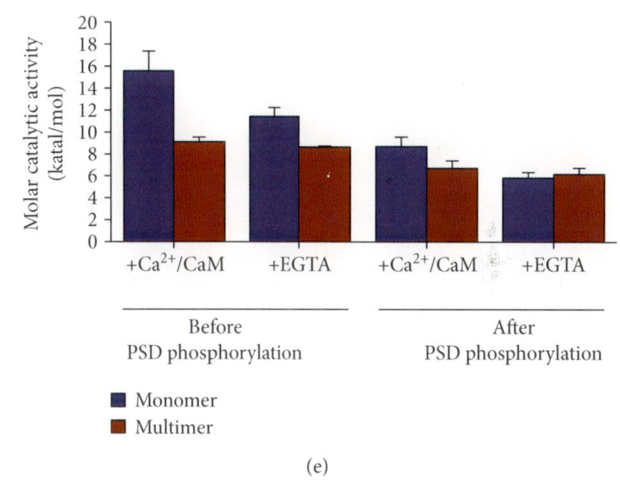

FIGURE 2: Maximally active CaMKII holoenzymes enhance the phosphorylation of PSD proteins over monomeric CaMKII. (a–d) Isolated rat PSDs were phosphorylated in low (EGTA) or high calcium (Ca^{2+}/CaM) to assess endogenous, copurified kinases. PSDs were also phosphorylated with the addition of equal molar catalytic subunits of T^{287} autophosphorylated CaMKII multimer ($CaMKII_{holo}^{+P}$ = diamond) or monomer ($CaMKII_{m}^{+P}$ = circle). (a) Coomassie-stained gel illustrating the PSD profile and the purified proteins used in the reaction. Square indicates CaM. (b) Phosphorimaging of the SDS-PAGE showing ^{32}P-phosphoprotein bands. (c) Phosphorylation profile scaled to total Coomassie-stained protein. Molecular weight markers indicated along the scaled axis (pixels) representing the scaled lane of the SDS-PAGE. (d) Total phosphorylation for each condition assessed using the area under the curve (AUC) as arbitrary intensity units. (e) Quantitation of Ca^{2+}-dependent (Ca^{2+}/CaM) and Ca^{2+}-independent (EGTA) enzymatic activity (katal/mol) of CaMKII measured via soluble peptide assays with radioactive ($\gamma^{32}P$) ATP. CaMKII, monomer or multimer, was autophosphorylated at T^{287} prior to the PSD phosphorylation (and activity measurement) (see Materials and Methods) ($n = 3$). Error bars denote ± s.d.

scaffolding, and other regulatory proteins within the PSD could complicate our analysis; therefore, we created a multiple substrate SPOT array in order to explore how graded levels of CaMKII activity influence substrate utilization (see Materials and Methods). An obvious advantage of this immobilized peptide assay is that diverse substrates can be exposed to identical conditions without high-affinity substrates dominating mixed soluble substrate reactions [37]. We selected four well-studied CaMKII substrates studied with varying affinities as determined by standard solution kinetics—a high-affinity substrate ($GluN2B_{S1303}$, $K_m = 4.6 \pm 1.1$ μM) and three lower-affinity, weak substrates (Syntide, $K_m = 43.5 \pm 2.3$ μM; $Vimentin_{S83}$ and $GluA1_{S849}$, $K_m > 1$ mM). All peptide sequences are denoted in Materials and Methods.

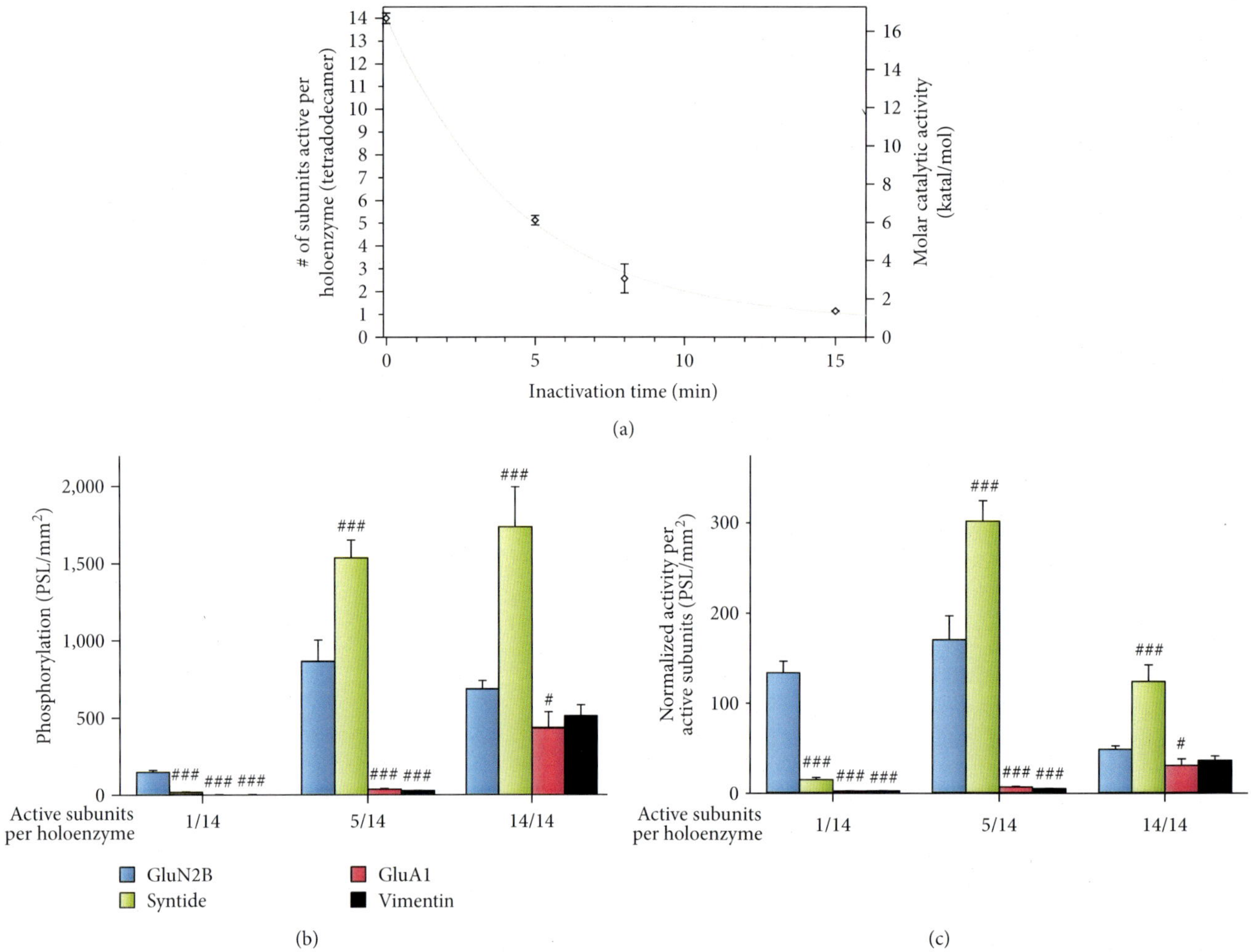

Figure 3: Enhanced phosphorylation of intermediate and weak SPOT substrates with increasing number of active subunits per holoenzyme. (a) Time-dependent inactivation of CaMKII by basal autophosphorylation. Ca^{2+}/CaM-stimulated activity of $CaMKII_{holo}$ expressed in molar terms (katal/mol) and measured via standard soluble peptide (AC-2) assays with radioactive ($\gamma^{32}P$) ATP. Enzymatic activity was measured following preinactivation reactions of various times (see Materials and Methods); mean ± s.d. ($n = 3$). By calculating the average enzymatic activity per subunit in a fully activatable tetradecameric holoenzyme (i.e., 0 min of inactivation), the average number of activated subunits per holoenzyme was determined for each condition. (b, c) Phosphorylation ([^{32}P] phosphate incorporation) of immobilized CaMKII substrates (GluN2B, Syntide, GluA1, and Vimentin synthesized via SPOTs) by $CaMKII_{holo}$ exhibiting 1, 5, or 14 activated subunits per holoenzyme. Substrates ranked from the lowest to the highest K_m. (b) Raw SPOT phosphorylation (PSL/mm^2) represented as mean ± s.d. ($n = 3$). (c) SPOT phosphorylation normalized by the number of subunits activated per holoenzyme and represented as mean ± s.d. ($n = 3$). One-way ANOVA of log-normalized data with Holm-Šidák posttest compared to GluN2B within each group ($^{\#}P < 0.05$, $^{\#\#\#}P < 0.001$).

To create graded levels of CaMKII activity and T^{286} autophosphorylation in conditions of saturating Ca^{2+}/CaM, we took advantage of the basal, inhibitory (Ca^{2+}/CaM-independent) autophosphorylation (i.e., capping) described previously [38]. Specifically, naïve multimeric CaMKII is exposed to Mg^{2+}/ATP for varying times in the absence of Ca^{2+}/CaM. This is a relatively slow intramolecular autophosphorylation reaction (complete in 15–20 mins) within the CaM-binding domain (T^{306} in CaMKIIδ) that blocks subsequent Ca^{2+}/CaM binding/activation [19, 38–40]. The degree of inactivation is measured by exposing the Mg^{2+}/ATP-treated CaMKII to saturating Ca^{2+}/CaM and AC-2 in a soluble kinase assay (see Materials and Methods). We expressed maximal catalytic activity as a function of the number of subunits in the holoenzyme (the human CaMKIIδ holoenzyme is tetradecameric [11]). This allowed for the determination of the molar catalytic activity associated with one catalytic subunit. Using this metric, the average number of activatable subunits per holoenzyme was calculated for each inactivation timepoint shown in Figure 3(a) (see Materials and Methods). Thus, by normalizing our treated or "capped" holoenzymes to naïve untreated CaMKII (14/14 subunits), we calculated that residual bulk kinase activity in solution as represented on average by holoenzymes with 1/14 or 5/14 subunits is available for Ca^{2+}/CaM activation.

Using this capping pretreatment strategy to limit the number of Ca^{2+}/CaM activatable subunits per holoenzyme, we observed that one active subunit per holoenzyme ($CaMKII_{holo}^{1/14}$) displays preferential phosphorylation for the high-affinity substrate GluN2B (Figure 3(b)). In

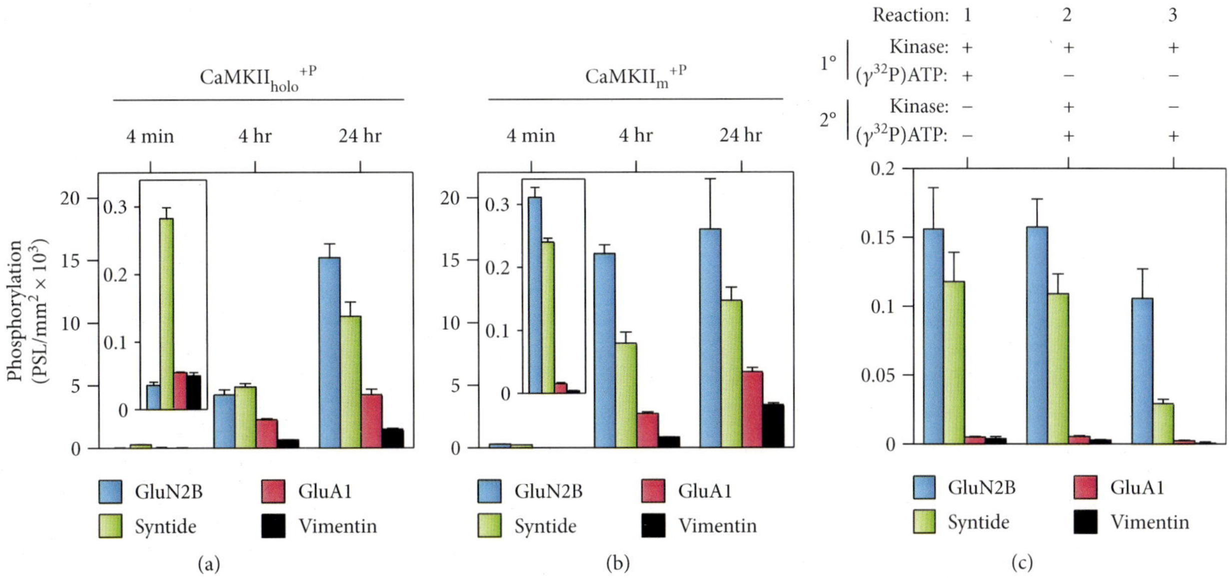

FIGURE 4: Substrate availability and reaction linearity for SPOT phosphorylation reactions. (a–c) Substrate phosphorylation profiles ([^{32}P] phosphate incorporation of SPOT peptides). Phosphorylation time course of $CaMKII_{holo}^{+P}$ (a) or $CaMKII_{m}^{+P}$ (b) with an expanded view of 4 min reaction (inset); mean ± s.d. ($n = 3$). (c) Phosphorylation by $CaMKII_{m}^{+P}$ comparing a normal 4 min SPOT reaction (c-1) to reactions with only radioactive secondary 4 min reactions with (c-2) or without (c-3) additional kinase in the secondary reaction; mean ± s.d. ($n = 3$).

Figure 3(c), the phosphorylation data was normalized to account for the different levels of "starting" kinase activity produced by the capping reaction in order to better evaluate substrate selectivity profiles. Unlike GluN2B, increasing the number of activatable subunits per holoenzyme significantly increases relative phosphorylation of Syntide (intermediate substrate affinity) and GluA1 and Vimentin (weak substrates) (Figure 3(c)). While minimal changes in GluN2B phosphorylation were observed, a 20-fold increase in Syntide phosphorylation by submaximally activated $CaMKII_{holo}^{5/14}$ was measured (Figure 3(c)). Maximally activated $CaMKII_{holo}^{14/14}$ produced the greatest increase (12-fold) in phosphorylation of the weakest substrates, GluA1 and Vimentin (Figure 3(c)). These data indicate that intermediate- and low-affinity substrates require multiple activated subunits within the holoenzyme for phosphorylation. In contrast, high-affinity substrates are preferentially phosphorylated when the number of subunits per holoenzyme is limited. The reduced phosphorylation of high-affinity substrates seen in Figure 3(c) may result from substrates like NR2B possessing T-Site (i.e., targeting mode) characteristics [41], which allow substrates mimicking the ARD of CaMKII to bind in a mode that is biochemically distinct from the substrate binding pocket [42]. These stable, high-affinity interactions may punish substrate utilization via avidity effects as discussed further below.

We elected to use the SPOTs immobilized peptide approach as it has the obvious advantage that multiple defined substrates can be examined simultaneously without having the high-affinity substrates dominate the diffusion-limited solution assay. However, it is still important for these interfacial reactions to obey specific requirements for any enzyme analysis, including a nonsaturating reaction (Figure 4). We observed that less than 2% of the available peptide for each substrate (as compared to a 24-hour reaction for GluN2B, Syntide, GluA1, and Vimentin) was phosphorylated by $CaMKII_{holo}^{+P}$ in our standard reactions (Figure 4(a)). While we did not extend the phosphorylation reactions longer than 24 hrs, this time point is likely at equilibrium as the extent of phosphorylation follows an expected ranking based on substrate affinity (GluN2B > Syntide > GluA1/Vimentin). Furthermore, we observed minimal differences between maximally activated (14/14 subunits) holoenzymes at 60 nM versus 5 nM (Figures 3(b) and 4(a)—inset, resp.), indicating that while the extent of phosphorylation is sensitive to kinase concentration, changes in the substrate phosphorylation profile are not. Thus, for our standard SPOT reactions (4 mins), changes in the phosphorylation profile are not due to differential substrate availability.

One caveat of using SPOT arrays for enzyme analysis is that they can be negatively influenced by avidity effects created by multivalent contacts [43]. For example, the binding affinity of a protein with its immobilized peptide target increased by over 1000-fold when a dimeric protein is compared to a monomeric variant [44]. Consistent with avidity effects contaminating CaMKII phosphorylation of the high-affinity substrates in the SPOT assays, we observed that phosphorylation for the high- (GluN2B) and intermediate-affinity (Syntide) substrates was suppressed as the number of activated subunits within the holoenzyme increased from 5/14 to 14/14. This becomes readily apparent when CaMKII substrate phosphorylation is normalized to the number of activated subunits in the capping experiments (Figure 3(c)). This avidity effect was not seen with monomeric CaMKII, as substrate phosphorylation profile for $CaMKII_m^{+P}$ follows the expected profile (i.e., higher affinity, greater substrate phosphorylation (Figure 4(b))). Again, linearity for the monomer CaMKII reaction rates was supported by the observation that in our standard SPOT reactions, less than 2% of the available peptide for each substrate (as compared to a 24-hour reaction for GluN2B, Syntide, GluA1, and Vimentin) was phosphorylated by $CaMKII_m^{+P}$ (Figure 4(b)). Conclusive support for a linear kinase-substrate reaction is supported by a pulse-chase style reaction in which nearly identical levels of ^{32}P incorporation are obtained when a secondary reaction occurs on the same SPOT membrane immediately after an initial nonradioactive reaction (Figure 4(c)—reaction 1 versus 2). A modification of this assay whereby $CaMKII_m^{+P}$ is applied to the SPOT membrane in the absence of ATP^{32} reveals that bound kinase continues to form product over time when the membrane is washed and ATP^{32} is added during the chase without additional kinase (Figure 3(c)). In total, our standard SPOT reactions are not limited by substrate availability nor are they outside of a linear reaction range. However, because the reduced substrate phosphorylation of higher affinity substrates with maximally activated $CaMKII_{holo}^{+P}$ is likely contaminated by multivalent avidity effects, we employed the monomeric kinase to directly evaluate the contribution of T^{287} autophosphorylation on substrate selectivity.

$CaMKII_m$ autophosphorylation at T^{287} is a well-controlled, second-order reaction under saturating Ca^{2+}/CaM conditions [15]. Like with $CaMKII_{holo}^{+P}$, the percentage of autophosphorylated subunits can be detected using the high-affinity substrate AC-2 (Figure 5(a)) which exhibits a 1 : 1 correlation in the number of T^{287} autophosphorylated subunits and maximal autonomous activity ([Ca^{2+}/CaM-independent]/[Ca^{2+}/CaM-stimulated]) [45]. Therefore, we generated populations of $CaMKII_m$ containing varying ratios of $CaMKII_m^{-P}$ and $CaMKII_m^{+P}$ using temperature and time to vary the extent of autophosphorylated subunits (see Materials and Methods) (Figures 5(a) and 5(b)). Importantly, for each condition (i.e., extent of autophosphorylated CaMKII), the number of $CaMKII_m^{+P}$ subunits generated in the prereaction does not change during our standard SPOT assays, as the level of autonomous activity measured in a solution assay using the AC-2 substrate is the same pre- and post-SPOTs (Figure 5(c)). We observed a direct relationship between the extent of substrate phosphorylation and the percentage of T^{287} autophosphorylated subunits in the SPOT assay (Figure 5(d)). However, intermediate- and low-affinity substrates (Figure 5(d)) displayed the greatest increases in their phosphorylation in response to T^{287} autophosphorylation. Interestingly, the phosphorylation profile of the non-T^{287} autophosphorylated $CaMKII_m$ (Figure 5(b)) was highly similar to the minimally activated $CaMKII_{holo}$ (one subunit/holoenzyme condition in Figure 3(b), suggesting that inactivation (via T^{306} capping) can allow holoenzymes with limited activatable subunits to behave as non-T^{287}-autophosphorylated monomers. Overall, our data support the hypothesis that the extent of activation and T^{287} autophosphorylation within the CaMKII holoenzyme functions to broaden the substrate specificity of CaMKII.

3. Discussion

Like other multifunctional protein kinases, CaMKII exhibits broad substrate specificity, targeting substrates involved in carbohydrate, amino acid and lipid metabolism, neurotransmitter synthesis and release, ion channels, receptors, transcription and translation, cytoskeletal organization and dynamics, cell cycle control, and Ca^{2+} homoeostasis [8]. In the nervous system, the role of CaMKII in synaptic plasticity has been intensively studied from both its role as a structural protein and as kinase [4–7]. In fact, while a number of different proteins and effector pathways have been implicated in regulating LTP over the years, CaMKII is considered to be a key mediator of this plasticity [46]. CaMKII is best known for signaling in the postsynaptic neuron for regulating the macromolecular signaling complex known as the PSD, a cytoskeletal organelle important for postsynaptic function. CaMKII translocation to the PSD is thought to be a critical feature of its function [47–51], a process that presumably functions to sequester and localize CaMKII activated with postsynaptic activity. The NMDA-R complex is a critical targeting molecule for CaMKII localization to the PSD and a substrate [27]. CaMKII phosphorylation of S^{1303} on the GluN2B subunit of the NMDA-R [52] reduces desensitization of the channel and hypothesized to serve as a feed-forward mechanism to sustain Ca^{2+} entry during learning and memory [53]. In addition to NMDA-R targeting, densin-180 and alpha-actinin also serve to recruit CaMKII to the PSD, possibly to simultaneously interact with CaMKII via multivalent contacts to nucleate and create a defined signaling complex [54] for the >40 CaMKII substrates identified at the PSD [55–57]. Thus, CaMKII translocation to the PSD appears to involve complex interactions that function to restrict CaMKII signaling to active postsynaptic sites. However, once targeted to the PSD, it is unknown how different substrates are selected to create specific functional outputs, including opposing forms of synaptic plasticity LTP and LTD. Thus, the purpose of our study was to determine how graded activity and T^{287} autophosphorylation impact the output of CaMKII, substrate phosphorylation, and selectivity.

We reasoned that for graded levels of CaMKII activation to be important for its signaling, then there should be an intrinsic advantage for multiple subunits to be activated within the holoenzyme versus a similar catalytic level of individual or monomeric CaMKII molecules in phosphorylating PSD substrates. Our studies revealed that while we began our phosphorylation reactions with ~2-fold monomeric CaMKII activity (as measured via a soluble assay) compared to multimeric CaMKII, the native form displays a catalytic advantage at phosphorylating purified PSDs *in vitro*. Thus, while the early work by Cline and colleagues using viral expression of monomeric constitutively active CaMKII (T^{286}D) [58–60] clearly shows that monomeric CaMKII modulates axonal growth, glutamatergic synapse maturation and stabilization of dendritic arbors, our work demonstrates that the native holoenzyme has an advantage over the monomer in PSD phosphorylation *in vitro*. We reasoned that the diffusion-restricted substrate environment like the PSD with many

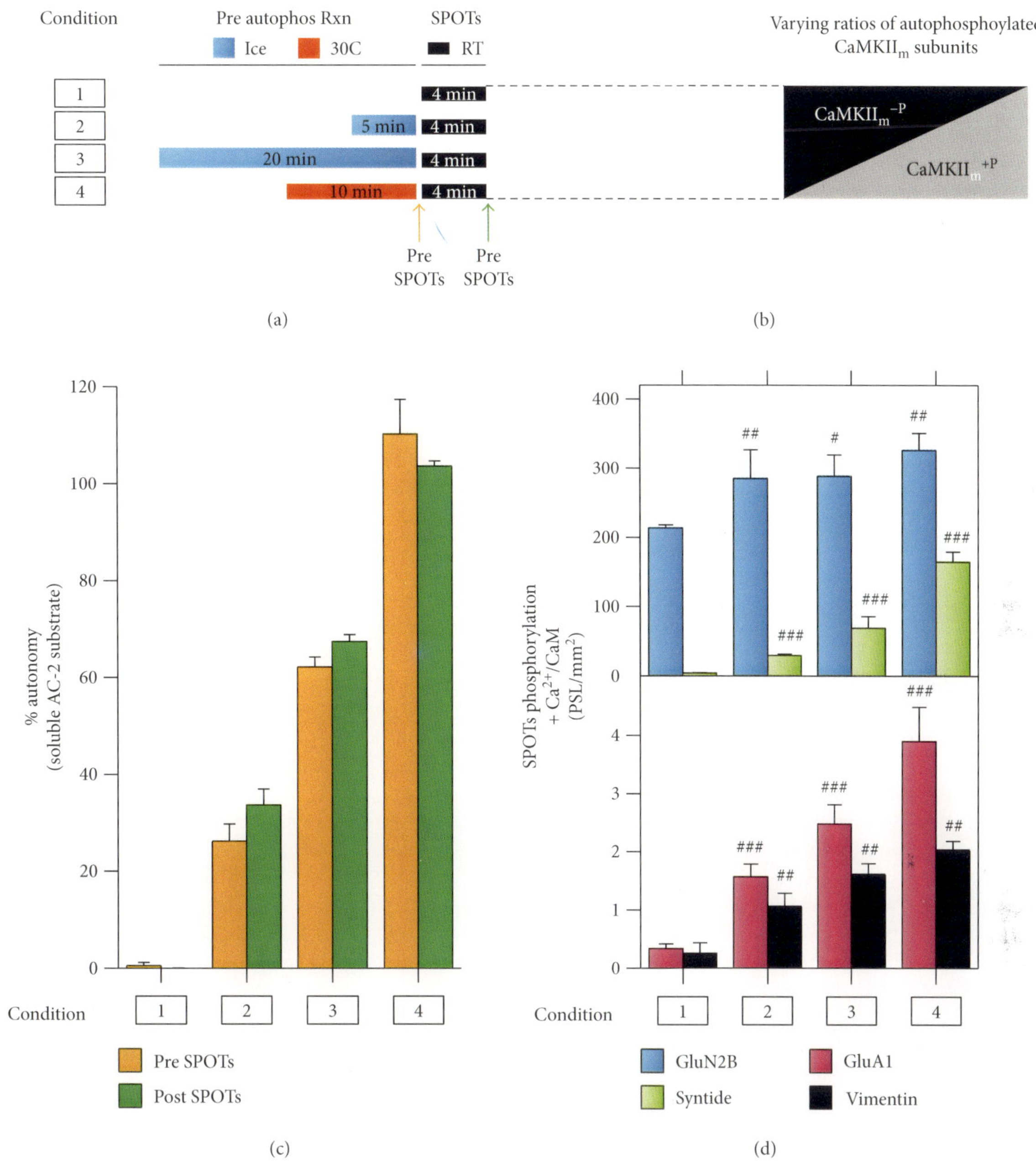

FIGURE 5: CaMKII substrate utilization and selectivity are differentially altered by T^{287} autophosphorylation. (a) Schematic representation of various conditions used to preautophosphorylate CaMKII$_m$ prior to Ca^{2+}/CaM-stimulated substrate phosphorylation reactions on SPOT arrays (see Materials and Methods). Essentially, time and/or temperature was altered to generate different extents of T^{287} autophosphorylation (i.e., varying ratios of CaMKII$_m^{-P}$/CaMKII$_m^{+P}$) as graphically illustrated in (b). (c) As a readout of T^{287} autophosphorylation, the % autonomy (i.e., [Ca^{2+}/CaM-independent]/[Ca^{2+}/CaM-stimulated] activity) was measured in separate soluble kinase assays using the high-affinity CaMKII substrate AC-2. Autonomous activity was measured immediately after the prereaction (pre-SPOTs) and following the SPOT reaction (post-SPOTs); mean ± s.e.m. ($n = 3$). (d) Ca^{2+}/CaM-stimulated SPOT substrate phosphorylation for various T^{287} autophosphorylation conditions; mean ± s.d. ($n = 3$). Results represent one-way ANOVA of log-normalized data with Holm-Šídák posttest compared to 0% autonomy. $^{\#}P < 0.05$; $^{\#\#}P < 0.01$; $^{\#\#\#}P < 0.001$.

different CaMKII substrates (and targeting proteins) takes advantage of the multivalent structure of CaMKII [54], a process that could also take advantage of graded activity within the same CaMKII holoenzyme. Multivalent interactions between CaMKII and its targeting proteins and substrates [54] may contribute to the catalytic advantage observed for native CaMKII over monomeric CaMKII. Future studies are required to explore the interplay between autophosphorylation-dependent substrate gating and the contribution of known PSD targeting proteins (e.g., NR2B, actin, and actinin) in this enhanced PSD phosphorylation by autophosphorylated CaMKII.

We explored this idea directly using multisubstrate SPOT membranes with peptide substrates synthesized from well-known CaMKII substrates. The four model substrates we selected differed in affinity ($GluN2B_{S1303}$ > Syntide > $Vimentin_{S83}$ and $GluA1_{S849}$), possessed divergent phosphorylation motifs, and have been previously characterized *in vivo* and *in vitro* as protein and peptide substrates. Unlike the other three substrates, the $GluN2B_{S1303}$ is a classic example of a T-site-interacting substrate (i.e., mimics CaMKII's ARD) which allows for this substrate to form high-affinity stable interactions to influence targeting [42] and catalytic activity [41, 61]. We elected to use the multisubstrate SPOT array approach because like isolated PSDs, we can explore CaMKII phosphorylation of diverse substrates simultaneously in a diffusion-restricted environment; however, unlike the PSD, the SPOT arrays avoid the intrinsic complexity produced by endogenous CaMKII, scaffolding, and regulatory proteins, factors that can be envisioned to influence our enzymatic analysis of substrate specificity.

To create graded levels of CaMKII activity autophosphorylation, we considered the following. First, the intraholoenzyme-intermolecular T^{287} autophosphorylation reaction is rapid (i.e., seconds) under saturating Ca^{2+}/CaM conditions [15]. Second, while limiting Ca^{2+}/CaM used to restrict the activation process, it will ultimately produce a heterogeneous mixture of activation states in CaMKII ($\pm T^{287}$ autophosphorylation, $\pm T^{306}$ autophosphorylation, and/or $\pm Ca^{2+}$/CaM activation) that will be difficult to interpret. Third, creating mixed holoenzymes of dead or T^{287}A mutants in our insect expression system has an obvious limitation in that quantitatively controlling the mutant to wild-type subunit ratios within individual holoenzymes will be difficult. Fourth, inhibitory autophosphorylation is used by CaMKII *in vivo* to create "capped" or Ca^{2+}/CaM-insensitive subunits [4]. Thus, we elected to create graded levels of CaMKII activation by using this intrinsic property of CaMKII whereby inhibitory (Ca^{2+}/CaM-independent) basal autophosphorylation inactivates CaMKII subunits [19, 38–40]. We created holoenzyme populations with varying ratios of capped subunits (nonresponsive to Ca^{2+}/CaM and inactive) by incubating naïve multimeric CaMKII with Mg^{2+}/ATP. This intramolecular subunit reaction [62] occurs in the absence of Ca^{2+}/CaM as the autophosphorylation event leading to capping occurs within the CaM-binding domain (T^{306} in $\delta/\beta/\gamma$ CaMKII and T^{305} in α CaMKII) [38]. Using this strategy, we created CaMKII holoenzymes with graded levels of activity in the presence of saturating Ca^{2+}/CaM to reveal dramatic shifts in the substrate specificity of the kinase. Higher affinity substrates appear to be preferentially phosphorylated when limited subunits are available for activation per holoenzyme (1/14). However, intermediate and weak substrates become utilized as multiple subunits are available for activation within the holoenzyme (5/15 and 14/14). This analysis requires the assumption that the capping protocol limiting subunit availability to Ca^{2+}/CaM is stochastic at the microscopic level (i.e., individual subunit). The substrate phosphorylation profile for the CaMKII multimer (1/14) looks very similar to monomeric CaMKII in the absence of T^{287} autophosphorylation, suggesting that at the macroscopic level (bulk holoenzymes in solution), the theoretical 1/14 condition functionally approximates a single non-T^{287} autophosphorylated state. While we did have success in creating CaMKII with graded levels of activity (under saturating Ca^{2+}/CaM), this protocol does not have sufficient control to separate different activation states ($\pm T^{287}$ autophosphorylation in the capped CaMKII holoenzymes). Therefore, we employed monomeric CaMKII to explore the specific question of whether T^{287} autophosphorylation impacts substrate selectivity.

The role of autophosphorylation in regulating substrate accessibility was examined more recently and found to have mild [32] or no effect [33] on substrate phosphorylation. While differences in our conclusions may be attributable to different species of CaMKII (human versus rat) and isoforms (α versus δ), we do not favor these possibilities as the catalytic domain of all four CaMKII isoforms is highly conserved [9]. Historically, early structure-function studies demonstrated a lag in substrate catalysis that was relieved by CaMKII autophosphorylation [63]. Our substrate reactions used preautophosphorylated CaMKII and sufficiently dilute monomeric CaMKII in order to minimize this caveat. Our studies with monomer and native multimeric CaMKII indicate that graded levels of activation and/or T^{287} autophosphorylation are important determinants of intermediate and weak substrate phosphorylation. While high-affinity substrate phosphorylation is also enhanced by T^{287} autophosphorylation in $CaMKII_m^{+P}$, the effect was not seen in native CaMKII due to avidity effects. Whether this $CaMKII_{holo}^{+P}$ phenomenon is simply an artifact of peptide density generated in our SPOT membranes or operates in complex substrate environments like the PSD requires additional studies. However, our studies suggest that high-affinity substrates do not have the same requirement for T^{287} autophosphorylation as intermediate- or low-affinity substrates. In total, our data consistent with PSD substrates are tuned for phosphorylation by the multivalent structure of CaMKII and T^{287} autophosphorylation specifically broadens substrate specificity by enhancing intermediate and weak substrate utilization.

4. Conclusions

The unique structure and autoregulation make CaMKII an ideal sensor to encode Ca^{2+}-spike frequency into graded levels of activity and T^{287} autophosphorylation within the holoenzyme. While this process is influenced by Ca^{2+}-spike duration and amplitude [20] as well as phosphatase activity [21], alternative spliced linker length and CaM availability [22, 23], how the number of activated subunits and/or extent of T^{287} autophosphorylation elicits different functional outputs is unknown. Our studies indicate that the activation state of CaMKII, and specifically T^{287} autophosphorylation, is critical drivers of substrate selectivity. Furthermore, our studies suggest a mechanistic explanation for how CaMKII signaling could regulate even opposing functional outputs like LTP and LTD via alterations in substrate selectivity. Future studies are required to determine if graded activity and autophosphorylation operates within complex heterogeneous compartments like the PSD. Furthermore, while our highly reduced biochemical studies suggest that the substrate gating effect of T^{287} autophosphorylation is an intrinsic property of the catalytic domain (and independent of the holoenzyme), further studies are required to illuminate how this mechanism differentially regulates substrate accessibility.

5. Materials and Methods

5.1. Expression and Purification of CaMKII and Calmodulin. Recombinant human CaMKIIδ (NCBI RefSeq: NP_742113.1) with an N-terminal 6xHN tag was integrated into a baculoviral construct (BacPAK9-6xHN), amplified in Sf9 insect cells (expression systems), and expressed in Hi5 (*T. ni;* (Expression Systems)) insect cells [64]. Site-directed mutagenesis was used to generate monomeric hCaMKIIδ_{1-317} (i.e., CaMKII$_m$) (by truncation through the addition of stop codon at aa318). Kinases were purified under reducing conditions by affinity chromatography (NiNTA resin) followed by size exclusion chromatography (Sephacryl S-400 [holoenzyme] or S-300 [CaMKII$_m$]) using an Äkta Purifier (Amersham). SDS-PAGE of the purified proteins revealed a single band with purities > 98%. Recombinant calmodulin was expressed and purified in E.coli as described previously [12, 65] via boiling, ammonium sulfate precipitation, and phenyl-sepharose affinity chromatography.

5.2. Postsynaptic Density Purification. PSDs were acquired from male/female adult rats (Sprague-Dawley) using previously defined procedures involving differential centrifugation with various sucrose gradients followed by Triton X-100 extraction and collection of the Triton-insoluble fraction [34, 35]. Several steps were taken to limit and reduce the Ca^{2+}/CaM-stimulated and autonomous activity of endogenous CaMKII within the PSDs. Rat brains were extracted and snap frozen in liquid nitrogen within 90 secs after sacrificing the animal, as CaMKII is known to activate and translocate to the PSDs within minutes in response to cell death [36].

5.3. Postsynaptic Density Phosphorylation. The PSDs were dephosphorylated to prevent autonomous activity of endogenous CaMKII (resulting from prior T^{287} autophosphorylation), as well as to reduce the phosphorylation state of endogenous substrates. This was accomplished with 1.5 μM PP1α (6xHis purified) overnight at 4°C or at RT for 2 hours with shaking in the presence of 50 mM HEPES pH 7.4, 100 mM NaCl, 1 mM $MnCl_2$, 0.015 Brij 35, 2.5 mM DTT, 10 μM KN-93, and 2x calbiochem protease inhibitor cocktail set V. Phosphorylation reactions were carried out on dephosphorylated PSDs in the presence of 2x phosphatase inhibitor cocktail (Calbiochem) as well as the small molecule CaMKII inhibitor KN93 which only inhibits the autoinhibited kinase (naïve). PSD phosphorylation reactions were carried out on ~50 μg of dephosphorylated PSDs (see above) in the presence of 20 mM HEPES pH 7.4, 100 mM NaCl, 10 mM $MgCl_2$, 0.5 mM $CaCl_2$, 5 μM CaM, 100 μM cold ATP, 120 μCi/ml [γ-^{32}P]-ATP, and 350 nM CaMKII (per subunit). For reactions involving T^{287} autophosphorylated CaMKII, a prereaction was performed in the presence of 20 mM HEPES pH 7.4, 100 mM NaCl, 10 mM $MgCl_2$, 0.5 mM $CaCl_2$, 5 μM CaM, 500 μM ATPγS, and 3.5 μM kinase for 10 min at 30°C (for monomer) or on ice (for the holoenzyme). PSD phosphorylation reactions (60 μl total) were incubated at room temperature for 4 min unless otherwise noted. Reactions were terminated with the addition of 500 μl of 100 mM sodium phosphate pH 7.0, 1 M NaCl, and 10 mM EDTA) followed by centrifugation to obtain a PSD pellet. Pellet was three times in the same termination buffer. The PSD pellet was resuspended in 2x LDS sample buffer and resuspended using a horn sonicator. SDS-PAGE was performed followed by Coomassie staining and drying of the gel. Total protein was assessed by densitometry of the Coomassie signal while the extent of radioactive phosphate incorporation was quantified using a Fujifilm phosphorimager and profiles measured as photostimulated luminescence (PSL/mm^2). The densitometric intensity data was converted to area under the curve (AUC) to determine to protein or total phosphorylation.

5.4. Soluble Peptide Assays. Soluble peptide substrates (generally 15mers) were obtained (Biopeptide Co. Inc.) and utilized in standard radioactive activity assays. In typical Ca^{2+}/CaM-dependent reactions, 50-200 μM substrate was used in the presence of 50 mM HEPES pH 7.4, 100 mM NaCl, 10 mM $MgCl_2$, 0.2 mM $CaCl_2$, 1 μM CaM, 100 μM cold ATP, 60 μCi/ml [γ-^{32}P] ATP, and 5–10 nM CaMKII (per subunit). In Ca^{2+}/CaM-independent reactions, 5 mM EGTA (or BAPTA) was used to chelate free Ca^{2+}. This constitutive (i.e., autonomous) activity in the absence of Ca^{2+} was expressed, a percentage of the Ca^{2+}/CaM-dependent activity. Reactions were carried out at 30°C for 1 minute and quenched by spotting onto Whatman Grade P81 ion exchange chromatography paper (Whatman, GE Healthcare, Piscataway, NJ). The filter papers were washed with 75 mM phosphoric acid 3 times for 5 minutes each and subsequently quantified in a scintillation counter (Beckman) via the Cerenkov counting method [66, 67]. AC-2 (KKALRRQEtVDAL), a CaMKII substrate derived from the CaMKII T^{287} autophosphorylation site was used for standard soluble peptide substrate reactions as described previously [64, 68].

5.5. Holoenzyme Inactivation. CaMKII$_{holo}$ (600 nM) was exposed to inhibitory autophosphorylation ($T^{306/7}$ capping) for 0, 5, or 15 minutes in the presence of 50 mM HEPES pH 7.4, 100 mM NaCl, 10 mM $MgCl_2$, and 500 μM ATP. Inactivated states of CaMKII were then diluted to 60 nM for SPOT substrate phosphorylation reactions (described below). For all states of preinactivation (0, 5, 8, or 15 min), the SPOT phosphorylation was normalized to the number of active subunits per holoenzyme (assuming each holoenzyme is tetradecameric). The number of active subunits per holoenzyme was assessed by measuring the Ca^{2+}/CaM-dependent activity of each inactivation condition in standard soluble peptide substrate phosphorylation assays using AC-2 peptide. These activity assays were performed at the beginning and end (4 min) of the SPOT phosphorylation assay, their values averaged together. The activity from naïve

$CaMKII_{holo}$ (i.e., 0 min preinactivation) was considered to maximal (i.e., all 14 subunits activated) and was thus used to calculate the average enzymatic activity per subunit.

5.6. Preautophosphorylation Reactions. For reactions involving T^{287} autophosphorylated CaMKII, a prereaction was performed in the presence of 20 mM HEPES pH 7.4, 100 mM NaCl, 10 mM $MgCl_2$, 0.5 mM $CaCl_2$, 5 μM CaM, 500 μM cold ATP, and 500 nM kinase for 10 minutes on ice. To achieve varying numbers/percentages of T^{287} autophosphorylated subunits (%AutoP), similar prereactions were used with 50 nM kinase incubation times of 0, 5, or 20 minutes on ice, or 10 minutes at 30°C (Figure 5; preconditions 1–4, resp.).

5.7. In Vitro SPOT Phosphorylation Assay. Peptides (generally 15mers) were synthesized using the SPOT method [69, 70] onto β-alanine derivatized cellulose membranes via a MultiPep synthesizer (Intavis AG, Cologne, Germany). The peptide blots were blocked with 5% BSA in 50 mM HEPES pH 7.4, 100 mM NaCl, 1 mM EDTA, and 0.02% NP-40 for 30 minutes followed by three washes in 100 mM Tris–HCl pH 7.4. Membranes were subjected to a kinase phosphorylation assay in the presence of 50 mM HEPES pH 7.4, 100 mM NaCl, 10 mM $MgCl_2$, 0.2 mM $CaCl_2$, 1 μM CaM, 0.2 mg/ml BSA, 1 mM DTT, 100 μM cold ATP, 6–12 μCi/ml (γ-^{32}P) ATP, and 5–10 nM CaMKII (per subunit). The reactions were incubated at room temperature for 4 minutes unless otherwise noted, terminated with three washes (100 mM sodium phosphate pH 7.0, 1 M NaCl, and 10 mM EDTA), and dried. The extent of radioactive phosphate incorporation was quantified using a Fujifilm phosphoimager and expressed as photostimulated luminescence (PSL/mm^2) for a 1.5 mm × 1.5 mm circle centered on each spot. Three to four replicate spots were averaged for each peptide for a given condition with error bars indicating s.d., unless otherwise noted. $GluN2B_{S1303}$ = RNKLRRQHsYDTFVD; Syntide = PLARTLsVAGLPGKK; $GluA1_{S849}$ = GFCLIPQQsINEAIR; $Vimentin_{S83}$ = PGVRLLQDsVDFSLA.

5.8. Data and Statistical Analysis. One-way analysis of variance (ANOVA) with subsequent Holm-Šídák posttest was performed on log transformed to account for mean-dependent variances, compared to control (#). Statistical analyses were performed using SigmaPlot 12.5. Statistical significance is denoted by the number of symbols for different P values (e.g., $^{\#}P < 0.05$, $^{\#\#}P < 0.01$, and $^{\#\#\#}P < 0.001$).

Abbreviations

CaMKII: Calcium/calmodulin-dependent protein kinase II
AUC: Area under the curve
PSD: Postsynaptic density.

Disclosure

A. Hudmon's present address is Department of Medicinal Chemistry and Molecular Pharmacology, College of Pharmacy, Purdue University, West Lafayette, IN 47907, USA. D. E. Johnson present address is AIT Bioscience, 7840 Innovation Blvd, Indianapolis, IN 46278, USA.

Conflicts of Interest

The authors declare no conflicts of interest. The authors declare no competing financial interests.

Acknowledgments

The authors thank N. M. Ashpole, J. M. Bradshaw, H. Schulman, M. C. Sousa, and M. N. Waxham for valuable suggestions and insightful comments during various iterations of this manuscript. This work was supported by the National Institutes of Health Grant NS078171 to A. Hudmon.

References

[1] J. D. Sweatt, "Neural plasticity and behavior - sixty years of conceptual advances," *Journal of Neurochemistry*, vol. 139, Supplement 2, pp. 179–199, 2016.

[2] P. K. Stanton, "LTD, LTP, and the sliding threshold for long-term synaptic plasticity," *Hippocampus*, vol. 6, no. 1, pp. 35–42, 1996.

[3] J. Lisman, "The CaM kinase II hypothesis for the storage of synaptic memory," *Trends in Neurosciences*, vol. 17, no. 10, pp. 406–412, 1994.

[4] S. J. Coultrap and K. U. Bayer, "CaMKII regulation in information processing and storage," *Trends in Neurosciences*, vol. 35, no. 10, pp. 607–618, 2012.

[5] B. C. Shonesy, N. Jalan-Sakrikar, V. S. Cavener, and R. J. Colbran, "CaMKII: a molecular substrate for synaptic plasticity and memory," *Progress in Molecular Biology and Translational Science*, vol. 122, pp. 61–87, 2014.

[6] J. W. Hell, "CaMKII: claiming center stage in postsynaptic function and organization," *Neuron*, vol. 81, no. 2, pp. 249–265, 2014.

[7] B. E. Herring and R. A. Nicoll, "Long-term potentiation: from CaMKII to AMPA receptor trafficking," *Annual Review of Physiology*, vol. 78, no. 1, pp. 351–365, 2016.

[8] A. Hudmon and H. Schulman, "Structure-function of the multifunctional Ca2+/calmodulin-dependent protein kinase II," *Biochemical Journal*, vol. 364, no. 3, pp. 593–611, 2002.

[9] A. Hudmon and H. Schulman, "Neuronal CA2+/calmodulin-dependent protein kinase II: the role of structure and autoregulation in cellular function," *Annual Review of Biochemistry*, vol. 71, no. 1, pp. 473–510, 2002.

[10] J. Lisman, H. Schulman, and H. Cline, "The molecular basis of CaMKII function in synaptic and behavioural memory," *Nature Reviews Neuroscience*, vol. 3, no. 3, pp. 175–190, 2002.

[11] P. Rellos, A. C. W. Pike, F. H. Niesen et al., "Structure of the CaMKIIdelta/calmodulin complex reveals the molecular mechanism of CaMKII kinase activation," *PLoS Biology*, vol. 8, no. 7, article e1000426, 2010.

[12] T. R. Gaertner, S. J. Kolodziej, D. Wang et al., "Comparative analyses of the three-dimensional structures and enzymatic properties of alpha, beta, gamma and delta isoforms of Ca2+-calmodulin-dependent protein kinase II," *Journal of Biological Chemistry*, vol. 279, no. 13, pp. 12484–12494, 2004.

[13] L. H. Chao, M. M. Stratton, I. H. Lee et al., "A mechanism for tunable autoinhibition in the structure of a human Ca2+/calmodulin- dependent kinase II holoenzyme," *Cell*, vol. 146, no. 5, pp. 732–745, 2011.

[14] R. C. Rich and H. Schulman, "Substrate-directed function of calmodulin in autophosphorylation of Ca^{2+}/calmodulin-dependent protein kinase II," *Journal of Biological Chemistry*, vol. 273, no. 43, pp. 28424–28429, 1998.

[15] P. I. Hanson, T. Meyer, L. Stryer, and H. Schulman, "Dual role of calmodulin in autophosphorylation of multifunctional cam kinase may underlie decoding of calcium signals," *Neuron*, vol. 12, no. 5, pp. 943–956, 1994.

[16] A. J. Baucum 2nd, B. C. Shonesy, K. L. Rose, and R. J. Colbran, "Quantitative proteomics analysis of CaMKII phosphorylation and the CaMKII interactome in the mouse forebrain," *ACS Chemical Neuroscience*, vol. 6, no. 4, pp. 615–631, 2015.

[17] T. Meyer, P. I. Hanson, L. Stryer, and H. Schulman, "Calmodulin trapping by calcium-calmodulin-dependent protein kinase," *Science*, vol. 256, no. 5060, pp. 1199–1202, 1992.

[18] C. M. Schworer, R. J. Colbran, J. R. Keefer, and T. R. Soderling, "Ca2+/calmodulin-dependent protein kinase II. Identification of a regulatory autophosphorylation site adjacent to the inhibitory and calmodulin-binding domains," *The Journal of Biological Chemistry*, vol. 263, no. 27, pp. 13486–13489, 1988.

[19] L. L. Lou and H. Schulman, "Distinct autophosphorylation sites sequentially produce autonomy and inhibition of the multifunctional Ca2+/calmodulin-dependent protein kinase," *Journal of Neuroscience*, vol. 9, no. 6, pp. 2020–2032, 1989.

[20] P. De Koninck and H. Schulman, "Sensitivity of CaM kinase II to the frequency of Ca^{2+} oscillations," *Science*, vol. 279, no. 5348, pp. 227–230, 1998.

[21] R. J. Colbran, "Protein phosphatases and calcium/calmodulin-dependent protein kinase II-dependent synaptic plasticity," *Journal of Neuroscience*, vol. 24, no. 39, pp. 8404–8409, 2004.

[22] A. Persechini and P. M. Stemmer, "Calmodulin is a limiting factor in the cell," *Trends in Cardiovascular Medicine*, vol. 12, no. 1, pp. 32–37, 2002.

[23] R. P. Estep, K. A. Alexander, and D. R. Storm, "Regulation of free calmodulin levels in neurons by neuromodulin: relationship to neuronal growth and regeneration," *Current Topics in Cellular Regulation*, vol. 31, pp. 161–180, 1989.

[24] D. J. Grab, R. K. Carlin, and P. Siekevitz, "Function of a calmodulin in postsynaptic densities. II. Presence of a calmodulin-activatable protein kinase activity," *The Journal of Cell Biology*, vol. 89, no. 3, pp. 440–448, 1981.

[25] P. T. Kelly and P. R. Montgomery, "Subcellular localization of the 52,000 molecular weight major postsynaptic density protein," *Brain Research*, vol. 233, no. 2, pp. 265–286, 1982.

[26] P. T. Kelly, T. L. McGuinness, and P. Greengard, "Evidence that the major postsynaptic density protein is a component of a Ca2+/calmodulin-dependent protein kinase," *Proceedings of the National Academy of Sciences of the United States of America*, vol. 81, no. 3, pp. 945–949, 1984.

[27] M. Sanhueza and J. Lisman, "The CaMKII/NMDAR complex as a molecular memory," *Molecular Brain*, vol. 6, no. 1, p. 10, 2013.

[28] K. Kim, T. Saneyoshi, T. Hosokawa, K. Okamoto, and Y. Hayashi, "Interplay of enzymatic and structural functions of CaMKII in long-term potentiation," *Journal of Neurochemistry*, vol. 139, no. 6, pp. 959–972, 2016.

[29] B. G. Mockett, D. Guevremont, M. Wutte, S. R. Hulme, J. M. Williams, and W. C. Abraham, "Calcium/calmodulin-dependent protein kinase II mediates group I metabotropic glutamate receptor-dependent protein synthesis and long-term depression in rat hippocampus," *Journal of Neuroscience*, vol. 31, no. 20, pp. 7380–7391, 2011.

[30] K. C. Marsden, J. B. Beattie, J. Friedenthal, and R. C. Carroll, "NMDA receptor activation potentiates inhibitory transmission through GABA receptor-associated protein-dependent exocytosis of $GABA_A$ receptors," *Journal of Neuroscience*, vol. 27, no. 52, pp. 14326–14337, 2007.

[31] S. J. Coultrap, R. K. Freund, H. O'Leary et al., "Autonomous CaMKII mediates both LTP and LTD using a mechanism for differential substrate site selection," *Cell Reports*, vol. 6, no. 3, pp. 431–437, 2014.

[32] S. J. Coultrap, K. Barcomb, and K. U. Bayer, "A significant but rather mild contribution of T286 autophosphorylation to Ca2+/CaM-stimulated CaMKII activity," *PLoS One*, vol. 7, no. 5, article e37176, 2012.

[33] S. J. Coultrap, I. Buard, J. R. Kulbe, M. L. Dell'Acqua, and K. U. Bayer, "CaMKII autonomy is substrate-dependent and further stimulated by Ca2+/calmodulin," *Journal of Biological Chemistry*, vol. 285, no. 23, pp. 17930–17937, 2010.

[34] M. D. Ehlers, "Activity level controls postsynaptic composition and signaling via the ubiquitin-proteasome system," *Nature Neuroscience*, vol. 6, no. 3, pp. 231–242, 2003.

[35] M. T. Swulius, Y. Kubota, A. Forest, and M. N. Waxham, "Structure and composition of the postsynaptic density during development," *The Journal of Comparative Neurology*, vol. 518, no. 20, pp. 4243–4260, 2010.

[36] T. Suzuki, K. Okumura-Noji, R. Tanakå, and T. Tada, "Rapid translocation of cytosolic Ca2+/calmodulin-dependent protein-kinase-II into postsynaptic density after decapitation," *Journal of Neurochemistry*, vol. 63, no. 4, pp. 1529–1537, 1994.

[37] J. A. Ubersax and J. E. Ferrell Jr., "Mechanisms of specificity in protein phosphorylation," *Nature Reviews. Molecular Cell Biology*, vol. 8, no. 7, pp. 530–541, 2007.

[38] R. J. Colbran, "Inactivation of Ca^{2+}/calmodulin-dependent protein kinase II by basal autophosphorylation," *Journal of Biological Chemistry*, vol. 268, no. 10, pp. 7163–7170, 1993.

[39] R. J. Colbran and T. R. Soderling, "Calcium/calmodulin-independent autophosphorylation sites of calcium/calmodulin-dependent protein kinase II. Studies on the effect of phosphorylation of threonine 305/306 and serine 314 on calmodulin binding using synthetic peptides," *Journal of Biological Chemistry*, vol. 265, no. 19, pp. 11213–11219, 1990.

[40] B. L. Patton, S. G. Miller, and M. B. Kennedy, "Activation of type II calcium/calmodulin-dependent protein kinase by Ca2+/calmodulin is inhibited by autophosphorylation of threonine within the calmodulin-binding domain," *Journal of Biological Chemistry*, vol. 265, no. 19, pp. 11204–11212, 1990.

[41] K. U. Bayer, P. de Koninck, A. S. Leonard, J. W. Hell, and H. Schulman, "Interaction with the NMDA receptor locks CaMKII in an active conformation," *Nature*, vol. 411, no. 6839, pp. 801–805, 2001.

[42] S. Strack, R. B. McNeill, and R. J. Colbran, "Mechanism and regulation of calcium/calmodulin-dependent protein kinase II targeting to the NR2B subunit of the N-methyl-D-aspartate receptor," *Journal of Biological Chemistry*, vol. 275, no. 31, pp. 23798–23806, 2000.

[43] X. Liao, J. Su, and M. Mrksich, "An adaptor domain-mediated autocatalytic interfacial kinase reaction," *Chemistry*, vol. 15, no. 45, pp. 12303–12309, 2009.

[44] J. L. Naffin, Y. Han, H. J. Olivos, M. M. Reddy, T. Sun, and T. Kodadek, "Immobilized peptides as high-affinity capture agents for self-associating proteins," *Chemistry & Biology*, vol. 10, no. 3, pp. 251–259, 2003.

[45] A. Ikeda, S. Okuno, and H. Fujisawa, "Studies on the generation of Ca2+/calmodulin-independent activity of calmodulin-dependent protein kinase II by autophosphorylation. Autothiophosphorylation of the enzyme," *Journal of Biological Chemistry*, vol. 266, no. 18, pp. 11582–11588, 1991.

[46] J. R. Sanes and J. W. Lichtman, "Can molecules explain long-term potentiation?," *Nature Neuroscience*, vol. 2, no. 7, pp. 597–604, 1999.

[47] K. Shen and T. Meyer, "Dynamic control of CaMKII translocation and localization in hippocampal neurons by NMDA receptor stimulation," *Science*, vol. 284, no. 5411, pp. 162–167, 1999.

[48] K. Shen, M. N. Teruel, J. H. Connor, S. Shenolikar, and T. Meyer, "Molecular memory by reversible translocation of calcium/calmodulin-dependent protein kinase II," *Nature Neuroscience*, vol. 3, no. 9, pp. 881–886, 2000.

[49] M. R. Gleason, S. Higashijima, J. Dallman, K. Liu, G. Mandel, and J. R. Fetcho, "Translocation of CaM kinase II to synaptic sites *in vivo*," *Nature Neuroscience*, vol. 6, no. 3, pp. 217-218, 2003.

[50] N. Otmakhov, J. H. Tao-Cheng, S. Carpenter et al., "Persistent accumulation of calcium/calmodulin-dependent protein kinase II in dendritic spines after induction of NMDA receptor-dependent chemical long-term potentiation," *Journal of Neuroscience*, vol. 24, no. 42, pp. 9324–9331, 2004.

[51] A. R. Halt, R. F. Dallapiazza, Y. Zhou et al., "CaMKII binding to GluN2B is critical during memory consolidation," *The EMBO Journal*, vol. 31, no. 5, pp. 1203–1216, 2012.

[52] R. V. Omkumar, M. J. Kiely, A. J. Rosenstein, K. T. Min, and M. B. Kennedy, "Identification of a phosphorylation site for calcium/calmodulindependent protein kinase II in the NR2B subunit of the N-methyl-D-aspartate receptor," *Journal of Biological Chemistry*, vol. 271, no. 49, pp. 31670–31678, 1996.

[53] S. J. Tavalin and R. J. Colbran, "CaMKII-mediated phosphorylation of GluN2B regulates recombinant NMDA receptor currents in a chloride-dependent manner," *Molecular and Cellular Neurosciences*, vol. 79, pp. 45–52, 2017.

[54] A. J. Robison, M. A. Bass, Y. Jiao et al., "Multivalent interactions of calcium/calmodulin-dependent protein kinase II with the postsynaptic density proteins NR2B, densin-180, and alpha-actinin-2," *Journal of Biological Chemistry*, vol. 280, no. 42, pp. 35329–35336, 2005.

[55] H. Jaffe, L. Vinade, and A. Dosemeci, "Identification of novel phosphorylation sites on postsynaptic density proteins," *Biochemical and Biophysical Research Communications*, vol. 321, no. 1, pp. 210–218, 2004.

[56] Y. Yoshimura, C. Aoi, and T. Yamauchi, "Investigation of protein substrates of Ca(2+)/calmodulin-dependent protein kinase II translocated to the postsynaptic density," *Brain Research. Molecular Brain Research*, vol. 81, no. 1-2, pp. 118–128, 2000.

[57] Y. Yoshimura, T. Shinkawa, M. Taoka, K. Kobayashi, T. Isobe, and T. Yamauchi, "Identification of protein substrates of Ca(2+)/calmodulin-dependent protein kinase II in the postsynaptic density by protein sequencing and mass spectrometry," *Biochemical and Biophysical Research Communications*, vol. 290, no. 3, pp. 948–954, 2002.

[58] D. J. Zou and H. T. Cline, "Expression of constitutively active CaMKII in target tissue modifies presynaptic axon arbor growth," *Neuron*, vol. 16, no. 3, pp. 529–539, 1996.

[59] G. Wu, R. Malinow, and H. T. Cline, "Maturation of a central glutamatergic synapse," *Science*, vol. 274, no. 5289, pp. 972–976, 1996.

[60] G. Y. Wu and H. T. Cline, "Stabilization of dendritic arbor structure in vivo by CaMKII," *Science*, vol. 279, no. 5348, pp. 222–226, 1998.

[61] M. Praseeda, M. Mayadevi, and R. V. Omkumar, "Interaction of peptide substrate outside the active site influences catalysis by CaMKII," *Biochemical and Biophysical Research Communications*, vol. 313, no. 4, pp. 845–849, 2004.

[62] S. Mukherji and T. R. Soderling, "Regulation of Ca2+/calmodulin-dependent protein kinase II by inter- and intrasubunit-catalyzed autophosphorylations," *Journal of Biological Chemistry*, vol. 269, no. 19, pp. 13744–13747, 1994.

[63] A. P. Kwiatkowski, D. J. Shell, and M. M. King, "The role of autophosphorylation in activation of the type II calmodulin-dependent protein kinase," *Journal of Biological Chemistry*, vol. 263, no. 14, pp. 6484–6486, 1988.

[64] N. M. Ashpole and A. Hudmon, "Excitotoxic neuroprotection and vulnerability with CaMKII inhibition," *Molecular and Cellular Neurosciences*, vol. 46, no. 4, pp. 720–730, 2011.

[65] S. I. Singla, A. Hudmon, J. M. Goldberg, J. L. Smith, and H. Schulman, "Molecular characterization of calmodulin trapping by calcium/calmodulin-dependent protein kinase II," *Journal of Biological Chemistry*, vol. 276, no. 31, pp. 29353–29360, 2001.

[66] A. Hudmon, J. Aronowski, S. J. Kolb, and M. N. Waxham, "Inactivation and self-association of Ca2+/calmodulin-dependent protein kinase II during autophosphorylation," *Journal of Biological Chemistry*, vol. 271, no. 15, pp. 8800–8808, 1996.

[67] R. Roskoski Jr., "Assays of protein kinase," *Methods in Enzymology*, vol. 99, pp. 3–6, 1983.

[68] M. L. Bangaru, J. Meng, D. J. Kaiser et al., "Differential expression of CaMKII isoforms and overall kinase activity in rat dorsal root ganglia after injury," *Neuroscience*, vol. 300, pp. 116–127, 2015.

[69] R. Frank, "The SPOT-synthesis technique. Synthetic peptide arrays on membrane supports—principles and applications," *Journal of Immunological Methods*, vol. 267, no. 1, pp. 13–26, 2002.

[70] R. Frank and H. Overwin, "SPOT synthesis. Epitope analysis with arrays of synthetic peptides prepared on cellulose membranes," *Methods in Molecular Biology*, vol. 66, pp. 149–169, 1996.

[71] J. Zheng, E. A. Trafny, D. R. Knighton et al., "2.2 A refined crystal structure of the catalytic subunit of cAMP-dependent protein kinase complexed with MnATP and a peptide inhibitor," *Acta Crystallographica Section D Biological Crystallography*, vol. 49, no. 3, pp. 362–365, 1993.

[72] L. H. Chao, P. Pellicena, S. Deindl, L. A. Barclay, H. Schulman, and J. Kuriyan, "Intersubunit capture of regulatory segments is a component of cooperative CaMKII activation," *Nature Structural & Molecular Biology*, vol. 17, no. 3, pp. 264–272, 2010.

Acoustical Enrichment during Early Development Improves Response Reliability in the Adult Auditory Cortex of the Rat

Zbyněk Bureš,[1,2] **Kateryna Pysanenko**,[1] **Jiří Lindovský**,[1] **and Josef Syka**[1]

[1]*Department of Auditory Neuroscience, Institute of Experimental Medicine, Czech Academy of Sciences, Vídeňská 1083, 14220 Prague 4, Czech Republic*
[2]*Department of Technical Studies, College of Polytechnics, Tolstého 16, 58601 Jihlava, Czech Republic*

Correspondence should be addressed to Zbyněk Bureš; buresz@biomed.cas.cz

Academic Editor: Preston E. Garraghty

It is well known that auditory experience during early development shapes response properties of auditory cortex (AC) neurons, influencing, for example, tonotopical arrangement, response thresholds and strength, or frequency selectivity. Here, we show that rearing rat pups in a complex acoustically enriched environment leads to an increased reliability of responses of AC neurons, affecting both the rate and the temporal codes. For a repetitive stimulus, the neurons exhibit a lower spike count variance, indicating a more stable rate coding. At the level of individual spikes, the discharge patterns of individual neurons show a higher degree of similarity across stimulus repetitions. Furthermore, the neurons follow more precisely the temporal course of the stimulus, as manifested by improved phase-locking to temporally modulated sounds. The changes are persistent and present up to adulthood. The results document that besides basic alterations of receptive fields presented in our previous study, the acoustic environment during the critical period of postnatal development also leads to a decreased stochasticity and a higher reproducibility of neuronal spiking patterns.

1. Introduction

For the auditory system of rats, the early postnatal developmental period (the so-called critical period, CP) represents the epoch of increased plasticity and susceptibility [1–3]. Progressive refinements taking place during this time substantially modulate the structure and function of the auditory centers, often leaving a lifelong trace. An important message brought by recent research is that the final maturation of the system and development of its proper response characteristics are heavily influenced by ongoing auditory stimulation [4–6]. Interventions such as sensory deprivation, monotonous stimulation, or excessive sound exposure result in impairments of neuronal responsiveness both in the auditory cortex (AC) and in subcortical structures such as the inferior colliculus (IC) [5, 7–10]. On the other hand, a richer and stimulating environment may improve the response properties of the system by, for example, more favorable shaping of the neuronal receptive fields [6, 11, 12]. In the simplest case, when the augmented stimulation comprises an elementary sound like pure tone or click train, the outcome is usually characterized by selective enhancement of responses related to that specific stimulus [3, 4, 13]. A more beneficial situation, however, is when the responses of the auditory system are amended globally in a nonspecific manner. To achieve this, the enriched environment has to be more complex and possibly contain a positive feedback to motivate the animals to attend to the stimulation [6, 14, 15]. Our previous results have shown that application of a complex acoustically enriched environment (AEE) during the period of development nonselectively and permanently improves the representations of tonal frequency and intensity in IC and AC neurons by increasing their sensitivity and frequency selectivity and by lowering the number of nonmonotonic rate-intensity functions [6, 16]. Advancing one step further from the basic evaluation of neuronal receptive fields performed in our previous work, the aim of the current study is to address the ability of neurons to precisely encode a given stimulus using either the rate code or the temporal code. Employing mostly complex temporally modulated stimuli, we focus on the assessment of the reliability, stability, and temporal acuity of individual responses. By providing more stable and repeatable response patterns that could be more easily detected in a background spiking noise, the acoustical enrichment during the developmental period, complemented with an active stimulus-reward paradigm, may ultimately enhance the stimulus discrimination ability of the animals.

2. Materials and Methods

2.1. Experimental Groups. In total, 51 female rats were used in the experiment (strain Long-Evans, obtained from the local breeding facility). One group of rats ($n = 27$) denoted as *enriched* was exposed to an acoustically enriched environment reinforced with active feedback for two weeks starting on postnatal day 14. The acoustic environment was based on a broadband (983 Hz–48461 Hz) amplitude-modulated (low-pass exponential noise envelope with cut-off frequency 2 Hz) rippled noise (depth of the spectral ripples 30 dB) presented at 55 dB SPL. To draw the animals' attention to the overall acoustic stimulation, the continuous background was complemented with several types of randomly appearing embedded target sounds (60 dB SPL, 500 ms duration, spectral contents centered near 6 kHz): pure tone, sawtooth signal, sinusoidally frequency-modulated tone (modulation frequency 10 Hz), and 1/3-octave noise. The frequency-modulated tone triggered the release of reward, which was slightly delayed relative to the triggering sound. The drop was always available for approximately 2 s and then fell out of reach of the animals. The presence and identity of animals at the reward-delivering spout were monitored by a custom-made system based on an infrared gate (Coulbourn Instruments), an Arduino RFID reader, and a MATLAB script. The RFID chips (kindly donated by LUX-IDent, Czech Republic) were subcutaneously implanted on the neck under temporary isoflurane anesthesia. More details about the AEE can be found in [6, 16].

An age-matched group of rats denoted as controls ($n = 24$) was raised in standard conditions with no acoustical enrichment. The responses of AC neurons were recorded later, at the age of 3 to 6 months. A schematic illustration of the experimental paradigm is shown in Figure 1. The care and use of animals were approved by the Ethics Committee of the Institute of Experimental Medicine, Academy of Sciences of the Czech Republic, and followed the guidelines of the EU Directive 2010/63/EU for animal experiments.

2.2. Recording of the Neuronal Activity in the AC. Recording of the neuronal activity in the AC was carried out in a sound-proof anechoic room. The rats were anaesthetized with an intramuscular injection of a mixture of 35 mg/kg ketamine (Calypsol 50 mg/ml; Gedeon Richter, Budapest, Hungary) and 6 mg/kg xylazine (Xylapan 20 mg/ml; Vetoquinol SA., Lure Cedex, France). Supplementary subcutaneous injections of one-half of the original dose of the ketamine-xylazine mixture were administered approximately every hour to maintain a sufficient level of anesthesia. The body temperature was maintained at 37-38 deg C using a heating pad. Respiratory and heart rates, along with pedal

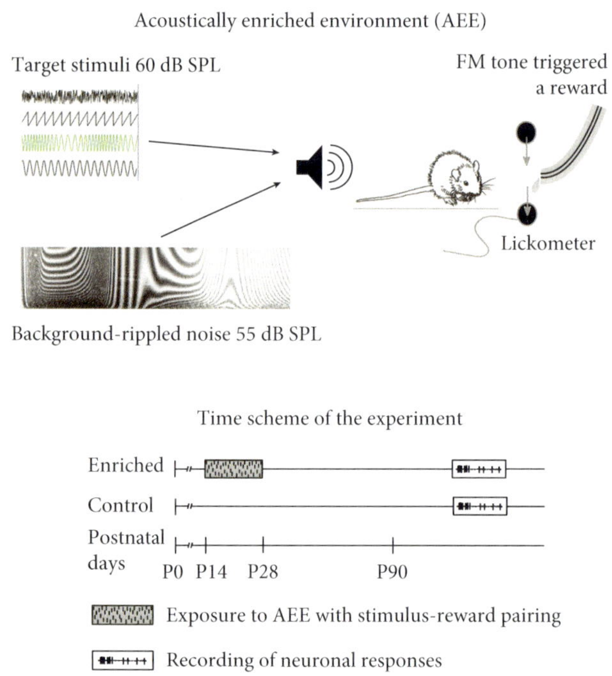

FIGURE 1: Schematic illustration of the experimental paradigm.

reflex (toe pinch) or eye blink reflex, were monitored. The skin and muscles above the right temporal region of the skull were removed, and a craniotomy with a diameter of approximately 5 mm was performed above the AC area. The base of an S-shaped holder was screwed into the skull above the frontal part of the right hemisphere. After placing the rat in a stereotaxic apparatus and fixing the head with the previously screwed holder, the dura mater was removed. The A1 location was determined by recording tone-evoked responses at the cortical surface using a custom-made multichannel low-impedance electrode array. The responses of single neurons or small groups of adjacent neurons were recorded using a 16-channel electrode array (NeuroNexus Technologies, single shank probe, 50 μm or 100 μm distance between electrode spots) inserted into the AC using an electronic driver. The recording depths varied between 100 and 1200 μm beneath the cortex surface, and the recordings thus originated from all layers of the AC. The amplified and bandpass-filtered (300 Hz–10 kHz) signal processed by a TDT System III, RX5-2 Pentusa Base Station was subsequently recorded and analyzed with BrainWare software (Tucker Davis Technologies, Alachua, FL, USA). The discrimination of individual action potentials was performed online based on amplitude thresholding.

2.3. Test Stimuli and Data Analyses. Acoustic stimuli were generated with a TDT System III using the RP 2.1 Enhanced Real-Time Processor and delivered in free-field conditions via a two-way loudspeaker system (Selenium 6W4P woofer and RAAL70-20 tweeter) placed 70 cm in front of the animal's head.

To quantify the stability and precision of the rate coding, we measured the variability of noise-evoked responses. White noise bursts (60 ms in duration, 5 ms rise/fall times) with a variable intensity (10 dB step) were presented in a random order, each stimulus appearing at least fifty times. For each stimulus, the variance of evoked spike rates was computed for each neuron. To better judge the level discrimination ability, detection distance at a given sound level was computed as follows:

$$d(I) = \frac{\mu(I+10) - \mu(I-10)}{\sigma(I)}, \quad (1)$$

where I is the sound level in dB, $\mu(I)$ is the mean spike count at sound level I, and $\sigma(I)$ is the standard deviation of the spike count at sound level I.

To assess the properties of the temporal coding, amplitude-modulated (AM) white noise, frequency-modulated (FM) tones, and a series of clicks were used. In the case of amplitude modulation, white noise bursts (500 ms in duration) were modulated by a sinusoidal envelope ranging from 0% to 100%. The modulation frequencies ranged from 2 Hz to 24 Hz with a 2 Hz step. The equivalent (time-averaged) SPL was set to 60 dB. In the case of frequency modulation, pure tone pulses (1000 ms in duration, frequency matching the best frequency of the measured neuron) were modulated sinusoidally with logarithmically spaced modulation frequencies ranging from 2 Hz to 100 Hz. The mean frequency shift was set to 0.23 octaves, and the equivalent SPL was set to 60 dB. In the case of click trains, short rectangular pulses (0.1 ms pulse duration, 2000 ms click train duration) were presented with a variable repetition rate. The repetition rate varied logarithmically from 2 Hz to 100 Hz. All three temporally structured stimuli (i.e., the AM noise, the FM tones, and the click trains) were used to determine the amount of synchronization of neuronal responses with the stimulus. Vector strength values along with the Rayleigh statistics were computed for each sound-evoked spike pattern; only responses having Rayleigh statistics of at least 5.991 were considered as significantly phase-locking [17]. The vector strength value quantifies how well a spike train is synchronized with a periodic stimulus waveform and is computed as follows:

$$\mathrm{VS} = \frac{\sqrt{\left(\sum_{i=1}^{n} \sin\theta_i\right)^2 + \left(\sum_{i=1}^{n} \cos\theta_i\right)^2}}{n}, \quad (2)$$

where n is the number of spikes and θ_i is the phase of each spike, given as

$$\theta_i = 2\pi \frac{t_i \bmod T}{T}, \quad (3)$$

where t_i is the spike time relative to the stimulus onset and T is the period of the modulation frequency (both in milliseconds). The Rayleigh statistics was computed as

$$R = 2n(\mathrm{VS})^2. \quad (4)$$

In addition, the FM tones and click trains were used to determine the similarity of spike trains evoked by the same stimulus. The van Rossum distance [18, 19] was computed for each pair of responses of the same neuron to the same stimulus. The van Rossum distance quantifies the similarity of two spike trains $X(k)$ and $Y(k)$ and is computed as follows: first, each discrete spike train is transformed to continuous function $x(t)$ and $y(t)$, respectively, using convolution of the spike train with exponential function.

$$H(t)\exp\left(-\frac{t}{\tau}\right), \quad (5)$$

where τ is the time constant (set here to 10 ms) and $H(t)$ is the Heaviside step function which is zero for $t < 0$ and one otherwise. Then, the van Rossum distance is computed as

$$D^2 = \frac{1}{\tau}\int_0^{\infty} [x(t) - y(t)]^2 dt. \quad (6)$$

Both vector strength values and van Rossum distances were computed from the complete response (including onset and sustained portions of the evoked response).

2.4. Statistical Analysis. Normality of distributions of the data sets was tested using Shapiro-Wilk test prior to subsequent analyses. Due to the fact that many of the data sets were found to have distribution significantly deviating from normality, two-sided Wilcoxon rank sum tests were computed for comparisons of the medians of two data sets. Chi-square tests were employed to compare the percentual occurrences of certain phenomenon (e.g., percentages of phase-locking neurons). Possible relationship between synchronization index (vector strength) and response magnitude was tested using Spearman's linear correlation coefficient. In all cases, the alpha level was set to 0.05. Statistical analyses were performed using Prism (GraphPad Software Inc., La Jolla, California, USA) and MATLAB (Mathworks Inc., Massachusetts, USA).

3. Results

In our previous work [16], we explored basic neuronal response properties in the animals enriched during early development. In the current study, we did not focus on the direct relationship between an acoustic parameter of interest and its neuronal representation but rather on stability and reproducibility of that representation, which relates to the precision of the code and possibly also to behavioral stimulus-discrimination ability. The first type of neuronal informational code tested was the rate code in which information is carried by the number of discharges during a time window. The stability of the rate code was measured in 2051 units of enriched animals (20 animals, numbers of units: 150, 150, 120, 165, 195, 165, 135, 75, 135, 120, 30, 60, 90, 45, 75, 74, 56, 84, 71, and 56) and 1714 units of control animals (17 animals, numbers of units: 107, 168, 195, 165, 165, 45, 165, 30, 45, 90, 90, 30, 120, 75, 98, 70, and 56), by computing the variances of spike counts for responses evoked by broadband noise pulses. To test the possible level-dependent behavior, the noise stimuli ranged in level from 30 to 70 dB SPL. As the neurons were previously divided to two groups according to monotonicity of their rate-intensity functions [16], the spike count variance was

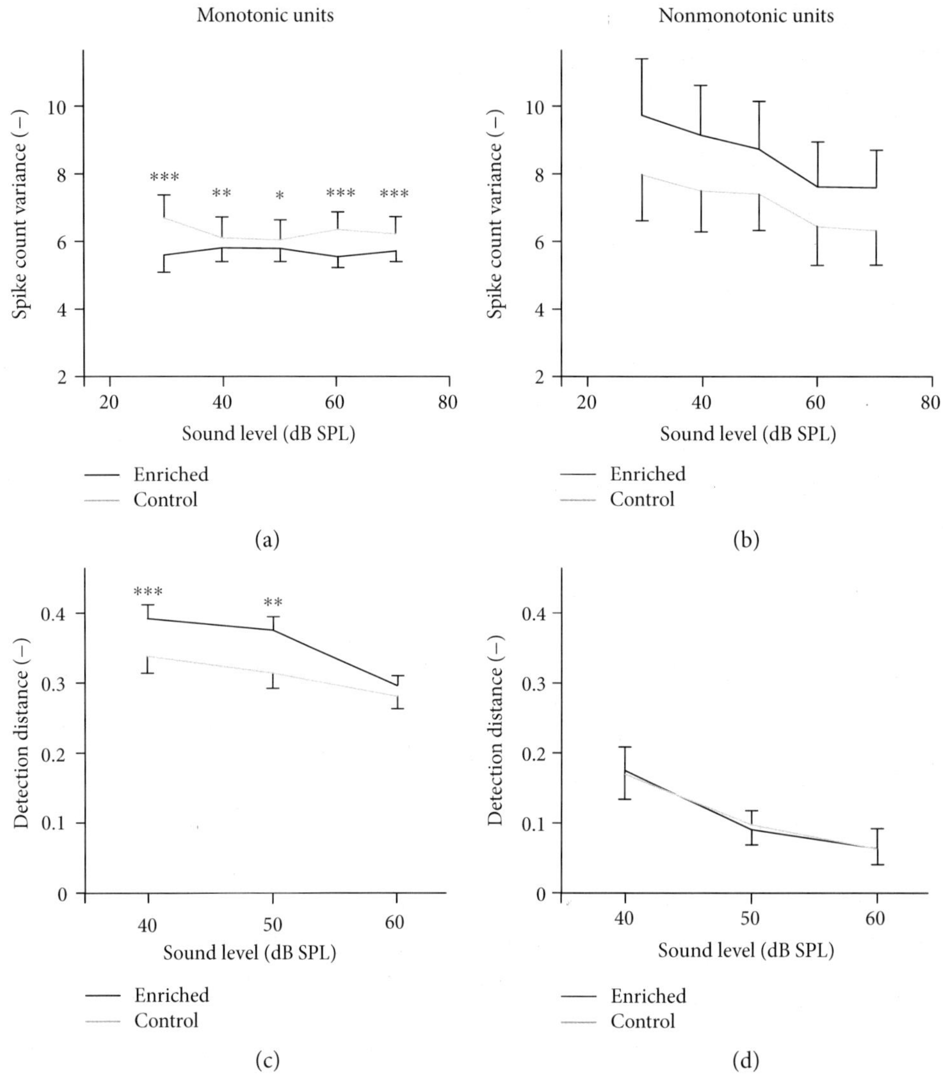

FIGURE 2: Spike count variances computed for noise-evoked responses in monotonic (a) and nonmonotonic (b) units. Detection distances computed for noise-evoked responses in monotonic (c) and nonmonotonic (d) units. The curves represent medians ±95% confidence intervals, and significant differences of individual data pairs are marked with asterisks (Wilcoxon rank sum tests, $^{***}p < 0.001$, $^{**}p < 0.01$, and $^{*}p < 0.05$).

computed separately in these two classes of neurons. As seen in Figure 2, the enriched animals exhibit significantly lower spike count variances in the monotonic neurons, indicating a higher stability of responses at all tested intensities (Wilcoxon rank sum tests, $p < 0.001$ at 30, 60, and 70 dB SPL; $p < 0.01$ at 40 dB SPL; and $p < 0.05$ at 50 dB SPL). In the nonmonotonic units, on the other hand, the spike count variances tend to be higher in the enriched animals; however, the differences are not statistically significant (Wilcoxon rank sum tests, $p > 0.7$ at all intensities).

Signal detection theory [20, 21] states that the smallest detectable change of firing rate depends not only on the spike count variance but also on the differences of firing rates evoked by the two sounds of different intensities. For this reason, we also computed detection distances where possible by combining the current data with the firing rate data from [16]. Figure 2 illustrates that in the monotonic neurons, the detection distances are significantly higher in the enriched animals at 40 and 50 dB SPL (Wilcoxon rank sum tests, $p < 0.001$ at 40 dB SPL; and $p < 0.01$ at 50 dB SPL), while in nonmonotonic neurons, the detection distances do not differ between the animal groups (Wilcoxon rank sum tests, $p > 0.3$ at all intensities).

Synchronization of the responses with temporally varying stimuli was tested first using the amplitude-modulated white noise. In this case, the fine structure of the signal was random and the neurons synchronized only with the envelope. We analyzed 593 units of enriched animals (8 animals, numbers of units: 96, 48, 80, 65, 64, 96, 80, and 64) and 640 units of controls (8 animals, numbers of units: 48, 96, 32, 128, 80, 112, 80, and 64), and only significantly phase-locking responses were considered. Typical responses to amplitude-modulated noise in the enriched and control animals are plotted in Figure 3(b). It is obvious that the neuron

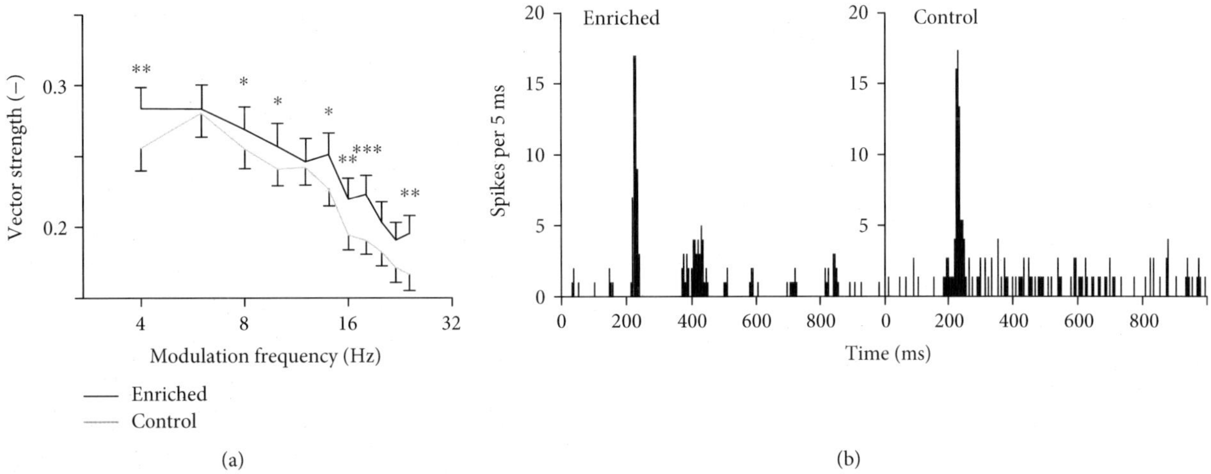

FIGURE 3: Synchronization of units with amplitude modulated noise. (a) Vector strength computed for responses to AM noise. The curves represent medians ±95% confidence intervals, and significant differences of individual data pairs are marked with asterisks (Wilcoxon rank sum tests, $^{***}p < 0.001$, $^{**}p < 0.01$, and $^{*}p < 0.05$). (b) Typical responses of neurons from enriched and control animals to AM noise with 10 Hz modulation frequency (peristimulus time histograms).

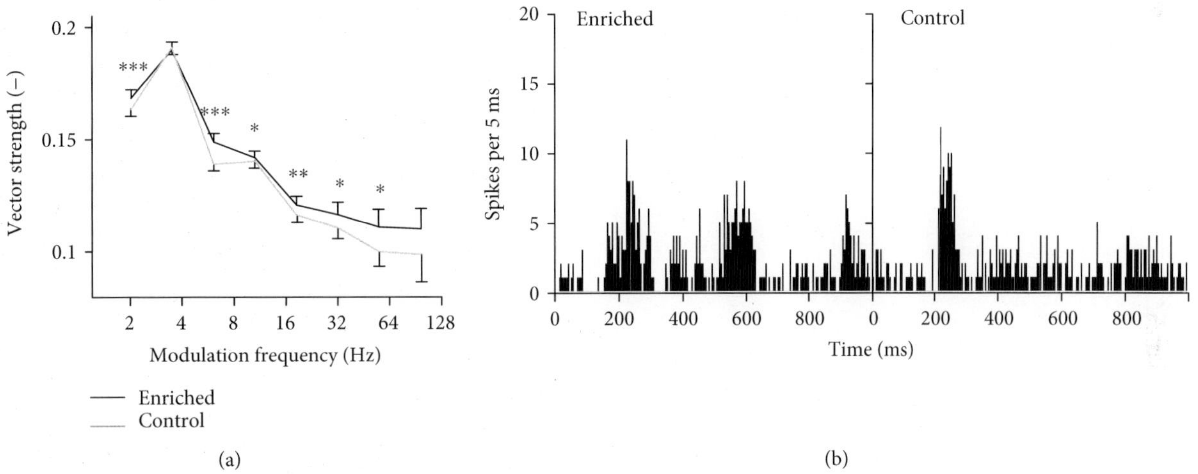

FIGURE 4: Synchronization of units with frequency modulated tones. (a) Vector strength computed for responses to FM tones. The curves represent medians ±95% confidence intervals, and significant differences of individual data pairs are marked with asterisks (Wilcoxon rank sum tests, $^{***}p < 0.001$, $^{**}p < 0.01$, and $^{*}p < 0.05$). (b) Typical responses of neurons from enriched and control animals to FM tones with 10 Hz modulation frequency (peristimulus time histograms).

from the enriched animal responds with better synchronization than the control neuron. The dependence of vector strength (VS) values on the modulation frequency is plotted in Figure 3(a). The vector strength quantifies how well the individual spikes are synchronized (phase-locked) with a periodic signal. The enriched animals exhibit a significantly higher degree of synchronization at most modulation frequencies (Wilcoxon rank sum tests, significant differences occur at 4, 8, 10, 14, 16, 18, and 24 Hz). The percentages of phase-locking neurons given by the Rayleigh statistics are not significantly different in the two experimental groups (enriched: 76.4%; control: 75.3%; chi-squared test, $p > 0.05$); however, when quantifying the percentage of units with VS values higher than 0.3, the enriched animals show significantly higher values (enriched: 28%; control: 22%; chi-squared test, $p < 0.001$).

Neurons can respond to temporal modulation either by changes in their firing rate or by phase-locking to the temporal structure. To see whether the neurons with good synchronization also show changes in firing rate, we correlated the vector strength values with the firing rate in individual neurons. The results indicate that the phase-locking and changes in firing rate are largely independent, as the correlation coefficients were −0.35 in the enriched rats and −0.26 in the controls, respectively.

Next, synchronization with a deterministic and stationary stimulus was measured using frequency-modulated tones in 288 units of enriched animals (6 animals, numbers of units: 48, 52, 45, 47, 52, and 44) and 259 units of controls (6 animals, numbers of units: 25, 50, 38, 42, 44, and 60). Typical neuronal responses to frequency-modulated tones are depicted in Figure 4(b). Despite that the modulation

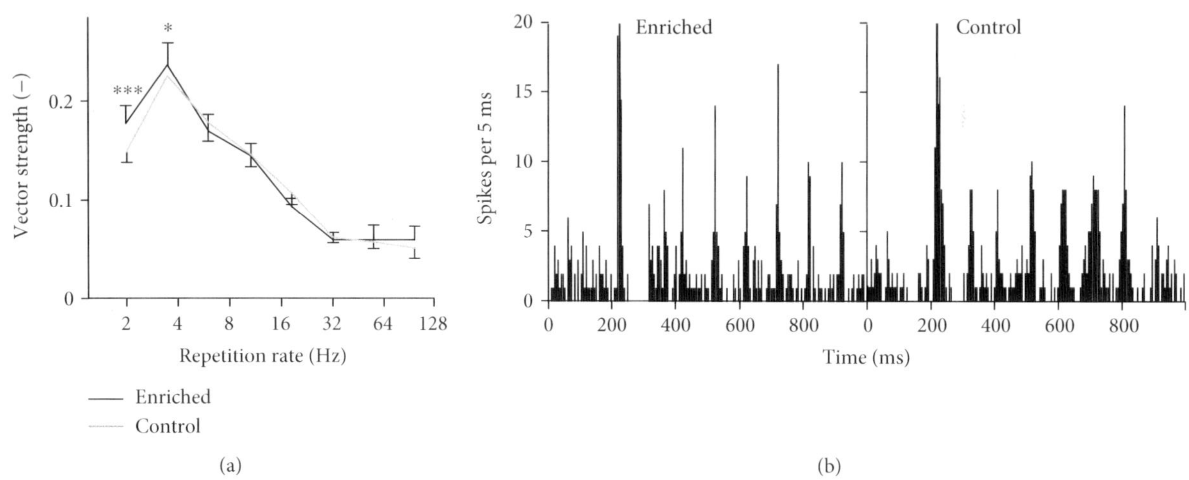

FIGURE 5: Synchronization of units with click trains. (a) Vector strength computed for responses to click trains. The curves represent medians ±95% confidence intervals, and significant differences of individual data pairs are marked with asterisks (Wilcoxon rank sum tests, $^{***}p < 0.001$, and $^{*}p < 0.05$). (b) Typical responses of neurons from enriched and control animals to click trains with 10 Hz repetition rate (peristimulus time histograms).

period was 100 ms, the periodicity of the peristimulus time histogram indicates that the enriched neuron reacts to every second or fourth period, while the control neuron responds rather with a sustained activity. The dependence of VS values of significantly phase-locking responses on the modulation frequency is shown in Figure 4(a). As in the case of the amplitude-modulated noise, the enriched animals exhibit significantly higher VS values at most modulation frequencies (Wilcoxon rank sum tests, significant differences occur at all frequencies except 4 and 100 Hz). The percentages of phase-locking neurons are not significantly different in the two experimental groups (enriched: 42.5%; control: 42.1%; chi-squared test, $p > 0.05$); however, the percentage of units with VS values above 0.3 is higher in the enriched animals (enriched: 6%; control: 3%; chi-squared test, $p < 0.001$). As with the amplitude-modulated noise, we tried to correlate the vector strength values with the firing rate. This time the correlation is even weaker (correlation coefficients: −0.15 in the enriched rats and −0.08 in the controls, resp.); the phase-locking and changes in firing rate can be thus considered as independent for the frequency modulation.

Finally, phase-locking ability to a series of clicks with different repetition rates was tested in 290 units of enriched animals (6 animals, numbers of units: 48, 56, 46, 44, 51, and 45) and 255 units of controls (6 animals, numbers of units: 25, 50, 38, 40, 42, and 60). Typical neuronal responses to click trains are depicted in Figure 5(b). Apparently, for this type of stimulus, the neurons of both groups of animals have a similar phase-locking ability: enriched animals show higher VS values only at low repetition rates, see Figure 5(a) (Wilcoxon rank sum tests, $p < 0.001$ at 2 Hz and $p < 0.05$ at 4 Hz). The percentages of phase-locking neurons are not significantly different in the two experimental groups (enriched: 66.6%; control: 67.8%; chi-squared test, $p > 0.05$); however, the percentage of units with VS values above 0.3 is higher in the enriched animals (enriched: 12%; control: 9%; chi-squared test, $p < 0.01$). The correlation of vector strength values and firing rates is again very low (correlation coefficients: 0.16 in the enriched rats and 0.19 in the controls, resp.); the phase-locking and changes in firing rate can be thus considered as independent.

The vector strength measure evaluates the position of each spike within the period of the signal. Simply put, to achieve high VS, most spikes have to lie near a specific phase of the periodic signal. The VS thus indicates the ability of the neuron to capture the periodicity of the signal. However, it means neither that a spike has to appear in every signal period nor that the response patterns as a whole have to be similar. In order to see whether the individual neurons give response patterns that are similar to each other, we computed the van Rossum distances of different responses to the same stimulus. As the noise-based stimuli are inherently random, we used the deterministic frequency-modulated tones and click trains. For both types of stimuli, the van Rossum distances were nearly independent on the modulation frequency or repetition rate, as seen in Figure 6. Clearly, the enriched animals express a higher degree of similarity of responses across multiple stimulus repetitions both for the FM tones (Wilcoxon rank sum tests, $p < 0.001$ at all modulation frequencies) and for the series of clicks (Wilcoxon rank sum tests, $p < 0.05$ at 18, 32, and 55 Hz repetition rates, $p < 0.01$ elsewhere).

4. Discussion

The current study adds another piece to the mosaic of knowledge about environmental effects during hearing development. It is known from previous studies that maturation of the central auditory system is shaped by input to the developing nuclei. The sound-evoked activity controls the refinements of the structure of neuronal network [22–25], which in turn results in functional refinements and maturation of neuronal responsiveness and representation of the stimulus [4, 6, 9, 26]; hence, altering the input will also alter the

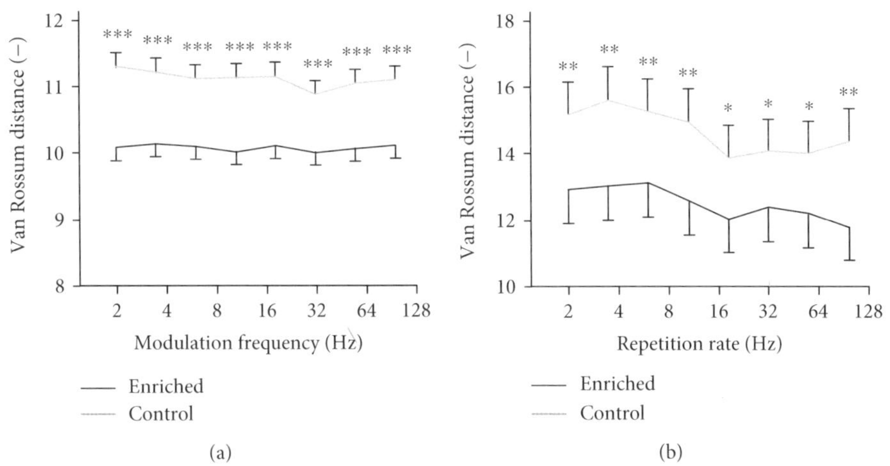

FIGURE 6: van Rossum distances of responses to a repetitive stimulus computed for responses to frequency-modulated tones (a) and click trains (b). The curves represent medians ±95% confidence intervals, and significant differences of individual data pairs are marked with asterisks (Wilcoxon rank sum tests, $^{***}p < 0.001$, $^{**}p < 0.01$, and $^{*}p < 0.05$).

development of the system. Despite considerable uncertainty as to what effect a specific stimulation will have, it appears that the resulting state of the system relates to spectral and temporal characteristics of the acoustic input. Studies that used a simple and basic stimulus often report an expanded representation of that stimulus in the AC [3, 4], while a complex environment may lead to nonspecific changes spanning the entire hearing range [6, 11, 16, 27]. The issue is mostly explored by evaluation of the neuronal receptive fields and tonotopical arrangement—a description of the system based on averaging multiple responses over time. Here, we show that besides modifications of integrated receptive fields, environmental conditions also affect the detailed structure of the spiking patterns.

Most of the works investigating developmental plasticity exposed the animals during a period starting shortly before the onset of hearing (often on P7 or P9) and lasting for two to four weeks [3, 4, 7, 12, 13, 28, 29]. The period between P11 and P13 is often stressed out as the most important period for the development of AC, and in particular, for tonotopy. However, numerous works showed that also exposure which starts markedly later (e.g., on P21) profoundly influences development of the auditory system [11, 30–34]. Our recent works have focused on the period after P14 in which the basic tonotopical arrangement is mostly final and the sensory experience shapes other properties of the auditory system: sensitivity, frequency selectivity, sound level coding, or morphology of AC neurons [6, 8, 10, 22, 35–37]. Previous studies reported that the sensitive phase of postnatal development (the so-called critical period) is not homogenous and uniform but rather that it may be divided in a series of distinct time windows during which different features of the auditory system develop consecutively [2, 38, 39]. From this viewpoint, the sound exposure used in most of the works on developmental plasticity covers several phases of the critical period. Hence, it is not currently possible to clearly identify which phase of the critical period is responsible for maturation of the spiking patterns, as reported in the current study.

In our experiments, we are interested in global changes that would not be stimulus specific but rather influence general response characteristics of auditory neurons. To accomplish this, we have developed a scenario in which the neuronal responses are mostly measured using different stimuli than those contained in the acoustic-enriching environment. This approach makes the results independent on the chosen enriching environment and makes them more comparable to other studies. In our previous studies on the inferior colliculus [6] and auditory cortex [16], we showed that developmentally enriched animals exhibited permanent changes of neuronal responsiveness; in particular, the neurons of the enriched animals were on average more sensitive (lower excitatory thresholds), more frequency selective (higher quality factor), and less nonmonotonic with respect to intensity coding (lower percentage of nonmonotonic rate-level functions). The changes were present across the entire range of tonotopical sites and were not directly linked to the properties of the acoustical stimulation. Extending and confirming these data, the current results show that an acoustical enrichment during the sensitive phase of postnatal development also influences the stability and precision of the rate code and the accuracy and reproducibility of the temporal code in the auditory cortex neurons. Importantly, the effect can still be seen in adult animals; that is, the developmental intervention introduces long-lasting consequences rather than temporary alterations which disappear shortly after the return of the organism to standard conditions.

Our experimental paradigm involves active discrimination of randomly occurring acoustic stimuli embedded in a complex modulated background noise. Previous studies show that the effects of a given acoustic stimulation may be different depending on the attention of the subjects [6, 14, 40]. Our idea was to attract the animals' attention to the acoustic environment and to motivate them to listen to it. It is conceivable that the outcomes presented in the current study are a consequence of a combination of the acoustic stimulation and the active behavioral task.

As a first outcome, we presented the improved stability of the rate-based stimulus representation. The principle of the rate code lies in representation of quantity (sound level in our case) by the number of neuronal discharges, or, when normalized by time, the spike-rate. Due to the inherent randomness and variability of neuronal firing, the evoked spike count is different for each stimulus presentation; the information on sound level is thus encoded in a mean spike count averaged over several stimulus repetitions. Stimuli of different sound levels will result in different evoked spike counts; however, for the difference to be detectable, it must be large enough not to be masked by the spiking variability [21, 41]. In the enriched animals, reduced spike count variances were observed, which suggests an improved discrimination ability of sound level changes. On the other hand, the neurons in the enriched animals may have lower evoked spike counts at the same time [16]. With regard to level discrimination ability, these two facts operate in opposite directions; thus to better quantify the level discrimination ability, detection distance (sometimes also called sensitivity index) was computed. We found that detection distances were larger in the enriched animals. According to signal detection theory [20, 21], this fact corresponds to lower theoretical just-noticeable differences of sound level, that is, better level discrimination ability. Nevertheless, to determine the influence on subjective perception of sound, an additional behavioral experiment would be necessary. Interestingly, the described changes occurred only in neurons with monotonic rate-intensity functions; detection distances of nonmonotonic neurons did not differ significantly between enriched and control animals. This indicates that monotonic and nonmonotonic neurons might play different roles with respect to sound level coding.

Information carried by the firing rate is usually based on integration (or averaging) across the interval of around 100 ms long [42, 43], thus discarding the information on events occurring at shorter time scales. Unlike the rate-based code, temporal coding employs precise positioning of individual spikes in time [44], which may potentially carry larger information content than the rate code, and furthermore, the information is conveyed almost immediately [45]. Considering also the neuronal populations, if a group of neurons projecting to another neuron produces spike patterns that are well-aligned in time, the higher synchrony will improve the detection of the signal. We studied the temporal acuity using two measures: the vector strength quantifying the synchronization of spikes with sound period and the van Rossum distance quantifying the similarity of individual-evoked patterns.

The neurons in the enriched animals exhibited an improved synchronization with temporally structured stimuli—amplitude-modulated noise, frequency-modulated tones, and click trains. The observed higher vector strength values indicate that the evoked spikes are positioned more precisely within the period of the signal modulation (in the case of amplitude-modulated noise and frequency-modulated tones) or repetition (in the case of click trains). The dependence of vector strength on the modulation frequency or repetition rate is similar in both animal groups and has the character of a shallow bandpass filter. In the case of the amplitude-modulated noise, the modulation VS function peaks around 6 Hz while for the FM tones and click trains, the peak lies slightly lower, around 4 Hz. These values are somewhat lower than those observed by Chang et al. [26] and Zhou and Merzenich [17], around 10 to 12 Hz; the difference is probably due to different measuring stimuli (noise or tone pulses) and different time of exposure. The proportion of significantly phase-locking neurons is not different in the two groups; however, the percentage of neurons with high VS values is significantly higher in the enriched rats. Taken together, the AEE used in the current study did not change the overall VS tuning properties of AC neurons; it instead increased the temporal acuity of the responses. This fact suggests that the enriched animals might have a better ability to detect and discriminate temporally varying stimuli; furthermore, the regularity of firing patterns may influence neural computations [46]. In our previous study [16], we showed that the enriched animals exhibited also different shapes or shifts of modulation-transfer functions, which again shows that both rate and temporal codes were affected by the enrichment.

Both the number of evoked potentials and the vector strength represent measures that are based on summation and averaging or pooling over time; hence, they provide limited information on the temporal spiking patterns. Yet, the reproducibility and self-consistency of firing patterns as a response to a given stimulus may play an important role in stimulus detection and discrimination tasks, particularly in complicated listening conditions such as a noisy environment. The smaller van Rossum distances of firing patterns to a repetitive stimulus in the enriched group indicate that the individual neuronal responses are more similar to each other, thus encoding more precisely or reliably the respective stimulus. This fact may relate to the experimental paradigm in which the enriched animals were motivated to discriminate several similar stimuli to obtain a reward. Smaller van Rossum distances after an acoustic training have also been observed by Cheng et al. [19].

While the developmental alterations of neuronal receptive fields after enrichment as reported, for example, in Bureš et al. [6, 16], can be explained by influencing the formation of detailed topographic maps and neuronal projections, such structural changes are probably not completely responsible for the changes of reliability and precision of spiking patterns. Partly, the changes in discharge characteristics can be influenced by an altered function of inhibitory circuits, which may develop after neonatal sound exposure [8, 10, 29, 47]. However, the observed improvements most likely result from changes at the subcellular and synaptic level. Tao et al. [48] reported that amplitude and timing of events at the synaptic input highly influence the generation and timing of output spikes in the auditory cortex. According to Rodriguez-Molina and Aertsen [49], timing and reliability of firing patterns depend on the synaptic potential kinetics, temporal jitter of excitatory inputs, and background synaptic noise. Zhou et al. [50] found that the temporal diversity of responses in the dorsal cochlear nucleus is dependent on the properties of the excitatory and inhibitory inputs and excitatory/inhibitory balance. It thus appears that the environmental conditions during the critical period of development also influence the properties of the synaptic transmission. As learning, training, and attention were shown to affect neural synchrony [19, 51] and modulate neural coding of attended stimuli [52], the stimulus discrimination task which was included in the enriching environment of the current study probably also contributed to the presented results.

5. Conclusions

Reliability and precision of neuronal firing is a key aspect determining the ability to detect and/or discriminate acoustic signals. Here, we have shown that this aspect is influenced by the acoustic environment that encompasses the organism during its postnatal development. An enriched environment presented shortly after the onset of hearing has the power to improve the stability of evoked cortical responses and to lower the variance of spike rates in response to a repetitive stimulus. Furthermore, the temporal acuity of individual spikes expressed by synchronization and similarity indexes (vector strength and van Rossum distance, resp.) was significantly amended compared to the control animals. The changes were retained to adulthood, suggesting that they had their origin in developmental processes, presumably shaping the properties of excitatory and inhibitory synaptic transmission. As neuronal synchrony and ability to capture the temporal changes of an acoustic stimulus are important prerequisites of speech understanding, particularly in demanding listening conditions, the results of this study again emphasize the importance of a rich and stimulating acoustic environment during hearing development.

Abbreviations

AC: Auditory cortex
AEE: Acoustically enriched environment
AM: Amplitude-modulated
CP: Critical period
FM: Frequency-modulated
IC: Inferior colliculus
SPL: Sound pressure level
VS: Vector strength.

Conflicts of Interest

The authors declare that there is no conflict of interest regarding the publication of this article.

Authors' Contributions

Josef Syka, Zbyněk Bureš, and Jiří Lindovský designed the study. Kateryna Pysanenko and Jiří Lindovský performed the experiments. Kateryna Pysanenko, Jiří Lindovský, and Zbyněk Bureš performed the data processing and statistical analysis. Zbyněk Bureš and Kateryna Pysanenko interpreted the data and wrote the manuscript. Zbyněk Bureš and Josef Syka performed the experiment guidance and manuscript supervision.

Acknowledgments

This work was supported by the Grantová Agentura České Republiky (Grant no. P304/12/G069).

References

[1] N. Rybalko and J. Syka, "Susceptibility to noise exposure during postnatal development in rats," *Hearing Research*, vol. 155, no. 1-2, pp. 32–40, 2001.

[2] M. N. Insanally, H. Kover, H. Kim, and S. Bao, "Feature-dependent sensitive periods in the development of complex sound representation," *Journal of Neuroscience*, vol. 29, no. 17, pp. 5456–5462, 2009.

[3] E. de Villers-Sidani, E. F. Chang, S. Bao, and M. M. Merzenich, "Critical period window for spectral tuning defined in the primary auditory cortex (A1) in the rat," *Journal of Neuroscience*, vol. 27, no. 1, pp. 180–189, 2007.

[4] L. I. Zhang, S. Bao, and M. M. Merzenich, "Persistent and specific influences of early acoustic environments on primary auditory cortex," *Nature Neuroscience*, vol. 4, no. 11, pp. 1123–1130, 2001.

[5] X. Zhou, N. Nagarajan, B. J. Mossop, and M. M. Merzenich, "Influences of un-modulated acoustic inputs on functional maturation and critical-period plasticity of the primary auditory cortex," *Neuroscience*, vol. 154, no. 1, pp. 390–396, 2008.

[6] Z. Bureš, J. Bartošová, J. Lindovský, T. Chumak, J. Popelář, and J. Syka, "Acoustical enrichment during early postnatal development changes response properties of inferior colliculus neurons in rats," *European Journal of Neuroscience*, vol. 40, no. 11, pp. 3674–3683, 2014.

[7] E. Chang and M. Merzenich, "Environmental noise retards auditory cortical development," *Science*, vol. 300, no. 5618, pp. 498–502, 2003.

[8] Z. Bureš, J. Grécová, J. Popelář, and J. Syka, "Noise exposure during early development impairs the processing of sound intensity in adult rats," *European Journal of Neuroscience*, vol. 32, no. 1, pp. 155–164, 2010.

[9] Z. Bureš, J. Popelář, and J. Syka, "The effect of noise exposure during the developmental period on the function of the auditory system," *Hearing Research*, vol. 352, pp. 1–11, 2017.

[10] J. Grécová, Z. Bureš, J. Popelář, D. Šuta, and J. Syka, "Brief exposure of juvenile rats to noise impairs the development of the response properties of inferior colliculus neurons," *European Journal of Neuroscience*, vol. 29, no. 9, pp. 1921–1930, 2009.

[11] N. D. Engineer, C. R. Percaccio, P. K. Pandya, R. Moucha, D. L. Rathbun, and M. P. Kilgard, "Environmental enrichment improves response strength, threshold, selectivity, and latency of auditory cortex neurons," *Journal of Neurophysiology*, vol. 92, no. 1, pp. 73–82, 2004.

[12] D. L. Oliver, M. A. Izquierdo, and M. S. Malmierca, "Persistent effects of early augmented acoustic environment on the auditory brainstem," *Neuroscience*, vol. 184, pp. 75–87, 2011.

[13] A. Miyakawa, R. Gibboni, and S. Bao, "Repeated exposure to a tone transiently alters spectral tuning bandwidth of neurons in the central nucleus of inferior colliculus in juvenile rats," *Neuroscience*, vol. 230, pp. 114–120, 2013.

[14] D. Polley, E. Steinberg, and M. Merzenich, "Perceptual learning directs auditory cortical map reorganization through top-down influences," *Journal of Neuroscience*, vol. 26, no. 18, pp. 4970–4982, 2006.

[15] C. R. Percaccio, A. L. Pruette, S. T. Mistry, Y. H. Chen, and M. P. Kilgard, "Sensory experience determines enrichment-induced plasticity in rat auditory cortex," *Brain Research*, vol. 1174, pp. 76–91, 2007.

[16] K. Pysanenko, Z. Bureš, J. Lindovský, and J. Syka, "The effect of complex acoustic environment during early development on the responses of auditory cortex neurons in rats," *Neuroscience*, vol. 371, pp. 221–228, 2018.

[17] X. Zhou and M. M. Merzenich, "Enduring effects of early structured noise exposure on temporal modulation in the primary auditory cortex," *Proceedings of the National Academy of Sciences*, vol. 105, no. 11, pp. 4423–4428, 2008.

[18] M. C. W. van Rossum, "A novel spike distance," *Neural Computation*, vol. 13, no. 4, pp. 751–763, 2001.

[19] Y. Cheng, G. Jia, Y. Zhang et al., "Positive impacts of early auditory training on cortical processing at an older age," *Proceedings of the National Academy of Sciences of the United States of America*, vol. 114, no. 24, pp. 6364–6369, 2017.

[20] D. M. Green and J. A. Swets, *Signal Detection Theory and Psychophysics*, Wiley, New York, 1966.

[21] H. Steven Colburn, L. H. Carney, and M. G. Heinz, "Quantifying the information in auditory-nerve responses for level discrimination," *Journal of the Association for Research in Otolaryngology*, vol. 4, no. 3, pp. 294–311, 2003.

[22] L. Ouda, J. Burianová, Z. Balogová, H. P. Lu, and J. Syka, "Structural changes in the adult rat auditory system induced by brief postnatal noise exposure," *Brain Structure and Function*, vol. 221, no. 1, pp. 617–629, 2016.

[23] K. Kandler and D. C. Gillespie, "Developmental refinement of inhibitory sound-localization circuits," *Trends in Neurosciences*, vol. 28, no. 6, pp. 290–296, 2005.

[24] D. H. Sanes and C. Takács, "Activity-dependent refinement of inhibitory connections," *European Journal of Neuroscience*, vol. 5, no. 6, pp. 570–574, 1993.

[25] H. P. Lu, J. Syka, T. W. Chiu, and P. W. F. Poon, "Prolonged sound exposure has different effects on increasing neuronal size in the auditory cortex and brainstem," *Hearing Research*, vol. 314, pp. 42–50, 2014.

[26] E. F. Chang, S. Bao, K. Imaizumi, C. E. Schreiner, and M. M. Merzenich, "Development of spectral and temporal response selectivity in the auditory cortex," *Proceedings of the National Academy of Sciences*, vol. 102, no. 45, pp. 16460–16465, 2005.

[27] C. Jiang, X. Xu, L. Yu, J. Xu, and J. Zhang, "Environmental enrichment rescues the degraded auditory temporal resolution of cortical neurons induced by early noise exposure," *European Journal of Neuroscience*, vol. 42, no. 5, pp. 2144–2154, 2015.

[28] E. de Villers-Sidani, K. L. Simpson, Y.-F. Lu, R. C. S. Lin, and M. M. Merzenich, "Manipulating critical period closure across different sectors of the primary auditory cortex," *Nature Neuroscience*, vol. 11, no. 8, pp. 957–965, 2008.

[29] A. L. Dorrn, K. Yuan, A. J. Barker, C. E. Schreiner, and R. C. Froemke, "Developmental sensory experience balances cortical excitation and inhibition," *Nature*, vol. 465, no. 7300, pp. 932–936, 2010.

[30] C. R. Percaccio, N. D. Engineer, A. L. Pruette et al., "Environmental enrichment increases paired-pulse depression in rat auditory cortex," *Journal of Neurophysiology*, vol. 94, no. 5, pp. 3590–3600, 2005.

[31] M. Bose, P. Muñoz-llancao, S. Roychowdhury et al., "Effect of the environment on the dendritic morphology of the rat auditory cortex," *Synapse*, vol. 64, no. 2, pp. 97–110, 2010.

[32] J. Xu, L. Yu, R. Cai, J. Zhang, and X. Sun, "Early auditory enrichment with music enhances auditory discrimination learning and alters NR2B protein expression in rat auditory cortex," *Behavioural Brain Research*, vol. 196, no. 1, pp. 49–54, 2009.

[33] J. García-Estrada, Y. Ruvalcaba-Delgadillo, S. Luquín et al., "Early-life exposure to noise reduces mPFC astrocyte numbers and T-maze alternation/discrimination task performance in adult male rats," *Noise & Health*, vol. 17, no. 77, pp. 216–226, 2015.

[34] J. A. Nichols, V. P. Jakkamsetti, H. Salgado, L. Dinh, M. P. Kilgard, and M. Atzori, "Environmental enrichment selectively increases glutamatergic responses in layer II/III of the auditory cortex of the rat," *Neuroscience*, vol. 145, no. 3, pp. 832–840, 2007.

[35] N. Rybalko, Z. Bureš, J. Burianová, J. Popelář, J. Grécová, and J. Syka, "Noise exposure during early development influences the acoustic startle reflex in adult rats," *Physiology & Behavior*, vol. 102, no. 5, pp. 453–458, 2011.

[36] N. Rybalko, T. Chumak, Z. Bureš, J. Popelář, D. Šuta, and J. Syka, "Development of the acoustic startle response in rats and its change after early acoustic trauma," *Behavioural Brain Research*, vol. 286, pp. 212–221, 2015.

[37] D. Šuta, N. Rybalko, D.-W. Shen, J. Popelář, P. W. F. Poon, and J. Syka, "Frequency discrimination in rats exposed to noise as juveniles," *Physiology & Behavior*, vol. 144, pp. 60–65, 2015.

[38] M. N. Insanally, B. F. Albanna, and S. Bao, "Pulsed noise experience disrupts complex sound representations," *Journal of Neurophysiology*, vol. 103, no. 5, pp. 2611–2617, 2010.

[39] D. B. Polley, J. H. Thompson, and W. Guo, "Brief hearing loss disrupts binaural integration during two early critical periods of auditory cortex development," *Nature Communications*, vol. 4, 2013.

[40] J. Fritz, S. Shamma, M. Elhilali, and D. Klein, "Rapid task-related plasticity of spectrotemporal receptive fields in primary auditory cortex," *Nature Neuroscience*, vol. 6, no. 11, pp. 1216–1223, 2003.

[41] R. A. Silver, "Neuronal arithmetic," *Nature Reviews Neuroscience*, vol. 11, no. 7, pp. 474–489, 2010.

[42] H. Fastl and E. Zwicker, *Psychoacoustics: Facts and Models*, Springer, Berlin Heidelberg, 2007.

[43] Z. Bureš and P. Maršálek, "On the precision of neural computation with interaural level differences in the lateral superior olive," *Brain Research*, vol. 1536, pp. 16–26, 2013.

[44] P. Cariani, "Temporal coding of periodicity pitch in the auditory system: an overview," *Neural Plasticity*, vol. 6, no. 4, pp. 147–172, 1999.

[45] P. Tiesinga, J.-M. Fellous, and T. J. Sejnowski, "Regulation of spike timing in visual cortical circuits," *Nature Reviews Neuroscience*, vol. 9, no. 2, pp. 97–107, 2008.

[46] Z. Bureš, "The stochastic properties of input spike trains control neuronal arithmetic," *Biological Cybernetics*, vol. 106, no. 2, pp. 111–122, 2012.

[47] A. E. Takesian, V. C. Kotak, and D. H. Sanes, "Age-dependent effect of hearing loss on cortical inhibitory synapse function," *Journal of Neurophysiology*, vol. 107, no. 3, pp. 937–947, 2012.

[48] C. Tao, G. Zhang, C. Zhou et al., "Synaptic basis for the generation of response variation in auditory cortex," *Scientific Reports*, vol. 6, no. 1, article 31024, 2016.

[49] V. M. Rodriguez-Molina, A. Aertsen, and D. H. Heck, "Spike timing and reliability in cortical pyramidal neurons: effects of EPSC kinetics, input synchronization and background noise on spike timing," *PLoS One*, vol. 2, no. 3, article e319, 2007.

[50] M. Zhou, Y.-T. Li, W. Yuan, H. W. Tao, and L. I. Zhang, "Synaptic mechanisms for generating temporal diversity of auditory representation in the dorsal cochlear nucleus," *Journal of Neurophysiology*, vol. 113, no. 5, pp. 1358–1368, 2015.

[51] R. Yokota, K. Aihara, R. Kanzaki, and H. Takahashi, "Learning-stage-dependent plasticity of temporal coherence in the auditory cortex of rats," *Brain Topography*, vol. 28, no. 3, pp. 401–410, 2015.

[52] I. P. Jaaskelainen and J. Ahveninen, "Auditory-cortex short-term plasticity induced by selective attention," *Neural Plasticity*, vol. 2014, Article ID 216731, 11 pages, 2014.

6

Progress in Gene Therapy to Prevent Retinal Ganglion Cell Loss in Glaucoma and Leber's Hereditary Optic Neuropathy

Sara E. Ratican,[1,2] Andrew Osborne,[1] and Keith R. Martin[1,3,4,5]

[1]*John van Geest Centre for Brain Repair, Department of Clinical Neurosciences, University of Cambridge, Cambridge, UK*
[2]*Geisel School of Medicine, Dartmouth College, Hanover, NH, USA*
[3]*Eye Department, Addenbrooke's Hospital, Cambridge, UK*
[4]*Cambridge NIHR Biomedical Research Centre, Cambridge, UK*
[5]*Wellcome Trust-MRC Cambridge Stem Cell Institute, University of Cambridge, Cambridge, UK*

Correspondence should be addressed to Keith R. Martin; krgm2@cam.ac.uk

Academic Editor: Joost Verhaagen

The eye is at the forefront of the application of gene therapy techniques to medicine. In the United States, a gene therapy treatment for Leber's congenital amaurosis, a rare inherited retinal disease, recently became the first gene therapy to be approved by the FDA for the treatment of disease caused by mutations in a specific gene. Phase III clinical trials of gene therapy for other single-gene defect diseases of the retina and optic nerve are also currently underway. However, for optic nerve diseases not caused by single-gene defects, gene therapy strategies are likely to focus on slowing or preventing neuronal death through the expression of neuroprotective agents. In addition to these strategies, there has also been recent interest in the potential use of precise genome editing techniques to treat ocular disease. This review focuses on recent developments in gene therapy techniques for the treatment of glaucoma and Leber's hereditary optic neuropathy (LHON). We discuss recent successes in clinical trials for the treatment of LHON using gene supplementation therapy, promising neuroprotective strategies that have been employed in animal models of glaucoma and the potential use of genome editing techniques in treating optic nerve disease.

1. Introduction

In the last two decades, human gene therapy has advanced significantly. As our understanding of optic nerve disease pathologies has improved, the eye has become a particularly appealing clinical target for gene therapy and genome editing studies. The eye as a model organ for testing gene therapies has always been attractive. Firstly, the eye is largely immune privileged [1, 2] and vectors delivered to the eye are relatively isolated from the rest of the body. The size and ease of access to the eye is also favourable allowing small volumes of drug to be precisely delivered. Furthermore, testing the effectiveness of treatments via both electrophysiological and psychophysical testing is well-established, quick, and reliable [3]. Both Leber's hereditary optic neuropathy (LHON) and glaucoma are diseases resulting in permanent, irreversible loss of vision. With an undeniable need to treat and manage these diseases with novel therapeutic approaches, gene therapy may hold significant benefits in the coming years [4].

A prerequisite for a successful gene therapy in the eye is a vector system that leads to long, sustained levels of therapeutic gene expression within a select target cell with minimal side effects [5, 6]. This is particularly important for chronic, long-term pathologies such as glaucoma. Of the various non-viral and viral vector systems that have been used for retinal gene therapy (i.e., adenovirus, lentivirus, and nanoparticles), recombinant adeno-associated viral vectors (AAVs) have proven the most promising. Hundreds of clinical trials have been performed using AAV vectors spanning back 25 years [7] with 25 trials currently registered to test AAVs in retinal diseases (http://clinicaltrials.gov).

AAVs are composed of a 4.7 kb single-stranded genome packaged within a nonenveloped icosahedral capsid. After removal of 4.4 kb of the viral genome, vectors can be packaged with a similar-sized foreign piece of DNA that

TABLE 1: Promoters typically chosen for transduction of retinal ganglion cells (RGCs) within the eye.

Promoter	Specificity for RGCs	Strength of expression in RGCs	Off-target labelling	Size (bp) % of AAV cargo	References
CMV	+	+++	Muller glia Amacrine cells Bipolar cells	(508–800) *(10–17%)*	[10–14]
CAG	+	++++	Muller glia Amacrine cells Bipolar cells	(584–1132) *(12–24%)*	[15–17]
SYN1	+++	++	Amacrine cells	(400–469) *(8–10%)*	[20, 21]
Nefh	++++	+++		(2251) *(48%)*	[22]
Thy1	++++	++		(6500) (exceeds limit)	[23]
Mcp-1	++	+++	injured cells	560 (mouse only) *(12%)*	[24]

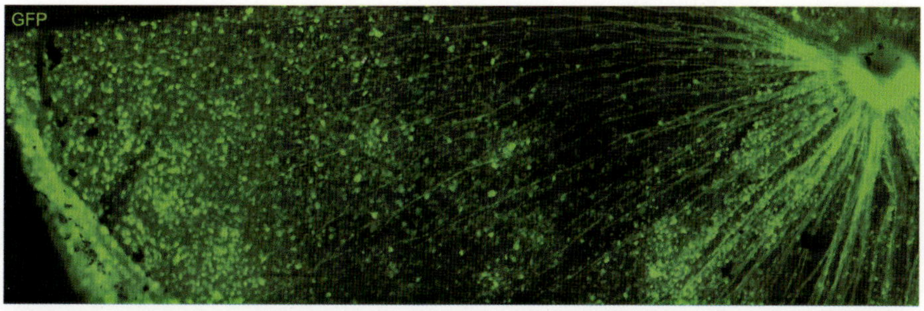

FIGURE 1: GFP expression throughout the mouse retina three weeks after intravitreal injection of AAV2-CAG GFP. Image courtesy of Dr. Andrew Osborne and Dr. Tasneem Khatib.

can be adjusted and optimized to improve cell-specific targeting and transgene expression via a series of cassette elements [8]. Various AAV serotypes exist whereby the vector capsid determines tissue specificity, with AAV2 regarded as the most efficient serotype for RGC transduction [9, 10]. In particular, vectors possessing an AAV2 backbone, cross packed into capsids from another serotype such as AAV2/2 and AAV2/6, have been shown to have the highest transduction efficiency in the retina [9]. AAV2/2 has been shown to transduce RGC more than any other cell type, while AAV2/6 displays the most diverse tropism profile, transducing Müller glia and many neuronal cell types [9].

Promoter choice is also important for cell-specific expression and the strength of transgene expression within the targeted cell. While several RGC-specific promoters exist (Table 1), many vectors designed for optic neuropathies employ a ubiquitous CMV [10–14] or a hybrid CMV early enhancer/chicken b-actin promoter (CAG) [15–17] due to their small size and high levels of transgene expression [18, 19]. Promoter size is particularly important when looking to incorporate larger genes into an AAV. For optic neuropathies in particular, there is a reduced necessity for a selective promoter due to the method of delivery into the eye, which is a compartmentalized structure. The largely cell void vitreous means that the first cells which the vector particles come into contact with are of the inner retina, leading to a significant transduction of RGCs in the presence of an appropriate promoter. CMV and CAG promoters have been shown to facilitate transduction of around 85% of RGCs in the adult rat eye [10, 16] with similar expression seen in mice (Figure 1).

Numerous studies support this observation, with both CMV and CAG promoters increasing expression primarily in RGCs, although some amacrine, Müller glial, and bipolar cells are also transduced [10, 14, 25] (Figure 2). Interestingly, a different profile of transduction is observed when the AAV2-CMV vector is injected at birth as opposed to adulthood. When intravitreally injected at P0, transduction is predominantly observed on rat photoreceptors (50%) compared to largely RGCs (60–70%) if injected in adults [10].

Depending on the gene therapy product and expected level of expression, careful consideration needs to be taken to ensure that off-target transduction does not have adverse effects on retinal function and health.

There is some limitation to AAV therapies, in particular the relatively small cargo capacity of AAV vectors for foreign DNA. Therefore, large genes are not suitable for use in a standard AAV vector, although dual vector [26] and more recently triple vector [27] approaches are being designed to overcome the coding capacity. Splitting large genes into two

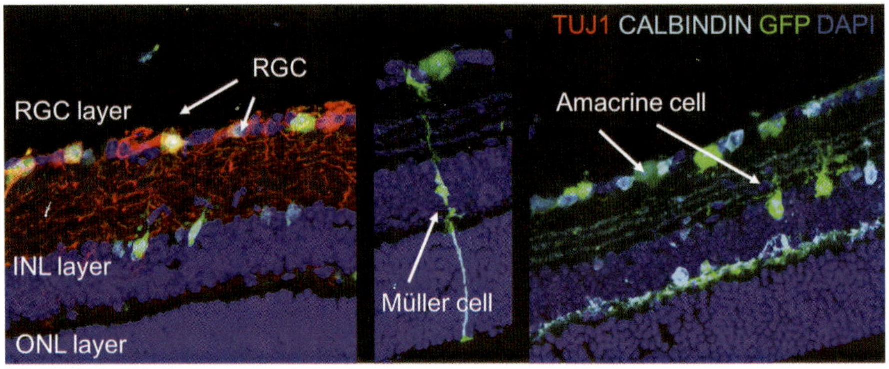

FIGURE 2: GFP expression and colocalization with retinal markers three weeks after intravitreal injection of AAV2-CAG GFP into the mouse eye. TUJ1 = retinal ganglion cells; CALBINDIN = amacrine cells. Image courtesy of Dr. Andrew Osborne.

halves and packing them into two independent AAV vectors has made it possible to treat mouse models of Stargardt's disease and Usher syndrome type IB whereby the full-length, large gene is reconstituted in photoreceptors or the retinal pigment epithelium via splicing or homologous recombination [26]. Admittedly, this method is less effective than single AAV-mediated gene delivery and at present has not been used to address any genetic defects for glaucoma or LHON, but it removes a significant hurdle in the possible advancement of larger gene therapies.

For inherited optic nerve diseases where a specific genetic defect has been well defined, gene supplementation therapies have gained considerable ground. Recently, the U.S. FDA approved the first gene therapy for vision loss, created by Spark Therapeutics Inc., who utilized this approach in clinical trials for Leber's congenital amaurosis (LCA), a disease characterized by severe childhood visual loss. In their studies carried out by Bennett et al. [28], AAV-meditated gene supplementation was used to compensate for a deficiency in retinal pigment epithelium, caused by a mutation in the RPE65 gene. One year following phase 3 trials, the mean bilateral multiluminance mobility test (MLMT) change score was 1.8 (SD 1.1) light levels in the intervention group and only 0.2 (1.0) in the control group [29]. The results of this trial mark a significant improvement in functional vision in patients with RPE65 mutations, a condition that was previously medically untreatable.

While still unproven, rapid advances in precise genome editing technologies have provided the possibility of new gene therapy approaches to optic nerve diseases that have a clear genetic basis. RNA-guided nucleases (i.e., CRISPR/Cas9) and designer endonucleases (i.e., TALENs or ZFNs) [30] have been of particular interest and over the coming decade are likely to replace many of the current gene supplementation methods.

While still early in its development, CRISPR/Cas9-based therapies have already been demonstrated for the treatment of optic diseases [31, 32]. With this technique, the CRISPR-associated protein Cas9 creates site-specific double-stranded breaks in DNA [33], which can stimulate host DNA repair mechanisms [34]. In its most widely used form, this system requires that two components are expressed in cells: the Cas9 nuclease and a guide RNA (gRNA), consisting of a fusion of a crRNA and a fixed tracrRNA. The first 20 nucleotides of the gRNA correspond to the DNA sequence targeted for editing and direct Cas9 to this site using standard RNA–DNA complementarity base-pairing [35]. Gene knockouts can be created through nonhomologous end joining (NHEJ), which creates small nucleotide insertions or deletions (indels) resulting in a frameshift mutation and termination [36, 37]. Alternatively, site-specific integration of transgenes is typically achieved by homology-directed repair (HDR) in the presence of a donor DNA template [31]. While this pathway is not available to nondividing cells, a homology-independent targeted integration (HITI) strategy has recently been developed which achieves robust DNA knock-in in both dividing and nondividing cells *in vitro* and *in vivo* [38].

CRISPR/Cas9 can be efficiently delivered to select cell populations in the eye using a dual AAV system. In a proof-of-concept study by Hung et al. [39], a dual AAV2 system was used to introduce CRISPR/Cas9 into mouse RGCs *in vivo* and achieve knockout of a YFP transgene. With this dual-vector system, one AAV2 delivered SpCas9, while the other contained a single guide RNA (sgRNA) against YFP, achieving a knockout rate of 84% in YFP-sgRNA-infected retinal cells. Similarly, Yu et al. [31]. delivered CRISPR/Cas9 using a dual AAV system to therapeutically target the *Nrl* gene in postmitotic photoreceptors in mice. Deep sequencing of the targeted region indicated that 98% of total reads included changes almost exclusively at the targeted genome site.

Before CRISPR/Cas9 approaches can be transitioned to clinical use, the frequency of off-target activity and modification remains a major concern that will need to be assessed [35]. Possible long-term consequences may include Cas9 activation or repression, and possible epigenetic editing, although while long-term AAV-mediated gene expression is beneficial for gene supplementation therapies, CRISPR/Cas9 only requires a short period of expression [40]. Studies by Chew et al. [41] found that the editing frequency of CRISPR/Cas9 and its off-target effects had dose dependency. It is therefore likely that continuous AAV expression could contribute to a rise in off-target modification and should be considered when assessing these therapies.

Conditions with an unclear or heterogeneous etiology, however, will still require a gene therapy such as AAV that focuses on enhancing survival of neurons by manipulating molecular pathways in the host cell rather than by correcting a primary genetic defect. The rest of this review will focus on current strategies for the optic neuropathies glaucoma and LHON with a focus on AAV-mediated protection and the possibility of genome editing as a potential future treatment.

2. Gene Therapy to Treat Adult-Onset Glaucoma

Glaucoma is a group of eye diseases characterized by progressive and irreversible degeneration of retinal ganglion cells whose axonal projections constitute the optic nerve [42–44]. It is currently the leading cause of irreversible blindness worldwide [45] and by the year 2020 is projected to affect more than 76 million people [46]. Currently, the standard clinical treatment for glaucoma is based solely on lowering the intraocular pressure (IOP) of those affected through pharmacology, laser treatment, or surgery. However, surgery and laser treatment carry risks and often require further intervention or a combinational approach supplementing with additive topical therapies throughout a patient's life [46]. The need for such regular treatment, often with multiple different eye drops administered several times per day, means patient compliance is a challenge, and even in those adhering to treatment, a significant fraction continues to experience progressive visual loss even after their IOP is reduced [47, 48]. Therefore, there exists a great deal of interest in new therapeutic approaches which can be offered as a single injection directly into the eye and that lead to long-lasting or permanent beneficial outcomes.

Much of adult glaucoma has an unclear, heterogeneous etiology involving multiple genetic factors, individual risk factors, and environmental factors [43, 46, 49]. For these reasons, gene therapies for adult-onset glaucoma have focused primarily on neuroprotection, which involves slowing the loss of RGCs by altering their physiology to limit the pathogenesis of the disease. This can be accomplished in two ways: (1) by enhancing the activity of innate survival pathways in RGC or (2) by inhibiting the progression of cell death.

2.1. Enhancing the Activity of Innate Survival Pathways. Neurotrophic factors are known to promote neuron survival through activation of prosurvival pathways or inhibition of default apoptotic pathways when a cell experiences pathophysiological stress [50–52]. During development of the central nervous system, immature neurons require trophic factors to survive, differentiate, and establish synaptic connections. To control these developmental processes, some neurotrophic factors are expressed in limited quantities by target tissues and only neurons exposed to optimal neurotrophic levels survive and establish synaptic connections [53]. Neurotrophic factors have also been studied as potential neuroprotective factors in neurodegenerative diseases, with brain-derived neurotrophic factor (BDNF) and ciliary-derived neurotrophic factor (CNTF) both having been shown to protect axotomized RGC [54–56] and RGC in animal models of glaucoma [16, 57–61].

The biological effects of neurotrophins are mediated by cell surface receptors. BDNF acts by binding to the receptor tropomyosin-related kinase B (TrkB), which stimulates multiple signalling pathways within RGC, including extracellular signal-regulated kinases 1/2 (Erk 1/2) and the phosphatidylinositol-3 kinase (PI3K)/Akt pathways [12, 44, 62]. These pathways have been shown to play a key role in promoting neuronal survival and regeneration. Additionally, RGC are trophically dependent on BDNF with BDNF strongly expressed in the superior colliculus [63, 64] and transported retrogradely by RGC axons to ganglion cell bodies in the retina during both development and into adult life [65–69]. There is also substantial evidence that depletion of BDNF plays a central role in the onset of glaucoma, with evidence for impaired retrograde BDNF transport found in experimental models of ocular dysfunction [58, 70, 71].

Research conducted over the past two decades has consistently shown that intraocular injection of BDNF protein or AAV-mediated BDNF expression provides a robust but temporary neuroprotective effect on RGC after optic nerve transection or crush [54–56] or following ablation of the superior colliculus [72]. While these results offer promise for the use of neuroprotective strategies in glaucoma, overexpression of BDNF can cause tachyphylaxis of the survival response through downregulation of TrkB and its subsequent degradation [73]. Studies by Cheng et al. [12] have also found that mRNA levels of TrkB were reduced to 40% of their normal level following optic nerve transection in rats, and more recently, Guo et al. [74] used RGC-enriched mRNA samples from glaucomatous retinas and demonstrated a 97% decrease in TrkB message indicating that supplementation alone may not be sufficient in the long term.

Interestingly, combining AAV-CMV TrkB transduction with an intraocular injection of exogenous BDNF *in vivo* showed markedly increased neuronal survival compared to expressing TrkB alone [12]. At 2 weeks after axotomy, AAV TrkB with BDNF protected 76% of RGCs, whereas independent administration of BDNF or AAV TrkB promoted 38% or 27% neuronal survival, respectively [12]. This would imply a gene therapy strategy to increase both ligand and receptor expression which may provide a more potent, long-term treatment.

CNTF, which is expressed in all retinal cell layers, has also been identified as a potential neuroprotective agent for glaucoma gene therapy. Intravitreal injection of CNTF and adenoviral-mediated CNTF expression has been shown to increase STAT3 in RGC, implicating the JAK-STAT pathways as the pathway responsible for its survival effect [75]. In a study by Leaver et al. [57], intravitreal injection of AAV-CAG CNTF significantly increased RGC survival at 7 weeks after optic nerve crush and regenerating axons were visible in the distal optic nerve. Another study by Pease et al. [59] also found that AAV-CAG CNTF reduced axonal loss by 15% compared to control groups following laser-induced IOP elevation [55]. A potential limitation of CNTF is that exogenous gene transfer of CNTF impairs visual function in a dose-dependent manner [76], adversely affecting photoreceptor function [77–79]. It has also been shown to cause increased aberrant dendritic growth and a significant reduction in the complexity of the RGC dendritic arbor in both transduced and nontransduced RGC populations [80, 81].

Neurotech Pharmaceuticals has recently commenced a phase 2 clinical for its NT-501 encapsulated cell therapy, based on the therapeutic benefits of CNTF (http://clinicaltrials.gov/ct2/show/NCT02862938). This experimental treatment for glaucoma consists of surgically implanting small capsules into the eye, which are filled with human cells modified to secrete a steady stream of CNTF. Subjects will be followed for two years following implantation and will give greater insight into the therapeutic potential of sustained CNTF signalling.

2.2. Strategies to Inhibit Cell Death Pathways. Other approaches to gene therapy for glaucoma have explored the therapeutic potential of antiapoptotic proteins that inhibit the progression of RGC apoptosis. RGC have been shown to die by apoptosis in both experimental [82] and human glaucoma [83]. Caspase activity is the final common element central to the implementation of apoptosis in RGC, making caspase inhibitors an appealing prospect for neuroprotective glaucoma therapies. Taking this approach, McKinnon et al. [84] injected an AAV-CAG vector expressing a known caspase inhibitor, baculoviral IAP repeat-containing protein-4 (BIRC4), into one eye on rat models of glaucoma. BIRC4 was shown to significantly promote RGC survival, although significant differences in IOP exposure among treatment groups were observed. However, it should be noted that apoptosis plays an important role in controlling cell populations throughout the body and inhibitors of apoptosis have had limited success as therapies to date.

Affected by many proapoptotic stimuli, mitochondria also play a key role in determining the cell's fate, making them important therapeutic targets [85]. Proteins of the Bcl-2 family have been of particular interest as important mediators of mitochondrial integrity. In particular, Bcl-XL has been shown to repress apoptosis through the sequestration of proapoptotic proteins [86]. Malik et al. [85] showed that AAV2-SYN1-mediated overexpression of Bcl-XL in RGC of adult rat retinas provided a significant neuroprotective affect to optic nerve transections. 94% of transduced RGC survived the lesion compared to 15% of control RGC, and after 8 weeks, 46% of Bcl-XL overexpressing RGC remained viable. Modest improvements have also been observed with AAV2 neuron-specific enolase overexpression of Bcl-2-associated athanogene-1 (BAG1), an Hsp70/Hsc70-binding protein, which has been shown to suppress apoptosis and enhance neuronal differentiation through interaction with the MAPK cascade [87].

It has also been suggested that RGC experience greater metabolic stress than other retinal neurons. A study by Williams et al. [88] hypothesized that RGC go through a period of mitochondrial stress and metabolite depletion, which causes them to undergo greater fatty acid metabolism. Fatty acid beta-oxidation in particular can increase free-radical generation leading to a greater consumption of NAD^+ [89], reducing its levels and leaving RGC vulnerable to damage from elevated IOP. To test this theory, an NAD^+ precursor nicotinamide (vitamin B3) was orally administered at a high dose (2000 mg/kg per day) to DBA/2J mouse models of chronic, age-related, inherited glaucoma. At this high dose, 93% of eyes tested did not develop glaucoma over the 12-month study. As a single-dose therapy, AAV2-CMV expressing Nmnat1, a terminal enzyme involved in the last step of NAD^+ production, was administered to DBA/2J mice. This protein was expressed in 83% of RGC at 2 weeks, and its overexpression was thought to drive further NAD^+ production, thus preventing axon and soma loss, preserving axon transport and electrical activity in RGC and preventing glaucomatous nerve damage in more than 70% of treated eyes [88]. While further studies are needed to validate these findings in other models, combining this single molecule supplement with current glaucoma treatment may have a substantial impact on preventing progressive RGC death in glaucoma and could demonstrate therapeutic potential in other age-related diseases.

While neuroprotective approaches have shown promise, further developments will need to be made before these gene therapies can reach clinical use. Due to the slow progression of glaucoma, prolonged gene expression may be necessary to produce significant clinical benefit. However, prolonged expressions of BDNF and CNTF have been shown to alter the dendritic structure of both transduced and nontransduced RGC populations [81], although the functional importance of these changes remains uncertain. Additionally, long-term AAV-mediated secretion of BDNF or CNTF has been shown to significantly change the expression of endogenous retinal genes in transduced and nontransduced retinal tissue [90]. An analysis of unfixed whole retinal tissue infected with either AAV2-BDNF-GFP or AAV2-CNTF-GFP showed that 56% of the 93 retinal genes tested had significantly altered expression compared to control AAV2-GFP retinas with greatest fold changes in the RGC layer. Three times as many genes were altered after receiving CNTF treatment in comparison to BDNF treatment [90]. Long-term studies will need to be carried out to account for potentially adverse effects resulting from extended manipulation of gene expression and alterations in endogenous gene expression.

3. Gene Therapy to Treat Early-Onset Glaucoma

Unlike most forms of adult-onset glaucoma, early-onset glaucoma more frequently has a single genetic cause. Myocilin- (MYOC-) dominant gain-of-function mutations have been reported in approximately 4% of all primary open-angle glaucoma (POAG) cases, but 10–33% of juvenile open-angle glaucoma cases harbour a MYOC mutation [91, 92]. While they do not directly disrupt RGC function, these mutations have been shown to affect trabecular meshwork (TM) functioning and lead to elevated IOP [93]. Mutations in the genes encoding cytochrome P450 have also been identified in 40% of individuals with primary congenital glaucoma [92, 94]. With advances in the specificity and efficiency of genome editing tools, there exists the possibility that these mutations can be targeted therapeutically. In a recent study by Jain et al. [91], adenoviruses expressing CRISPR/Cas9 components (Ad5-cas9 and Ad5-cr*MYOC*) were used to target dominant MYOC mutations in a mouse model of myocilin-associated POAG. Cas9 was shown to effectively disrupt the mutant MYOC gene, lowering IOP in treated mouse eyes and preventing further glaucomatous damage to RGC. In the same study, these constructs were used to treat trabecular meshwork tissue in human ex vivo cultured eyes [91]. A reduction of myocilin mRNA was observed, suggesting the feasibility of translating this technology to patients with MYOC mutations.

4. Gene Therapy to Treat Leber's Hereditary Optic Neuropathy

Leber's hereditary optic neuropathy (LHON) is an optic nerve disorder characterized by rapid, painless visual loss in one eye, shortly followed by successive visual loss in the remaining eye [95]. The disease is seen more predominantly in men, and symptoms appear in the second to third decades of life [65]. LHON is caused by point mutations in mitochondrial DNA (mtDNA). Three of the most common mutations, causing approximately 95% of LHON cases, lead to decreased NADH dehydrogenase activity in complex I of the mitochondrial respiratory chain and a reduction in energy production by the mitochondria [96–98]. In particular, mutation of the NADH dehydrogenase subunit 4 complex I (*ND4*) gene (G11778A) is present in 60% of LHON cases worldwide [99]. Though these genes are expressed in all mitochondria, the disease phenotype is limited to loss of RGC and degeneration of the optic nerve [100], possibly due to increased RGC energy demands. The majority of individuals with LHON are homoplasmic, meaning they carry only mutant mtDNA. Approximately 15% of LHON patients are heteroplasmic for the primary LHON mutation, with varying proportions of mutated and wild-type mtDNA present in peripheral blood leukocytes [101].

There is currently no definitive treatment for LHON. While current interventions of idebenone and vitamin B12 therapy have been effective in some patients, they have no effect in others [102]. Within the last decade, gene therapy research for LHON has advanced significantly, from the first LHON animal model by Qi et al. [103] to recent clinical trials supporting the feasibility of using gene therapy to treat this disorder through allotropic expression of the corrected mitochondrial gene sequences. The future treatment for LHON is likely to be through (1) incorporating new mitochondrial DNA via AAV or (2) CRISPR/Cas9 technology for mtDNA editing which may provide potentially novel avenues to treat heteroplasmic LHON mutation.

4.1. Incorporating Mitochondrial DNA via AAV. How LHON disease pathology develops is determined by the balance between the amounts of mutant and normal protein (typically ND4) expressed in RGC [100]. As a result, gene therapy studies have focused on promoting expression of the normal protein in a degree high enough to prevent RGC degeneration. Currently, viral vectors can only transfer genes to the nucleolus and not directly to mammalian mitochondria. To overcome this limitation, Guy et al. [104] developed what has become the foundation for allotropic expression of LHON mitochondrial genes. AAV-CAG were used to construct a nuclear version of the mitochondrial gene which codes for cytoplasmically expressed proteins. The proteins generated contain a mitochondrial targeting sequence, which allows for effective trafficking to their target site in the mitochondria [104]. This method was validated *in vivo* using a rat model of LHON, where electroporation of a construct carrying the wild-type ND4 allele effectively protected against RGC degeneration using allotropic expression [105].

Validating this method has led to rapid advances in LHON gene therapy. In 2015, Cwerman-Thibault et al. [106] introduced a recombinant AAV2 containing ND4 into a rat model of LHON, demonstrating both the safety and efficacy of allotropic ND4 expression in treating LHON. This approach suppressed RGC degeneration and preserved visual function in mutant ND4 rodents, making it an appealing candidate for human LHON clinical trials.

Recently, the results of the first three clinical trials of LHON gene therapy were released and provide promising prospects for the future. A study by Wan et al. [96] carried out at Tongji Hospital in Wuhan, China, evaluated the safety and efficacy of AAV2-mediated allotropic expression of ND4 in nine patients with the G11778A mutation. AAV-ND4 was injected in one eye each in each of nine patients, all of whom had been diagnosed for over a year. Each patient was followed for nine months. Over that period, none of the patients showed local or systemic adverse side effects from the treatment and visual acuity of 6 of the 9 patients showed significant improvement. In particular, patient 1 improved from 2 to 1.1 log MAR and was able to read newspaper headlines after treatment and patient 6 (a 9-year-old female) improved her visual acuity from 1.2 to 0.4 log MAR, allowing her to return to school and study with her classmates [96].

The results of phase I clinical trials performed in the United States by Guy et al. [107] also showed modest but statistically significant improvements of visual acuity following allotropic LHON gene therapy. 14 patients in three groups with varying durations of vision loss were recruited for this study, which administered low and medium doses of the gene therapy. Similar to the Chinese study, no serious safety concerns were associated with allotropic gene therapy of LHON [96, 107]. Following intravitreal injection, improvements in treated eyes were observed within 7 to 30 days [107], a duration when expression was observed in 90% of rodent RGC as reported by Koilkonda et al. [108]. High-dose cohorts are now being established for the next phase of clinical testing.

Similar to the previous studies, Vignal et al. [109] conducted a single-centre phase 1/2 clinical trial of rAAV2/2-ND4 that included 15 subjects and 4 dose-escalation cohorts (9×10^9 vector genomes [vg]/eye, 3×10^{10} vg/eye, 9×10^{10} vg/eye, and 1.8×10^{11} vg/eye). The study found that rAAV2/2-ND4 was safe and well tolerated 2 years after a single intravitreal administration with an observed between-eye difference in visual acuity change from baseline noted at week 96, favouring the treated eye.

While still in its early stages, the findings of these studies support the development of further clinical studies on allotropic gene therapies for LHON, but with larger patient cohorts. With mild improvements reported, it is reasonable to assume that normal ND4 was effectively targeted to the mitochondria and was able to increase energy supply to the optic nerve in both studies [96, 107]. Initial findings suggest that the degree of response to treatment is highest when treatment is administered at 1 year of visual loss [107]. In future studies, the duration of visual loss and degree of remaining optic nerve function will be important considerations to determine the timing of administration and clinical efficacy of each LHON gene therapy.

4.2. CRISPR/Cas9 Gene Shifting. Gene shifting describes the process of selectively destroying mutant mtDNA while preserving normal mtDNA in heteroplasmic mitochondrial diseases, which make up approximately 15% of LHON cases [110]. As described previously, the development of LHON is the result of the balance between the amount of normal and mutant protein [100]. The majority of mtDNA mutations cause disease when the level of heteroplasmy exceeds 70–80% [111].

Advances in the CRISPR/Cas9 system for efficient genome editing in mammals have opened up new avenues for intervention of inherited diseases. Studies by Hung et al. [39] have demonstrated that CRISPR/Cas9 components can efficiently target RGCs and achieve high levels of gene knockout *in vivo* using a dual AAV2 system. While CRISPR/Cas9 has been widely used to edit nuclear DNA, it has been unclear whether this system could be applied to edit mtDNA, with the mitochondrial inner membrane presenting a substantial entry barrier to AAVs. In a recent study, Jo et al. [112] demonstrated that FLAG-Cas9 is able to localize to the mitochondria with sgRNAs to edit mitochondrial DNA in a site-specific manner. To overcome nonspecific distribution of FLAG-Cas9, a mitochondria-targeted Cas9 (mitoCas9) was also created which localizes only to the mitochondria to produce site-specific cleavage of mtDNA. While further validation of this approach and analysis of off-target editing would be necessary, advances in CRISPR/Cas9 technology for mtDNA editing presents an opportunity to study the effects of gene shifting through knockout of mtDNA. With continued advances in this technology, future studies on AAV-mediated genome editing in heteroplasmic LHON cases may be possible.

Taking a different approach, the concept of gene shifting could potentially be applied to reduce mutant mtDNA copies in the oocytes of women carrying LHON mutations. In a recent study by Reddy et al. [113], mitochondrial targeted endonucleases known as mitoTALENs were able to eliminate mutant mitochondrial haplotypes in both mice oocytes and one-cell embryos, leaving only the selected mtDNA haplotype. This heteroplasmy shift resulted in phenotypically normal animals and prevented transmission of the eliminated mtDNA haplotypes to future offspring [113]. Additionally, mitoTALENs targeting the 14459G>A human LHON mutation were able to successfully reduce mutant mtDNA in mouse oocytes 24 hours after infection [113].

While there is a long way to go in further developing these technologies, genome-editing techniques are advancing at an astonishing rate. The development of CRISPR/Cas9 in particular demonstrates several advantages in comparison to ZFNs or TALENs. CRISPR/Cas9 has been shown to be more efficient at inducing genetic modifications [114] and can be easily adapted to target different DNA sites requiring only a simple modification to the 20 bp protospacer region of the gRNA, whereas ZFNs and TALENs require recoding of proteins using large 500–1500 bp DNA segments [115]. Cas9 also has the unique advantage of being able to induce double-stranded breaks at numerous sites in parallel using multiple RNA guides [37]. Ensuring the elimination of off-target cleavage with these editing techniques remains a primary concern [35] and justifiable barrier to clinical use. Additional consideration is also needed regarding when or if these types of intervention are necessary. Only 50% of male and 10% of female patients with the G11778A LHON mutation actually develop visual loss [99]. While predictions of susceptibility to disease can be made, making unnecessary modifications could pose a significant risk to what might be otherwise healthy eyes.

5. Conclusion

Substantial developments in technology over the past two decades have made glaucoma and LHON exciting potential targets for gene therapy. While further trials with larger patient cohorts are needed, initial results of LHON gene therapy clinical trials demonstrate the progress made and prospects for future clinical use of gene therapy. Future research will need to determine the ideal timing of gene therapy administration and whether a "critical window" for effective treatment exists either before or after symptoms occur. While many hurdles will need to be overcome before glaucoma gene therapy treatments reach routine clinical use, our advances in understanding the disease's pathology and our achievements in RGC neuroprotection in animal models provide grounds for optimism. Moving forward, the most challenging aspect of translating these findings will be determining the best avenue for RGC neuroprotection. Several different animal models of glaucoma and optic nerve disease are currently used in research, with each having advantages and limitations. Clinically, the presentation of glaucoma pathology also varies significantly. Determining the most effective pathway to target will depend heavily on the specific features of each case. In some patients, multiple pathways may contribute to the onset of the disease. Nevertheless, these rapid developments and successes achieved thus far give reason to believe that novel clinical therapies are on the horizon.

Conflicts of Interest

Keith R. Martin is a cofounder of Quethera Ltd, a company currently working to develop gene therapy approaches for glaucoma.

Acknowledgments

Original work described in this article was supported by Fight for Sight, the Cambridge Eye Trust, and the Jukes Glaucoma Research Fund.

References

[1] A. W. Taylor, "Ocular immune privilege and transplantation," *Frontiers in Immunology*, vol. 7, 2016.

[2] J. V. Forrester and H. Xu, "Good news-bad news: the Yin and Yang of immune privilege in the eye," *Frontiers in Immunology*, vol. 3, 2012.

[3] A. Auricchio and F. Rolling, "Adeno-associated viral vectors for retinal gene transfer and treatment of retinal diseases," *Current Gene Therapy*, vol. 5, no. 3, pp. 339–348, 2005.

[4] L. H. Vandenberghe, "What is next for retinal gene therapy?," *Cold Spring Harbor Perspectives in Medicine*, vol. 5, no. 10, 2015.

[5] T. Borrás, C. R. Brandt, R. Nickells, and R. Ritch, "Gene therapy for glaucoma: treating a multifaceted, chronic disease," *Investigative Ophthalmology & Visual Science*, vol. 43, no. 8, pp. 2513–2518, 2002.

[6] W. Hauswirth and L. Beaufrere, "Ocular gene therapy: quo vadis?," *Investigative Ophthalmology & Visual Science*, vol. 41, no. 10, pp. 2821–2826, 2000.

[7] J. E. Rabinowitz, F. Rolling, C. Li et al., "Cross-packaging of a single adeno-associated virus (AAV) type 2 vector genome into multiple AAV serotypes enables transduction with broad specificity," *Journal of Virology*, vol. 76, no. 2, pp. 791–801, 2002.

[8] S. Powell, R. Rivera-Soto, and S. Gray, "Viral expression cassette elements to enhance transgene target specificity and expression in gene therapy," *Discovery Medicine*, vol. 19, no. 102, pp. 49–57, 2015.

[9] M. Hellström, M. J. Ruitenberg, M. A. Pollett et al., "Cellular tropism and transduction properties of seven adeno-associated viral vector serotypes in adult retina after intravitreal injection," *Gene Therapy*, vol. 16, no. 4, pp. 521–532, 2009.

[10] A. Harvey, W. Kamphuis, R. Eggers et al., "Intravitreal injection of adeno-associated viral vectors results in the transduction of different types of retinal neurons in neonatal and adult rats: a comparison with lentiviral vectors," *Molecular and Cellular Neurosciences*, vol. 21, no. 1, pp. 141–157, 2002.

[11] K.-T. Tshilenge, B. Ameline, M. Weber et al., "Vitrectomy before intravitreal injection of AAV2/2 vector promotes efficient transduction of retinal ganglion cells in dogs and nonhuman primates," *Human Gene Therapy Methods*, vol. 27, no. 3, pp. 122–134, 2016.

[12] L. Cheng, P. Sapieha, P. Kittlerová, W. W. Hauswirth, and A. di Polo, "TrkB gene transfer protects retinal ganglion cells from axotomy-induced death in vivo," *The Journal of Neuroscience*, vol. 22, no. 10, pp. 3977–3986, 2002.

[13] J. Y. Lee, Y. Hwang, J. H. Kim et al., "In vivo fluorescence retinal imaging following AAV2-mediated gene delivery in the rat retina," *Investigative Ophthalmology & Visual Science*, vol. 57, no. 7, p. 3390, 2016.

[14] R. W. Nickells, H. M. Schmitt, M. E. Maes, and C. L. Schlamp, "AAV2-mediated transduction of the mouse retina after optic nerve injury," *Investigative Ophthalmology & Visual Science*, vol. 58, no. 14, pp. 6091–6104, 2017.

[15] L. Yin, K. Greenberg, J. J. Hunter et al., "Intravitreal injection of AAV2 transduces macaque inner retina," *Investigative Ophthalmology & Visual Science*, vol. 52, no. 5, pp. 2775–2783, 2011.

[16] K. R. G. Martin, H. A. Quigley, D. J. Zack et al., "Gene therapy with brain-derived neurotrophic factor as a protection: retinal ganglion cells in a rat glaucoma model," *Investigative Opthalmology & Visual Science*, vol. 44, no. 10, p. 4357, 2003.

[17] Y. Zhou, V. Pernet, W. W. Hauswirth, and A. di Polo, "Activation of the extracellular signal-regulated kinase 1/2 pathway by AAV gene transfer protects retinal ganglion cells in glaucoma," *Molecular Therapy*, vol. 12, no. 3, pp. 402–412, 2005.

[18] A. R. Harvey, M. Hellström, and J. Rodger, "Gene therapy and transplantation in the retinofugal pathway," *Progress in Brain Research*, vol. 175, pp. 151–161, 2009.

[19] C. Schön, M. Biel, and S. Michalakis, "Retinal gene delivery by adeno-associated virus (AAV) vectors: strategies and applications," *European Journal of Pharmaceutics and Biopharmaceutics*, vol. 95, Part B, pp. 343–352, 2015.

[20] Z. Shevtsova, J. M. I. Malik, U. Michel, M. Bähr, and S. Kügler, "Promoters and serotypes: targeting of adeno-associated virus vectors for gene transfer in the rat central nervous system in vitro and in vivo," *Experimental Physiology*, vol. 90, no. 1, pp. 53–59, 2005.

[21] S. Kügler, P. Lingor, U. Schöll, S. Zolotukhin, and M. Bähr, "Differential transgene expression in brain cells in vivo and in vitro from AAV-2 vectors with small transcriptional control units," *Virology*, vol. 311, no. 1, pp. 89–95, 2003.

[22] K. S. Hanlon, N. Chadderton, A. Palfi et al., "A novel retinal ganglion cell promoter for utility in AAV vectors," *Frontiers in Neuroscience*, vol. 11, no. 521, 2017.

[23] E. Spanopoulou, V. Giguere, and F. Grosveld, "The functional domains of the murine Thy-1 gene promoter," *Molecular and Cellular Biology*, vol. 11, no. 4, pp. 2216–2228, 1991.

[24] K. Fujita, K. M. Nishiguchi, Y. Shiga, and T. Nakazawa, "Spatially and temporally regulated NRF2 gene therapy using Mcp-1 promoter in retinal ganglion cell injury," *Molecular Therapy - Methods & Clinical Development*, vol. 5, pp. 130–141, 2017.

[25] J. Pang, A. Lauramore, W. T. Deng et al., "Comparative analysis of in vivo and in vitro AAV vector transduction in the neonatal mouse retina: effects of serotype and site of administration," *Vision Research*, vol. 48, no. 3, pp. 377–385, 2008.

[26] I. Trapani, P. Colella, A. Sommella et al., "Effective delivery of large genes to the retina by dual AAV vectors," *EMBO Molecular Medicine*, vol. 6, no. 2, pp. 194–211, 2014.

[27] A. Maddalena, P. Tornabene, P. Tiberi et al., "Triple vectors expand AAV transfer capacity in the retina," *Molecular Therapy*, vol. 26, no. 2, pp. 524–541, 2018.

[28] J. Bennett, J. Wellman, K. A. Marshall et al., "Safety and durability of effect of contralateral-eye administration of AAV2 gene therapy in patients with childhood-onset blindness caused by RPE65 mutations: a follow-on phase 1 trial," *The Lancet*, vol. 388, no. 10045, pp. 661–672, 2016.

[29] S. Russell, J. Bennett, J. A. Wellman et al., "Efficacy and safety of voretigene neparvovec (AAV2-hRPE65v2) in patients with RPE65-mediated inherited retinal dystrophy: a randomised,

controlled, open-label, phase 3 trial," *The Lancet*, vol. 390, no. 10097, pp. 849–860, 2017.

[30] M. Yanik, B. Müller, F. Song et al., "In vivo genome editing as a potential treatment strategy for inherited retinal dystrophies," *Progress in Retinal and Eye Research*, vol. 56, pp. 1–18, 2017.

[31] W. Yu, S. Mookherjee, V. Chaitankar et al., "Nrl knockdown by AAV-delivered CRISPR/Cas9 prevents retinal degeneration in mice," *Nature Communications*, vol. 8, article 14716, 2017.

[32] K. A. Schaefer, W.-H. Wu, D. F. Colgan, S. H. Tsang, A. G. Bassuk, and V. B. Mahajan, "Unexpected mutations after CRISPR-Cas9 editing in vivo," *Nature Methods*, vol. 14, no. 6, pp. 547-548, 2017.

[33] J. A. Doudna and E. Charpentier, "Genome editing. The new frontier of genome engineering with CRISPR-Cas9," *Science*, vol. 346, no. 6213, article 1258096, 2014.

[34] R. O. Bak and M. H. Porteus, "CRISPR-mediated integration of large gene cassettes using AAV donor vectors," *Cell Reports*, vol. 20, no. 3, pp. 750–756, 2017.

[35] J. D. Sander and J. K. Joung, "CRISPR-Cas systems for editing, regulating and targeting genomes," *Nature Biotechnology*, vol. 32, no. 4, pp. 347–355, 2014.

[36] P. Mali, L. Yang, K. M. Esvelt et al., "RNA-guided human genome engineering via Cas9," *Science*, vol. 339, no. 6121, pp. 823–826, 2013.

[37] L. Cong, F. A. Ran, D. Cox et al., "Multiplex genome engineering using CRISPR/Cas systems," *Science*, vol. 339, no. 6121, pp. 819–823, 2013.

[38] K. Suzuki, Y. Tsunekawa, R. Hernandez-Benitez et al., "In vivo genome editing via CRISPR/Cas9 mediated homology-independent targeted integration," *Nature*, vol. 540, no. 7631, pp. 144–149, 2016.

[39] S. S. C. Hung, V. Chrysostomou, F. Li et al., "AAV-mediated CRISPR/Cas gene editing of retinal cells in vivo," *Investigative Ophthalmology & Visual Science*, vol. 57, no. 7, p. 3470, 2016.

[40] A. Keeler, M. ElMallah, and T. Flotte, "Gene therapy 2017: progress and future directions," *Clinical and Translational Science*, vol. 10, no. 4, pp. 242–248, 2017.

[41] W. L. Chew, M. Tabebordbar, J. K. W. Cheng et al., "A multifunctional AAV-CRISPR-Cas9 and its host response," *Nature Methods*, vol. 13, no. 10, pp. 868–874, 2016.

[42] D. Lee and E. Higginbotham, "Glaucoma and its treatment: a review," *American Journal of Health-System Pharmacy*, vol. 62, no. 7, pp. 691–699, 2005.

[43] H. A. Quigley, "Glaucoma," *The Lancet*, vol. 377, no. 9774, pp. 1367–1377, 2011.

[44] M. Almasieh, A. M. Wilson, B. Morquette, J. L. Cueva Vargas, and A. di Polo, "The molecular basis of retinal ganglion cell death in glaucoma," *Progress in Retinal and Eye Research*, vol. 31, no. 2, pp. 152–181, 2012.

[45] Y.-C. Tham, X. Li, T. Y. Wong, H. A. Quigley, T. Aung, and C.-Y. Cheng, "Global prevalence of glaucoma and projections of glaucoma burden through 2040: a systematic review and meta-analysis," *Ophthalmology*, vol. 121, no. 11, pp. 2081–2090, 2014.

[46] J. B. Jonas, T. Aung, R. R. Bourne, A. M. Bron, R. Ritch, and S. Panda-Jonas, "Glaucoma," *The Lancet*, vol. 390, no. 10108, pp. 2183–2193, 2017.

[47] A. Heijl, P. Buchholz, G. Norrgren, and B. Bengtsson, "Rates of visual field progression in clinical glaucoma care," *Acta Ophthalmologica*, vol. 91, no. 5, pp. 406–412, 2013.

[48] L. Rossetti, M. Digiuni, G. Montesano et al., "Correction: blindness and glaucoma: a multicenter data review from 7 academic eye clinics," *PLoS One*, vol. 11, no. 3, article e0151010, 2016.

[49] R. W. Nickells, "Retinal ganglion cell death in glaucoma," *Journal of Glaucoma*, vol. 5, no. 5, pp. 345–356, 1996.

[50] M. Raff, B. Barres, J. Burne, H. Coles, Y. Ishizaki, and M. Jacobson, "Programmed cell death and the control of cell survival: lessons from the nervous system," *Science*, vol. 262, no. 5134, pp. 695–700, 1993.

[51] M. Bibel and Y. A. Barde, "Neurotrophins: key regulators of cell fate and cell shape in the vertebrate nervous system," *Genes & Development*, vol. 14, no. 23, pp. 2919–2937, 2000.

[52] A. Baltmr, J. Duggan, S. Nizari, T. E. Salt, and M. F. Cordeiro, "Neuroprotection in glaucoma - is there a future role?," *Experimental Eye Research*, vol. 91, no. 5, pp. 554–566, 2010.

[53] H. Levkovitch-Verbin, N. Harizman, R. Dardik, Y. Nisgav, S. Vander, and S. Melamed, "Regulation of cell death and survival pathways in experimental glaucoma," *Experimental Eye Research*, vol. 85, no. 2, pp. 250–258, 2007.

[54] S. Mansour-Robaey, D. B. Clarke, Y. C. Wang, G. M. Bray, and A. J. Aguayo, "Effects of ocular injury and administration of brain-derived neurotrophic factor on survival and regrowth of axotomized retinal ganglion cells," *Proceedings of the National Academy of Sciences*, vol. 91, no. 5, pp. 1632–1636, 1994.

[55] A. Di Polo, L. J. Aigner, R. J. Dunn, G. M. Bray, and A. J. Aguayo, "Prolonged delivery of brain-derived neurotrophic factor by adenovirus-infected Muller cells temporarily rescues injured retinal ganglion cells," *Proceedings of the National Academy of Sciences*, vol. 95, no. 7, pp. 3978–3983, 1998.

[56] D. B. Clarke, G. M. Bray, and A. J. Aguayo, "Prolonged administration of NT-4/5 fails to rescue most axotomized retinal ganglion cells in adult rats," *Vision Research*, vol. 38, no. 10, pp. 1517–1524, 1998.

[57] S. G. Leaver, Q. Cui, G. W. Plant et al., "AAV-mediated expression of CNTF promotes long-term survival and regeneration of adult rat retinal ganglion cells," *Gene Therapy*, vol. 13, no. 18, pp. 1328–1341, 2006.

[58] M. E. Pease, S. J. McKinnon, H. A. Quigley, L. A. Kerrigan-Baumrind, and D. J. Zack, "Obstructed axonal transport of BDNF and its receptor TrkB in experimental glaucoma," *Investigative Ophthalmology & Visual Science*, vol. 41, no. 3, pp. 764–774, 2000.

[59] M. E. Pease, D. J. Zack, C. Berlinicke et al., "Effect of CNTF on retinal ganglion cell survival in experimental glaucoma," *Investigative Ophthalmology & Visual Science*, vol. 50, no. 5, pp. 2194–2200, 2009.

[60] H. Chen and A. Weber, "BDNF enhances retinal ganglion cell survival in cats with optic nerve damage," *Investigative Ophthalmology & Visual Science*, vol. 42, no. 5, pp. 966–974, 2001.

[61] R. Ren, Y. Li, Z. Liu, K. Liu, and S. He, "Long-term rescue of rat retinal ganglion cells and visual function by AAV-mediated BDNF expression after acute elevation of intraocular pressure," *Investigative Ophthalmology & Visual Science*, vol. 53, no. 2, pp. 1003–1011, 2012.

[62] A. Kimura, K. Namekata, X. Guo, C. Harada, and T. Harada, "Neuroprotection, growth factors and BDNF-TrkB signalling in retinal degeneration," *International Journal of Molecular Sciences*, vol. 17, no. 9, p. 1584, 2016.

[63] K.-H. Herzog and C. S. von Bartheld, "Contributions of the optic tectum and the retina as sources of brain-derived neurotrophic factor for retinal ganglion cells in the chick embryo," *The Journal of Neuroscience*, vol. 18, no. 8, pp. 2891–2906, 1998.

[64] M. Hofer, S. R. Pagliusi, A. Hohn, J. Leibrock, and Y. A. Barde, "Regional distribution of brain-derived neurotrophic factor mRNA in the adult mouse brain," *The EMBO Journal*, vol. 9, no. 8, pp. 2459–2464, 1990.

[65] K. R. G. Martin and H. A. Quigley, "Gene therapy for optic nerve disease," *Eye*, vol. 18, no. 11, pp. 1049–1055, 2004.

[66] D. O. Frost, Y.-T. Ma, T. Hsieh, M. E. Forbes, and J. E. Johnson, "Developmental changes in BDNF protein levels in the hamster retina and superior colliculus," *Journal of Neurobiology*, vol. 49, no. 3, pp. 173–187, 2001.

[67] Y.-T. Ma, T. Hsieh, M. E. Forbes, J. E. Johnson, and D. O. Frost, "BDNF injected into the superior colliculus reduces developmental retinal ganglion cell death," *The Journal of Neuroscience*, vol. 18, no. 6, pp. 2097–2107, 1998.

[68] C. Moses, L. P. G. Wheeler, C. J. LeVaillant et al., "The acquisition of target dependence by developing rat retinal ganglion cells," *eNeuro*, vol. 2, no. 3, 2015.

[69] K. L. Spalding, R. A. Rush, and A. R. Harvey, "Target-derived and locally derived neurotrophins support retinal ganglion cell survival in the neonatal rat retina," *Journal of Neurobiology*, vol. 60, no. 3, pp. 319–327, 2004.

[70] S. Iwabe, N. A. Moreno-Mendoza, F. Trigo-Tavera, C. Crowder, and G. A. García-Sánchez, "Retrograde axonal transport obstruction of brain-derived neurotrophic factor (BDNF) and its TrkB receptor in the retina and optic nerve of American Cocker Spaniel dogs with spontaneous glaucoma," *Veterinary Ophthalmology*, vol. 10, Supplement 1, pp. 12–19, 2007.

[71] V. Gupta, Y. You, J. Li et al., "BDNF impairment is associated with age-related changes in the inner retina and exacerbates experimental glaucoma," *Biochimica et Biophysica Acta (BBA) - Molecular Basis of Disease*, vol. 1842, no. 9, pp. 1567–1578, 2014.

[72] K. L. Spalding, Q. Cui, and A. R. Harvey, "Retinal ganglion cell neurotrophin receptor levels and trophic requirements following target ablation in the neonatal rat," *Neuroscience*, vol. 131, no. 2, pp. 387–395, 2005.

[73] C. C. Proenca, M. Song, and F. S. Lee, "Differential effects of BDNF and neurotrophin 4 (NT4) on endocytic sorting of TrkB receptors," *Journal of Neurochemistry*, vol. 138, no. 3, pp. 397–406, 2016.

[74] Y. Guo, E. Johnson, W. Cepurna, L. Jia, J. Dyck, and J. C. Morrison, "Does elevated intraocular pressure reduce retinal TRKB-mediated survival signaling in experimental glaucoma?," *Experimental Eye Research*, vol. 89, no. 6, pp. 921–933, 2009.

[75] B. A. van Adel, J. M. Arnold, J. Phipps, L. C. Doering, and A. K. Ball, "Ciliary neurotrophic factor protects retinal ganglion cells from axotomy-induced apoptosis via modulation of retinal glia in vivo," *Journal of Neurobiology*, vol. 63, no. 3, pp. 215–234, 2005.

[76] T. J. McGill, G. T. Prusky, R. M. Douglas et al., "Intraocular CNTF reduces vision in normal rats in a dose-dependent manner," *Investigative Ophthalmology & Visual Science*, vol. 48, no. 12, pp. 5756–5766, 2007.

[77] W. M. Zein, B. G. Jeffrey, H. E. Wiley et al., "CNGB3-achromatopsia clinical trial with CNTF: diminished rod pathway responses with no evidence of improvement in cone function," *Investigative Ophthalmology & Visual Science*, vol. 55, no. 10, pp. 6301–6308, 2014.

[78] P. K. Buch, R. E. MacLaren, Y. Durán et al., "In contrast to AAV-mediated Cntf expression, AAV-mediated Gdnf expression enhances gene replacement therapy in rodent models of retinal degeneration," *Molecular Therapy*, vol. 14, no. 5, pp. 700–709, 2006.

[79] R. Wen, Y. Song, S. Kjellstrom et al., "Regulation of rod phototransduction machinery by ciliary neurotrophic factor," *The Journal of Neuroscience*, vol. 26, no. 52, pp. 13523–13530, 2006.

[80] E. R. Bray, M. Noga, K. Thakor et al., "3D visualization of individual regenerating retinal ganglion cell axons reveals surprisingly complex growth paths," *eNeuro*, vol. 4, no. 4, pp. ENEURO.0093–ENEU17.2017, 2017.

[81] J. Rodger, E. S. Drummond, M. Hellström, D. Robertson, and A. R. Harvey, "Long-term gene therapy causes transgene-specific changes in the morphology of regenerating retinal ganglion cells," *PLoS One*, vol. 7, no. 2, article e31061, 2012.

[82] H. Quigley, R. W. Nickells, L. A. Kerrigan, M. E. Pease, D. J. Thibault, and D. J. Zack, "Retinal ganglion cell death in experimental glaucoma and after axotomy occurs by apoptosis," *Investigative Ophthalmology & Visual Science*, vol. 36, no. 5, pp. 774–786, 1995.

[83] L. Kerrigan, D. J. Zack, H. A. Quigley, S. D. Smith, and M. E. Pease, "TUNEL-positive ganglion cells in human primary open-angle glaucoma," *Archives of Ophthalmology*, vol. 115, no. 8, pp. 1031–1035, 1997.

[84] S. J. McKinnon, D. M. Lehman, N. G. Tahzib et al., "Baculoviral IAP repeat-containing-4 protects optic nerve axons in a rat glaucoma model," *Molecular Therapy*, vol. 5, no. 6, pp. 780–787, 2002.

[85] J. M. I. Malik, Z. Shevtsova, M. Bähr, and S. Kügler, "Long-term in vivo inhibition of CNS neurodegeneration by Bcl-XL gene transfer," *Molecular Therapy*, vol. 11, no. 3, pp. 373–381, 2005.

[86] E. Yang, J. Zha, J. Jockel, L. H. Boise, C. B. Thompson, and S. J. Korsmeyer, "Bad, a heterodimeric partner for Bcl-XL and Bcl-2, displaces Bax and promotes cell death," *Cell*, vol. 80, no. 2, pp. 285–291, 1995.

[87] V. Planchamp, C. Bermel, L. Tönges et al., "BAG1 promotes axonal outgrowth and regeneration in vivo via Raf-1 and reduction of ROCK activity," *Brain*, vol. 131, no. 10, pp. 2606–2619, 2008.

[88] P. A. Williams, J. M. Harder, N. E. Foxworth et al., "Vitamin B3modulates mitochondrial vulnerability and prevents glaucoma in aged mice," *Science*, vol. 355, no. 6326, pp. 756–760, 2017.

[89] P. Schönfeld and G. Reiser, "Why does brain metabolism not favor burning of fatty acids to provide energy? Reflections on disadvantages of the use of free fatty acids as fuel for brain," *Journal of Cerebral Blood Flow & Metabolism*, vol. 33, no. 10, pp. 1493–1499, 2013.

[90] C. J. LeVaillant, A. Sharma, J. Muhling et al., "Significant changes in endogenous retinal gene expression assessed

1 year after a single intraocular injection of AAV-CNTF or AAV-BDNF," *Molecular Therapy - Methods & Clinical Development*, vol. 3, article 16078, 2016.

[91] A. Jain, G. Zode, R. B. Kasetti et al., "CRISPR-Cas9-based treatment of myocilin-associated glaucoma," *Proceedings of the National Academy of Sciences*, vol. 114, no. 42, pp. 11199–11204, 2017.

[92] A. M. Wilson and A. Di Polo, "Gene therapy for retinal ganglion cell neuroprotection in glaucoma," *Gene Therapy*, vol. 19, no. 2, pp. 127–136, 2012.

[93] M. Sarfarazi and I. Stoilov, "Molecular genetics of primary congenital glaucoma," *Eye*, vol. 14, no. 3b, pp. 422–428, 2000.

[94] K. R. G. Martin, R. L. Klein, and H. A. Quigley, "Gene delivery to the eye using adeno-associated viral vectors," *Methods*, vol. 28, no. 2, pp. 267–275, 2002.

[95] M. Yen, A. Wang, and Y. Wei, "Leber's hereditary optic neuropathy: a multifactorial disease," *Progress in Retinal and Eye Research*, vol. 25, no. 4, pp. 381–396, 2006.

[96] X. Wan, H. Pei, M.-J. Zhao et al., "Efficacy and safety of rAAV2-ND4 treatment for Leber's hereditary optic neuropathy," *Scientific Reports*, vol. 6, no. 1, 2016.

[97] P. F. Chinnery, M. A. Johnson, T. M. Wardell et al., "The epidemiology of pathogenic mitochondrial DNA mutations," *Annals of Neurology*, vol. 48, no. 2, pp. 188–193, 2000.

[98] W. J. Feuer, J. C. Schiffman, J. L. Davis et al., "Gene therapy for Leber hereditary optic neuropathy: initial results," *Ophthalmology*, vol. 123, no. 3, pp. 558–570, 2016.

[99] D. Wallace, G. Singh, M. Lott et al., "Mitochondrial DNA mutation associated with Leber's hereditary optic neuropathy," *Science*, vol. 242, no. 4884, pp. 1427–1430, 1988.

[100] A. J. Smith, J. W. B. Bainbridge, and R. R. Ali, "Gene supplementation therapy for recessive forms of inherited retinal dystrophies," *Gene Therapy*, vol. 19, no. 2, pp. 154–161, 2012.

[101] P. F. Chinnery, R. M. Andrews, D. M. Turnbull, and N. Howell, "Leber hereditary optic neuropathy: does heteroplasmy influence the inheritance and expression of the G11778A mitochondrial DNA mutation?," *American Journal of Medical Genetics*, vol. 98, no. 3, pp. 235–243, 2001.

[102] N. Barnils, E. Mesa, S. Muñoz, A. Ferrer-Artola, and J. Arruga, "Response to idebenone and multivitamin therapy in Leber's hereditary optic neuropathy," *Archivos De La Sociedad Espanola De Oftalmologia*, vol. 82, no. 6, pp. 377–380, 2007.

[103] X. Qi, L. Sun, A. S. Lewin, W. W. Hauswirth, and J. Guy, "The mutant human ND4 subunit of complex I induces optic neuropathy in the mouse," *Investigative Ophthalmology & Visual Science*, vol. 48, no. 1, pp. 1–10, 2007.

[104] J. Guy, X. Qi, F. Pallotti et al., "Rescue of a mitochondrial deficiency causing Leber hereditary optic neuropathy," *Annals of Neurology*, vol. 52, no. 5, pp. 534–542, 2002.

[105] S. Ellouze, S. Augustin, A. Bouaita et al., "Optimized allotopic expression of the human mitochondrial ND4 prevents blindness in a rat model of mitochondrial dysfunction," *American Journal of Human Genetics*, vol. 83, no. 3, pp. 373–387, 2008.

[106] H. Cwerman-Thibault, S. Augustin, C. Lechauve et al., "Nuclear expression of mitochondrial ND4 leads to the protein assembling in complex I and prevents optic atrophy and visual loss," *Molecular Therapy - Methods & Clinical Development*, vol. 2, article 15003, 2015.

[107] J. Guy, W. J. Feuer, J. L. Davis et al., "Gene therapy for Leber hereditary optic neuropathy: low- and medium-dose visual results," *Ophthalmology*, vol. 124, no. 11, pp. 1621–1634, 2017.

[108] R. Koilkonda, T. H. Chou, V. Porciatti, W. W. Hauswirth, and J. Guy, "Induction of rapid and highly efficient expression of the human ND4 complex I subunit in the mouse visual system by self-complementary adeno-associated virus," *Archives of Ophthalmology*, vol. 128, no. 7, pp. 876–883, 2010.

[109] C. Vignal, S. Uretsky, S. Fitoussi et al., "Safety of rAAV2/2-ND4 gene therapy for Leber hereditary optic neuropathy," *Ophthalmology*, 2018.

[110] J. H. Peragallo and N. J. Newman, "Is there treatment for Leber hereditary optic neuropathy?," *Current Opinion in Ophthalmology*, vol. 26, no. 6, pp. 450–457, 2015.

[111] P. Yu-Wai-Man, "Genetic manipulation for inherited neurodegenerative diseases: myth or reality?," *British Journal of Ophthalmology*, vol. 100, no. 10, pp. 1322–1331, 2016.

[112] A. Jo, S. Ham, G. H. Lee et al., "Efficient mitochondrial genome editing by CRISPR/Cas9," *BioMed Research International*, vol. 2015, Article ID 305716, 10 pages, 2015.

[113] P. Reddy, A. Ocampo, K. Suzuki et al., "Selective elimination of mitochondrial mutations in the germline by genome editing," *Cell*, vol. 161, no. 3, pp. 459–469, 2015.

[114] H. Liu, C. Liu, Y.-H. Zhao et al., "Comparing successful gene knock-in efficiencies of CRISPR/Cas9 with ZFNs and TALENs gene editing systems in bovine and dairy goat fetal fibroblasts," *Journal of Integrative Agriculture*, vol. 17, no. 2, pp. 406–414, 2018.

[115] R. M. Gupta and K. Musunuru, "Expanding the genetic editing tool kit: ZFNs, TALENs, and CRISPR-Cas9," *The Journal of Clinical Investigation*, vol. 124, no. 10, pp. 4154–4161, 2014.

7

Dance Training Shapes Action Perception and Its Neural Implementation within the Young and Older Adult Brain

Louise P. Kirsch,[1,2] Nadine Diersch,[3] Dilini K. Sumanapala,[1,4] and Emily S. Cross[1,5]

[1]Social Brain in Action Laboratory, Wales Institute for Cognitive Neuroscience, School of Psychology, Bangor University, Bangor, UK
[2]Research Department of Clinical, Educational, and Health Psychology, Division of Psychology and Language Sciences, Faculty of Brain Sciences, University College London, London, UK
[3]Aging & Cognition Research Group, German Center for Neurodegenerative Diseases (DZNE), Magdeburg, Germany
[4]Centre for Brain and Cognitive Development, Birkbeck College, University of London, London, UK
[5]Institute of Neuroscience and Psychology & School of Psychology, University of Glasgow, Glasgow, UK

Correspondence should be addressed to Emily S. Cross; emily.cross@glasgow.ac.uk

Academic Editor: Thierry Pozzo

How we perceive others in action is shaped by our prior experience. Many factors influence brain responses when observing others in action, including training in a particular physical skill, such as sport or dance, and also general development and aging processes. Here, we investigate how learning a complex motor skill shapes neural and behavioural responses among a dance-naïve sample of 20 young and 19 older adults. Across four days, participants physically rehearsed one set of dance sequences, observed a second set, and a third set remained untrained. Functional MRI was obtained prior to and immediately following training. Participants' behavioural performance on motor and visual tasks improved across the training period, with younger adults showing steeper performance gains than older adults. At the brain level, both age groups demonstrated decreased sensorimotor cortical engagement after physical training, with younger adults showing more pronounced decreases in inferior parietal activity compared to older adults. Neural decoding results demonstrate that among both age groups, visual and motor regions contain experience-specific representations of new motor learning. By combining behavioural measures of performance with univariate and multivariate measures of brain activity, we can start to build a more complete picture of age-related changes in experience-dependent plasticity.

1. Introduction

Throughout the lifespan, when learning a new skill such as riding a bicycle or dancing the tango, we benefit from not only physically practicing the new skill but also from watching others who can already perform that skill. Our ability to learn by physical practice as well as by observation is a key ingredient for acquiring new motor skills and is thus essential for us to survive and thrive within a social world. For over a century, it has been suggested that actions learned by physical or observational practice are represented within common cognitive and neural structures [1]. However, behavioural and brain-based investigations to date have not satisfactorily examined the extent to which this is actually the case. Moreover, how the aging process impacts our ability to learn via physical practice and observation remain underexplored. Such a lack of knowledge means that critical questions for understanding how best to facilitate new learning in educational and therapeutic contexts are ripe for exploration.

Prior work demonstrates the existence of an action observation network (AON), comprising sensorimotor brain regions including premotor, parietal, and occipitotemporal cortices [2–4]. These brain regions have been shown to be engaged when watching others in action and respond more robustly when observing actions that have been physically practiced [5–9] or visually experienced [10–14], compared with similar actions with which participants have had no prior experience.

Since the original work establishing the functionality of the action observation network, a rich literature examining how laboratory-based complex action training interventions shape the relationship between action and perception has emerged [5, 15–22]. As mentioned above, what many of these studies demonstrate is that the more familiar an action is, the stronger the response is within core AON regions [5, 6, 18, 23, 24]. On the other hand, an increasing number of studies report findings demonstrating that AON activity does not *necessarily* follow this linear trend of increasing engagement with increasing familiarity [17, 25–28]. These studies demonstrate equivalent or greater AON activity when participants observe *less* familiar actions (compared to more familiar actions), which is often interpreted as increases in neural efficiency [29–32].

Such marked differences in how the response amplitude of sensorimotor cortices changes after learning have been well documented in the motor control literature more broadly (see [33–35] for reviews). This has led to the suggestion that human neuroimaging investigations of sensorimotor learning are limited by the blunted sensitivity of traditional magnitude-based blood oxygen level-dependent (BOLD) approaches [36, 37]. An increasing number of studies are moving beyond univariate approaches of examining sensorimotor learning in the human brain, by attempting to evaluate *representations* of learning, as evidenced by more subtle modulations of the voxel-by-voxel activity patterns within the same area of cortex (e.g., [38, 39]). The ability to more closely evaluate learning representations is made possible using multivoxel pattern analyses (MVPA), an analytic approach we use in the present study to not only address how complex action learning shapes engagement of sensorimotor cortices but also how the same complex action training paradigm shapes brain responses within both young and older adults. Through combining training interventions with the increased analytical sophistication of MVPA, the present study explores how physical and observational learning impacts behaviour and the corresponding neural representations of actions.

With advancing age, sensorimotor and cognitive resources needed for learning a new motor skill decline and the efficacy of the matching process between observed and executed actions appear to be compromised [40]. However, this is modulated by the type of action observed. Evidence from studies investigating age-related changes in biological motion perception, motor imagery, and action observation suggests that forming an internal action representation may remain relatively preserved with advancing age for simple movement sequences, whereas it appears to become more imprecise in conditions with higher task complexity or when flexible adaptations to changes in the environment are required [41–43]. Such changes in behavioral performance are typically accompanied by a loss of neural selectivity in relevant regions of the aging brain [44, 45]. Overactivations, particularly in sensory cortices, are frequently reported leading to the assumption that older adults might be less adept at embodying new actions compared to younger adults [46, 47]. Thus, their ability to form an action representation based on physical and observational training might be limited, particularly compared to younger adults.

However, it remains unknown how learning complex whole-body actions, such as those that might be required in a fitness or social dance class, shapes behavioural and brain responses in young compared to older adults. In the present study, we aimed to explore this question by manipulating the type of sensorimotor experience that young and older adults received with dance sequences to determine how experience shapes responses at behavioural and brain levels. We attempt to address three main questions: (i) How do different types of training influence complex action performance among young compared to older adults? (ii) How do different types of training shape brain responses at a global level during action observation among young compared to older adults? (iii) How does physical training shape brain responses at the level of action representations? To address the first two questions, we implemented similar behavioural and univariate functional magnetic neuroimaging (fMRI) procedures reported in previous training studies [3, 18, 48] and studies that have compared the impact of complex action experience among young and older adults [43, 49]. To address the third aim, we used multivariate decoding procedures [50] to determine whether distributed voxel activity could be used to discriminate between patterns associated with viewing physically trained and untrained movements in the brains of young compared to older adult participants.

2. Methods

2.1. Participants. Twenty-three physically and neurologically healthy young adults were recruited from the Bangor University student population, and nineteen physically and neurologically healthy older adults were recruited from the local community. Older adults were screened for any past medical history, and we excluded any participants who reported any prior neurological diseases or use of medication that might alter their performance during the task or fMRI scanning. In addition, they were asked to complete the MMSE [51] to assess any cognitive impairment ($M = 28.9$, range = 26.5–30.0, maximum score: 30) and an fMRI safety screening questionnaire. The older adult participants were also invited to perform one dance sequence from the Dance Central Kinect Game before the study began, to ensure they felt comfortable with the technical equipment and were able to take part in all the procedures that would be required in the full study. Only those older adults who enjoyed this experience and were eager to take part after this prestudy trial were selected to take part. All participants (young and older adults) were dance naïve, meaning they had limited or no experience performing or observing dance, and none reported prior experience playing dance video games. All participants were right-handed or ambidextrous (ranging from moderately right-handed to strong right-handed; young adults $M = 60.78$, $SD = 22.20$; older adults $M = 86.58$, $SD = 20.91$, range 33–100), as assessed by the Edinburgh Handedness Inventory [52]. Two younger adult participants were excluded from the final sample due to excessive head motion artefacts whilst undergoing fMRI scanning, and one younger adult dropped out of the study half way through the training phase and thus was excluded due to having an

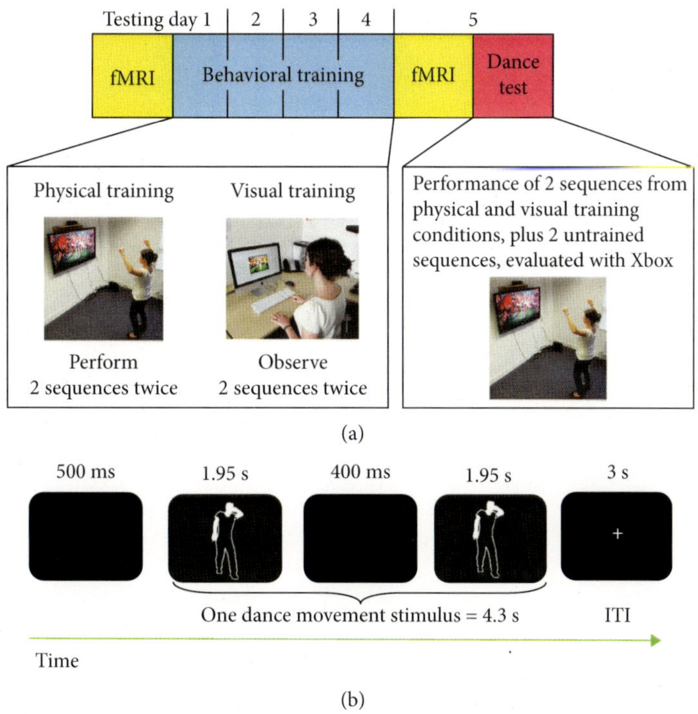

Figure 1: (a) Overview of experimental procedures. Participants of both age group underwent the exact same procedure. First they underwent a scanning session on day 1 and then started the behavioural training on that same day and the following 3 days. During each training day (days 1–4), participants physically trained with 2 long sequences and visually trained with other long sequences. Two other long sequences remained untrained. On day 5, participants underwent the same scanning session as on day 1. After scanning on day 5, participants had to physically perform all the long sequences (physically, visually trained, and untrained). (b) Schematic of an example fMRI trial. Each typical fMRI trial consisted of a 500 ms fixation cross, one dance movement stimulus lasting for 4.3 s, and an intertrial interval (ITI) of 3 s.

incomplete dataset. The final sample comprised 20 younger participants (12 females) with a mean age of 19.5 years (SD = 1.54 years, range 18–23 years) and 19 older participants (11 females) with a mean age of 63.6 years (SD = 4.4 years, range 55–69 years). All participants provided a written informed consent prior to taking part in any study procedures and were reimbursed for their involvement with either cash or course credit. The Bangor University School of Psychology Research Ethics Committee approved all components of this study (protocol number 2014-13123-A12806).

2.2. Stimuli and Apparatus. Six dance sequences from the dance game "Dance Central 2" (Harmonix Music Systems, 2011) for the Xbox 360 Kinect™ console were chosen that featured gender-neutral dance movements. The six chosen dance sequences were specifically selected so as to contain no overlapping dance moves between songs (i.e., each move was uniquely associated to one song/dance sequence). Each dance sequence was set to a popular song (e.g., *Like a G6* by Far East Movement or *What is love* by Haddaway) and varied in length from 2:20 to 2:29 minutes (average length = 2.22 s; SD = 10 s) and in tempo between 105 and 129 bpm (average tempo = 118.83 bpm; SD = 11.21). To focus participants' attention on the avatar whose moves they were learning, the same background setting was selected for all dance videos, which had a minimal amount of extraneous movement. The difficulty of the dance sequences (complexity and amplitude of dance movements) was set to a minimum level to ensure participants across both age groups could perform them to some degree from the very first training day but would still have ample room for improvement. The six dance sequences were paired to create three groups whose composition was matched for number and complexity of specific dance movements, as well as tempo. Each pair of sequences was assigned to one of the three training conditions: physical training, visual training, and no experience/untrained (Figure 1). A total of three different training groups were assembled, meaning that each pair of dance sequences was trained in all three training conditions across participants.

Animated silhouettes from the game depicting individual movements from the preselected dance sequences were captured and used as stimuli during both pre- and post-training fMRI sessions. The use of silhouettes, instead of original game footage, was specifically chosen to reduce visual cues associated with the original training context and to focus attention on the movements alone [48]. In this way, brain activity recorded when observing these pared-down dance movements should be more attributable to sensorimotor experience. 18 short animated silhouettes dance segments without music were extracted using iMovie '11 (Apple Inc.) and edited using Adobe Premiere Pro (Version 7.1 for Microsoft Windows 7), three sequences from each full dance sequence. The resultant 18 stimuli were matched for length to all be 1.95 seconds. Each stimulus was edited so that it featured one complete, coherent dance move involving whole-body motion and significant spatial displacement of the limbs (cf. [53]). All stimuli were novel to the participants during the pre-training fMRI scan.

2.3. Behavioural Training Procedure and Analysis. Both age groups underwent identical training and testing procedures. Participants were randomly assigned to one of three training groups in which they experienced the same pairs of sequences assigned to the two training conditions (place between the pre- and post-training fMRI scanning sessions) (Figure 1). For each training session, participants completed physical and visual training on the set of sequences to which they had been randomly assigned. Participants physically practiced the same two sequences twice (once with a female and once with a male avatar) and observed two different sequences twice. The order in which participants completed the training conditions was counterbalanced within and between participants across training days. Each training session lasted approximately 30 minutes.

2.3.1. Physical Training. For sequences of which participants physically practiced, they stood approximately 2 meters away from a 52″ Sharp flat screen television mounted on the wall in front of them. Participants' task was to mirror the dance movements of the avatar in the *Dance Central 2* Xbox 360 game as closely as possible and concentrate on improving their performance during subsequent sessions. The Kinect motion capture system compared participants' movements to the avatar's movements and assigned a score based on accuracy of mirroring the avatar. The Kinect's scoring system is based on how closely participants match the temporal and spatial features of the avatar's movements, including the avatar's movement amplitude. As the Kinect is a closed system consumer product, further details about how scores are assigned are not available. Similar procedures using this system were successfully applied in previous studies measuring the neural effects of dance training in young adults (see also [18, 48, 54, 55]). The game provides on-screen feedback about performance accuracy in the form of a final score after each sequence. However, to make the physical training condition as comparable as possible to the visual training condition (where no performance feedback was given), we covered the side margin of the TV screen (where the score is displayed after performance) so that participants were not aware of their dance scores after performing each sequence. These participant dance scores were recorded by the researcher and used as an objective measure of dance performance ability for the behavioural analyses.

The four overall dance scores participants received each day for the dance sequences in the physical training condition were averaged so that each participant had a single score representing dance performance for each training day. A mixed ANOVA with training day assigned as a within-subjects factor with four levels (training days 1–4), and age group as between-subject factor (young adults, older adults) was conducted on these scores in order to determine how performance across consecutive days of training compared between age groups. Additionally, we performed a repeated measure ANOVA for each age group separately to confirm the training manipulation worked and that physical performance increased across the daily training sessions.

2.3.2. Visual Training. For the sequences for which participants acquired visual experience, they sat comfortably in front of a computer running Psychophysics Toolbox 3 in MATLAB R2010a (MathWorks Inc.), which presented the full dance videos. Each video was shown twice, once for each avatar (male, female), in a random order. The dimensions of the dance videos were 640×480 mm, which reflected perceptually similar scaling to the physical training condition. As well as visual information, participants listened to the soundtrack that accompanied each sequence via the computer speakers. Participants were instructed to pay close attention to the dance sequences and were told that they would have to perform the sequences at the end of the week, so they should try to learn the movements as best as they could. To test that they were paying close attention, at the end of each music video, ten short dance segments (five from the videos they had just watched) were displayed, without music, each followed by the question "Did you see this movement in the video you just watched?". Participants had to respond "yes" or "no" using the keyboard arrow keys. All test videos were presented silently (as the task would have been too easy if the accompanying soundtracks were also presented).

An accuracy score for each participant for each of the four days of training was calculated based on their performance on this task. Similar analyses done for the physical dance scores were performed on the visual accuracy scores.

2.3.3. Post-Training Performance Assessment. On the final day of the study (day 5), participants returned to the laboratory to perform the four full dance sequences used in training (two physically trained sequences and two visually trained sequences) as well as the two untrained sequences (segments that they had observed during both fMRI sessions only). The test followed the same paradigm as the physical training phase of the study: participants physically performed the dance sequences from all six songs, mirroring the avatar's dance movements as closely as possible whilst the Kinect system captured and scored their movements. The six sequences were randomised and balanced for the gender of the avatar. Objective performance scores were obtained in the same way as for the physical training condition.

Raw scores from both exemplars from each training category were averaged within training conditions to produce an average score per participant for each of the three test conditions. We first performed a mixed-design ANOVA using an age group as a between-groups factor to compare dance performance between young and older adults on day 5. To further investigate performance in each age group independently, we next performed repeated-measures ANOVAs on these scores to investigate the impact of different kinds of experience on physical performance. Pairwise comparisons (Bonferroni corrected for multiple comparisons, with adjusted alpha levels of 0.025) were subsequently evaluated to investigate differences between conditions in more detail.

Degrees of freedom reflect the Greenhouse-Geisser correction where sphericity has been violated.

2.3.4. Training Modality Categorization Task. On day 5, immediately following the post-training fMRI scan and before the post-training performance assessment, participants performed a short control task, similar to the one in Sumanapala et al. [48]. In this task, participants watched again each dancing silhouette stimulus they observed during scanning (18 in total; 6 per training category). After each stimulus, participants were asked to categorize the movement as being either "physically trained," "visually trained," or "untrained", using the 1, 2, and 3 keys on a computer keyboard. Answers were untimed. Accuracy scores for each training condition were computed for each age group.

2.4. Neuroimaging Procedure. Each participant completed one fMRI session prior to the training procedures and an identical session immediately following the four days of training (Figure 1(a)). Participants completed 6 runs within each scanning session, lasting an average of 9 min and containing 60 trials each. In each run, participants watched three times 18 stimuli featuring short dance segments taken from the three training conditions (physically trained, visually trained, and untrained; 6 stimuli per training condition). Unlike the video footage used during training, the videos used during scanning featured the silhouette of an avatar performing each dance movement, which lasted 1.95 seconds. Each individual dance movement was presented twice in a row with a 400 ms black screen between each presentation (see Figure 1(b)). Each stimulus was preceded by a green fixation cross presented for 500 milliseconds, to announce the next trial. Each dance stimulus was followed by a fixation cross presented for a fixed duration of 3 seconds. After this, the next trial started. Finally, six additional video stimuli (featuring dance movements that were not part of the full set of 18 videos taken from the training conditions—these dance movements were never encountered outside of scanning) were included for attentional control questions. After each of these six test trials, participants were asked a question that required a yes or no response (button responses were counterbalanced across participants, with an index finger press corresponding to a yes response and a middle finger press corresponding to a no response for half of the participants and the inverse response schedule for the other half of participants). Participants had 4 seconds to provide a response via a four-button fibre optic response box placed on their lap on which they rested the index finger and middle fingers of both hands over the buttons. The question that appeared was randomly selected to be one of the following four: "Did the dancer place at least one arm above his head?," "Did the dancer reproduced the same movement on the left and on the right?," "Did the dancer take a step forward?," or "Did the dancer move his legs?." These questions appeared in a random order and were designed to ensure participants paid full attention to the dancer's movement in each stimulus. Each test trial was followed by a 12-second fixation cross that served as implicit baseline. Participants were familiarized outside the scanner prior to the pre-training scan with all features of the experiment and what they would be asked to do whilst in the scanner.

Stimulus presentation and response recording was done via a Mac desktop computer running MATLAB R2013a (MathWorks, Natick, MA) and Psychophysics Toolbox 3 [56–58]. The video stimuli were presented on a 24$''$ LCD BOLDscreen (Cambridge Research Systems), which was visible to participants via a mirror mounted on the head coil. The experiment was carried out in a 3 T Philips MRI scanner using a SENSE phased-array 32-channel head coil. For functional imaging, a single-shot echo planar imaging (EPI) sequence was used (T2$*$-weighted, gradient echo sequence; echo time TE = 30 ms; flip angle, 90°). The scanning parameters were set as follows: repetition time TR = 2500 ms; 38 transverse slices; voxel dimensions, 2.3×2.3 mm with voxel slice thickness = 3 mm; slice gap = 0.1 mm; field of view, $224 \times 224 \times 118$ mm; matrix size, 96×95 mm $\times$ 38 slices; and anterior-posterior phase encoding. Parameters for T1-weighted anatomical scans were $240 \times 224 \times 175$ mm; voxel dimensions, $1 \times 1 \times 1$ mm; TR = 12 ms; TE = 3.5 ms; and flip angle = 8°. All the scans were collected in an ascending order. For each run of each scanning session, the first two brain volumes were discarded to reduce saturation effects. 224 volumes per functional run were collected for each participant.

2.5. fMRI Data Analysis

2.5.1. Univariate Analyses. Neuroimaging data from each scanning session (before and after training) were preprocessed together to facilitate the construction of first-level design matrices including data from both scanning sessions. When there are several sessions, data can be either preprocessed separately or together. We decided to combine neuroimaging data from both scan sessions at the first level of analyses, for several reasons: (i) this leads to both days sharing the same implicit baseline, subsequently reducing the likelihood of results emerging simply due to differences between the two scanning sessions that are not result of the training manipulation, per se; (ii) the smoothness estimation on the data should be better with more data points, thereby reducing the threshold for multiple comparison correction using random field theory; and (iii) this preprocessing method was necessary for the subsequent RSA analyses.

Using SPM12 (Wellcome Department of Imaging Neuroscience, London, UK), data were realigned and unwarped, coregistered to the individual participants' T1 scans, and normalized to the Montreal Neurological Institute (MNI) template. Slice timing correction was performed after realignment, and all images were finally spatially smoothed using an 8 mm FWHM Gaussian kernel. A design matrix was fitted for each participant with a high-pass filter cut-off of 128 s, with each type of dance video (physical training, visual training, and untrained conditions), as well as attentional control videos and button presses associated, modelled together as a boxcar function convolved with the hemodynamic response function with temporal and dispersion derivatives. Additionally, participant-specific movement parameters were modelled as separate regressors of no interest.

The univariate analyses were designed to achieve three aims:

(i) To test both direct matching and neural efficiency accounts of experience-dependent plasticity, we first examined both increases and decreases in training-related brain activity among young and older adults separately. The most rigorous test of these effects involves evaluating scanning session by training experience interactions (i.e., to assess physical training experience, e.g., this would involve contrasting physical training > untrained on the post-training scan session compared to the pre-training scan session and the inverse (e.g., [18, 27, 59])). However, when evaluating these analyses in both directions, for physical and visual training experience separately, and among young and older adults independently, no brain regions survived a $p < 0.05_{\text{FWEcorrected}}$ threshold. This is not necessarily a cause for concern, as the type of manipulation and stimuli we have used in the present study could reasonably be expected to have subtle effects that do not meet the most stringent imaging threshold criteria (see, e.g., [3, 16]).

    In order to probe more subtle influences of our training manipulation and visual task in the scanner, we also evaluate direct contrasts comparing each training condition to itself in the pre- and post-training scans. We therefore examined brain regions that showed either increases or decreases in BOLD responses after compared to before training, for physical and visual training separately. These analyses were performed at the whole brain level while focusing on activations that survived a FWE-corrected threshold of $p < 0.001$ at the cluster level. This was achieved by contrasting pre- and post-training brain activity separately for dancing silhouettes that were associated with physical training or visual training at the 1st level for each participant and then conducting one-sample t-tests at the group level. The identical procedures were repeated for the young and older adults' data.

(ii) The second set of univariate analyses directly compared neural responses between young and older adults from the physical training condition. We focused on this training condition in particular as this was the most intensive type of training where we would reasonably expect the most robust effects to emerge [16, 18, 39]. This was achieved by using a two-sample t-test at the group level, which compared the 1st-level contrasts evaluating physical training before and after training, among young adults compared to older adults. To avoid any contamination of brain findings due to differences in physical performance scores/abilities between young and older adults, physical performance gains (calculated as the difference between physical performance scores on day 5 – day 1) were included as a covariate.

(iii) Finally, similarities between young and older adults when observing sequences that have been physically trained were examined through a customised conjunction analysis based on that reported in [18]. This analysis examined brain regions that showed increases or decreases after four days of physical training when both young adults and older adults observed these sequences after physical training compared to pre-training.

2.5.2. Multivariate Analyses. After evaluating magnitude-based univariate analyses, we next performed multivariate analyses to ascertain with finer detail on how sensorimotor training experience shapes neural representations during action observation among young and older adults. Specifically, this approach enabled us to explore how young and older brains distinguish between different types of training experience. Using The Decoding Toolbox scripts [50], we performed whole-brain searchlight decoding to assess the degree of outcome adaptation in local fMRI patterns surrounding each voxel (radius 8 mm) for each participant using the unsmoothed, realigned, and normalized imaging data.

This procedure involves extracting voxel pattern information from individual subject beta values generated during first-level preprocessing within SPM. Pattern information is specifically extracted from these beta values using support vector machine (SVM) algorithms that maximise mathematically defined representational distances within a shared coordinate space between different classes of data [50, 60]. To achieve this distinction, a data set is usually split into "training sets" and "test sets" before being introduced to SVM pattern recognition algorithms for classification. The algorithms are trained to identify patterns of data associated with specific classes within a training set before being tested on their ability to identify class membership on an unknown "test" set. Within neuroimaging, training sets and test sets can be shuffled in a leave-one-out cross-validation procedure [61], which limits the likelihood that spurious noise within specific subsets of data may lead to biases in pattern classification accuracy.

Following this, we implemented GLM analyses similar to the ones described for the univariate analyses. This involved modelling each training condition separately (physical, visual, and untrained) as well as attentional control videos and button presses. Also included in this model were participant-specific movement parameters, modelled as separate regressors of no interest. Physical and untrained events served as inputs for the classifiers and were labelled according to the model. Data were then split into different training and testing subsets depending on the model, using in turn each separate run as training and test runs [62]. Classification accuracy values (corresponding to observed prediction accuracy minus chance prediction for each voxel, with chance being 50%) for each analysis were entered into second-level t-tests for group-level analysis on a voxel-by-voxel basis. We decided to take "to be physically trained" and "to remain untrained" sequences as input for the classifiers, as previous literature [17, 39] documents that the most robust differences emerge after physical training, a finding corroborated by the univariate analyses from this study as well.

The multivariate analyses were designed to achieve two distinct aims:

(i) The first set of analyses is aimed at identifying brain regions that can distinguish between physical and untrained movement sequences after training compared to before training, among young and older adults separately. Naturally, we would predict this between-category classification accuracy to be better overall after training compared to before training, when all stimuli were equally unfamiliar. This was achieved by running the searchlight decoding scripts on the 1st-level data from pre-training and post-training scans separately, taking as the two classifiers the "physically trained" movement sequences and the "untrained" movement sequences, and then running paired-sample t-tests at the group level, separately for young and older adults.

(ii) The aim of the second set of analyses was to compare classification accuracies between the two age groups. We were particularly interested in accuracy to distinguish between physically trained and untrained sequences after physical training (which entails examination of the post-training scan data only). To achieve this, we first ran a separate whole-brain decoding analysis to determine which brain regions distinguish between physically trained and untrained sequences after training, separately for each age group. The results of this analysis for both age groups are presented in Supplementary Table 1. Then, contrasts from post-training classification for young and older adults were entered into a two-sample t-test. Finally, we explored which regions in young and older adults could similarly distinguish between physically trained and untrained movements after training by running a conjunction analysis, similarly to the one done for the univariate analysis above (and in [18]).

3. Results

3.1. Behavioural Results

3.1.1. Physical and Visual Training. For each participant, physical performance was assessed each day by averaging performance scores across both dance sequences assigned to the physical training condition (Figure 2(a)). When evaluating young and older adults' physical performance across days of training, a main effect of training day was observed ($F_{(2.086,75.088)} = 79.476$, $p < 0.001$, $\eta_p^2 = 0.688$) as well as an interaction between age group and performance across days, with younger adults performing better than older adults ($F_{(2.086,75.088)} = 14.320$, $p < 0.001$, $\eta_p^2 = 0.285$). In both age groups, a main effect of training day was observed whereby physical performance significantly improved across the four days of training (young adults: $F_{(2.026,36.47)} = 50.218$, $p < 0.001$, $\eta_p^2 = 0.736$; older adults: $F_{(3,54)} = 33.417$, $p < 0.001$, $\eta_p^2 = 0.748$). Pairwise comparisons indicate that significant differences were observed between all possible pairs of days (young adults: day 1 versus day 2: $t_{(18)} = -5.430$, $p < 0.001$; day 2 versus day 3: $t_{(18)} = -3.960$, $p = 0.001$; and day 3 versus day 4: $t_{(18)} = -3.375$, $p = 0.003$; older adults: day 1 versus day 2: $t_{(18)} = -5.225$, $p < 0.001$; day 2 versus day 3: $t_{(18)} = -2.981$, $p = 0.008$; and day 3 versus day 4: $t_{(19)} = -3.375$, $p = 0.003$).

Participants' performance on the visual training task was assessed through a movement recognition task after observing two different sequences (Figure 2(b)). A main effect of visual training was found across groups ($F_{(2.311,83.201)} = 17.224$, $p < 0.001$, $\eta_p^2 = 0.324$); however, no interaction emerged between training scores and age group, yielding no differences in the visual training manipulation among young and older adults ($F_{(2.311,83.201)} = 1.376$, $p = 0.258$, $\eta_p^2 = 0.037$). Average response accuracy appeared to improve across the four days of training for both age groups (young adults: $F_{(1.799,32.376)} = 5.846$, $p = 0.008$, $\eta_p^2 = 0.245$; older adults: $F_{(3,54)} = 11.856$, $p < 0.001$, $\eta_p^2 = 0.397$), indicating that participants were consistently able to recognize movements that had appeared in the visually trained videos. This effect was driven by a significant improvement from day 1 to day 2 (young adults: $t_{(18)} = -2.851$, $p = 0.011$; older adults: $t_{(18)} = -4.237$, $p < 0.001$) and no further significant improvements between any other pairs of consecutive days (all p values > 0.05: young adults: day 2 versus day 3: $t_{(18)} = -0.498$, $p = 0.624$; day 3 versus day 4: $t_{(19)} = -1.299$, $p = 0.210$; older adults: day 2 versus day 3: $t_{(18)} = 0$, $p = 1$; day 3 versus day 4: $t_{(18)} = -0.137$, $p = 0.893$). This suggests that the performance level of participants in both age groups reached ceiling after the second day of training.

3.1.2. Physical Performance on Day 5. On the final day of testing, after the second fMRI session was completed, participants were asked to perform all six dance sequences (two from each training category: physically trained, visually trained, and untrained conditions) in order to generate an objective measure of their ability to perform each of the dance movements they observed during both fMRI sessions and assess the impact of differentiated sensorimotor experience on motor performance (Figure 2(c)).

A main effect of training type was observed across groups ($F_{(1.684,62.307)} = 46.048$, $p < 0.001$, $\eta_p^2 = 0.554$) as well as an interaction between age group and training condition ($F_{(1.684,62.307)} = 8.139$, $p = 0.001$, $\eta_p^2 = 0.180$), and a main effect of age confirming that young adults performed better overall than older adults ($F_{(1,37)} = 15.013$, $p < 0.001$, $\eta_p^2 = 0.289$). A one-way ANOVA ran within each age group separately revealed a main effect of training type on dance performance in both groups (young adults: $F_{(2,38)} = 40.802$, $p < 0.001$, $\eta_p^2 = 0.682$; older adults: $F_{(2,36)} = 9.284$, $p = 0.001$,

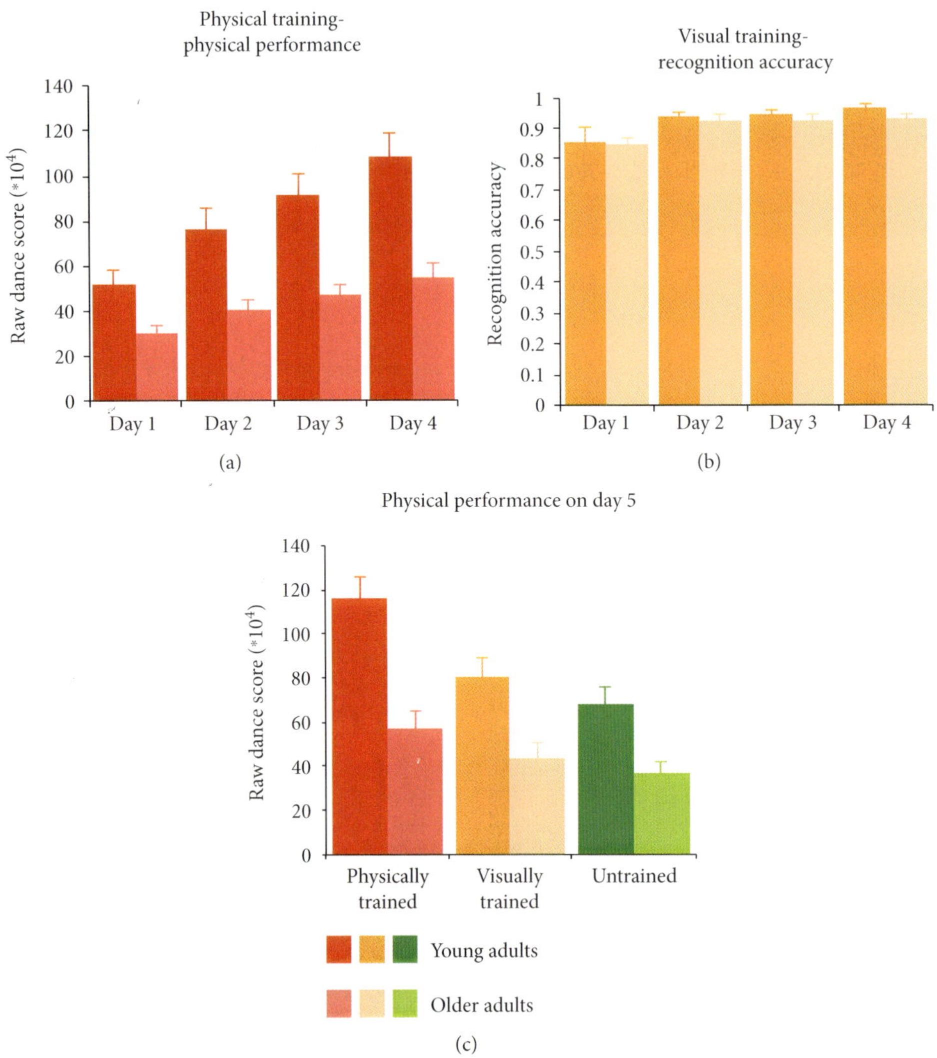

FIGURE 2: Training performances for both age groups. (a) Physical performance across the 4 consecutive days of physical training, for both younger (bright red) and older adults (pale red). (b) Recognition accuracy after each day of visual training, for both younger (bright orange) and older adults (pale orange). (c) Average physical performance on day 5, for each training condition (physical, visual, and untrained sequences), for both younger (darker bars) and older adults (lighter bars).

$\eta_p^2 = 0.340$). Pairwise comparisons indicate that physically trained sequences were performed significantly better than visually trained or untrained sequences, among both young and older adults (young adults: physically versus visually trained: $t_{(19)} = 7.556$, $p < 0.001$; physically trained versus untrained: $t_{(19)} = 7.251$, $p < 0.001$; older adults: physically versus visually trained: $t_{(18)} = 3.275$, $p = 0.008$; physically trained versus untrained: $t_{(18)} = 3.551$, $p = 0.004$). Differences in performance between observed and untrained sequences did not reach significance, with the Bonferroni-corrected alpha level of 0.025 (young adults: $t_{(19)} = 2.331$, $p = 0.031$; older adults: $t_{(18)} = 1.613$, $p = 0.124$).

3.1.3. Training Modality Categorization Task Performance. As a follow-up task, immediately following the post-training scan on day 5 of the study, participants were asked to watch each silhouette stimulus again (6 per training condition) and to categorize each stimulus as either being physically trained, visually trained, or untrained (see Supplementary Figure 1). Overall, young adults were better than older adults in identifying the training category to which each stimulus belonged ($F_{(1,36)} = 65.560$, $p < 0.001$). Moreover, we observed a main effect of the training type ($F_{(2,56.315)} = 25.501$, $p < 0.001$) and a nonsignificant trend towards an interaction between training category and age group ($F_{(2,56.315)} = 3.093$, $p = 0.065$). This marginal interaction suggests that older adults are overall not performing poorly at recognizing the training category for those videos that have been physically or visually trained (all above chance level). However, they do perform particularly poorly at categorizing the untrained videos (categorizing them as trained in 79% of cases). It is to note that this task was not designed to definitively determine how well participants can match specific movements with a prior training condition (as was the aim in [48]), as participants only performed a total of 18 trials in this follow-up test (one trial for each stimulus). However, this exploratory follow-up task was designed to give us an indication of how well young and older adults can explicitly categorize the training condition associated with the different moves they observed in the scanner.

3.2. Effect of Sensorimotor Training among Young and Older Adults at the Whole Brain Level. Our first neuroimaging objective was to examine the effects of physical and visual training on whole brain activity. We did this first within each age group separately and then comparing young with older adults. As a reminder, we always evaluated contrasts to explore both increases and decreases in BOLD responses after training (comparing post and pre-training scans in both directions).

All of the following analyses were run with both days modelled in the same design matrix at the 1st level (and pre-processed together). All contrasts were evaluated at $p_{\text{unc}} < 0.001$, $k = 10$ voxels, and here, we focus on those results that survive correction of $p_{\text{FWEcorr}} < 0.05$ at the cluster level.

3.2.1. Brain Regions Involved in Physical and Visual Learning in Younger Adults

(1) Effects of Physical Training: Younger Adults. Among young adults, the observation of body movements after physical training compared to before (post-training > pre-training) did not yield any significant increases in neural activity. However, this same contrast did reveal several brain regions that demonstrated a decreased response after training, including areas associated with sensorimotor processing, such as the left paracentral lobule and postcentral gyrus and right precentral gyrus and inferior temporal gyrus. In addition, the amygdala and middle occipital gyrus also demonstrated decreased response amplitude when observing those movements that had been physically trained (Table 1(a)).

(2) Effects of Visual Training: Younger Adults. Among younger adults, the observation of body movements encountered after visual training compared to before did not lead to any significant increases in activation. In comparison, several brain regions in the right hemisphere showed a marked decrease in response amplitude after four days of visual training, including the fusiform gyrus, postcentral gyrus, and middle temporal gyrus (Table 1(b)).

3.2.2. Brain Regions Involved in Physical and Visual Learning in Older Adults

(1) Physical Training: Older Adults. Among older adults, the observation of body movements after physical training compared to before physical training resulted in increased activation in the right precuneus, and activity decreases within the right superior and inferior parietal lobules (SPL and IPL) and the right thalamus (Table 2(a)).

(2) Visual Training: Older Adults. In older adults, the observation of body movements after visual training compared to before four days of visual training resulted in an increase of activation of the right precuneus, similarly than after physical training but with no significant decrease of activity in any region (Table 2(b)).

3.2.3. Differences and Similarities between Age Groups, by Training Experience

(1) Differences between Young and Older Adults. In order to evaluate regions in which activation varied as a function of the age group, young and older adults were compared to each other while the factor performance gain was included as covariate of no interest. These contrasts were evaluated as two-sample t-tests. Compared to older adults, young adults showed decreased recruitment of the left inferior parietal lobule after training compared to before physical training (Figure 3). No other contrasts yielded any significant difference between young and older adults when comparing pre- and post-training scans (including the positive effect of performance). It is to note that running the same contrasts with performance on day 5 as the covariate of no interest (instead of performance gain) lead to a nearly identical pattern of activation, with the only significant activation emerging within the left inferior parietal lobule ($x = -50$, $y = -28$, $z = 48$, $p_{\text{FWE-corr}} = 0.001$, $t = 4.8$) when comparing young adults to older adults.

(2) Common Regions Influenced by Training among Young and Older Adults. When analysed separately, training effects among young and older adults mainly resulted in decreased activity after physical training compared to before. For this reason, we focused on this contrast to see which regions were similarly showing a decrease of activity in both age groups after physical training compared to before. This conjunction analysis (using $t > 3.5$ as the threshold) yielded overlapping activation across 87 voxels, in three main regions, namely, the left fusiform gyrus, the right inferior temporal gyrus, and the right inferior parietal lobule (Figure 4).

3.3. Effects of Training on Neural Representations of Actions

3.3.1. Regions That Discriminate Better between Dance Movements after Compared to before Training in Each Age Group. This first set of decoding analyses is aimed at identifying which brain regions were better able to distinguish between physically trained and untrained movement sequences after compared to before training, among young and older adults separately.

All results reported are $p_{\text{FWEcorr}} < 0.05$ at the cluster level, with a threshold at $p_{\text{unc}} < 0.005$, $k = 20$ voxels.

(1) Younger Adults. When comparing regions that could better distinguish between physically trained and untrained sequences after training compared to before training, the left angular gyrus (IPC) and right middle frontal gyrus (close to IFS) were the two only regions that could discriminate accurately (i.e., above chance) after training between physically trained and untrained sequences (Figure 5(a) and Table 3(a)).

(2) Older Adults. When comparing regions that could distinguish between physically trained and untrained sequences after training better than before training, left SMA and primary somatosensory cortex were the only regions that came

Table 1: Regions associated with an increase and decrease of activity post-training compared to pre-training among younger adults, depending on the type of training.

(a) Physical training

Region	BA	MNI coordinates			t value	Cluster size	$pFWE_{corr}$ value
		x	y	z			
(i) Increase post-training compared to pre-training							
No cluster survived the threshold							
(ii) Decrease post-training compared to pre-training							
L paracentral lobule	**5**	**−10**	**−34**	**58**	**7.17**	**233**	**<0.001**
L postcentral gyrus	1	−28	−36	56	4.50		
L superior parietal lobule	3b	−20	−42	58	4.13		
R precentral gyrus	**4**	**34**	**−28**	**58**	**6.02**	**706**	**<0.001**
R postcentral gyrus	1	38	−38	56	5.07		
R postcentral gyrus	1	26	−32	58	5.06		
R inferior temporal gyrus	**37**	**50**	**−50**	**−16**	**5.89**	**380**	**<0.001**
R inferior temporal gyrus	37	40	−52	−14	5.51		
R inferior temporal gyrus		36	−60	−4	3.85		
R hippocampus		**26**	**−4**	**−24**	**5.65**	**168**	**0.003**
R hippocampus		34	−4	−22	5.05		
R middle temporal gyrus	21	46	−4	−20	4.55		
L postcentral gyrus	**1**	**−40**	**−30**	**56**	**5.00**	**94**	**0.048**
L postcentral gyrus	1	−44	−22	56	4.26		
R middle occipital gyrus	**19**	**46**	**−76**	**18**	**4.63**	**153**	**0.005**
R middle occipital gyrus	19	40	−84	14	4.59		
R middle occipital gyrus	19	52	−64	14	4.55		

(b) Visual training

Region	BA	MNI coordinates			t value	Cluster size	$pFWE_{corr}$ value
		x	y	z			
(i) Increase post-training compared to pre-training							
No cluster survived the threshold							
(ii) Decrease post-training compared to pre-training							
L inferior temporal gyrus	20	−40	−32	−18	6.30	83	0.081
L inferior temporal gyrus	37	−42	−40	−18	4.68		
L fusiform gyrus	37	−38	−56	−18	4.14		
R amygdala		30	−2	−24	5.68	80	0.092
R parahippocampal gyrus	36	24	−26	−24	4.44		
R parahippocampal gyrus	36	20	−12	−24	4.36		
R fusiform gyrus	**37**	**42**	**−42**	**−16**	**5.58**	**394**	**<0.001**
R inferior temporal gyrus	37	40	−52	−14	4.86		
R inferior temporal gyrus	37	50	−50	−16	4.46		
R postcentral gyrus	**1**	**30**	**−32**	**58**	**5.40**	**498**	**<0.001**
R postcentral gyrus	1	28	−40	66	4.86		
R postcentral gyrus	1	36	−34	66	4.69		
R middle temporal gyrus	**19**	**52**	**−66**	**12**	**5.36**	**180**	**0.002**
R middle occipital gyrus	19	46	−80	12	4.88		
R middle occipital gyrus	39	40	−58	12	3.91		

BA: Brodmann's area; R: right; L: left. Analysis performed at $p < 0.001$, uncorrected, $k = 10$ voxels, and regions in bold font are FWE cluster corrected at the $p < 0.05$ level. Up to three local maxima are listed when a cluster has multiple peaks more than 8 mm apart.

TABLE 2: Regions associated with increases and decreases of activity post-training compared to pre-training in older adults, depending on the type of training.

(a) Physical training

Region	BA	MNI coordinates x	y	z	t value	Cluster size	pFWEcorr value
(i) Increase post-training compared to pre-training							
R precuneus	**7**	**4**	**−68**	**30**	**6.68**	**510**	**<0.001**
R precuneus	31	10	−66	24	5.45		
L cuneus	18	−6	−66	22	4.98		
(ii) Decrease post-training compared to pre-training							
R thalamus		**8**	**−26**	**6**	**5.88**	**314**	**<0.001**
L thalamus		−2	−24	6	5.66		
L thalamus		−12	−32	2	5.26		
R superior parietal lobule	**39**	**32**	**−56**	**48**	**5.55**	**187**	**0.002**
R superior occipital gyrus	7	22	−62	48	4.72		
R superior parietal lobule	7	26	−50	46	4.31		
R inferior temporal gyrus	37	50	−50	14	5.22	69	0.147
R inferior temporal gyrus		44	−54	−6	4.53		
R fusiform gyrus		34	−54	−12	3.97		
R inferior parietal lobule	**1**	**60**	**−20**	**36**	**4.92**	**182**	**0.002**
R supramarginal gyrus	40	60	−30	38	4.83		
R supramarginal gyrus	40	54	−28	48	4.05		

(b) Visual training

Region	BA	MNI coordinates x	y	z	t value	Cluster size	pFWEcorr value
(i) Increase post-training compared to pre-training							
R precuneus	**31**	**10**	**−66**	**24**	**5.67**	**220**	**<0.001**
R precuneus	31	18	−62	22	4.34		
L precuneus	31	−2	−66	28	4.33		
(ii) Decrease post-training compared to pre-training							
No cluster survived the threshold (all pFWEcorr > 0.1)							

BA: Brodmann's area; R: right, L: left. $p < 0.001$, uncorrected; $k = 10$ voxels. Regions in bold font are FWE cluster corrected at the $p < 0.05$ level. Up to three local maxima are listed when a cluster has multiple peaks more than 8 mm apart.

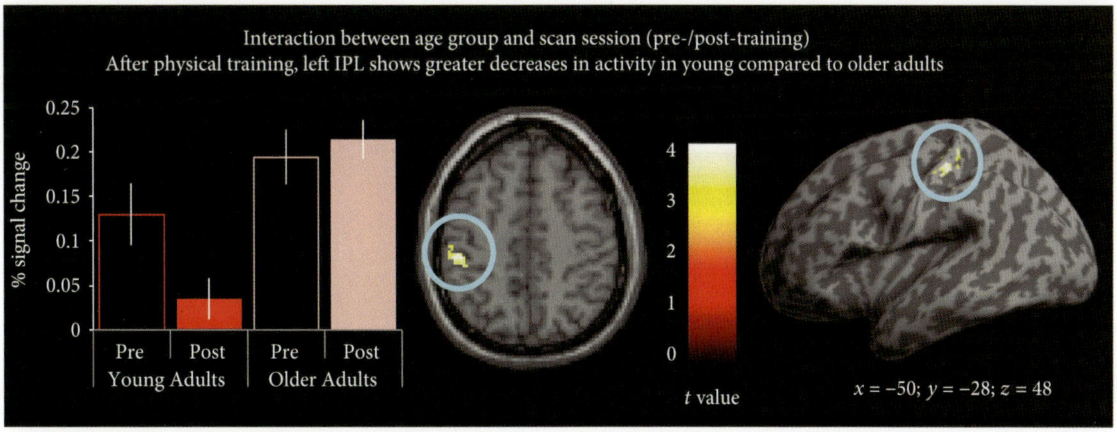

FIGURE 3: Training experience by age group interaction. The left inferior parietal lobule (IPL) demonstrates more marked decreases in engagement after physical training among the young adult participant sample compared to the older adults ($p_{\text{FWE-corr}} = 0.01$, $t = 4.3$).

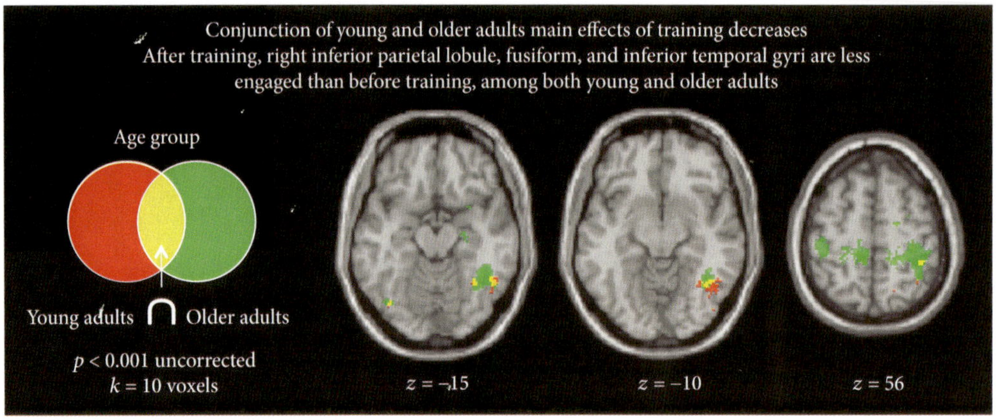

FIGURE 4: Common regions among young and older adults demonstrating a decreased response after physical training.

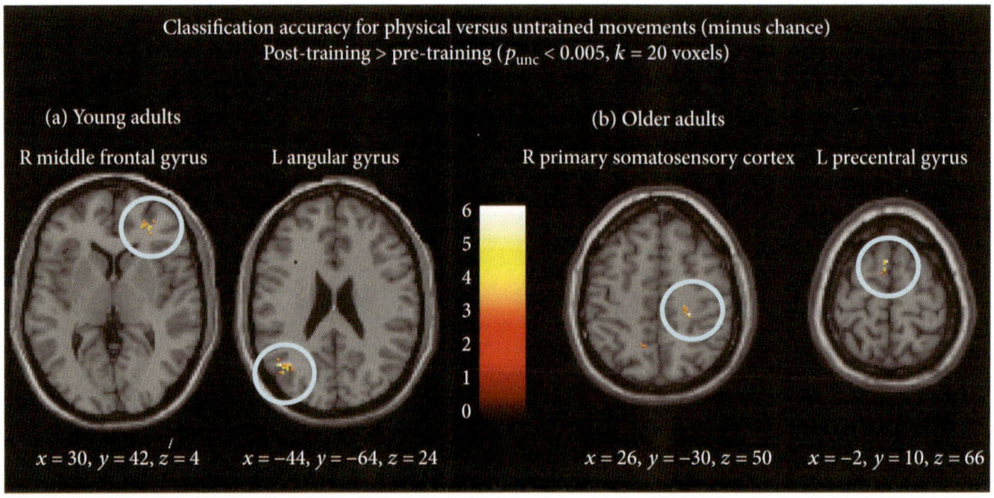

FIGURE 5: Regions that can accurately discriminate better between physically trained and untrained movements after training compared to before training. (a) In young adults. (b) In older adults. Coordinates of the centre of the cluster are given for all cluster-corrected regions (x, y, and z in MNI coordinates).

close to the FWEcorr threshold criteria ($p_{\text{FWEcorr}} = 0.05$ and $p_{\text{FWEcorr}} = 0.07$, resp.; Figure 5(b) and Table 3(b)).

3.3.2. Effect of Age on Discrimination Accuracy after Physical Training. In the following analyses, only accuracy maps from post-training scans were taken into account, to explore which regions can accurately discriminate between physically trained sequences and untrained sequences after training, comparing younger and older adults. When evaluating this contrast on the post-training data, the right superior parietal lobule and the right cerebellum discriminate between physically trained and untrained sequences more accurately in young adults compared to older adults (Figure 6(a) and Table 4(a)). In contrast, the inverse contrast, evaluating brain regions that discriminate between physically trained and untrained sequences better in older adults compared to young adults, yielded the right angular gyrus and left middle occipital gyrus (Figure 6(b) and Table 4(b)).

Finally, we conducted an exploratory conjunction analysis on the accuracy maps (using $t > 3.5$ as the threshold), to determine whether there were any common brain regions among young and older adults that could distinguish between physically trained and untrained sequences after training (for full results of these maps on day 5 for young and older adults separately, please see Supplementary Materials). This conjunction analysis yielded overlap across 794 voxels, including multiple subregions within the occipital cortex, as well as sensorimotor areas, including the left paracentral gyrus (Figure 7).

4. Discussion

In the present study, we manipulated the type of sensorimotor experience that young and older adults received with dance sequences to determine how experience shapes responses at behavioural and brain levels, during early and later adulthood. We set out to address three main questions: (i) How do different types of training influence complex action performance among young compared to older adults? (ii) How do different types of training shape brain responses at a global level during action observation among young compared to older adults? (iii) How does physical training shape brain responses at the level of action representations?

TABLE 3: Regions that can accurately discriminate better between physically trained and untrained movements after training compared to before training. (a) Young adults. (b) Older adults.

Region	BA	MNI coordinates x	y	z	t value	Cluster size	pFWEcorr value
(a) Physically trained versus untrained in younger adults							
L angular gyrus	**39**	**−44**	**−64**	**24**	**6.05**	**69**	**<0.001**
L angular gyrus	39	−34	−66	26	4.00		
L middle occipital gyrus	19	−38	−68	18	3.94		
R middle frontal gyrus	**10**	**30**	**42**	**4**	**4.68**	**40**	**0.048**
R middle frontal gyrus	10	28	48	−2	4.21		
R middle frontal gyrus		28	40	12	3.35		
(b) Physically trained versus untrained in older adults							
R postcentral gyrus	3	26	−30	50	6.12	46	0.053
R middle cingulate cortex		16	−28	46	4.38		
L precentral gyrus	6	−2	10	66	5.68	43	0.078
L precentral gyrus	6	−8	2	60	3.75		

BA: Brodmann's area; R: right, L: left. $p < 0.001$, uncorrected; $k = 10$ voxels. Regions in bold font are FWE cluster corrected at the $p < 0.05$ level. Up to three local maxima are listed when a cluster has multiple peaks more than 8 mm apart.

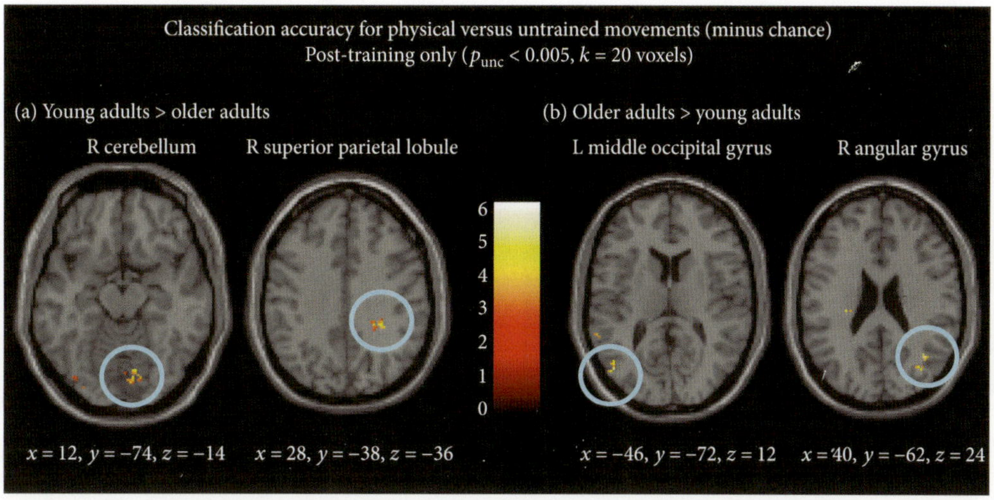

FIGURE 6: Direct comparison of classification accuracy for physical versus untrained sequences, minus chance, comparing young and older adults. (a) Brain regions that are better able to discriminate between physical and untrained movements in young adults compared to older adults. (b) Brain regions better able to discriminate between physical and untrained movements in older adults compared to young adults. Coordinates are reported in MNI space (x, y, and z).

Overall, participants' behavioural performance on motor and visual tasks improved across the training period, with younger adults showing greater performance gains than older adults. At the brain level, both age groups demonstrated overall *decreases* in sensorimotor cortical engagement after physical training, with younger adults showing more pronounced decreases in the inferior parietal lobule (IPL) activity compared to older adults. However, it is of note that the older adult population also showed an *increase* in precuneus activity after training. Neural decoding results show that among both young and older adults, visual and motor cortices contain experience-specific representations of new motor learning. In the following, we consider each of these findings, including how they relate to prior work and how they might form a foundation for future research.

4.1. Behavioural Differences between Younger and Older Adults. Both young and older adults' performance on both behavioural tasks (physical and visual learning tasks) improved across the four days of training. However, young adults outperformed older adults overall in terms of physical performance, and as Figure 2(a) shows, this performance discrepancy was present from the first day of training. This pattern of findings is likely explained by overall better physical condition and motor learning abilities among younger adults, whose movements are also more fluid than those made by individuals in advanced age [46, 63, 64]. However, the young adults did not outperform older adults in terms of recognition accuracy on the visual training task. This might be driven by the fact that participants in both age groups found the recognition task very easy, and the plots

TABLE 4: Physical versus untrained classification accuracy minus chance comparing young and older adults. (a) Young adults > older adults. (b) Older adults > young adults.

Region	BA	MNI coordinates x	y	z	t value	Cluster size	pFWEcorr value
(a) Young adults > older adults							
R superior parietal lobule		**28**	**−38**	**36**	**4.62**	**46**	**0.039**
R cerebellum		**12**	**−74**	**−14**	**4.43**	**81**	**<0.001**
R calcarine gyrus	18	14	−70	−6	4.35		
R lingual gyrus	17	8	−82	−12	3.86		
(b) Older adults > young adults							
R angular gyrus	**39**	**40**	**−62**	**24**	**4.28**	**46**	**0.039**
R middle occipital gyrus		34	−70	26	4.07		
L middle occipital gyrus	**19**	**−46**	**−72**	**12**	**4.24**	**47**	**0.034**
L middle temporal gyrus	39	−50	−62	18	4.15		
L middle temporal gyrus	39	−40	−60	20	3.62		

BA: Brodmann's area; R: right, L: left. $p < 0.001$, uncorrected; $k = 10$ voxels. Regions in bold font are FWE cluster corrected at the $p < 0.05$ level. Up to three local maxima are listed when a cluster has multiple peaks more than 8 mm apart.

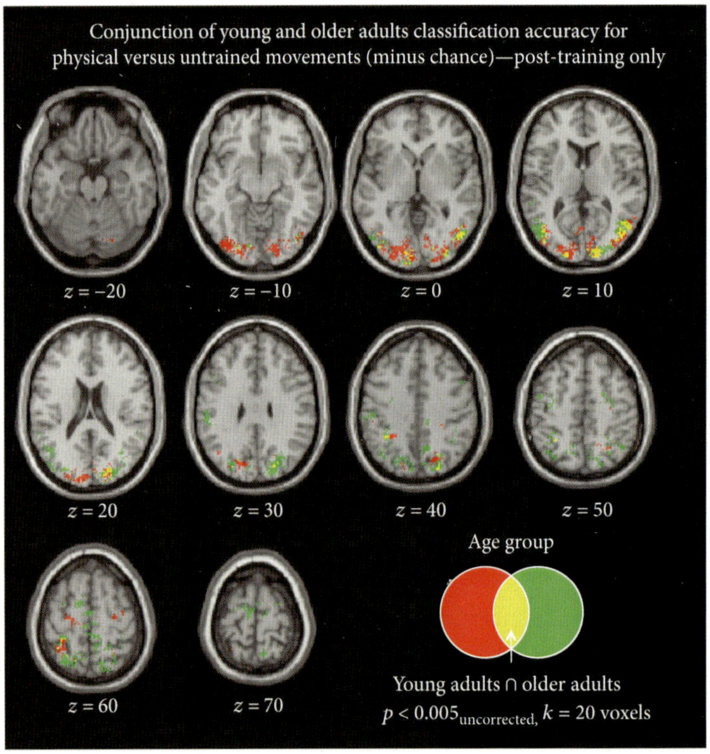

FIGURE 7: Conjunction analysis: common regions among young and older adults for accurately discriminating between physical and untrained sequences, on day 5.

of behavioural performance on this task (Figure 2(b)) document that participants from both age groups were more or less performing at ceiling from day 2 onwards.

When considering physical performance score discrepancies between young and older adults, it is also worth noting that the Kinect motion tracking system and the Xbox scoring system take into account the fluidity or smoothness of a performer's movements and participants have the potential to score many extra "bonus points" when they reproduce a move being performed by the avatar on screen in a particularly smooth manner. This aspect of the video game design might have penalized older adults' physical performance scores, as research demonstrates that gross bodily movements become less fluid/smooth with advancing age [46]. However, such differences between young and older adults' general kinematics should not affect the overall improvements across days within each age group, but here again, we also see more marked improvements among younger adults. To better understand the underlying neural basis for these differences between the two age groups, we investigated our main hypotheses by means of fMRI.

4.2. Effect of Training at a Global Brain Level during Action Observation. Taken together, the univariate analyses show a similar pattern of results among both young and older adults, characterised by activity decreases post-training. Specifically, evidence emerges that the right ITG and IPL, brain regions associated with the AON, show decreased response amplitude after physical training among both groups of participants. The left fusiform gyrus demonstrates a similar response profile in both groups. It thus appears that, regardless of age, physical training results in less recruitment of these sensorimotor and higher-order visual association cortices that are robustly recruited when observing unfamiliar or novel actions [26, 27, 65]. In a recent meta-analysis, Hardwick and colleagues [34] report similar decreases in activity among these same brain regions following motor learning, even though many of the studies included in this meta-analysis report increases in activity after training. This line of results helps to further illuminate how physical training influences brain regions recruited during observation of complex whole-body movements, with no other cue than a pared-down silhouetted representation of the movement.

The only increase of activity found after training in the present study emerged from the older adults group in the right precuneus, after both physical and visual training. This finding suggests that in advanced age, the precuneus is sensitive to the type of visuomotor training examined in the present study. More generally, the precuneus has been implicated in higher-order cognitive processes such as episodic memory, motor imagery, and spatial aspects of motor behaviour control [66–68] and has also been shown to respond more robustly during motor tasks in advanced age [69]. However, as this region did not emerge from the direct contrast comparing older and younger adults, it is not possible to conclude that its increased engagement when observing movements that have been associated with visuomotor or visual experience is due to age, per se. Further investigation, perhaps taking a longitudinal approach, would be beneficial for clarifying the relationship between precuneus activity, aging, and visuomotor learning.

The fact that we fail to find robust increases of activity within brain regions classically associated with the AON after physical training, as we report previously with similar training paradigm [3, 18], might seem surprising at first, until a number of factors are taken into consideration. First, the pattern of results we report here is broadly consistent with the fine movement motor learning literature [39, 59], which reliably documents decreases in whole brain activity after training as a signature of neural efficiency [17, 37, 70, 71]. For example, Higuchi and colleagues [71] report that for both observation and execution of guitar chords, reliable neural efficiency effects emerged across training days. The field would benefit from studies using complex, multisensory training paradigms looking more systematically at both increases and decreases of activity. A recent study by Gardner and colleagues has attempted to explore the issue of post-training increases and decreases in neural response amplitude by using guitar training to probe the subjective nature of the prediction error signal [17]. These authors report results consistent with a predictive coding account of AON engagement during action observation and execution that also takes into account effects of changes in neural efficiency, providing a promising theoretical grounding for taking this work further.

It is also important to consider how the training and testing approach used in the present study differs from prior work that reports increased response amplitude with increased experience (e.g., [5, 6, 19, 22, 49]). First, many prior studies look at effects of years, if not decades, of training experience on perception [5, 6, 22], while those examining the effects of aging often study how physical skills that older adults learned when they were still young are perceived [43, 49]. Such a short-term training intervention, like the one used in the present study, might thus be suboptimal for generating robust age-related differences in brain activity. In addition, the movements observed during brain scanning were far simpler in the present study than those used in many previous studies [6, 18, 19, 22, 53]. As such, the kind of learning examined in the present study might be quite different from what our group and others have previously found [18, 49]. In further contrast to previous studies, the pared-down action silhouettes used here revealed no further information about each action beyond its kinematics [48]. This means that any training effect found at the brain level should be linked to pure motor learning and visual movement processing, which might further contribute to subtle findings compared to previous work in this vein. Moreover, in contrast to recent work by our group [18], it is important to note that the task participants performed in the scanner was also markedly different and very likely contributed to the different pattern of results we report here. In Kirsch and Cross's earlier study [18], each trial was followed by one of two questions: "How much did you *like* the movement you just watched?" and "How well could you *reproduce* the movement you just watched?" It should be evident that these two questions required much deeper kinematic, visual, and aesthetic processing than what was required in the present study (participants watch closely each movement and respond to occasional probe questions about very simple kinematic features of the previously viewed movement). For this reason, it is imperative to consider the different tasks and stimuli when evaluating discrepant results reported by previous studies that have used similar training paradigms, such as Kirsch and Cross [18], and the present study. These different patterns of findings also provide a useful consideration for future studies, namely, future work can examine the extent to which decreases in sensorimotor engagement following training are due to strengthened purely 'kinematic' representations or to observers' not being prompted to think about their physical abilities to reproduce observed moves during action observation.

Even though the right IPL was found to be less activated after training among both age groups (Figure 4), the left IPL was the only region to demonstrate more marked decreases in engagement after physical training among young compared to older adults (Figure 3). The parameter estimate plot on this figure suggests that this finding is being driven by decrease in IPL engagement among young adults, while this region's response profile remains relatively unchanged among older adults. This could be indicative of processing efficiency gains among young adults that are simply not present among older adults. It is to note that no regions showed a greater decrease or increase after training in older adults compared to younger adults, when we control for physical gain performance. The IPL is one of the core regions of the AON, and its activity has been shown to be modulated by training [6, 16, 18].

In terms of visual training effects, we observed decreased engagement of sensorimotor and visual processing regions among young adults, similar to physical training. This is in line with previous literature showing common regions sensitive to observational and physical training [1–3, 14, 18]. However, among older adults, no regions showed decreased activity after visual training. This raises the possibility that visual training effects among older adults are either subtler or perhaps altogether different, perhaps due to declines in attentional and visual processing decline with advancing age [34]. A challenge for future research will be to examine in more depth age-related differences in observational training effects, possibly using a different task that can better capture performance and improvement via observation (which our task clearly failed to capture, as all participants were performing at ceiling by day 2).

Moreover, taking into account the results from the training modality categorization task participants completed after the post-training scan session, one could argue that the differences seen between young and older adults' brain activity is due to older adults not being able to accurately identify the training modality of the observed movements. Our results show that older adults performed more poorly than young adults on this task overall and that they were more likely to categorize untrained moves as trained. This finding of a carry-over effect is consistent with previous studies showing that older adults frequently show this tendency to misclassify new material as being familiar, which has been interpreted as showing that internal representations of events become more rigid with age [72]. However, as this categorization task did not include multiple trials for each stimulus (thus reducing its power) and our main aim was to examine differences before and after training within one training category (physical practice), we are reluctant to place too much stock in age differences on this task in our particular study. One final reason to be cautious with how we interpret young and older adults' performance on the categorization task is because even if older adults do not explicitly recognize the training category to which each stimulus belongs as well as younger adults, our main interest was in the neural implementation of the training, where we do see differences.

4.3. Examining the Impact of Physical Training on a Representational Level. The present study was designed to enable investigation of how physical training shapes brain responses not just at the level of magnitude differences but also at the level of more fine-grained action representations. The aim of our first set of pattern analyses was to identify brain regions that can distinguish between physical and untrained movement sequences after training compared to pre-training, among young and older adults separately. We predicted this between-category classification accuracy to be better overall after training compared to before training, when all stimuli were equally unfamiliar. Among younger adults, we found that the left angular gyrus and MFG could discriminate better after training between physically trained and untrained sequences, whereas among older adults, the left supplementary motor area and sensorimotor cortex could discriminate better after training between physically trained and untrained sequences.

The second set of analyses compared classification accuracies between the age groups, in particular their accuracy at distinguishing between physically trained and untrained sequence after physical training. These analyses yielded clear age-related differences, with better discrimination within the right superior parietal lobule and cerebellum in young compared to that in older adults. In contrast, older adults showed better discrimination in visual processing areas and multisensory integration areas such as the right angular gyrus and left MOG, compared to young adults.

This broad pattern of results is consistent with literature documenting that older adults rely more on sensory cortices during action observation than younger adults, even if the observed actions are familiar to them [47]. Computational models of cognitive aging posit that neural representations become less distinctive in old age [73]. Recent work by Carp and colleagues [74] reported that neural distinctiveness was reduced in older adults throughout the motor network. Neuroimaging studies of visual perception support this view, indicating that distributed patterns of brain activation evoked by different visual stimuli are less distinctive among older adults compared to young adults [75, 76]. In the present study, our findings do not speak to reductions in neural distinctiveness in advanced age per se, but instead we find different regions involved in distinguishing between different categories of stimuli (physically trained versus untrained) in young compared to older adults. As such, our findings suggest that the kind of training manipulation we used here has a specific effect that goes beyond the natural dedifferentiation that occurs with aging and instead leads to distinct networks mediating training-induced neural representations among young compared to older adults. While this part of the study was exploratory in nature, it provides useful point of departure for continued investigation of the changing nature of the representation of new sensorimotor learning across the lifespan. Moreover, one might speculate that older adults process the stimuli differently than younger adults or are at a different stage of learning when being scanned (as the behavioural data might suggest). These factors could also explain some of the differences seen with young adults. Older adults might still be in the consolidation phase on day 5, whereas in young adults, the top-down modulation of sensory regions has possibly already taken place [45, 47, 77]. Future studies could add scanning sessions at more time points (or include longer training manipulations with scanning sessions interspersed regularly throughout them), in order to explore whether older adults achieve the same performance as young adults, which is also reflected as (more) similar patterns of brain activation.

Finally, we explored which brain regions among young and older adults similarly distinguish between physically trained and untrained movements post-training. This conjunction analysis yielded common regions in occipital and motor cortices, demonstrating finer motor representations on day 5 for both age groups. This suggests that physical training plays an important role in the coding of fine movements in higher-order visual and motor areas, lending further support to the neural efficiency theory and findings in the motor domain [39].

4.4. Limitations and Future Directions. As with any study and with exploratory studies in particular, this work has several important limitations and has raised a number of possibilities for future research that warrant consideration. Since the present study was the first to tackle questions of complex action learning at brain and behavioural levels among young and older adults, we chose to investigate age group differences when both groups attempt to learn initially novel actions for the same amount of time. In this way, performance at the end of training was consequently not matched between the age groups. Thus, we cannot clearly disentangle whether our between-age group results are related to the way participants learn and represent dance sequences or due to the fact that young and older adults are at different stages of the learning process. An alternative design could have continued training the older adults until they performed at the same level as the younger adults and then compared brain activity. Future studies might explore this possibility and implement paradigms in which performance is better matched at the end of training. However, with respect to physically trained sequences in particular, general changes in motor control might prevent older adults from reaching the same performance level as younger adults irrespective of the amount of training provided [63].

Moreover, the technology used for our training intervention might have had an impact on participants' dance experience and the extent to which they perceive the task as "real" dancing. Similarly, age differences could possibly impact participants' willingness to dance in front of a large TV with avatars. However, devices such as the Kinect system have become more and more common in many households in recent years. Consequently, more on more people, including older generations, are becoming accustomed to interacting with them (and indeed, several of our older participants mentioned at the conclusion of the study that they had seen their grandchildren playing games with the Xbox Kinect in the past and had never participated as they thought the technology was not for them, but their minds had been changed since taking part in our study). In addition, we asked older adults to try the Kinect dance set up in a separate session before actual testing, and only those older adults who felt comfortable to do the training took part in the main experiment. Finally, as all participants also reported having enjoyed the experience, we believe that our results are not biased due to differences in the perception of the training set-up between young and older adults.

5. Conclusions

To our knowledge, this is the first study to combine a complex, whole-body training paradigm with univariate and multivariate analyses to investigate the impact of sensorimotor learning on action representations among young and older adults. While this study was exploratory in nature, our results should contribute to building a more complete picture of age-related changes in experience-dependent plasticity. Ultimately, we hope that insights gained from this approach will inform visuomotor learning and rehabilitation interventions for those in early and advanced adulthood.

Conflicts of Interest

The authors declare no competing financial interests.

Acknowledgments

The authors would like to thank Jörn Diedrichsen for outstanding MVPA advice and support at the start of this project, as well as our young and older adult participants for their commitment to the training procedures. This work was supported by the following funding to Emily S. Cross: Economic and Social Research Council Future Research Leaders award (ES/K001892/1); Marie Curie Career Integration award (CIG11-2012-322256), and European Research Council starting Grant (ERC-2015-677270).

Supplementary Materials

Supplementary Table 1: regions that can accurately discriminate better between physically trained and untrained movements on day 5. (a) Younger adults. (b) Older adults. Supplementary Figure 1: recognition accuracy average scores in young and older adults. After the post-training scan on day 5, participants watched each dance movie stimulus again (6 training conditions) and were asked to categorize them as either being physically trained, visually trained, or untrained. *(Supplementary Materials)*

References

[1] W. Prinz, "A common coding approach to perception and action," in *Relationships between Perception and Action: Current Approaches*, O. Neumann and W. Prinz, Eds., pp. 167–201, Spring-Verlag, Berlin, 1990.

[2] S. H. Frey and V. E. Gerry, "Modulation of neural activity during observational learning of actions and their sequential orders," *The Journal of Neuroscience*, vol. 26, no. 51, pp. 13194–13201, 2006.

[3] E. S. Cross, D. J. M. Kraemer, A. F. C. Hamilton, W. M. Kelley, and S. T. Grafton, "Sensitivity of the action observation network to physical and observational learning," *Cerebral Cortex*, vol. 19, no. 2, pp. 315–326, 2009.

[4] S. Vogt and R. Thomaschke, "From visuo-motor interactions to imitation learning: behavioural and brain imaging

studies," *Journal of Sports Sciences*, vol. 25, no. 5, pp. 497–517, 2007.

[5] B. Calvo-Merino, D. E. Glaser, J. Grèzes, R. E. Passingham, and P. Haggard, "Action observation and acquired motor skills: an FMRI study with expert dancers," *Cerebral Cortex*, vol. 15, no. 8, pp. 1243–1249, 2005.

[6] E. S. Cross, A. F. C. Hamilton, and S. T. Grafton, "Building a motor simulation de novo: observation of dance by dancers," *NeuroImage*, vol. 31, no. 3, pp. 1257–1267, 2006.

[7] H. Lee and U. Noppeney, "Long-term music training tunes how the brain temporally binds signals from multiple senses," *Proceedings of the National Academy of Sciences of the United States of America*, vol. 108, no. 51, pp. E1441–E1450, 2011.

[8] S. L. Liew, T. Sheng, and L. Aziz-Zadeh, "Experience with an amputee modulates one's own sensorimotor response during action observation," *NeuroImage*, vol. 69, pp. 138–145, 2013.

[9] N. N. Rüther, E. C. Brown, A. Klepp, and C. Bellebaum, "Observed manipulation of novel tools leads to mu rhythm suppression over sensory-motor cortices," *Behavioural Brain Research*, vol. 261, pp. 328–335, 2014.

[10] E. S. Cross, A. F. C. Hamilton, D. J. M. Kraemer, W. M. Kelley, and S. T. Grafton, "Dissociable substrates for body motion and physical experience in the human action observation network," *The European Journal of Neuroscience*, vol. 30, no. 7, pp. 1383–1392, 2009.

[11] J. Jastorff, Z. Kourtzi, and M. A. Giese, "Visual learning shapes the processing of complex movement stimuli in the human brain," *The Journal of Neuroscience*, vol. 29, no. 44, pp. 14026–14038, 2009.

[12] C. Jola, A. Abedian-Amiri, A. Kuppuswamy, F. E. Pollick, and M. H. Grosbras, "Motor simulation without motor expertise: enhanced corticospinal excitability in visually experienced dance spectators," *PLoS One*, vol. 7, no. 3, article e33343, 2012.

[13] A. A. G. Mattar and P. L. Gribble, "Motor learning by observing," *Neuron*, vol. 46, no. 1, pp. 153–160, 2005.

[14] S. Torriero, M. Oliveri, G. Koch, C. Caltagirone, and L. Petrosini, "The what and how of observational learning," *Journal of Cognitive Neuroscience*, vol. 19, no. 10, pp. 1656–1663, 2007.

[15] E. S. Cross, N. R. Cohen, A. F. C. Hamilton, R. Ramsey, G. Wolford, and S. T. Grafton, "Physical experience leads to enhanced object perception in parietal cortex: insights from knot tying," *Neuropsychologia*, vol. 50, no. 14, pp. 3207–3217, 2012.

[16] E. S. Cross, A. F. C. Hamilton, N. R. Cohen, and S. T. Grafton, "Learning to tie the knot: the acquisition of functional object representations by physical and observational experience," *PLoS One*, vol. 12, no. 10, article e0185044, 2017.

[17] T. Gardner, A. Aglinskas, and E. S. Cross, "Using guitar learning to probe the Action Observation Network's response to visuomotor familiarity," *NeuroImage*, vol. 156, pp. 174–189, 2017.

[18] L. P. Kirsch and E. S. Cross, "Additive routes to action learning: layering experience shapes engagement of the action observation network," *Cerebral Cortex*, vol. 25, no. 12, pp. 4799–4811, 2015.

[19] B. Calvo-Merino, J. Grèzes, D. E. Glaser, R. E. Passingham, and P. Haggard, "Seeing or doing? Influence of visual and motor familiarity in action observation," *Current Biology*, vol. 16, no. 19, pp. 1905–1910, 2006.

[20] J. F. Christensen, A. Gomila, S. B. Gaigg, N. Sivarajah, and B. Calvo-Merino, "Dance expertise modulates behavioral and psychophysiological responses to affective body movement," *Journal of Experimental Psychology. Human Perception and Performance*, vol. 42, no. 8, pp. 1139–1147, 2016.

[21] L. P. Kirsch, K. A. Drommelschmidt, and E. S. Cross, "The impact of sensorimotor experience on affective evaluation of dance," *Frontiers in Human Neuroscience*, vol. 7, p. 521, 2013.

[22] G. Orgs, J. H. Dombrowski, M. Heil, and P. Jansen-Osmann, "Expertise in dance modulates alpha/beta event-related desynchronization during action observation," *The European Journal of Neuroscience*, vol. 27, no. 12, pp. 3380–3384, 2008.

[23] G. Buccino, F. Lui, N. Canessa et al., "Neural circuits involved in the recognition of actions performed by nonconspecifics: an fMRI study," *Journal of Cognitive Neuroscience*, vol. 16, no. 1, pp. 114–126, 2004.

[24] S. Shimada, "Deactivation in the sensorimotor area during observation of a human agent performing robotic actions," *Brain and Cognition*, vol. 72, no. 3, pp. 394–399, 2010.

[25] V. Gazzola, H. van der Worp, T. Mulder, B. Wicker, G. Rizzolatti, and C. Keysers, "Aplasics born without hands mirror the goal of hand actions with their feet," *Current Biology*, vol. 17, no. 14, pp. 1235–1240, 2007.

[26] S.-L. Liew, T. Sheng, J. L. Margetis, and L. Aziz-Zadeh, "Both novelty and expertise increase action observation network activity," *Frontiers in Human Neuroscience*, vol. 7, p. 541, 2013.

[27] E. S. Cross, R. Liepelt, A. F. d. C. Hamilton et al., "Robotic movement preferentially engages the action observation network," *Human Brain Mapping*, vol. 33, no. 9, pp. 2238–2254, 2012.

[28] C. M. Tipper, G. Signorini, and S. T. Grafton, "Body language in the brain: constructing meaning from expressive movement," *Frontiers in Human Neuroscience*, vol. 9, p. 450, 2015.

[29] C. Babiloni, C. del Percio, P. M. Rossini et al., "Judgment of actions in experts: a high-resolution EEG study in elite athletes," *NeuroImage*, vol. 45, no. 2, pp. 512–521, 2009.

[30] C. Babiloni, N. Marzano, F. Infarinato et al., ""Neural efficiency" of experts' brain during judgment of actions: a high-resolution EEG study in elite and amateur karate athletes," *Behavioural Brain Research*, vol. 207, no. 2, pp. 466–475, 2010.

[31] C. del Percio, C. Babiloni, N. Marzano et al., ""Neural efficiency" of athletes' brain for upright standing: a high-resolution EEG study," *Brain Research Bulletin*, vol. 79, no. 3-4, pp. 193–200, 2009.

[32] V. B. Penhune and J. Doyon, "Cerebellum and M1 interaction during early learning of timed motor sequences," *NeuroImage*, vol. 26, no. 3, pp. 801–812, 2005.

[33] E. Dayan and L. G. Cohen, "Neuroplasticity subserving motor skill learning," *Neuron*, vol. 72, no. 3, pp. 443–454, 2011.

[34] R. M. Hardwick, C. Rottschy, R. C. Miall, and S. B. Eickhoff, "A quantitative meta-analysis and review of motor learning in the human brain," *NeuroImage*, vol. 67, pp. 283–297, 2013.

[35] V. B. Penhune and C. J. Steele, "Parallel contributions of cerebellar, striatal and M1 mechanisms to motor sequence learning," *Behavioural Brain Research*, vol. 226, no. 2, pp. 579–591, 2012.

[36] N. N. Oosterhof, A. J. Wiggett, and E. S. Cross, "Testing key predictions of the associative account of mirror neurons in humans using multivariate pattern analysis," *Behavioral and Brain Sciences*, vol. 37, no. 2, pp. 213–215, 2014.

[37] C. J. Steele and V. B. Penhune, "Specific increases within global decreases: a functional magnetic resonance imaging investigation of five days of motor sequence learning," *The Journal of Neuroscience*, vol. 30, no. 24, pp. 8332–8341, 2010.

[38] N. N. Oosterhof, S. P. Tipper, and P. E. Downing, "Viewpoint (in)dependence of action representations: an MVPA study," *Journal of Cognitive Neuroscience*, vol. 24, no. 4, pp. 975–989, 2012.

[39] T. Wiestler and J. Diedrichsen, "Skill learning strengthens cortical representations of motor sequences," *eLife*, vol. 2, article e00801, 2013.

[40] J. A. Bernard and R. D. Seidler, "Moving forward: age effects on the cerebellum underlie cognitive and motor declines," *Neuroscience & Biobehavioral Reviews*, vol. 42, pp. 193–207, 2014.

[41] A. Saimpont, F. Malouin, B. Tousignant, and P. L. Jackson, "The influence of body configuration on motor imagery of walking in younger and older adults," *Neuroscience*, vol. 222, pp. 49–57, 2012.

[42] J. F. Norman, S. M. Payton, J. R. Long, and L. M. Hawkes, "Aging and the perception of biological motion," *Psychology and Aging*, vol. 19, no. 1, pp. 219–225, 2004.

[43] N. Diersch, E. S. Cross, W. Stadler, S. Schütz-Bosbach, and M. Rieger, "Representing others' actions: the role of expertise in the aging mind," *Psychological Research*, vol. 76, no. 4, pp. 525–541, 2012.

[44] L. Zapparoli, P. Invernizzi, M. Gandola et al., "Mental images across the adult lifespan: a behavioural and fMRI investigation of motor execution and motor imagery," *Experimental Brain Research*, vol. 224, no. 4, pp. 519–540, 2013.

[45] N. Diersch, A. L. Jones, and E. S. Cross, "The timing and precision of action prediction in the aging brain," *Human Brain Mapping*, vol. 37, no. 1, pp. 54–66, 2016.

[46] M. C. Costello and E. K. Bloesch, "Are older adults less embodied? A review of age effects through the lens of embodied cognition," *Frontiers in Psychology*, vol. 8, p. 267, 2017.

[47] E. Kuehn, M. B. Perez-Lopez, N. Diersch, J. Döhler, T. Wolbers, and M. Riemer, "Embodiment in the aging mind," *Neuroscience & Biobehavioral Reviews*, vol. 86, pp. 207–225, 2018.

[48] D. K. Sumanapala, L. A. Fish, A. L. Jones, and E. S. Cross, "Have I grooved to this before? Discriminating practised and observed actions in a novel context," *Acta Psychologica*, vol. 175, pp. 42–49, 2017.

[49] N. Diersch, K. Mueller, E. S. Cross, W. Stadler, M. Rieger, and S. Schütz-Bosbach, "Action prediction in younger versus older adults: neural correlates of motor familiarity," *PLoS One*, vol. 8, no. 5, article e64195, 2013.

[50] M. N. Hebart, K. Görgen, and J. D. Haynes, "The decoding toolbox (TDT): a versatile software package for multivariate analyses of functional imaging data," *Frontiers in Neuroinformatics*, vol. 8, p. 88, 2015.

[51] M. F. Folstein, S. E. Folstein, and P. R. McHugh, ""Mini-mental state": a practical method for grading the cognitive state of patients for the clinician," *Journal of Psychiatric Research*, vol. 12, no. 3, pp. 189–198, 1975.

[52] R. C. Oldfield, "The assessment and analysis of handedness: the Edinburgh inventory," *Neuropsychologia*, vol. 9, no. 1, pp. 97–113, 1971.

[53] B. Calvo-Merino, C. Jola, D. E. Glaser, and P. Haggard, "Towards a sensorimotor aesthetics of performing art," *Consciousness and Cognition*, vol. 17, no. 3, pp. 911–922, 2008.

[54] C. Giacosa, F. J. Karpati, N. E. V. Foster, V. B. Penhune, and K. L. Hyde, "Dance and music training have different effects on white matter diffusivity in sensorimotor pathways," *NeuroImage*, vol. 135, pp. 273–286, 2016.

[55] F. J. Karpati, C. Giacosa, N. E. V. Foster, V. B. Penhune, and K. L. Hyde, "Sensorimotor integration is enhanced in dancers and musicians," *Experimental Brain Research*, vol. 234, no. 3, pp. 893–903, 2016.

[56] D. H. Brainard, "The psychophysics toolbox," *Spatial Vision*, vol. 10, no. 4, pp. 433–436, 1997.

[57] D. G. Pelli, "The VideoToolbox software for visual psychophysics: transforming numbers into movies," *Spatial Vision*, vol. 10, no. 4, pp. 437–442, 1997.

[58] M. Kleiner, D. H. Brainard, D. G. Pelli, A. Ingling, R. Murray, and C. Broussard, "What's new in Psychtoolbox-3," *Perception*, vol. 36, no. 14, pp. 1–6, 2007.

[59] C. Bellebaum, M. Tettamanti, E. Marchetta et al., "Neural representations of unfamiliar objects are modulated by sensorimotor experience," *Cortex*, vol. 49, no. 4, pp. 1110–1125, 2013.

[60] C. Cortes and V. Vapnik, "Support-vector networks," *Machine Learning*, vol. 20, no. 3, pp. 273–297, 1995.

[61] N. Kriegeskorte, *Crossvalidation in Brain Imaging Analysis*, BioRxiv, 2015.

[62] K. R. Muller, S. Mika, G. Ratsch, K. Tsuda, and B. Scholkopf, "An introduction to kernel-based learning algorithms," *IEEE Transactions on Neural Networks*, vol. 12, no. 2, pp. 181–201, 2001.

[63] R. D. Seidler, J. A. Bernard, T. B. Burutolu et al., "Motor control and aging: links to age-related brain structural, functional, and biochemical effects," *Neuroscience & Biobehavioral Reviews*, vol. 34, no. 5, pp. 721–733, 2010.

[64] M. E. Tinetti, "Performance-oriented assessment of mobility problems in elderly patients," *Journal of the American Geriatrics Society*, vol. 34, no. 2, pp. 119–126, 1986.

[65] E. S. Cross, W. Stadler, J. Parkinson, S. Schütz-Bosbach, and W. Prinz, "The influence of visual training on predicting complex action sequences," *Human Brain Mapping*, vol. 34, no. 2, pp. 467–486, 2013.

[66] A. E. Cavanna and M. R. Trimble, "The precuneus: a review of its functional anatomy and behavioural correlates," *Brain*, vol. 129, no. 3, pp. 564–583, 2006.

[67] C. Grefkes, A. Ritzl, K. Zilles, and G. R. Fink, "Human medial intraparietal cortex subserves visuomotor coordinate transformation," *NeuroImage*, vol. 23, no. 4, pp. 1494–1506, 2004.

[68] N. Wenderoth, F. Debaere, S. Sunaert, and S. P. Swinnen, "The role of anterior cingulate cortex and precuneus in the coordination of motor behaviour," *The European Journal of Neuroscience*, vol. 22, no. 1, pp. 235–246, 2005.

[69] P. Linortner, M. Jehna, H. Johansen-Berg et al., "Aging associated changes in the motor control of ankle movements in the brain," *Neurobiology of Aging*, vol. 35, no. 10, pp. 2222–2229, 2014.

[70] T. Wu, K. Kansaku, and M. Hallett, "How self-initiated memorized movements become automatic: a functional MRI study," *Journal of Neurophysiology*, vol. 91, no. 4, pp. 1690–1698, 2004.

[71] S. Higuchi, H. Holle, N. Roberts, S. B. Eickhoff, and S. Vogt, "Imitation and observational learning of hand actions: prefrontal involvement and connectivity," *NeuroImage*, vol. 59, no. 2, pp. 1668–1683, 2012.

[72] P. Vieweg, M. Stangl, L. R. Howard, and T. Wolbers, "Changes in pattern completion—a key mechanism to explain

age-related recognition memory deficits?," *Cortex*, vol. 64, pp. 343–351, 2015.

[73] K. Z. H. Li, U. Lindenberger, A. M. Freund, and P. B. Baltes, "Walking while memorizing: age-related differences in compensatory behavior," *Psychological Science*, vol. 12, no. 3, pp. 230–237, 2016.

[74] J. Carp, J. Park, A. Hebrank, D. C. Park, and T. A. Polk, "Age-related neural dedifferentiation in the motor system," *PLoS One*, vol. 6, no. 12, article e29411, 2011.

[75] J. Carp, J. Park, T. A. Polk, and D. C. Park, "Age differences in neural distinctiveness revealed by multi-voxel pattern analysis," *NeuroImage*, vol. 56, no. 2, pp. 736–743, 2011.

[76] J. Park, J. Carp, A. Hebrank, D. C. Park, and T. A. Polk, "Neural specificity predicts fluid processing ability in older adults," *The Journal of Neuroscience*, vol. 30, no. 27, pp. 9253–9259, 2010.

[77] C. Lustig, P. Shah, R. Seidler, and P. A. Reuter-Lorenz, "Aging, training, and the brain: a review and future directions," *Neuropsychology Review*, vol. 19, no. 4, pp. 504–522, 2009.

8

Reorganization of the Action Observation Network and Sensory-Motor System in Children with Unilateral Cerebral Palsy: An fMRI Study

Giuseppina Sgandurra,[1,2] Laura Biagi,[3] Leonardo Fogassi,[4] Elisa Sicola,[1] Adriano Ferrari,[5,6] Andrea Guzzetta,[1,2] Michela Tosetti,[3] and Giovanni Cioni[1,2]

[1]*Department of Developmental Neuroscience, IRCCS Fondazione Stella Maris, Calambrone, Pisa, Italy*
[2]*Department of Clinical and Experimental Medicine, University of Pisa, Pisa, Italy*
[3]*Laboratory of Medical Physics and Biotechnologies for Magnetic Resonance, IRCCS Fondazione Stella Maris, Calambrone, Pisa, Italy*
[4]*Department of Neuroscience, University of Parma and Istituto Italiano di Tecnologia (RTM), Parma, Italy*
[5]*IRCCS S. Maria Nuova Hospital, Reggio Emilia, Italy*
[6]*University of Modena and Reggio Emilia, Modena, Italy*

Correspondence should be addressed to Laura Biagi; laura.biagi@fsm.unipi.it

Academic Editor: Sergio Bagnato

Little is known about the action observation network (AON) in children with unilateral cerebral palsy (UCP). Using fMRI, we aimed to explore AON and sensory-motor network (SMN) in UCP children and compare them to typically developed (TD) children and analyse the relationship between AON (re-)organization and several neurophysiological and clinical measures. Twelve UCP children were assessed with clinical scales and transcranial magnetic stimulation (TMS). For the fMRI study, they underwent a paradigm based on observation of complex and simple object-manipulation tasks executed by dominant and nondominant hand. Moreover, UCP and TD children carried out a further fMRI session to explore SMN in both an active motor and passive sensory task. AON in the UCP group showed higher lateralization, negatively related to performances on clinical scales, and had greater activation of unaffected hemisphere as compared to the bilateral representation in the TD group. In addition, a good congruence was found between bilateral or contralateral activation of AON and activation of SMN and TMS data. These findings indicate that our paradigm might be useful in exploring AON and the response to therapy in UCP subjects.

1. Introduction

Functional representation of actions, either observed or performed or even imagined, relies on the human action observation network (AON), constituted by the premotor, inferior frontal, parietal, and temporal regions. Its functionality is crucial for action understanding and for subserving imitation by observation of new motor skills [1, 2].

Some neurophysiological studies exploring the presence and functionality of AON networks in children have suggested that maturation of AON has an age-related course from a more bilateral to a more lateralized representation, indicating physiological plasticity [3–5]. These properties are very meaningful, and it would be important to know if similar mechanisms could also be observed in pathological conditions such as unilateral or asymmetrical early brain injuries in children with unilateral cerebral palsy (UCP). It has been extensively demonstrated that the type of lesion and reorganization, studied through functional magnetic resonance imaging (fMRI) and transcranial magnetic stimulation (TMS), of the central nervous system have an impact on severity of upper limb deficits [6, 7]. Types of lesion, underlying UCP, are often categorized into three groups, according to location and timing of insult: type I (prenatal): malformations or 1st and 2nd trimester patterns, presumed to occur in utero such as lissencephaly, focal cortical dysplasia, unilateral schizencephaly; type II (perinatal): periventricular white matter lesions mainly occurring in the early 3rd trimester and often in preterm born infants such as periventricular leukomalacia (PVL); type III (connatal): cortical or deep grey matter lesions that occur towards the end of gestation, that is, around term age, such as infarcts in the territory of the middle cerebral artery (MCA) [7–9].

Previous studies have shown that children with type II lesions demonstrated better upper limb sensorimotor functioning, compared to children with type III lesions [10, 11]. Regarding type of motor reorganization, there are two main types of (re-)organization: ipsilesional and contralesional [12]. In adults with stroke and in some children, the main mechanism for reconnection of the motor cortex to spinal cord consists of (re-)organization within the ipsilesional cortex. This mechanism is based on partial sparing of the primary motor cortex or on the possibility that functions may be taken over by intact nonprimary motor areas within the damaged hemisphere (ipsilesional (re-)organization). However, when lesions occur at an early development stage, either during intrauterine life or soon after birth, a different mechanism can be observed. This is based on the persistence of a significant component of monosynaptic fast-conducting ipsilateral motor projections, normally withdrawing within the first months of life, that may be permanently maintained if brain damage occurs early in life [6, 13, 14]. In this case, the unaffected hemisphere directly controls both upper limbs, giving rise to a pattern of reorganization unknown in adult pathologies (contralesional (re-)organization). It has been extensively demonstrated that ipsilesional motor projection is definitely correlated to better motor outcomes, measured by functional scales (e.g., Melbourne Unilateral Upper Limb Measurement [15] and Assisting Hand Assessment [16]), than contralesional reorganization [11]. The sensory system generally follows an ipsilesional reorganization; but when a dissociation of sensorimotor representation occurs, that is, a contralesional reorganization for motor function and an ipsilesional reorganization for sensory one, quality of motor function is usually more affected [6].

Regarding AON in UCP children, Dinomais et al. [17] have shown, in eighteen UCP patients, aged 7–21 years, that observation at rest of a simple opening-closing hand movement performed by either the left or the right hand of an actor produces large bilateral activations in the occipito-temporo-parieto-frontal network, including most AON nodes. Moreover, a stronger ipsilesional activation of primary motor cortex (M1) was shown when they viewed movement of the hand corresponding to the affected one. Finally, observation of hand movement engaged motor execution networks regardless of degree of motor impairment.

The fMRI paradigm in this latter study was created around the observation of a simple movement without an object. We have developed an fMRI paradigm to explore AON based on the observation of simple and complex object-manipulation tasks executed by both dominant and nondominant hand. This fMRI paradigm has been already tested on healthy adults [18] and in a sample TD children [5].

The aim of this fMRI study was to explore AON and sensory-motor network (SMN) in UCP children in comparison to age-matched TD children and analyse the relationship between AON (re-)organization and several neurophysiological and clinical measures.

2. Methods

2.1. Subjects. Twelve UCP patients (6 with left UCP, age range = 6.2 – 16.3 y, mean age ± standard deviation (SD) = 10.3 ± 2.9 y) were enrolled in this study. The sample included seven males (age range = 7.5 – 14.5 y; mean age ± SD = 10.7 ± 2.6 y) and five females (age range = 6.2 – 16.3 y; mean age ± SD = 10.5 ± 4.0 y). All UCP children had IQ > 70.

Dataset from 12 healthy right-handed children and adolescents (6 M, 6 F; age range = 7.0 – 15.3 y, mean age ± SD (SD) = 10.6 ± 2.1 y) already described in a previous study [5] were used as age-matched controls (TD children).

All subjects and their parents gave written informed consent in accordance with protocol approved by the Ethics Committee of the IRCCS Fondazione Stella Maris.

2.2. Clinical Tests. All children were classified according to the House Functional Classification System (HFCS) for assessing upper limb function. HFCS consists of nine grades ranging from a completely excluded hand (grade 0) to a spontaneous and independent one (grade 8) [19, 20]. In addition, they were clinically assessed with two standardized function tests, Assisting Hand Assessment (AHA, Version 4.4) [16] and Melbourne Assessment of Unilateral Upper Limb Function (MUUL) [15], in order to evaluate assisting hand use during bimanual performance and upper limb movement capacity, respectively.

AHA is a standardized, criterion-referenced test based on observations of affected hand/arm used during a videotaped 15-minute play session with toys from the AHA test kit. Video scoring produces raw values ranging from 22 (low ability) to 88 (high ability) that are converted to scaled scores ranging from 0 to 100. AHA was administered and scored by a certified rater.

MUUL is a standardized tool for measuring quality of upper limb movement capacity during 16 criterion-referenced items representative of reach, grasp, release, and manipulation. Performance is videotaped and scored using criteria for rating qualities of movement range, fluency, and dexterity [15, 21]. Scores vary from 0 to 100%, the latter indicating best performance.

Presence or absence of mirror movements in the unaffected hand during voluntary unimanual movements of the affected hand was evaluated by consensus by two experienced child physical therapists (ES and EB, 30 and 8 years of experience in clinical evaluation of UCP), analyzing the videotapes of the standardized clinical tests.

2.3. Transcranial Magnetic Stimulation. TMS was performed using a mapping procedure as described in Borghetti et al. [22], by using a Magstim 200® device (Magstim Company Ltd., Whitland, Wales, UK) connected to a figure-eight coil (diameter: 11 cm). Both hemispheres were searched

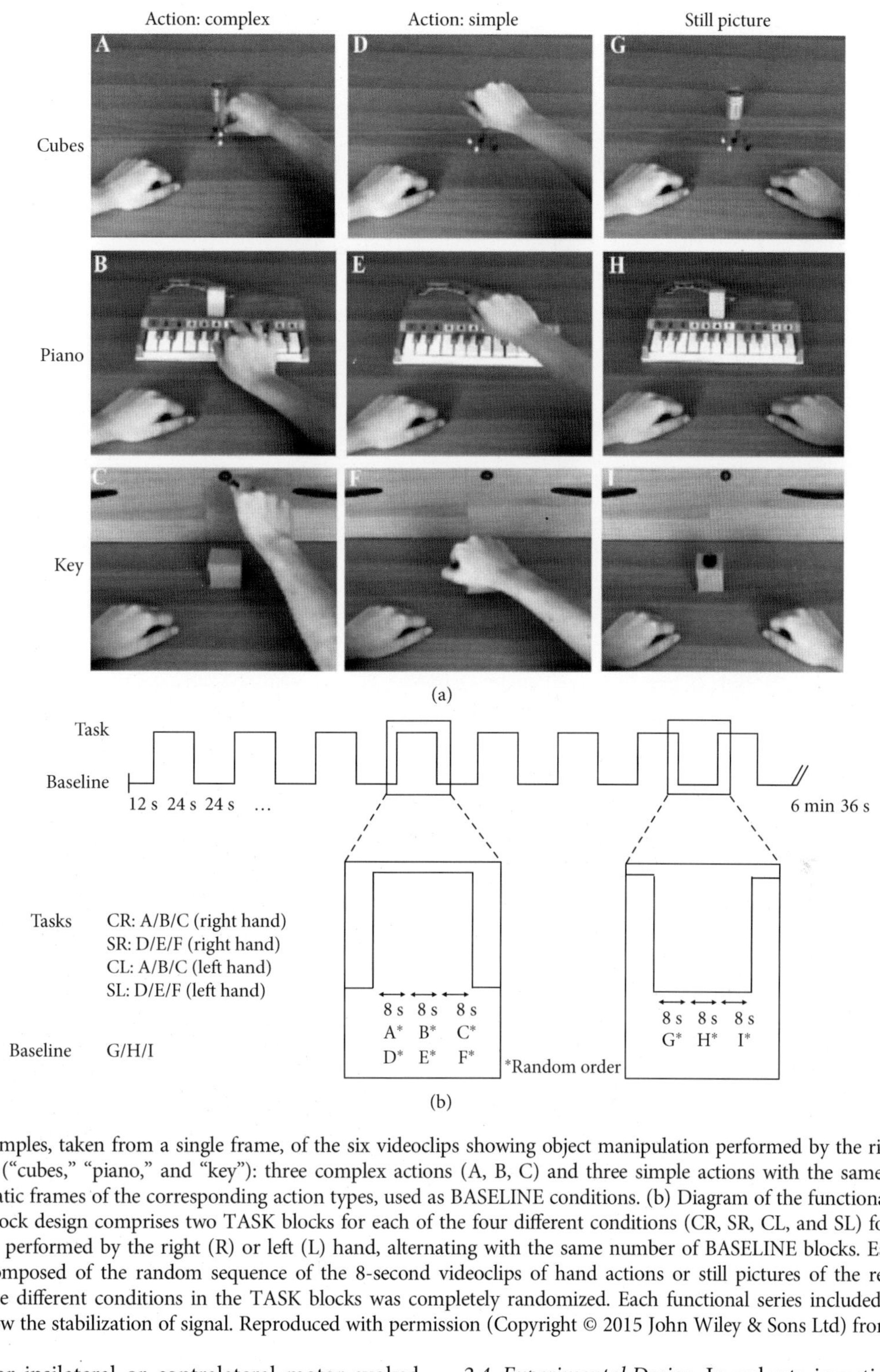

FIGURE 1: (a) Examples, taken from a single frame, of the six videoclips showing object manipulation performed by the right hand in three different contexts ("cubes," "piano," and "key"): three complex actions (A, B, C) and three simple actions with the same object (D, E, F). (G, H, I) Initial static frames of the corresponding action types, used as BASELINE conditions. (b) Diagram of the functional series presented to children: the block design comprises two TASK blocks for each of the four different conditions (CR, SR, CL, and SL) for complex (C) or simple (S) actions performed by the right (R) or left (L) hand, alternating with the same number of BASELINE blocks. Each block lasts 24 seconds and is composed of the random sequence of the 8-second videoclips of hand actions or still pictures of the resting hands. The presentation of the different conditions in the TASK blocks was completely randomized. Each functional series included four initial extra scans (12 s) to allow the stabilization of signal. Reproduced with permission (Copyright © 2015 John Wiley & Sons Ltd) from Biagi et al. [5].

systematically for ipsilateral or contralateral motor-evoked potentials, during a monitored low-level contraction of abductor digiti minimi (ADM) muscles. TMS results were used globally to establish the type of reorganization of sensorimotor system. In particular, contralesional (CL) reorganization was used to indicate a reorganization involving the unaffected hemisphere, and ipsilesional (IL) for a reorganization involving the lesioned hemisphere. Data acquisition was conducted following the international guidelines for TMS in children for aspects of safety [23].

2.4. Experimental Design. In order to investigate the relation of AON with reorganization of SMN, two different fMRI paradigms were used.

AON was explored as described by Biagi et al. [5]. Eight-second videoclips in a first-person perspective of three simple and three complex hand actions, performed by dominant and nondominant hand, were presented (Figure 1(a)). The three complex actions were grasping little cubes and putting them into a box (cubes), performing a simple scale on a piano keyboard (piano), and grasping a key, putting it into a lock, and turning it (key). The three simple actions consisted of a whole hand grasping a small box performed in the same visual contexts of the complex actions, in order to match luminance, colour, and visual information. Videoclips of the same type (hand, complexity) in the three contexts (cubes, piano, and key) were randomly combined to create four distinct conditions (TASKS), each lasting 24 seconds, corresponding to the presentation of a simple or a complex action performed by dominant or nondominant hand (simple-dominant (S-D), complex-dominant (C-D), simple-nondominant (S-ND), and complex-nondominant (C-ND)). The 24-second corresponding control condition (BASELINE) was created by combining a sequence of three still pictures of resting hands in the respective contexts. The paradigm of stimulus presentation was built on a block design scheme, with two blocks for each of the previous four TASKS intertwined with the same number of BASELINE blocks (16 blocks total). In each functional series, the order of TASKS blocks was randomly generated and four initial extra scans (dummies, 12 seconds) were added to allow for stabilization of signal, giving a total acquisition time of 6′36″ (Figure 1(b)). The AON experiment consisted of the acquisition of two functional series. Visual stimuli were presented through LCD goggles (Resonance Technology, USA). Subjects were asked to observe videos, staring at the middle of a screen. Gaze and attention to stimuli were continuously monitored using an eye tracker infrared camera mounted on goggles. Recorded eye movements were analysed to verify gaze and attention during AON stimuli.

For SMN localization, a block design paradigm was designed with both an active movement task (alternated hand opening and closing, MOTOR TASK) and a passive sensory task (palm and fingers passively brushed by an external operator by means of a wooden spatula, at a frequency of about 1 Hz, SENSORY TASK), in the same functional series. The series included eight blocks of 18 seconds each, alternating between motor and sensory tasks, each intertwined by an equivalent number of REST periods (REST-MOTOR TASK-REST-SENSORY TASK...). All subjects received detailed instructions before acquisition. They were asked to keep their eyes closed. During motor task, they were asked to repetitively open and close their hand at a frequency of 1 Hz; commands "move" and "stop" were given at the beginning and end of each block. During the sensory task and rest periods, they were asked simply to stay still. The examiner visually controlled the task performance. Each series included four initial extra scans (dummies, 12 seconds) for a total acquisition time of 5 minutes. Two sessions were performed, the first for the dominant hand and the second for the nondominant one, obtaining four conditions of interest (sensory-dominant (Sens-D), motor-dominant (Mot-D), sensory-nondominant (Sens-ND), and motor-nondominant (Mot-ND)).

During fMRI acquisitions, ambient scanner noise was constant and attenuated by ear plugs.

2.5. Imaging Acquisition and Processing. MR exams were performed on a 1.5 T MR scanner (HDx, GE Healthcare, Milwaukee, WI, USA). Standard MR protocol included FSE T2-weighted, SE T1-weighted, FLAIR, and DWI sequences. A whole brain, 3D high-resolution, T1-weighted series (FSPGR) was collected in an axial plane (TR/TE = 12.3 ms/2.4 ms; TI = 700 ms; voxel size = 1 mm^3 isotropic) for anatomic localization of activated regions and delineation and description of lesions.

MRI anatomical findings were classified retrospectively according to literature [7, 9] into three main forms related to timing of lesion: type I, brain malformations (early malformative); type II, abnormalities of periventricular white matter (prenatal); and type III, cortical-subcortical lesions, mainly due to middle cerebral artery infarction (connatal).

The fMRI session included four series, two functional series for AON task (each lasting 6′36″) and two series for sensory-motor task (5′00″), one for each hand. Blood oxygenation level-dependent (BOLD) responses were registered by using an echo planar imaging gradient-echo sequence (GRE-EPI) with the following parameters: TE/TE = 3000/50 ms, FA = 90°, field of view (FOV) = 240 × 240 mm, matrix = 64 × 64, slice thickness = 5 mm.

Data preprocessing, performed using BrainVoyager QX Software Package (BV, Brain Innovation, Maastricht, the Netherlands), included mean intensity adjustment to compensate for interscan intensity differences, temporal interpolation and resample to compensate for slice-dependent time differences (sinc function), 3D motion correction (sinc interpolation), and high-pass temporal filtering (GLM-Fourier approach, two cycles/time course).

Functional data were coregistered on the three-dimensional anatomical T1-weighted images by using an affine alignment with the standard BV nine parameters (three for translation, three for rotation, and three for FOV scale). Anatomical datasets were in turn transformed into standard Talairach's Space [24].

In order to combine data from UCP children in a group analysis, and considering that TD children were all right-handed, we designated the left hemisphere as the hemisphere contralateral to the dominant hand (unaffected hand in UCP, right hand in TD) and the right hemisphere as the hemisphere contralateral to the nondominant hand (affected hand in UCP, left hand in TD). To do this, we flipped the right-left (x) direction [17] of both functional and structural T1-weighted images of children with left hemisphere lesions (right hemiplegia), in order to have all lesioned hemispheres on the right side of the brain and all unaffected hemispheres on the left side.

2.6. fMRI and Statistical Analysis. BOLD responses were analysed using the general linear model (GLM) approach, using the same number of regressors as conditions of interest. Each regressor was obtained by convolving a box-car function for each stimulation block with the standard Boynton hemodynamic response function [25]. Four regressors were selected both for the AON stimulus (S-D, C-D, S-ND, and C-ND) and for the SMN task (Sens-D, Mot-D, Sens-ND, and Mot-ND). In all analyses, six spurious movement regressors (outputs of the 3D motion correction procedure) were included in GLM.

Table 1: Demographic and clinical data of children with UCP enrolled in fMRI study.

ID	Sex	Age (y)	Type of lesion	Side of hemiplegia	Type of reorganization	HFCS	MUUL	AHA	MM
1	M	7.5	I	RH	CL	5	72.13	65.15	Y
2	M	11.0	I	LH	CL	4	60	47	Y
3	M	11.5	I	LH	CL	5	74.59	60.61	Y
4	F	16.3	I	LH	CL	4	55	42	Y
5	M	8.1	II	RH	IL	7	90.98	86.36	N
6	M	10.6	II	RH	IL	8	93.58	77.27	N
7	F	12.0	II	LH	CL	5	79	53	Y
8	M	13.6	II	LH	CL	5	79.51	56.06	Y
9	F	6.2	II	RH	IL	6	81.15	63.64	Y
10	F	7.2	III	RH	IL	8	81.15	69.7	N
11	M	9.3	III	LH	IL	7	91	80.3	N
12	F	10.6	III	RH	CL	5	80.32	75.76	Y

F: female; M: male; y: years; I: early malformative; II: prenatal; III: connatal; RH: right hemiplegia; LH: left hemiplegia; IL: ipsilesional; CL: contralesional; HFCS: house functional classification system; MUUL: Melbourne Assessment of Unilateral Upper Limb Function; AHA: Assisting Hand Assessment; MM: mirror movements; Y: present; N: absent.

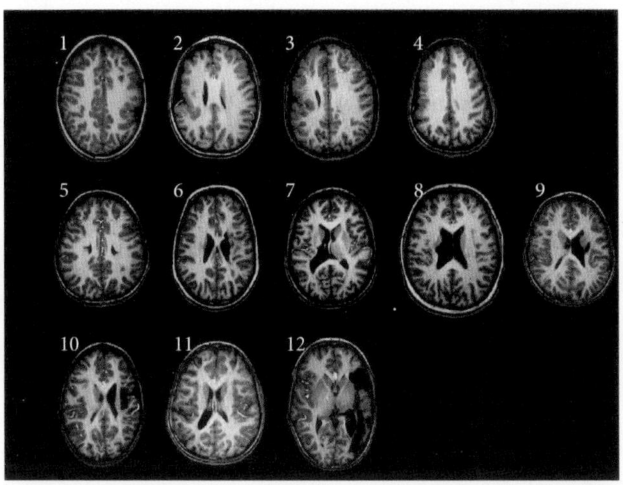

Figure 2: Representative slices of 3D T1-weighted images depicting the brain lesion of each UCP child. Numbers correspond to the ID of UCP children as reported in Table 1.

Multisubject analyses were conducted using random-effects (RFX) GLM-based analysis, for both groups (UCP and TD) in order to identify a group representation of cortical activations and to detect possible differences between groups. Threshold of statistical maps was $p < 0.05$ Bonferroni-corrected, and a minimum cluster size of 150 mm^3 was also applied. Group analyses were also used to reveal and define regions of interest (ROIs), to be selected subsequently in single-subject analysis.

For the AON stimulus, contrasted activity for all observed actions versus control condition was used (all TASKS > BASELINE) in order to identify possible differences in the representation of AON in UCP children with respect to their age-matched controls. Moreover, contrasted activities for observation of complex and simple actions performed by the dominant or nondominant hand versus control condition ((C-D + S-D) > BASELINE, (C-ND + S-ND) > BASELINE)) were also performed, in order to investigate hand identity properties in UCP children.

As in Biagi et al. [5, 18], a ROI analysis was conducted on activated areas in order to investigate possible differential responses to observation of both hands (laterality) and to observation of complex and simple actions (complexity). In particular, a 2×2 factorial design ANOVA was performed in specific areas (anterior intraparietal cortex (AIP), inferior temporal gyrus, MT, as control), considering as factors "hand" laterality (two levels: dominant and nondominant) and the "complexity" of action (two levels: simple and complex).

Finally, probabilistic functional maps were calculated to evaluate spatial consistency of activity patterns across subjects.

For the SMN task, two contrasts were employed, considering together sensory and motor stimuli of each hand, dominant or nondominant ((Sens-D + Mot-D) > REST and (Sens-ND + Mot-ND) > REST).

For the same contrasts, single-subject analyses were performed by using a fixed-effects (FFX) approach, with a lower, uncorrected statistical threshold ($p < 0.001$, minimum cluster size $\geq 150\ mm^3$) in order to extract, from each participant, coordinates of foci and number of activated voxels of areas identified by multisubject group analysis. Average and variability (defined as standard deviation divided by mean: SD/mean $\times$ 100) across subjects were also calculated. Moreover, a laterality index (LI) was calculated by comparing the size of homologous areas in both hemispheres. In particular, for the AON task, LI was obtained by computing the ratio $(N_{DS} - N_{nonDS})/(N_{DS} + N_{nonDS})$, where N_{DS} and N_{nonDS} are the number of activated voxels in the dominant side of the brain (DS, hemisphere contralateral to dominant hand) and in the nondominant side (non-DS, hemisphere contralateral to nondominant hand), respectively. For the SMN task, a laterality index was also calculated specifically for the primary sensorimotor cortex (pSMC), using the

Table 2: Areas elicited by observation of all object-related hand actions versus BASELINE condition in UCP children and age-matched TD children [5].

Area name	BA		UCP children					TD children				
			Talairach's coordinates			Cluster size	t-value	Talairach's coordinates			Cluster size	t-value
			x	y	z			x	y	z		
Inferior temporal gyrus	37	DS	−44	−65	0	8307	18.4	−44	−64	0	15,536	20.6
		Non-DS	47	−61	−2	8369	15.6	44	−61	1	18,659	18.7
Superior temporal gyrus	22	DS	−48	−35	12	1357	10.4	−51	−40	11	1531	8.2
		Non-DS	53	−33	9	1534	8.6	50	−40	11	2584	9.2
Inferior parietal lobule	40	DS	−44	−40	39	4278	7.6	−56	−31	30	3751	9.9
		Non-DS	48	−36	36	2281	7.7	57	−31	27	1669	6.9
Anterior IPS	40-7	DS	−36	−45	45	4231	12.7	−32	−44	50	4806	15.4
		Non-DS	37	−50	48	3023	7.3	33	−45	49	2265	10.6
Superior parietal lobule	7	DS	−16	−66	45	5112	11.9	−25	−67	46	11,593	15.7
		Non-DS	22	−62	45	3212	8.0	23	−64	47	8594	11.7
Precentral gyrus	6-4	DS	−35	−11	51	1688	6.2	−33	−16	52	3292	7.9
		Non-DS	35	−9	53	1458	7.2	32	−14	52	1865	5.3
	6-9	DS	−40	4	38	1260	8.3	−47	−2	32	2019	9.5
		Non-DS	43	6	39	1808	7.1	43	2	34	3242	9.7
Middle-superior frontal gyrus	9-10-46	DS	−50	14	24	925	5.0	−39	38	22	1180	5.0
		Non-DS	41	23	17	899	7.2	43	17	21	1154	5.1
Inferior frontal gyrus	45–47	DS						−33	23	2	441	5.2
		Non-DS	45	32	5	982	5.1	41	23	3	538	6.2
Middle occipital gyrus	18	DS	−23	−85	4	1465	10.3	−22	−83	3	3897	11.6
		Non-DS	22	−84	7	1417	7.4	24	−83	2	1369	14.9

BA = Brodmann area; UCP = unilateral cerebral palsy; TD = typically developing; DS = dominant side (controlateral to dominant hand); non-DS = nondominant side (controlateral to nondominant hand); IPS=inferior parietal sulcus. For convention, the dominant hand corresponds to the unaffected hand in UCP and to the right hand in TD children, while the nondominant hand corresponds to the plegic hand in UCP and to the left hand in TD children.

same formula, but considering only the number of activated voxels in the two pSMCs.

For hemispheric dominance [26], we assumed a standard threshold of 0.20 in absolute value: $LI > 0.20$ dominance in the hemisphere contralateral to the dominant hand, $LI < -0.20$ dominance in the hemisphere contralateral to the nondominant hand, and $-0.20 \leq LI \leq 0.20$ bilaterality.

Statistical analysis and data fitting were performed via the software package OriginPro 9.0 (OriginLab Corporation). For linear data fit, Pearson correlation coefficient and equivalent p value were calculated. For data comparison of both groups (UCP and TD) and for data regarding the two hands and respective hemispheres, a nonparametric Mann–Whitney U test was used.

3. Results

Table 1 shows demographic and clinical data of enrolled UCP children. According to type and timing of lesions, the sample was classified into three groups: the first one was composed of four children with early malformative lesions (type I), the second one of five children with white matter damage (type II) and the third group by three children with connatal stroke (type III). In all patients, except one, the lesion was strictly unilateral (see Figure 2). In patient 5, who had bilateral alterations on imaging, the more affected hemisphere was contralateral to the side of motor impairment.

Based on TMS results, all children with type I lesions showed a CL reorganization, while children with the other two types of lesion showed either CL or IL reorganization.

Mirror movements (MM) were present in all children with type I lesion, while they were variably present or not in children with the other two types of lesion.

In the fMRI experiment, all children were able to understand tasks and succeeded to collaborate and to maintain gaze in the middle of the screen for the AON task. For the SMN task, one child (number 4) in the UCP group was discarded from the following analysis because of the presence of excessive movement artefacts during functional acquisition, which were difficult to correct or compensate for.

3.1. AON in UCP and TD Children. As previously observed in TD children [5], also UCP children showed activation of areas belonging to the action observation network such as the inferior temporal gyrus (BA37), superior temporal sulcus (BA 22), anterior intraparietal sulcus (BA40-7), inferior

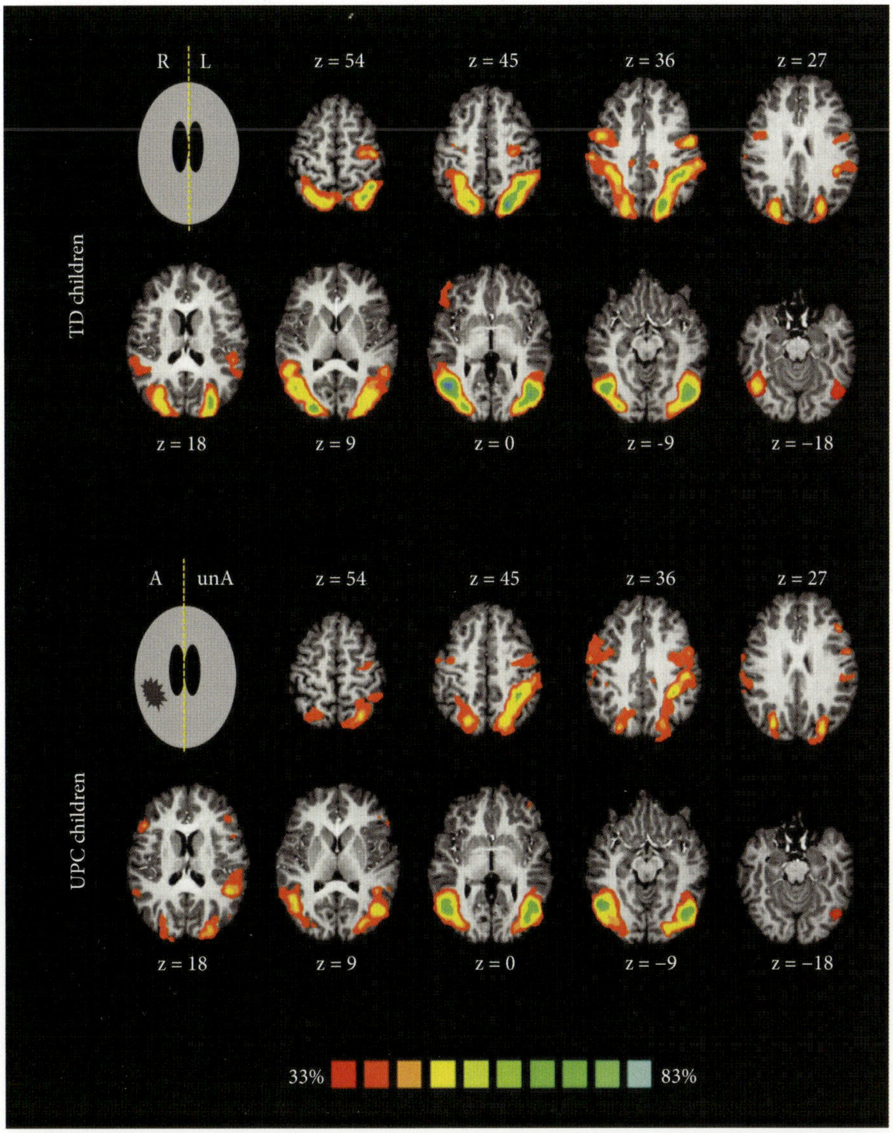

FIGURE 3: Probabilistic functional maps of the action observation circuit for the ALL TASKS > BASELINE contrast in TD children (as previously published in Biagi et al. 2015, top [5]) and in UCP children (bottom). Colour bar represents different levels of probability of activation for the action observation task from 33% (red, meaning that a brain region appeared in the map only if it was activated in at least 4 subjects) to 83% (cyan, equivalent to areas activated by more than 10 subjects). For each transversal slice, the z Tailarach's coordinate is indicated. On the right, we represent the left hemisphere for TD children (radiological convention; R = right, L = left) and the unaffected hemisphere, that is, the hemisphere contralateral to the unaffected hand, in UCP children (unA = unaffected, A = affected); on the left, the right hemisphere for TD and the hemisphere contralateral to the affected hand in UCP.

parietal lobule (BA40), superior parietal lobule (BA7), precentral gyrus (dorsolateral, BA6-9 and BA6-4), and inferior frontal gyrus (BA45-47). As in TD children, further activations were found in visual and somatosensory areas and in the middle frontal gyrus. Table 2 reports averages of Talairach's coordinates and of cluster sizes of activated areas, calculated across subjects of both groups, for the AON task.

Similarly, Figure 3 shows probabilistic maps about the contrast of all TASKS > BASELINE for UCP and TD children, allowing for a comparison of results between both groups.

Pattern of activations of AON in TD children presented higher levels of probability with respect to the UCP group, suggesting a more reproducible network. This was also confirmed by variability analysis conducted at the level of single-subject data, where the coefficient of variation of number of activated voxels across subjects was overall significantly different between TD children (67%) and UCP children (89%) (Mann Whitney U test, $p = 0.003$).

Regarding features of stimuli ("hand" laterality and "complexity" of action), a 2×2 factorial design ANOVA revealed a significant effect only for hand identity property

Table 3: Areas elicited by sensory-motor task for the dominant hand (DH) and nondominant hand (non-DH) in UCP children and in age-matched TD children.

		BA		UCP children: Talairach's coordinates x	y	z	Cluster size	t-value	TD children: Talairach's coordinates x	y	z	Cluster size	t-value
Motor-sensory task of DH	pSMC	2-3-4	CLH	−36	−27	53	8926	16.4	−40	−33	53	8811	17.9
			ILH	37	−29	48	1794	6.1	42	−30	54	1046	5.0
	IPL	40	CLH	−50	−29	26	1404	6.3	−50	−26	23	1212	5.5
			ILH	51	−24	25	1946	5.0	54	−20	22	931	6.0
	PrC gyrus	6	CLH	−56	−3	29	1430	5.1	−57	−4	36	712	5.0
			ILH										
	Insula	13	CLH	−44	−11	16	663	6.2					
			ILH										
	SMA	6–31	IH	−5	−17	48	1565	7.1	−4	−25	47	1024	6.9
	Cerebellum		CLH										
			ILH	14	−52	−23	1243	5.0	20	−52	−28	562	5.0
Motor-sensory task of non-DH	pSMC	2-3-4	CLH	35	−29	49	5928	10.1	38	−31	52	8645	18.3
			ILH	−41	−22	46	1032	7.5	−40	−25	55	621	5.8
	IPL	40	CLH	50	−20	27	1719	6.6	50	−25	22	1168	7.2
			ILH	−50	−29	25	502	5.1	−54	−30	28	1445	6.5
	PrC gyrus	6	CLH	48	3	31	878	5.3	42	−9	43	839	6.6
			ILH	−54	−5	29	554	5.7					
	Insula	13	CLH	33	−24	17	613	5.6					
			ILH	−46	−13	11	677	5.6					
	SMA	6–31	IH	0	−12	47	988	5.0	1	−18	52	788	6.1
	Cerebellum		CLH										
			ILH	−14	−52	−21	1495	7.3	−13	−61	−22	2288	7.0

BA = Brodmann area; UCP = unilateral cerebral palsy; TD = typically developing; pSMC = primary sensory-motor cortex; IPL = inferior parietal lobule; PrC gyrus = precentral gyrus; SMA = supplementary motor area; DH = dominant hand; non-DH = nondominant hand; CLH = contralateral hemisphere; ILH = ipsilateral hemisphere, IH = interhemispheric. For convention, the dominant hand corresponds to the unaffected hand in UCP and to the right hand in TD children, while the nondominant hand corresponds to the plegic hand in UCP and to the left hand in TD children.

("hand," $p < .001$) in AIP of the hemisphere contralateral to the nondominant hand. However, no significant effects were found for the "complexity" factor ($p = 0.23$) and the interaction effect ("hand" × "complexity," $p = 0.28$). No significant effect was found in either right or left MT, used as a control area.

3.2. Sensory-Motor Task in UCP and TD Children. BOLD responses to both sensory and motor tasks of both hands (contrasts: (Sens-D + Mot-D) > REST and (Sens-ND + Mot-ND) > REST) allowed for the identification of similar activity patterns in a number of cortical areas belonging to SMN in both groups.

In particular, the majority of subjects showed bilateral activations in the primary sensory motor cortex (pSMC, BA 1-2-3-4) and in inferior parietal lobule (BA 40). Other activations were found medially in the supplementary motor area (SMA), in a sector comprised between medial frontal gyrus and cingulate gyrus (BA 6-31), in the precentral gyrus of the hemisphere contralateral to the stimulated hand (BA 6), and in the cerebellar hemisphere ipsilateral to the stimulated hand. Differently from TD children, UCPs also showed activity in the insula (BA 13), contralaterally in the case of stimulation of the dominant hand, and bilaterally for the nondominant one. Table 3 reports averages of coordinates and number of activated voxels, calculated across subjects for both groups.

3.3. Lateralization of AON and of pSMC in UCP and TD Children. Concerning AON, Figure 3 shows bilateral brain activation in TD children, as previously reported in Biagi et al. [5]. On the contrary, UCP children presented a mildly lateralized circuit in the hemisphere contralateral to the dominant hand. This finding was obtained by computing global lateralization indices, using number of voxels in the two hemispheres obtained by multisubject analysis ($LI_{TD} = 0.01$, $LI_{UCP} = 0.23$).

Regarding the two hands separately, Figure 4 reports data on lateralization indices obtained in each subject for both stimuli. For AON, LIs were calculated considering the whole neuronal circuit identified by multisubject analysis, while for SMN, LIs referred more specifically to lateralization of the primary sensorimotor cortex (pSMC).

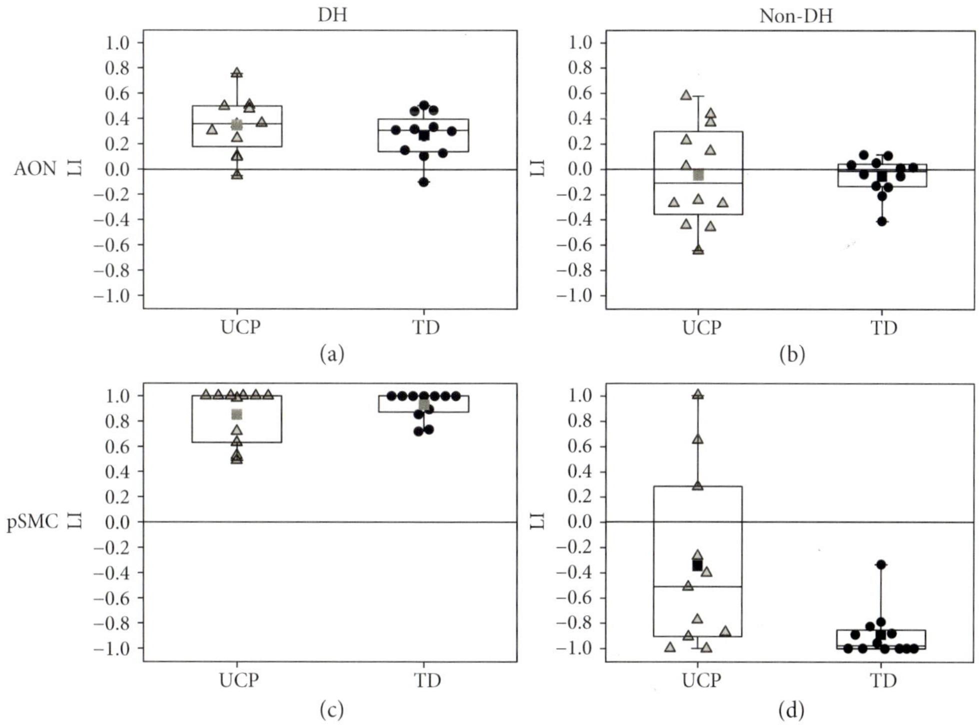

FIGURE 4: Box plots of the laterality indices of each single subject for AON (top row) of the dominant hand (DH) (a) and of the nondominant hand (non-DH) (b), as well as for the primary sensory-motor cortex, pSMC (bottom row), for the stimulation of the dominant hand (c) and of the nondominant hand (d). UCP children are indicated by light grey triangles, TD children by black circles. Each box is defined by the 25th and 75th percentiles. The whiskers are determined by the minimum and maximum values; the square indicates the mean value, while the line corresponds to the median value.

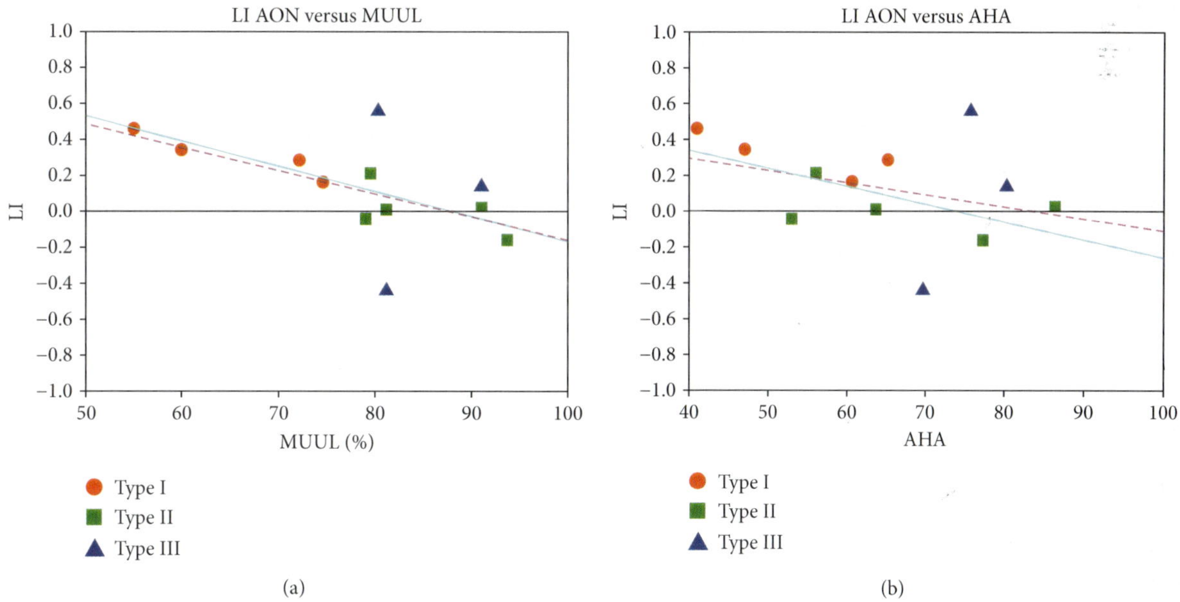

FIGURE 5: Lateralization index (LI) for the observation of all object-related actions versus BASELINE for each UCP child, plotted against his/her clinical scores (MUUL scale on panel a; AHA scale on b). Children were represented with different colours and symbols according to the classification of their lesions (type I = red circles, type II = green squares, type III = blue triangles). Data were fitted with a standard linear function. Considering all the subjects, the correlations are not significant (Pearson's value $R = -0.55$, $p = 0.06$ for MUUL; $R = -0.34$, $p = 0.28$ for AHA; pink dotted line). They become significant when only children with lesions of type I and type II are used in the fit ($R = -0.90$, $p = 0.0007$ for MUUL; $R = -0.68$, $p = 0.04$, for AHA; cyan solid line), due to big variability of data from children with type III lesion.

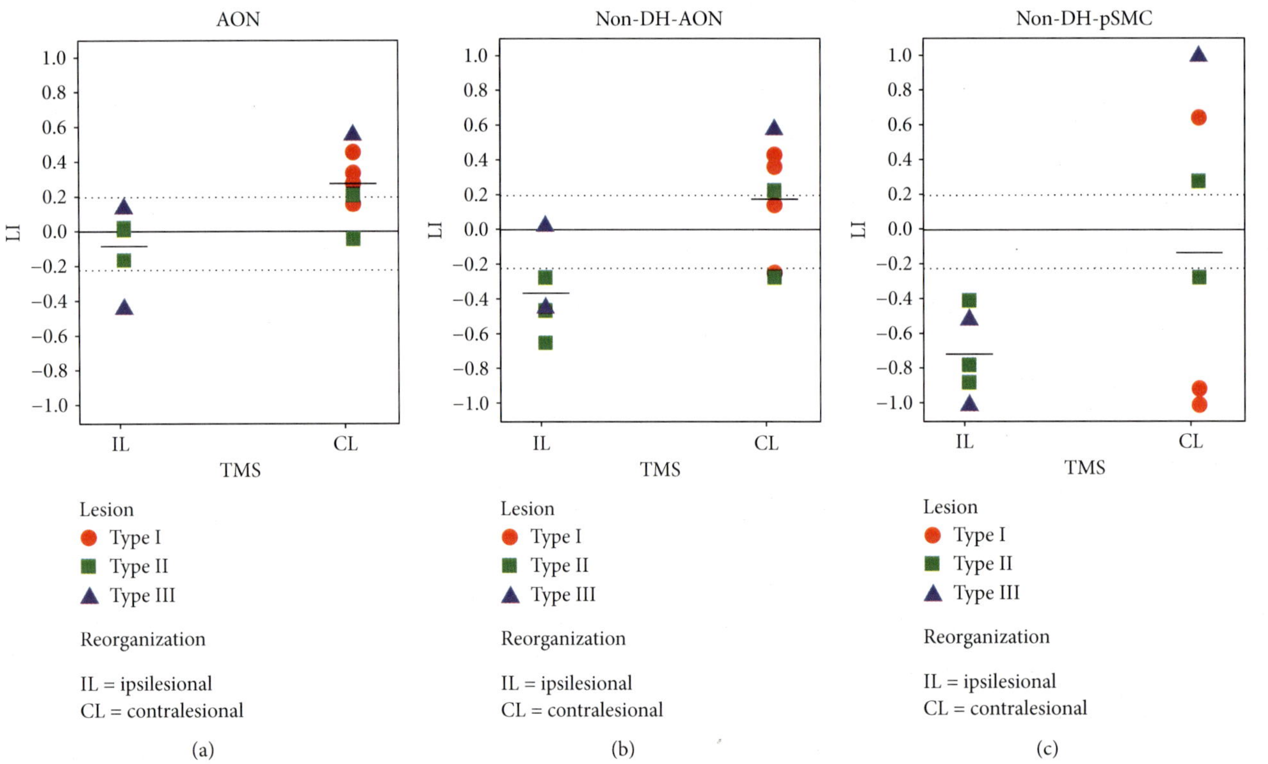

Figure 6: Box plots of LI values obtained by different contrasts (AON task: all TASK>BASELINE, panel a; AON task: (C-ND + S-ND) > BASELINE, panel b; and sensory-motor task: (Sens-ND + Mot-ND) > REST, panel c) in UCP children, grouped according to TMS data (CL = contralesional reorganization, IL = ipsilesional). As in Figure 5, children were represented with different colours and symbols with respect to the classification of their lesions (type I = red circles, type II = green squares, type III = blue triangles). Grey dotted lines represent the threshold value of |0.20| for hemispheric lateralization.

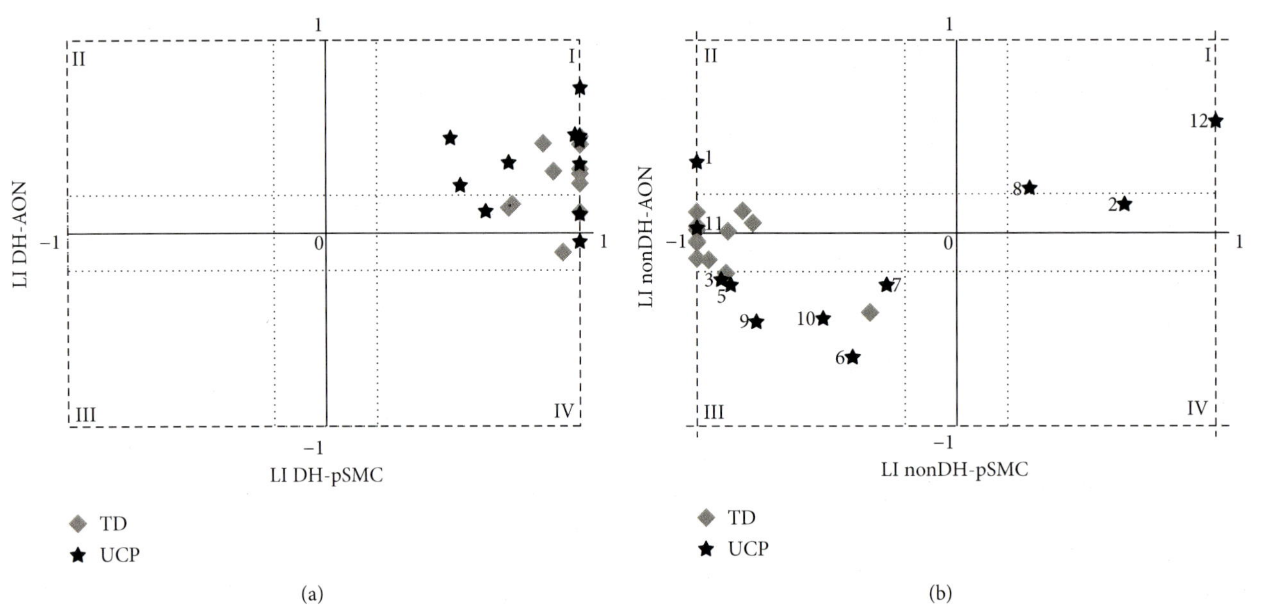

Figure 7: Four-quadrants charts of LI values of pSMC in the sensory motor task (abscissae) and of the AON (ordinates) of the two hands: dominant hand (DH) on panel a, nondominant hand (non-DH) on b. The first and third quadrants represent the congruence of the sign (both positive in the first, I; both negative in the third, III), while the second and the fourth represent the discordance of the sign (pSMC-negative and AON-positive in the second, II; pSMC-positive and AON-negative in the fourth, IV). TD children were represented by grey diamonds, UCP children by black stars. In the chart for the nondominant hand, labels on data of UCP children are used to identify subjects, according to Table 1.

Observation of simple and complex actions performed by the dominant hand ((C-D + S-D) > BASELINE) induced a slightly higher, but not significant, activation of contralateral hemisphere in UCP children ($LI_{UCP} = 0.35 \pm 0.22$) with respect to the TD group ($LI_{TD} = 0.27 \pm 0.17$) ($p = 0.35$, Figure 4(a)). LI mean values obtained from observation of actions performed by the nondominant hand ((C-ND + S-ND) > BASELINE) were very similar between the two groups ($LI_{UCP} = -0.04 \pm 0.40$; $LI_{TD} = -0.05 \pm 0.15$, $p = 0.98$) suggesting bilateral networks. However, in the UCP group there was a higher variability among children (LI_{UCP}range = $-0.64 \div 0.58$; LI_{TD}range = $-0.40 \div 0.12$), because single subjects presented very different lateralization indices. In particular, 4 subjects were lateralized to the hemisphere contralateral to the dominant hand, 6 subjects to the hemisphere contralateral to the nondominant hand, and only 2 subjects showed bilateral representation (Figure 4(b)). By comparing the two hands with an intragroup analysis, both groups presented significant differences in LI values between observation of the dominant and nondominant hand ($p = 0.02$ in the UCP group, $p = 4 \cdot 10^{-4}$ in TD).

For SMN, laterality indices of pSMC for stimulation of the dominant hand ((Sens-D + Mot-D) > REST) were similar between the two groups ($LI_{UCP} = 0.85 \pm 0.21$, $LI_{TD} = 0.93 \pm 0.11$, Figure 4(c)). On the contrary, there was a significant difference for values obtained with stimulation of the nondominant hand ((Sens-ND + Mot-ND) > REST; $LI_{UCP} = -0.35 \pm 0.7$; $LI_{TD} = -0.89 \pm 0.19$; $p = 0.02$; Figure 4(d)). Also for SMN, both groups presented significant differences in an intragroup analysis, when comparing LI values of both hands ($p = 0.001$ in UCP, $p < 1 \cdot 10^{-4}$ in TD).

3.4. Correlations between LI and Clinical Scores, Type of Lesion, and Reorganization in UCP Children. Due to great variability among subjects in the UCP group, a correlation analysis was performed between laterality indices and clinical scores, types of lesion, and type of reorganization.

For the AON task and all TASKS > BASELINE contrast, LIs of single UCP subjects were plotted against their respective values of clinical scales (Figure 5).

A negative correlation was found between LI and percentage MUUL and AHA scores. This finding is not significant, considering all subjects with three types of lesions in linear fit ($p = 0.06$ for MUUL; $p = 0.28$ for AHA). On the other hand, it is significant if only children with type I and type II lesions are included in the analysis ($p = 0.0007$ for MUUL; $p = 0.04$ for AHA). The same type of analysis was repeated considering only LI values obtained from observation of actions performed by the nondominant hand ((C-ND + S-ND) > BASELINE). Data showed similar trends, but statistical analysis was not significant ($p = 0.07$ for MUUL, $p = 0.08$ for AHA). No significant correlations were found in the same analysis using LI values of pSMC for sensory-motor stimulation of nondominant hand and clinical scales.

Figure 6 shows box plots of LI values of UCP children, grouped according to TMS results for different contrasts and different stimuli.

For all TASKS>BASELINE contrast of AON (Figure 6(a)), LI values of UCP children were significantly different when matched with the two types of reorganization revealed by TMS ($p = 0.023$, Mann–Whitney U test). In particular, children with IL reorganization at TMS (i.e., in the affected hemisphere) had bilateral AON activation ($LI_{IL} = -0.08 \pm 0.22$), except for one case (number 10), who presented a marked lateralization to the affected hemisphere. On the contrary, children with CL reorganization at TMS (i.e., in the unaffected hemisphere) presented either bilateral activation or higher activation in the hemisphere contralateral to the dominant hand ($LI_{CL} = 0.28 \pm 0.20$).

If the previous analysis is performed considering only observation of the nondominant hand (contrast: (C-ND + S-ND) > BASELINE, Figure 6(b)), both lateralization indices decrease accordingly (($LI_{IL} = -0.36 \pm 0.25$; $LI_{CL} = 0.18 \pm 0.33$) and their differences continue to be statistically significant ($p = 0.023$, Mann–Whitney U-test).

Regarding SMN of the nondominant hand (Figure 6(c)), UCP children with a different reorganization at TMS presented different trends of LI values of pSMC, even if globally their differences were not statistically significant ($p = 0.58$). Children with IL reorganization at TMS showed a greater activation of pSMC in the affected hemisphere ($LI_{IL} = -0.71 \pm 0.25$), in accordance to TMS. On the contrary, children with CL reorganization did not present a common behaviour, but rather a certain degree of variability ($LI_{CL} = -0.13 \pm 0.88$). Three cases (numbers 12, 2, and 8) showed lateralization of pSMC in the unaffected hemisphere (LI > 0), while the other three have it in the affected hemisphere (LI < 0): one (number 7) presented bilateral representation of pSMC, and two subjects (numbers 1 and 3) showed discordant reorganization with respect to TMS, showing an evident lateralization of pSMC to the affected hemisphere.

Similar results were found when this analysis was performed using the mirror movements data as discriminating factor (Figure in Supplementary Materials (available here)) .

3.5. Comparisons between AON and SMC in UCP and TD Children. In order to directly compare SMN and AON tasks, LI values were reported in a four-quadrants chart (SMN in *abscissae* and AON in *ordinates*), in which the first and third quadrants represent concordance of sign (both positive in the first, I, and both negative in the third, III), while the second and the fourth represent discordance of sign (one positive and one negative) (Figure 7).

In the case of stimuli performed by the dominant hand (Figure 7(a)), all subjects of both groups lie within the first or fourth quadrant, but very close to the zero axis, corresponding to a concordance between contralateral representation for pSMC and contralateral or bilateral representation for AON. Instead, scattered data were found in the case of stimuli performed by the nondominant hand (Figure 7(b)). All data of TD children are placed in the third, or second quadrant, but very close to the zero axis, meaning a contralateral representation for pSMC and contralateral or bilateral representation for AON, analogously to the dominant hand. For UCP children, the majority of data lies within the first and third quadrants, demonstrating a concordance in lateralization of pSMC and AON, with both representations in the unaffected (first quadrant, numbers 2, 8, and 12) or in the affected hemisphere (third quadrant, numbers 3, 5, 6, 7, 9, and 10). Subject number 11 is in line with the TD group, with contralateral representation for pSMC and bilateral representation for AON, while subject number 1 is the only exception with a shifted reorganization in the contralesional hemisphere for AON (as at TMS), but with a higher activation of ipsilesional pSMC for the sensory-motor task.

4. Discussion

This study explores for the first time AON of goal-directed actions in UCP children and its relation to type and timing of lesion, sensory-motor reorganization, and clinical assessment.

The first very relevant finding is that AON in UCP children engages brain activations similar to healthy age-matched children despite the presence of brain damage. However, neural networks activated by UCP children present a higher lateralization of maps with a higher activation of the unaffected hemisphere with respect to bilateral representation in the TD group. In our previous study [5], by comparing AON of TD children with that of healthy adults, we demonstrated that lateralization of AON is age-dependent and that adults have a more lateralized activated network in the dominant hemisphere while healthy children have more bilateral and widespread AON. This early lateralization, as a consequence of reorganization due to brain damage, could be reflective of unknown mechanisms that in turn determine an exclusion of natural development through a bilateral activation phase, affecting functioning in UCP children. Our results seem to confirm this hypothesis, because higher AON lateralization was correlated with lower performances on both scales (MUUL and AHA), while UCP children with bilateral AON activation similar to that of the TD group have better performances, reaching higher MUUL and AHA values (Figure 5). This finding is in line with examples of maladaptive plasticity in the context of reorganization of the sensory-motor system where contralateral (ipsilesional) reorganization is more effective in restoring good motor function as opposed to ipsilateral (contralesional) reorganization which is associated with lower grasping and manipulation skills [6, 7].

Another possible explanation could be related to the crucial role of the mirror neuron system in early motor learning by facilitating associations between action perception and corresponding motor programs [27–29]. An altered functioning of imitation capabilities, associated with limited motor system functioning, in early infancy, could contribute to determining maladaptive plasticity.

Regarding properties of observed actions, we found a significant "hand identity" effect in AIP of the hemisphere contralateral to the nondominant hand, similar to TD children [5]. However, contrarily to age-matched controls, this area did not present a significant effect for the "complexity" factor. Lack of significance for "complexity" could be related to the fact that all observed actions may be viewed as complex for UCP children. Another possible explanation could be that AON of UCP children processes mainly for goals rather than kinematics. These explorative hypotheses need further investigation.

For the first time, this study assessed in the same group of subjects both AON and SMN by using fMRI and correlated results with TMS data. Regarding fMRI results, we found a congruence between activation of contralateral pSMC during execution of the sensory-motor task and bilateral or contralateral activation of AON.

Moreover, a good correspondence was also found between AON and TMS data. In particular, observation of the nondominant hand elicited a greater activation of the affected hemisphere in children with ipsilesional reorganization at TMS, while children with contralesional reorganization at TMS had generally either bilateral activation or higher activation in the unaffected hemisphere (Figure 6(b)). However, relevant discrepancies between fMRI results of SMN and reorganization, measured by TMS, were found in two children (numbers 1 and 3, with type I lesion, Figure 6(c)) who presented a higher activation of pSMC of the affected hemisphere despite a TMS reorganization shifted to the contralesional hemisphere. The lateralization index for SMN should be driven by prevalence of sensory contribution to the activity in pSMC of the ipsilesional hemisphere, as confirmed by an explorative post hoc analysis of fMRI data for the sensory-motor task of the nondominant hand, using different regressors for sensory and motor blocks. Considering also clinical performances of the two patients, this finding could be related to a different reorganization of the motor and sensory system and to possible sensory-motor dissociation [6].

Concerning relationships between lateralization index, type of lesion, and type of reorganization evaluated with TMS, all type I UCPs have an ipsilateral (contralesional) reorganization, while type II and III UCPs are variable with lower abilities in children with ipsilateral (contralesional) reorganization and higher abilities in those with contralateral (ipsilesional) reorganization (Table 1). This finding is in line with current literature. In addition, this study shows that type I presents lower clinical scores than the other types do and higher values of lateralization indices, and type II has higher clinical scores and LI values similar to the TD group (bilateral representation), while type III has very high variability. In particular, there are two subjects with similar intermediate MUUL values but opposite LIs, one being more lateralized to the contralateral hemisphere and the other to the ipsilateral one. These diverse findings are related to the different clinical features of these two cases. In the child (number 10) with preferred AON lateralization in the affected hemisphere ($LI < 0$), also SMN activation and reorganization at TMS were present in the affected hemisphere and her functional level at HFCS was very good. On the contrary, the other child (number 12), with a lower level at HFCS, had greater activations in the contralateral unaffected hemisphere for AON and pSMC, in accordance also to reorganization at TMS.

Another interesting result is that observation of the dominant hand induced a higher, but not significant, activation of the contralateral hemisphere in UCP than the TD group (Figure 4(a)), suggesting a more lateralized circuit in UCP children. This is indirectly confirmed by observation of the nondominant (affected) hand which showed similar LIs between the two groups: although with bilateral activations, the UCP group showed higher variability among subjects, including single cases with high absolute LI values, indicating a specific lateralization in one of the two hemispheres (Figure 4(b)). This finding is in contrast with results of another study in which, for either side, observation of hand movements recruited the primary motor cortex contralateral to the viewed hand, while observation of the paretic side activated more strongly ipsilesional pSMC than viewing movement performed by the nonparetic side [17]. Moreover, in the same study, an engagement of AON was revealed regardless of degree of motor impairment assessed by a hand motor function Likert scale (1–4). These different findings could be related to a difference in the employed paradigm and in particular to non-goal-directed simple hand movements in the allocentric (third person) perspective of that study. Conversely, in the present study, simple and complex goal-directed movements were presented in the egocentric (first person) perspective. Concerning the issue of perspective from which action is observed, in monkeys it has been demonstrated that when comparing neural activation due to different points of view, such as first-person or third-person, first-person might be preferred [30]. An fMRI study in healthy adults showed that while the first-person perspective elicits activations in the hemisphere contralateral to the performing hand as if modelled action was mimicked with the same anatomical hand, in the third-person perspective, parietal activation ipsilateral to the modelled hand was found, indicating a specular strategy, rather than anatomical reproduction [31].

Moreover, the lack of correlation with degree of motor impairment in the study of [17] could be related to the narrower range of the Likert scale with respect to MUUL and AHA. The relationship between MUUL scale and type of sensory-motor reorganization has been previously reported [6], and both MUUL and AHA are highly correlated to lesion extension [32]. We have shown that not only the type of reorganization assessed with TMS but also the laterality index of AON (ALL TASKS > BASELINE) is related to MUUL and AHA scores if we consider type I and type II brain lesions (Figure 5). A similar result was found considering observation of actions performed by the nondominant hand ((C-ND + S-ND) > BASELINE); however, the lack of significance ($p = 0.07$) could be due to high variability of type III lesion (e.g., similar MUUL values with different types of reorganization and opposite laterality indices values).

As far as the relationship between SMN of each hand and laterality index is concerned, we have shown that in the TD group, beyond dominance, there is activation of pSMC of the contralateral hemisphere, reaching values of complete lateralization. In the UCP group, the dominant/unaffected hand induces similar activations while the nondominant/affected hand induces very variable activation with values varying from activation of the contralateral (lesioned) hemisphere to prevalent activation of the ipsilateral, unaffected hemisphere (Figure 4(d)). Another important finding is the lack of relationship between LI values of the nondominant hand and clinical scales, in contrast to the previous interesting relationship of clinical scales with LI of AON. This finding is in accordance with previous studies [33], and it could be related to different reorganization patterns among subjects that determine a huge variability of data with widespread values. All enrolled subjects did not undergo any intensive treatment for the upper limb, and from literature it seems that intensive treatments induce higher LI values with more lateralization in the affected hemisphere [34]. Another possible explanation could be related to the possibility of associated movements (e.g., mirror movements) that can alter SMN data. The solution of excluding UCP children with mirror movements from fMRI studies of SMN is not practicable since it would limit applicability to a small number of subjects. In our sample, the mirror movements, even if assessed with a nonstandardized method [35, 36], were present in 8 out of 12 UCP children. Further studies in UCP children with quantitative and standardized assessment of MM could shed light on the role of MM in SMN reorganization and clinical outcome.

Moreover, the sensorimotor tasks, especially for the affected hand, are often challenging for UCP children, and their execution can generate and be accompanied by an excessive head motion during fMRI sessions. In this study, we paid careful attention to the analysis and compensation of motion and we succeeded in obtaining fMRI data from all subjects for AON and from 11 out of 12 subjects for SMN. Taking into account these issues and considering the good concordance of lateralization indexes for pSMC and AON (Figure 7), the paradigm for exploring AON seems more reliable for studying the motor system in all UCP children, due to its greater feasibility. In fact, for AON tasks, children must only observe actions without doing any physical movement. Plasticity of the AON system with respect to the sensorimotor system still requires greater investigation.

5. Conclusion

This fMRI study explores, for the first time, AON of goal-directed actions and SMN in UCP children and their relation to type and timing of lesion, sensory-motor reorganization (TMS), and clinical assessment.

A good congruence was found between bilateral or contralateral activation of AON and SMN activation, TMS data, and clinical scores, suggesting that our paradigm might be useful in exploring AON and adaptive mechanisms or maladaptive plasticity. All these results, based on a small and variable group of UCP children, are necessarily exploratory and need to be extended to and confirmed by other studies. However, collectively, they indicate that, despite congenital and large brain lesions, AON is very active in these children, although with some characteristic differences when compared to TD children. These findings support clinical trials that have been carried out and are in line with numerous ones in progress using action observation therapy (AOT) as a tool to improve manual function, also in chronic phases of these children. Our explorative attempts to correlate manual proficiencies as shown by clinical scales and fMRI, TMS, and other findings may indicate ways to explain and predict efficacy of rehabilitation in UCP children. The fMRI paradigm could also be particularly suitable to investigate effects of plasticity induced by this specific rehabilitation program [37–39].

Conflicts of Interest

The authors declare that they have not conflict of interests.

Authors' Contributions

Giuseppina Sgandurra and Laura Biagi contributed equally to this work.

Acknowledgments

The authors would like to thank the children and parents who participated in this study and Vincent Corsentino for reviewing the English language of the manuscript. The authors would also like to thank Elena Beani for scoring the mirror movements. This trial has been partially funded by the Italian Ministry of Health to Giuseppina Sgandurra (GR-2011-02350053).

References

[1] L. Cattaneo and G. Rizzolatti, "The mirror neuron system," *Archives of Neurology*, vol. 66, no. 5, pp. 557–560, 2009.

[2] B. Calvo-Merino, D. E. Glaser, J. Grèzes, R. E. Passingham, and P. Haggard, "Action observation and acquired motor skills: an FMRI study with expert dancers," *Cerebral Cortex*, vol. 15, no. 8, pp. 1243–1249, 2005.

[3] D. J. Shaw, M. H. Grosbras, G. Leonard, G. B. Pike, and T. Paus, "Development of functional connectivity during adolescence: a longitudinal study using an action-observation paradigm," *Journal of Cognitive Neuroscience*, vol. 23, no. 12, pp. 3713–3724, 2011.

[4] D. J. Shaw, M. H. Grosbras, G. Leonard, G. B. Pike, and T. Paus, "Development of the action observation network during early adolescence: a longitudinal study," *Social Cognitive and Affective Neuroscience*, vol. 7, no. 1, pp. 64–80, 2012.

[5] L. Biagi, G. Cioni, L. Fogassi, A. Guzzetta, G. Sgandurra, and M. Tosetti, "Action observation network in childhood: a comparative fMRI study with adults," *Developmental Science*, vol. 19, no. 6, pp. 1075–1086, 2016.

[6] A. Guzzetta, P. Bonanni, L. Biagi et al., "Reorganisation of the somatosensory system after early brain damage," *Clinical Neurophysiology*, vol. 118, no. 5, pp. 1110–1121, 2007.

[7] M. Staudt, C. Gerloff, W. Grodd, H. Holthausen, G. Niemann, and I. Krageloh-Mann, "Reorganization in congenital hemiparesis acquired at different gestational ages," *Annals of Neurology*, vol. 56, no. 6, pp. 854–863, 2004.

[8] G. Cioni, G. Sgandurra, S. Muzzini, P. B. Paolicelli, and A. Ferrari, "Forms of hemiplegia," in *The Spastic Forms of Cerebral Palsy. A Guide to the Assessment of Adaptive Functions*, C. Ferrari, Ed., pp. 331–353, Springer-Verlag, Milan, 2009.

[9] G. Cioni, B. Sales, P. Paolicelli, E. Petacchi, M. Scusa, and R. Canapicchi, "MRI and clinical characteristics of children with hemiplegic cerebral palsy," *Neuropediatrics*, vol. 30, no. 5, pp. 249–255, 1999.

[10] E. Jaspers, H. Feys, H. Bruyninckx, J. Harlaar, G. Molenaers, and K. Desloovere, "Upper limb kinematics: development and reliability of a clinical protocol for children," *Gait & Posture*, vol. 33, no. 2, pp. 279–285, 2011.

[11] L. I. N. D. A. Holmström, B. Vollmer, K. Tedroff et al., "Hand function in relation to brain lesions and corticomotor-projection pattern in children with unilateral cerebral palsy," *Developmental Medicine & Child Neurology*, vol. 52, no. 2, pp. 145–152, 2010.

[12] M. Staudt, W. Grodd, C. Gerloff, M. Erb, J. Stitz, and I. Krageloh-Mann, "Two types of ipsilateral reorganization in congenital hemiparesis: a TMS and fMRI study," *Brain*, vol. 125, no. 10, pp. 2222–2237, 2002.

[13] J. A. Eyre, "Corticospinal tract development and its plasticity after perinatal injury," *Neuroscience & Biobehavioral Reviews*, vol. 31, no. 8, pp. 1136–1149, 2007.

[14] J. A. Eyre, M. Smith, L. Dabydeen et al., "Is hemiplegic cerebral palsy equivalent to amblyopia of the corticospinal system?," *Annals of Neurology*, vol. 62, no. 5, pp. 493–503, 2007.

[15] M. Randall, J. B. Carlin, P. Chondros, and D. Reddihough, "Reliability of the Melbourne assessment of unilateral upper limb function," *Developmental Medicine & Child Neurology*, vol. 43, no. 11, pp. 761–767, 2001.

[16] L. Krumlinde-Sundholm, M. Holmefur, A. Kottorp, and A. C. Eliasson, "The Assisting Hand Assessment: current evidence of validity, reliability, and responsiveness to change," *Developmental Medicine & Child Neurology*, vol. 49, no. 4, pp. 259–264, 2007.

[17] M. Dinomais, G. Lignon, E. Chinier, I. Richard, A. ter Minassian, and S. N.'. G. T. Tich, "Effect of observation of simple hand movement on brain activations in patients with unilateral cerebral palsy: an fMRI study," *Research in Developmental Disabilities*, vol. 34, no. 6, pp. 1928–1937, 2013.

[18] L. Biagi, G. Cioni, L. Fogassi, A. Guzzetta, and M. Tosetti, "Anterior intraparietal cortex codes complexity of observed hand movements," *Brain Research Bulletin*, vol. 81, no. 4-5, pp. 434–440, 2010.

[19] J. H. House, F. W. Gwathmey, and M. O. Fidler, "A dynamic approach to the thumb-in- palm deformity in cerebral palsy: evaluation and results in fifty-six patients," *The Journal of Bone & Joint Surgery*, vol. 63, no. 2, pp. 216–225, 1981.

[20] L. A. Koman, R. M. M. Williams, P. J. Evans et al., "Quantification of upper extremity function and range of motion in children with cerebral palsy," *Developmental Medicine & Child Neurology*, vol. 50, no. 12, pp. 910–917, 2008.

[21] M. Randall, L. Johnson, and D. S. Reddihough, *The Melbourne Assessment of Unilateral Upper Limb Function*, Occupational Therapy Department, Royal Children's Hospital, Melbourne, 1999.

[22] D. Borghetti, F. Sartucci, E. Petacchi et al., "Transcranial magnetic stimulation mapping: a model based on spline interpolation," *Brain Research Bulletin*, vol. 77, no. 2-3, pp. 143–148, 2008.

[23] S. Rossi, M. Hallett, P. M. Rossini, A. Pascual-Leone, and Safety of TMS Consensus Group, "Safety, ethical considerations, and application guidelines for the use of transcranial magnetic stimulation in clinical practice and research," *Clinical Neurophysiology*, vol. 120, no. 12, pp. 2008–2039, 2009.

[24] J. Talairach and P. Tournoux, *Co-Planar Stereotaxic Atlas of the Human Brain*, Thieme, New York, 1988.

[25] G. M. Boynton, S. A. Engel, G. H. Glover, and D. J. Heeger, "Linear systems analysis of functional magnetic resonance imaging in human V1," *The Journal of Neuroscience*, vol. 16, no. 13, pp. 4207–4221, 1996.

[26] M. L. Seghier, "Laterality index in functional MRI: methodological issues," *Magnetic Resonance Imaging*, vol. 26, no. 5, pp. 594–601, 2008.

[27] M. D. Giudice, V. Manera, and C. Keysers, "Programmed to learn? The ontogeny of mirror neurons," *Developmental Science*, vol. 12, no. 2, pp. 350–363, 2009.

[28] V. Burzi, G. Tealdi, R. N. Boyd, and A. Guzzetta, "Action observation in infancy: implications for neuro-rehabilitation," *Developmental Medicine & Child Neurology*, vol. 58, no. 4, pp. 74–77, 2016.

[29] V. Burzi, V. Marchi, R. N. Boyd et al., "Brain representation of action observation in human infants," *Developmental Medicine & Child Neurology*, vol. 57, no. 2, pp. 26–30, 2015.

[30] V. Caggiano, M. Giese, P. Thier, and A. Casile, "Encoding of point of view during action observation in the local field potentials of macaque area F5," *European Journal of Neuroscience*, vol. 41, no. 4, pp. 466–476, 2015.

[31] G. Vingerhoets, L. Stevens, M. Meesdom, P. Honoré, P. Vandemaele, and E. Achten, "Influence of perspective on the neural correlates of motor resonance during natural action observation," *Neuropsychological Rehabilitation*, vol. 22, no. 5, pp. 752–767, 2012.

[32] L. Mailleux, E. Jaspers, E. Ortibus et al., "Clinical assessment and three-dimensional movement analysis: an integrated approach for upper limb evaluation in children with unilateral cerebral palsy," *PLoS One*, vol. 12, no. 7, article e0180196, 2017.

[33] M. Weinstein, V. Myers, D. Green et al., "Brain plasticity following intensive bimanual therapy in children with hemiparesis: preliminary evidence," *Neural Plasticity*, vol. 2015, Article ID 798481, 13 pages, 2015.

[34] E. Inguaggiato, G. Sgandurra, S. Perazza, A. Guzzetta, and G. Cioni, "Brain reorganization following intervention in children with congenital hemiplegia: a systematic review," *Neural Plasticity*, vol. 2013, Article ID 356275, 8 pages, 2013.

[35] J. P. Kuhtz-Buschbeck, L. Krumlinde Sundholm, A.-C. Eliasson, and H. Forssberg, "Quantitative assessment of mirror movements in children and adolescents with hemiplegic cerebral palsy," *Developmental Medicine & Child Neurology*, vol. 42, no. 11, pp. 728–736, 2000.

[36] B. T. Woods and H.-L. Teuber, "Mirror movements after childhood hemiparesis," *Neurology*, vol. 28, no. 11, pp. 1152–1157, 1978.

[37] G. Sgandurra, A. Ferrari, G. Cossu, A. Guzzetta, L. Fogassi, and G. Cioni, "Randomized trial of observation and execution of upper extremity actions versus action alone in children with unilateral cerebral palsy," *Neurorehabilitation and Neural Repair*, vol. 27, no. 9, pp. 808–815, 2013.

[38] G. Sgandurra, A. Ferrari, G. Cossu et al., "Upper limb children action-observation training (UP-CAT): a randomised controlled trial in hemiplegic cerebral palsy," *BMC Neurology*, vol. 11, no. 1, p. 80, 2011.

[39] G. Sgandurra, F. Cecchi, E. Beani et al., "Tele-UPCAT: study protocol of a randomised controlled trial of a home-based Tele-monitored UPper limb Children Action observation Training for participants with unilateral cerebral palsy," *BMJ Open*, vol. 8, no. 5, article e017819, 2018.

9

Neural Mechanisms of Circadian Regulation of Natural and Drug Reward

Lauren M. DePoy,[1] Colleen A. McClung,[1,2,3,4] and Ryan W. Logan[1,2,3,4]

[1]Department of Psychiatry, University of Pittsburgh School of Medicine, Pittsburgh, PA, USA
[2]Translational Neuroscience Program, Department of Psychiatry, University of Pittsburgh School of Medicine, Pittsburgh, PA, USA
[3]Center for Neuroscience, University of Pittsburgh, Pittsburgh, PA, USA
[4]The Jackson Laboratory, Bar Harbor, ME, USA

Correspondence should be addressed to Ryan W. Logan; loganrw@upmc.edu

Academic Editor: Harry Pantazopoulos

Circadian rhythms are endogenously generated near 24-hour variations of physiological and behavioral functions. In humans, disruptions to the circadian system are associated with negative health outcomes, including metabolic, immune, and psychiatric diseases, such as addiction. Animal models suggest bidirectional relationships between the circadian system and drugs of abuse, whereby desynchrony, misalignment, or disruption may promote vulnerability to drug use and the transition to addiction, while exposure to drugs of abuse may entrain, disrupt, or perturb the circadian timing system. Recent evidence suggests natural (i.e., food) and drug rewards may influence overlapping neural circuitry, and the circadian system may modulate the physiological and behavioral responses to these stimuli. Environmental disruptions, such as shifting schedules or shorter/longer days, influence food and drug intake, and certain mutations of circadian genes that control cellular rhythms are associated with altered behavioral reward. We highlight the more recent findings associating circadian rhythms to reward function, linking environmental and genetic evidence to natural and drug reward and related neural circuitry.

1. Introduction

Circadian rhythms are near 24-hour oscillations in physiology and behavior, which help an organism adapt to changes in their internal or external environment to optimize function and promote survival. Synchrony or temporal coordination of circadian oscillators between central and peripheral tissues, in addition to alignment of those oscillators with the external environment, is important for maintaining organismal homeostasis. For example, disruptions to the circadian system are associated with poor health outcomes, including neurological diseases and psychiatric disorders. The circadian system is hierarchically organized in mammals, with the master circadian pacemaker of the suprachiasmatic nucleus (SCN) receiving photic (i.e., light) input from the eye and nonphotic inputs from disparate brain regions. The SCN relays timing information to other areas of the brain and the periphery through neural and humoral outputs. Coordination of these systems by the SCN is important for modulating the phases of peripheral oscillators. At the cellular level, timing information is kept by the molecular clock, a series of transcriptional and translational negative feedback loops. These feedback loops are driven primarily by circadian genes and their proteins. The transcription of *Period* (*Per1*, *Per2*, and *Per3*) and *cryptochrome* (*Cry1* and *Cry2*) genes are driven by CLOCK and BMAL1 heterodimers binding to enhancer elements (E-boxes) at their promoters. The accumulation of PERs and CRYs in the cytoplasm eventually translocate to the nucleus to interaction with CLOCK/BMAL1, effectively repressing their own transcription. Other genes form "auxiliary" loops providing stability and robustness to the core molecular clock loops.

Disruptions in sleep and circadian rhythms are observed across many psychiatric disorders (reviewed in [1]; reviewed in [2]), including addiction (reviewed in [3, 4]; reviewed in [5–7]). Moreover, polymorphisms in specific circadian genes are associated with drug intake and dependence in humans [8–12]. Evidence from animal studies suggests a bidirectional relationship between circadian rhythms and drugs of abuse. While circadian disruption, whether environmental or genetic, can impact "reward" function and drug-related behaviors, such as self-administration [13–16], exposure to drugs of abuse can also alter molecular, cellular, and behavioral rhythms [16–19], the expression of circadian genes [20], and sleep [21, 22].

After prolonged consistently timed exposure to drugs of abuse, rhythms may become entrained, as evident from anticipatory behavioral activity paralleled by temporal-specific changes of molecular rhythms in "reward" circuits [23–25]. Restricted feeding schedules may also entrain locomotor rhythms where anticipatory activity precedes feeding (reviewed in [26]), suggesting food, possibly acting a "natural reward," may be controlled or impacted by the circadian system. Natural and drug rewards seem to impact similar neural circuits (e.g., mesocorticolimbic dopamine system) with consequences on reward-related behaviors, such as behavioral anticipation. This review will examine the role of circadian rhythms in natural and drug reward, particularly the overlapping circuit, cellular, and molecular mechanisms of food and drug response. We also discuss the parallels between human and animal research within circadian rhythms and addiction, while highlighting key areas of future investigation.

2. Natural Reward

Eating behavior is driven by the need to maintain energy homeostasis, which is critical for survival and regulated by central and peripheral systems. Food is the most potent natural reward conserved across species. An organism must remember where, when, and how to obtain food to continue survival and improve reproduction, particularly during times of scarcity. Homeostatic and hedonic mechanisms may interact to regulate food intake, especially when food is abundant, since certain foods are more or less "rewarding." For example, palatable food has higher hedonic value than bland food and promotes greater activation within reward areas of the brain (see van der [27]). This activation closely parallels the activation pattern of drugs of abuse. Both drugs of abuse and food are potent reinforcers, which enhance dopamine release in reward-related brain regions (reviewed in [28]). Regardless of classification, rewards are powerful entraining forces, which can shift circadian rhythms.

2.1. Circadian Rhythms and Food. Beyond the hedonic value of food, organisms may use food and other stimuli to entrain, or adapt, to their environment to enhance survival; for example, the presence and consumption of food can shift circadian rhythms. Animals predominately eat during their active phase, with rhythms driving, seeking and feeding behavior at certain times of day. These feeding rhythms are in part regulated by circadian genes. Mutations in the *Per1* gene phase advances food intake into the sleep period, leading to obesity [29]. Similarly, *mPer2* knockout mice become obese after consuming food equally across the day and night (inactive and active phase, resp.) [30]. Day-night patterns of food intake are also abnormal in *ClockΔ19* mutants and BMAL1 null mice, with intake occurring more evenly across the 24-hour period [31, 32]. Moreover, metabolic homeostasis requires normal feeding rhythms, as shown by increased adiposity in rodents restricted to sleep phase feeding [33, 34]. On the other hand, active phase restriction of feeding prevents increased adiposity, glucose intolerance, and other measures typically induced by 24-hour access to high-fat diet [35].

Circadian rhythms are sensitive to changes in environmental stimuli, phase shifting (i.e., phase advance is the onset of the rhythm to an earlier time of day, while phase delay is the onset of the rhythm to a later time of day), and entraining across species to allow animals to adapt their behavior when necessary. Food is a potent stimulus of rhythm entrainment. Regardless of caloric restriction, locomotor rhythms will shift toward the time of a daily meal or a highly palatable snack (reviewed in [36]). For example, mice will begin to shift their activity into the light (inactive) phase, representing an advance of locomotor rhythms, when given chocolate without food restriction repeatedly during midday [37]. Furthermore, restricting feeding to a 12-hour period shifts the phase of circadian gene expression in peripheral cells, but not the SCN [38].

In addition to entraining circadian oscillators, food can reorganize temporal activity, for example, diurnality can be induced in rodents by a timed, daily palatable meal [37] or working for food while food restricted [39]. However, when mice are required to work to obtain chocolate with access to *ad libitum* chow, no shift in activity is observed [37]. This suggests that animals will continue to seek out food during their active phase, even when palatability is high if they are not energetically challenged. More importantly, these results indicate that an animal's metabolic state and the palatability of food play critical roles in how food shifts circadian rhythms. The shift seen in animals working for food seems to require an energetic challenge since it cannot be induced by increased running wheel activity or increased reward or palatability [37]. Furthermore, a daytime food reward is sufficient to induce a shift to diurnality even though this shift is smaller than that observed in the presence of food restriction ([39]; van der [40]).

Since metabolic state is important for inducing robust shifts in behavioral circadian rhythms, it is a fairly common practice to utilize food restriction [38, 41, 42]. However, when attempting to measure how food shifts and entrains rhythms in brain activity, the use of food restriction may be problematic. Hunger induced by food restriction could mask or artificially inflate the effects of a meal; therefore, it is important to include an *ad libitum* fed control group. Alternatively, a timed exposure to palatable food can be used alongside *ad libitum* access to chow. For example, a modest amount of entrainment in c-Fos expression occurs in the hypothalamus, which controls hunger, when a palatable food is present [43].

In addition to food entraining circadian rhythms, animals will learn to associate environmental cues, such as time of day with a food reward, or a scheduled meal. It is critical to account for time of day when studying food-related behaviors. The time of training and testing must overlap and be restricted to a certain circadian timeframe when studying conditioned place preference for food. Here, time is an internal circadian contextual cue that is critical for food-related behaviors in certain rat strains as well as marmosets [44, 45].

Anticipation, which is observed before a scheduled meal, particularly in rodents, is another example of a strong association between time of day and food. An increase in locomotion, core body temperature, and corticosterone usually precedes a timed meal (reviewed in [26]). The SCN does not appear to play a role in food entrainment since lesions fail to prevent the formation of anticipatory rhythms associated with restricted feeding schedules [46]. Although the brain regions responsible are largely unknown, the food-entrainable oscillator may be neuronal since anticipatory activity is resistant to adrenalectomy [47, 48] and cirrhosis [49]. Discovering the brain region, or regions, responsible for anticipation has been challenging. The food-entrainable oscillator could consist of a neuronal network, or circuit, and not a singular brain region [50], which is further complicated by the implication that the involvement of an oscillator could vary depending on the type of food.

In general, palatable food produces distinct effects compared to standard lab chow. Palatable food, such as chocolate, increases c-Fos expression, or activation, of corticolimbic regions including the prefrontal cortex (PFC) and nucleus accumbens (NAc) [51]. Moreover, the addition of palatable sucrose activates distinct neuronal networks in chow-restricted mice. Chow restriction entrains multiple subregions of the hypothalamus, activating the lateral, dorsomedial, and paraventricular nuclei during anticipation [42, 52]. The addition of palatable sucrose displaces most hypothalamic activity induced by restricted feeding, instead of activating the PFC, lateral septum, and NAc [42]. Relative to mice with restricted access to standard chow, mice with access to chocolate display a greater increase in amplitude and larger phase shift in rhythm of PER1 in corticolimbic structures, such as the amygdala, NAc, and PFC [41]. On the other hand, food restriction induces a higher amplitude of PER1 in the hypothalamus than chocolate [41]. These findings suggest that the mechanisms underlying anticipation of food may be distinct, depending on the type of food, and involve molecular rhythms.

Food-anticipatory activity is likely driven by both metabolic needs and reward. Accordingly, anticipation of palatable food entrains and/or activates the hypothalamus, even in the absence of food restriction, as well as reward-related brain circuitry (see Figure 1). Daily access to a palatable, fatty meal induces a modest amount of entrainment in c-Fos expression in the hypothalamus [43] and the anticipation of chocolate is associated with increased entrainment of PER1 expression in the dorsomedial hypothalamus [41]. Reward, motivation, or "wanting" also appear to contribute to anticipatory activity when limited access is given to a palatable food. For example, c-Fos expression is also induced in many corticolimbic structures, such as the PFC, NAc, and central amygdala [52].

Importantly, while ingesting, palatable food induces activation in reward-related brain regions such as the PFC and NAc and repeated presentations are required for these regions to become activated *during* anticipation [51]. Since repeated presentations are also required for anticipation to occur, anticipation-induced corticolimbic activation could underlie anticipatory activity. Furthermore, reward-related activation predating anticipation-related activation suggests that while the circuits mediating reward and anticipation may not be completely distinct, the underlying mechanisms may be different, but further study is needed. The transition from reward-induced activation to anticipation-induced activation in the case of food may extend to other rewarding substances, such as drugs of abuse, and importantly, could be a major contributor to relapse.

2.2. Potential Peripheral Mechanisms of Reward. In addition to the central mechanisms underlying reward and reward anticipation, peripheral oscillators may also impact reward. Primarily, peripheral hormones like estradiol and cortisol (corticosterone in the rodent) modulate neuronal activity, in turn altering circadian activity and reward. These peripheral hormones cycle in a daily rhythm. For example, estradiol cycles in an ultradian rhythm repeating approximately every 6 hours with an asymmetric peak in the early morning in humans [53]. Estrogen is known to modulate activity in circadian brain regions like the SCN where 17beta-estradiol administration increases firing frequency and miniature excitatory postsynaptic currents. This suggests that estrogen could be modulating and regulating circadian rhythms [54].

Fluctuations in circulating gonadal hormones, through treatment or normal menstrual cycling, also alter reward-related activity in the brain. In humans, when estrogen is unopposed by progesterone during the follicular phase of menses, reward-related brain regions are more active during anticipation, including the orbitofrontal cortex, amygdala, and striatum [55]. Hormone treatment early in menopause also increases anticipatory activity in the reward system, specifically the striatum and ventromedial PFC [56]. In non-human primates and rodents, the effects of estradiol on reward-related behavior are mixed. The reinforcing effects of cocaine do not vary across menstrual cycle phase in rhesus macaques [57], whereas estradiol treatment increases cocaine intake [58] and enhances acquisition for self-administration in rodents [59], while concurrent progesterone administration inhibits these effects. Together, these results suggest that estradiol plays an important role in reward, although some species differences exist. Generally, higher estradiol levels, whether through natural cycling or administration, promote reward-related behaviors as well as activity in reward-related brain regions.

Glucocorticoids, or stress hormones, which are released when the hypothalamic-pituitary-adrenal axis is activated by stress, also play a role in reward across species, but the results are mixed. These hormones also cycle over the 24-hour period, with a peak in the early morning during the daily shift to activity. In rodents, decreased glucocorticoids through adrenalectomy decrease reward through effects in the NAc, namely, decreased extracellular dopamine and Fos expression ([60]; reviewed in [61]). In humans, when high doses of cortisol are administered, activity in the striatum and basolateral amygdala decreases, but this is not specific to reward condition in a monetary incentive delay task [62].

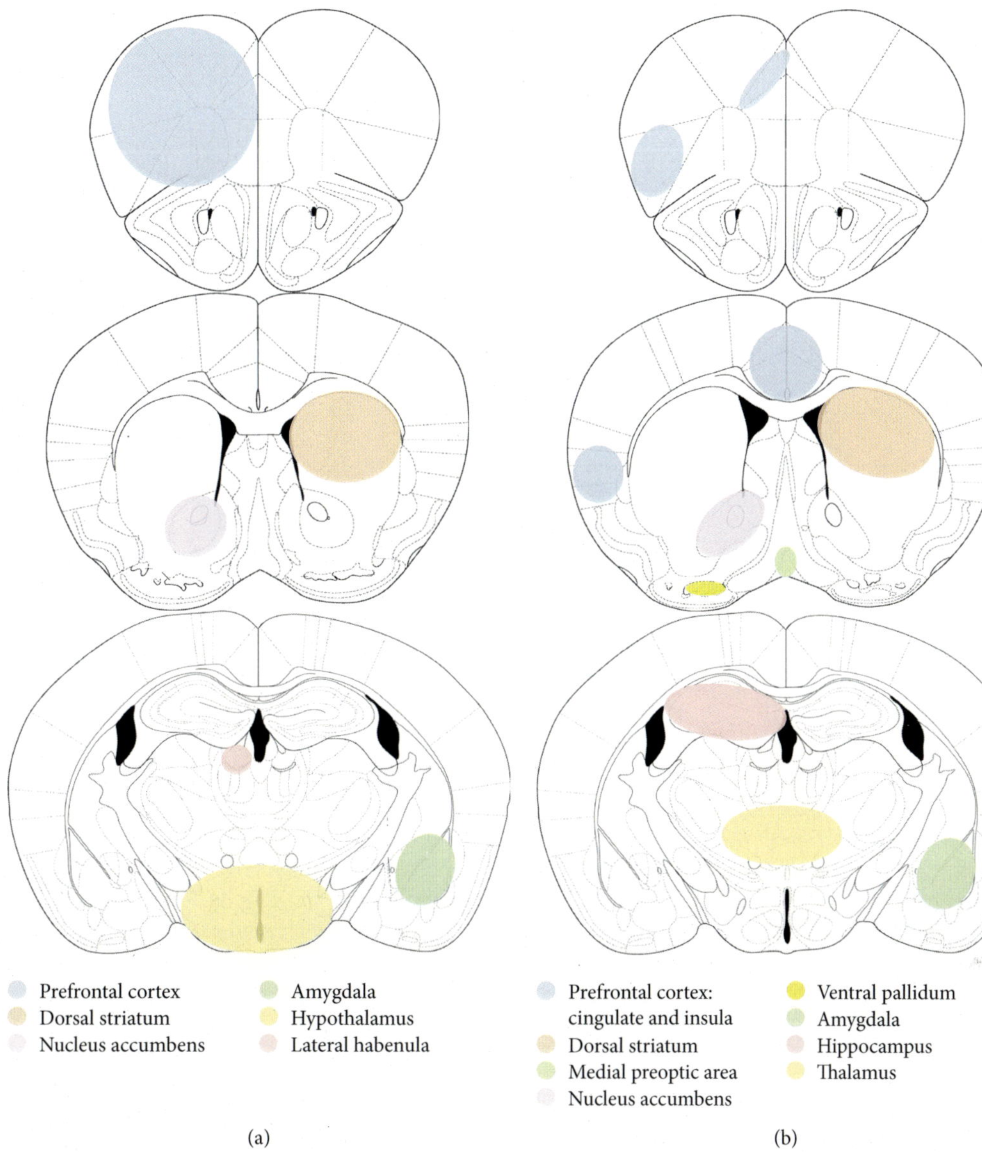

FIGURE 1: Multiple brain regions are activated or regulated by reward. Anticipation of (a) natural rewards, namely, food and (b) drugs of abuse activate discrete circuitry. The rhythmic expression of circadian genes in this and other brain regions is also altered by food or drugs of abuse demonstrating one potential mechanism by which reward influences circadian rhythms. (a) Anticipating a scheduled meal or palatable snack activates or increases c-Fos expression in the prefrontal cortex (PFC), nucleus accumbens (NAc), central amygdala, and hypothalamus. Furthermore, palatable food alters the expression of circadian genes in these and other brain regions. *Per1* rhythms are altered and shifted in the amygdala, NAc, and PFC, whereas the amplitude of *Per2* rhythms are intensified in the lateral habenula [116] as well as the suprachiasmatic nucleus (SCN not shown), cortex, and striatum [117] during anticipation of chocolate or after consumption of a high fat/high sugar diet or sucrose, respectively. (b) Anticipating drugs of abuse can activate multiple brain regions including the caudate, thalamus, insula, NAc, hippocampus, ventral pallidum, and cingulate. Similar to food, drugs of abuse also alter the expression of circadian genes. Specifically, cocaine alters the rhythm of *Npas2* and *Drd3* as well as the expression of numerous circadian genes in the NAc, most of which are upregulated. Circadian rhythms of period genes are also altered after withdrawal from morphine in the SCN, PFC, NAc, central and basolateral amygdala, hippocampus, and ventral tegmental area (not shown). Although it is beyond the scope of this figure to examine the differences in activation and circadian gene expression in various stages of addiction, it is important to note that acute versus chronic exposure to rewards have some distinct effects on the reward circuitry in the brain. For example, it is known that the role of various brain regions shifts during extended exposure to drugs of abuse (reviewed in [118]). It is thought that this shift contributes to the transition from use to abuse to dependence. Similarly, circadian genes may be contributing to this transition since mutations in these genes cause a loss of rhythmicity [16], which is also thought to contribute to loss of control over drug taking and the transition to addiction.

On the other hand, acute stress, which can increase cortisol, decreases activity in the dorsal striatum and orbitofrontal cortex during reward [63]. These results demonstrate that the effects of glucocorticoids on reward are still unclear. Species differences alone do not drive these mixed results, since the method of glucocorticoid induction (whether stress-induced or through exogenous administration) also appears to play an important role.

Together, it appears that peripheral hormones may play a key role in modulating reward-related brain regions and may bridge the gap between related changes in circadian rhythms and reward. Future research should focus on the importance of the oscillations of these peripheral hormones on reward since it is still unknown as to whether the circadian nature of these hormones is relevant to their roles in reward.

2.3. Neural Mechanisms of Food and Drug Reward. The long-standing question of whether any reward, whether "natural," such as food or sex, or drugs of abuse, has the same underlying mechanisms still remains largely unanswered. The brain evolved to respond to natural rewards, which are necessary for survival and reproduction. Both uncontrolled food intake, which is often compared to drug addiction, and drugs of abuse "hijack" reward and motivation associated neural circuitry (reviewed in [64]). Across species, both natural rewards and drugs of abuse predominately affect the corticolimbic reward system.

Palatable food, like drugs of abuse, has reinforcing effects mediated in part by enhanced dopamine release into reward-related areas of the brain (reviewed in [28]). For example, both sucrose and saccharin increase extracellular dopamine in the NAc of rats [65, 66], while palatability of food correlates with dopamine levels within the dorsal striatum [67]. Moreover, milkshakes, a highly palatable food, trigger striatal activation, whereas frequent ice cream consumption blunts striatal responses in humans [68]. The activation of reward circuits by repeated, restricted access to food, as discussed prior, can induce anticipatory activity. Similarly, exposure to drugs of abuse, such as methamphetamine and cocaine, induces anticipatory activity, potentially through entrainment of the circadian clock [23–25].

Although both food and drugs of abuse entrain rhythms, a single oscillator may not be responsible for generating reward-entrained rhythms. Rats are capable of entraining and showing anticipation, to both food and cocaine rewards separately, indicating that rewarding stimuli can be differentiated in a circadian fashion. Moreover, two separate free-running rhythms occurred after entrainment to food and cocaine rewards ceased. Together, these findings suggest that more than one oscillator generates reward-induced rhythms [23].

In addition to differences in circadian entrainment, anticipation of both food and drugs of abuse recruit corticolimbic brain regions (see Figure 1). Anticipation of nicotine due to the presentation of cues activates the caudate, thalamus, insula, NAc, and cingulate in humans [69]. In rats, anticipation of ethanol after the presentation of cues increases activity in the caudate, insula, hippocampus, ventral pallidum, NAc, and medial preoptic area [70]. This brain activity appears to be due to building anticipation induced by cues since repeated presentations over 5-6 days are required. This is similar to PFC and NAc activation induced by food anticipation, which requires 3–5 repeated presentations [51]. Although these studies did not use circadian entrainment of drug anticipation, they demonstrate that similar prefrontal cortical and striatal brain regions are active during anticipation of both food and drugs of abuse.

Interestingly, the hippocampus, medial preoptic area, and dorsal striatum appear to be activated by drug anticipation alone. These regions may have simply not been studied in food anticipatory experiments or these may be truly distinct effects. Future studies will need to examine additional brain regions of interest in order to determine which regions are universal, and which play a role in drug anticipation only. Another important consideration is that most experiments measuring brain activation induced by food anticipation investigate the PFC as one brain region [51, 52]. In future studies, it will be critical that distinct PFC subregions, such as the cingulate, orbitofrontal, prelimbic, and insula are examined separately. These various subregions of the PFC should be studied independently since they are critical for different features of addiction. Furthermore, this more specific analysis will allow for a better, more in-depth comparison of results between species and will paint a clearer picture of the roles of cortical subregions identified in human drug anticipation experiments, such as the insular and cingulate cortices.

On the other hand, the amygdala and the hypothalamus were only activated by food anticipation, even though both regions are believed to contribute to drug reward. The amygdala is critically important for the drug-related learning critical for associating cues with drugs of abuse [71], and studies suggest that the hypothalamus is involved in drug seeking. For example, hypothalamic orexin/hypocretin neurons play a role in cocaine seeking but do not appear to contribute to seeking motivated by a palatable food [72]. These results suggest that even though the hypothalamus is involved in metabolic regulation, food ingestion, and anticipatory activity in food-entrained rodents, distinct mechanisms likely underlie reward seeking between food and drugs of abuse. Taken together with findings that food and subsequently anticipation alone activate reward-related brain regions, these results suggest that although the brain regions mediating reward for food and drugs of abuse may be similar, how/when the regions are recruited and the underlying mechanisms by which those regions regulate reward may be very distinct.

In addition to parallels in brain circuitry, there are other fundamental differences in food and drug reward mechanisms. Palatable food is sometimes preferred over drugs of abuse, for example, rats tend to prefer saccharin and sucrose to cocaine [73]. Moreover, it has been shown that half of the mice tested prefer peanut butter compared to peanut butter mixed with methamphetamine [24]. From an evolutionary perspective, it is reasonable for food to be highly potent and rewarding since it is critical to survival. Since self-administration of highly palatable food, compared to drugs of abuse, is less time-consuming and complex, we should continue to leverage the potency of food to study the underlying processes giving rise to reward versus anticipation as well as increased and uncontrollable food intake. Despite food being a more potent reward in some circumstances, drugs of abuse have greater consequences in other regards. For example, associations between drugs of abuse and stimuli last longer than for natural reinforcers, indicating cues are especially powerful in the context of drug use (discussed in [64, 74]).

In the future, studies should continue to examine different types of reward in parallel. This will allow us to elucidate whether the mechanisms underlying the rewarding effects of drugs of abuse and natural rewards are different. Identifying the parallels and distinctions across types of reward could help us treat both obesity and drug addiction.

3. Loss of Rhythmicity and Loss of Control

3.1. Drugs of Abuse Alter Rhythms. Like natural rewards, there are diurnal variations in behavioral responses to drugs of abuse and drug taking in self-administration paradigms [19, 75]. For example, drug intake and self-administration of cocaine and ethanol are higher in rodents at night, during the active phase [19, 20, 76]. Not only are there natural rhythms to drug taking and reward, but exposure to drugs of abuse induces behavioral, anticipatory rhythms, potentially through entrainment of the circadian clock ([23–25]; reviewed in [77]).

Drugs of abuse induce behavioral rhythms, but drug exposure is also known to regulate circadian genes and alter circadian rhythms. Exposure to drugs of abuse alters expression of circadian genes, such as, *Period*, *Clock*, and *Npas2* ([15, 78]; reviewed in [77]). More importantly, volitional cocaine intake via self-administration regulates circadian genes, upregulating *Clock*, *Bmal1*, *cryptochrome1* (*Cry1*), and *Period2* (*Per2*) [20]. In addition, cocaine can induce phase shifts in circadian rhythms (reviewed in [77]). For example, even one acute injection of cocaine causes mice to phase advance 1 hour, and this effect is exacerbated in *Per2* mutant mice. These findings suggest that cocaine might also regulate free-running circadian rhythms.

3.2. Loss of Rhythmicity in Drug Self-Administration. Chronic exposure to drugs of abuse also causes a loss of rhythmicity in locomotor activity. These altered diurnal activity patterns are usually driven by increases in locomotor activity during the inactive period. For example, repeated amphetamine administration increases daytime locomotor activity in adolescent female rats [17]. Chronic alcohol exposure also increases daytime locomotor activity in mice, eliminating the typical rhythm as well as the peak in activity during the early night [79]. Over time, drugs of abuse also cause a loss of rhythmicity in self-administration and drug intake. Extended access or access to high doses of cocaine causes a loss of rhythmicity in drug taking, as evidenced by responding that continues well into the light phase, in lieu of predominating at night [19].

Drug exposure can alter rhythmicity, but mutations in circadian genes can also impact self-administration. Mice with a dominant negative mutation in the Clock gene self-administer cocaine equitably during the day and night. On the other hand, wild-type mice fail to acquire criteria for self-administration, but only during the day. This suggests that decreased Clock function increases vulnerability for cocaine use, at least in part by reducing rhythmicity and increasing drug use during the day [16]. Deletion of the circadian rhythm gene *Per1* also causes a loss of circadian rhythmicity in alcohol intake, again normalizing intake across time of day [80]. Loss of rhythmicity can also be seen for natural rewards, like palatable food. *mPer2* knockout mice eat the same amount of a high-fat diet during the day and night, which leads to obesity [30].

In addition to a loss of rhythmicity, chronic exposure to drugs of abuse can also cause an overall increase in, or loss of control over, drug intake. Increases in drug taking can be seen across species in extended access paradigms. In rodents, extended access to cocaine causes escalation and the development of excessive drug intake [81, 82]. In nonhuman primates, unlimited access produces erratic and rapid binge-like patterns of cocaine self-administration, which can ultimately lead to seizures and death [83, 84]. Escalated or excessive drug intake and as compulsive or habit-like drug seeking despite adverse consequences are primary features of drug addiction, which contribute to the development of substance dependence. Therefore, a loss of control over intake could model a transition to an addiction-like state.

Loss of control or escalation in drug taking appears to be closely paralleled by, and potentially driven by, a loss of rhythmicity and increased daytime responding in rodents [19]. When drug taking increases during the inactive phase, it reflects a loss of control in drug seeking and taking. In this case, animals are likely sacrificing time usually dedicated to sleep and rest. However, it is difficult to propose a causal or correlational relationship between loss of rhythmicity and loss of control because only a few key studies have examined rhythmicity or patterns of drug taking across a 24-hour period [19, 80]. Others, that do examine phase differences, do not always compare initial drug use to use after long-term exposure. Therefore, even if no differences in day-and-night responding are found, this cannot be correlated to an escalation of intake over time [85].

These questions are understudied because they are especially difficult and time-consuming experiments. Due to cost and space limitations, it is difficult to study self-administration over a 24-hour cycle. In addition to experimental challenges, unlimited access to drugs of abuse can cause death or health deterioration in animals. An alternative method is to use discrete trials spread out over a 24-hour period [19] or to use shorter access periods of self-administration and compare animals that self-administered during either the active or inactive phase.

In addition to being a key feature of addiction, escalation and loss of control over drug taking also contribute to other addiction-related behaviors. For example, paradigms which produce escalation also increase reinstatement of drug seeking, a model of relapse [86]. On the other hand, the role of rhythmicity in other addiction-related behaviors is less clear. In order to determine whether rhythmicity might play a role in other addiction-related behaviors, rhythms of self-administration can be correlated with measurements of reinforcement, motivation, and/or relapse-like behavior. If altered rhythmicity plays a critical role in the progression to substance dependence, it should contribute or at least correlate to other critical behaviors related to the overall phenotype of addiction.

In order to study the relationship between rhythmicity and loss of control, it is important to consider which parameters trigger escalation and compare those to parameters which do not: more versus fewer discrete trials, high versus low unit doses, and longer access sessions (approximately 6 versus 1 hour). Studies might successfully investigate the link between loss of rhythmicity and loss of control if these parameters are investigated further. For example, if we can slow down the progression of escalation, we can determine whether a loss of rhythmicity occurs prior to and is therefore potentially contributing to escalation.

Overall, parallels in loss of rhythmicity and loss of control have been difficult to connect. Future research should strive to complete and more elegant long-term studies examining patterns of self-administration. Future experiments should build on the existing literature and examine how other factors, such as mutations in circadian genes, previous drug or stressor exposure, or developmental stage, affect patterns and timing of self-administration. At the least, studies should attempt to investigate self-administration during both the active and inactive phases. It is possible that these phases will shed light onto the mechanisms underlying the development of different phases of addiction, with dark phase self-administration paralleling the development of substance use/abuse, and drug taking during the light cycle paralleling loss of control and the development of substance abuse/dependence.

3.3. Sleep Dysregulation and Circadian Rhythms. One parallel between loss of rhythmicity and loss of control in drug use is sleep deprivation. Increased drug intake during the inactive period is probably interrupting sleep, and excessive drug intake causes animals to neglect sleep. For example, a 24-hour access to cocaine causes rapid, erratic, and continuous self-administration across phase, which continues until the point of exhaustion in nonhuman primates, when drug taking is discontinued for a period of sleeping and eating [83]. Even in rats, self-administration of cocaine can cause generally deteriorated health and increased mortality [87].

Drug exposure also has direct effects on sleep across species. Cocaine self-administration during the day decreases sleep efficiency and increases sleep fragmentation in rhesus macaques [22]. This is very closely paralleled in rats, where withdrawal from cocaine self-administration reduces nonrapid-eye-movement (NREM) and REM sleep and increases sleep fragmentation [21]. In addition, withdrawal from long access cocaine self-administration reduces glucose utilization in both reward-related (caudate, NAc, amygdala, etc.) and sleep-related (dorsal raphe, locus coeruleus, and thalamus) brain regions in rats [82]. These findings can also be extended to other drugs of abuse. After ethanol withdrawal, mice show disruptions in sleep, with reduced NREM sleep and increased REM sleep [88]. These results parallel human findings, where addicts report sleep disturbances [7, 89, 90]. More specifically, a reduction in sleep and an increase in sleep fragmentation are reported during cocaine withdrawal ([91]; reviewed in [6, 92, 93]).

These symptoms closely resemble chronic insomnia, and it is thought that these sleep disruptions promote relapse. Recent studies have investigated the role of cocaine-induced sleep fragmentation in cocaine craving by augmenting or attenuating REM sleep fragmentation following cocaine self-administration in rats. Interestingly, as REM sleep fragmentation changes, the incubation of cocaine craving changes in parallel [21]. In addition, chronic sleep deprivation increased drug taking and incentive motivation for cocaine in high drug-taking rats [94]. Together, these findings demonstrate the cyclical relationship between drug exposure and sleep, with drug use affecting sleep and impaired sleep further perpetuating drug use.

It is important to note that although these studies examine sleep, they do not necessarily investigate circadian rhythms. Sleep and circadian rhythms are often not distinguished, being discussed interchangeably. It is important that studies attempt to measure both sleep and circadian phenotypes in order to gain insight about where sleep and circadian rhythms converge and diverge. Circadian rhythms and sleep can be studied concurrently by measuring sleep through electroencephalography (EEG) and electromyography (EMG) as well as circadian rhythms of locomotor activity, body temperature, and so forth [95, 96]. PiezoSleep mouse behavioral tracking systems have made this easier since they measure sleep/wake cycles through floor sensors, eliminating the EEG-/EMG-associated surgery. In addition, sleep/wake rhythms can be measured *in vivo* with circadian oscillations in gene expression or protein levels being examined in tissue ex vivo [95, 96].

It is particularly critical to investigate sleep and circadian rhythm disruptions in addiction research since sleep disturbances are a major symptom of addiction, which can trigger relapse. Using sleep boxes or measuring circadian rhythms, ex vivo are particularly important for studies examining addiction-related behaviors where limiting additional surgical exposures is critical. For example, mice self-administering drugs of abuse have already undergone an intravenous catheterization, and in many cases, an additional viral vector placement. If an additional surgery for measuring EEG/EMG is not absolutely required, it should be avoided. Furthermore, measuring activity rhythms with wheel running should be avoided because of the risk that the exteriorized self-administration port would catch on the wheel and injure the animal. Regardless, it is difficult to measure sleep and activity rhythms *during* active self-administration since mice typically self-administer drugs in an operant chamber. However, these measurements can be taken for a period before and/or after the length of drug exposure or daily during the drug self-administration paradigm if the hours of self-administration, when mice are out of the home cage, are excluded. Sleep disturbances in addicts might be more effectively treated once we better understand what causes them; understanding circadian rhythms might shed light onto how drugs of abuse alter sleep.

3.4. Rhythms of Drug Self-Administration and Treatment. Rhythms of drug self-administration will also be critical to study independently of escalation. Importantly, self-administration of cocaine under 3 discrete trials/hour (one infusion available during each trial) is tightly coupled during the dark phase of a normal light/dark cycle. In constant, dim light self-administration continues to be rhythmic in the absence of light-dark cues, although it is progressively phase delayed. On the other hand, in constant light, rhythms of self-administration become fragmented and animals take significantly less cocaine [97]. Taken together, these results suggest that cocaine intake is produced through a circadian mechanism and that circadian control of self-administration is influenced by light.

Determining the mechanisms by which various factors affect the rhythm of drug self-administration, and drug intake overall, will inform future treatment options. In the future, studies should continue to attempt to limit not only drug taking as above but also motivation and drug seeking with changes to light conditions, including lengthened or shortened light exposure. This paper suggests that light (or darkness in diurnal species) could be a useful therapy to suppress cocaine intake. In addition to changes in light/dark exposure, the appropriate phase-controlled timing of additional treatments, perhaps during the times of day with the highest periods of intake, could be critically important to the efficacy of treating addiction.

4. Circadian Rhythms and Drugs of Abuse: Human and Animal Parallels

4.1. Circadian Clock Genes. Drawing parallels between human and animal methods, mechanisms, and treatments is one of the most challenging necessities facing research today. Research focused on circadian genes, and drug use has been making strides in this vein, as indicated by a fairly large literature paralleling the role of circadian clock genes in addiction in both rodents and humans. Two of the genes that have been most extensively studied are *Period* and *Clock*.

Mutations in *Per1* and *Per2* have been extensively studied in rodents. For example, *mPer1* and *mPer2* null mutant mice increase ethanol intake and conditioned place preference [14]. In humans, various single nucleotide polymorphisms (SNP) within Per1 and Per2 are associated with alcohol drinking. For example, one SNP in Per1 is associated with alcohol dependence [13]. Per1 is also associated with drinking and stressor exposure. *mPer1* mice consumed more alcohol in response to social defeat stress [13], whereas a SNP in Per1 interacts with early life stress to predict problematic alcohol use in humans [8]. Two different SNPs in Per2 are associated with stressful events and alcohol drinking in young adults [10] as well as reward dysfunction in humans, respectively [11].

Mutations and variants in *Clock* are also associated with drug use across species. In rodents, *ClockΔ19* mice, with a dominant negative mutation in the Clock gene, have increased ethanol intake and self-administration of cocaine [15, 16]. In humans, variants in the CLOCK gene are associated with heavy cocaine use, although not DSM-IV diagnosis of dependence [9].

Even though there is extensive research on circadian rhythm genes and drug use across species, it is unclear whether these findings tell us something important. For example, on a mechanistic level, it is uncertain whether SNPs matter. The research is the most complete for alcohol, but SNPs have not been studied systematically across drugs of abuse. Furthermore, SNPs do not seem to always correlate with the severity of drug use and dependence. It is also unclear whether the mechanisms underlying the association between SNPs and drug use in humans actually contribute to the role of circadian genes in addiction. More technologies and mouse models are being created so we are now more capable of paralleling findings in humans and animals. With the advent of CRISPR, it is much easier to create humanized mouse lines with targeted changes to specific genes. Future studies should aim to identify whether the effects of SNPs associated with drug use or dependence in humans parallel the effects of mutations in *Period* or *Clock* genes in rodents. If effects are consistent across mutations and SNPs, that would suggest the mechanisms underlying these effects are similar and the parallel between human and rodent literature is stronger. These mouse lines can then be used to probe for underlying mechanisms and develop potential therapeutics based on those mechanisms and then the clinical researchers can build on these mechanisms to confirm they are paralleled in humans or test novel therapies.

4.2. Dopamine Receptors in the Striatum. Drugs of abuse, specifically psychostimulants, activate dopamine signaling, overriding natural reward circuitry. The ratio of D1 and D2 receptors plays an important role in the rewarding effects of cocaine; D1R signaling appears to enhance [98], while D2R signaling decreases cocaine reward [99]. In addition, future cocaine preference negatively correlates with D2-/D3R-binding availability in the ventral striatum in rats [100]. These results indicate that a predominance of D1R over D2R signaling must be present for the rewarding effects of cocaine. It has also been hypothesized that the transition to compulsive intake could result from this predominance.

In mice, acute cocaine causes both fast stimulation of D1R and slower stimulation of D2R containing neurons in the dorsal striatum [101]. This suggests that cocaine reward may be mediated by not only the abrupt activation of D1R neurons but also a longer-lasting, progressive deactivation of D2R neurons in the dorsal striatum [101]. Interestingly, in mice exposed to chronic cocaine, acute cocaine stimulates D1R and D2R neurons less, while inducing a slower, yet longer-lasting increase in D1R activation. This altered D1R neuron stimulation induced by acute cocaine extends the predominance of D1R over D2R signaling, which is typically rapid and short lasting [102]. Striatal D2R downregulation might contribute to the sustained signaling imbalance.

Similarly, cocaine abuse potently affects dopamine receptors in the striatum in humans, reducing D2/3 availability, which is associated with increased drug craving [103] and vulnerability to relapse [104]. Cocaine abusers show dampened stimulant-induced increases in dopamine, as shown by reduced D2/D3 receptor binding, in the striatum, despite the induction of intense craving [105]. Interestingly, reduced D2R signaling during intoxication is maintained even when cocaine-associated cues are present [106]. It has been

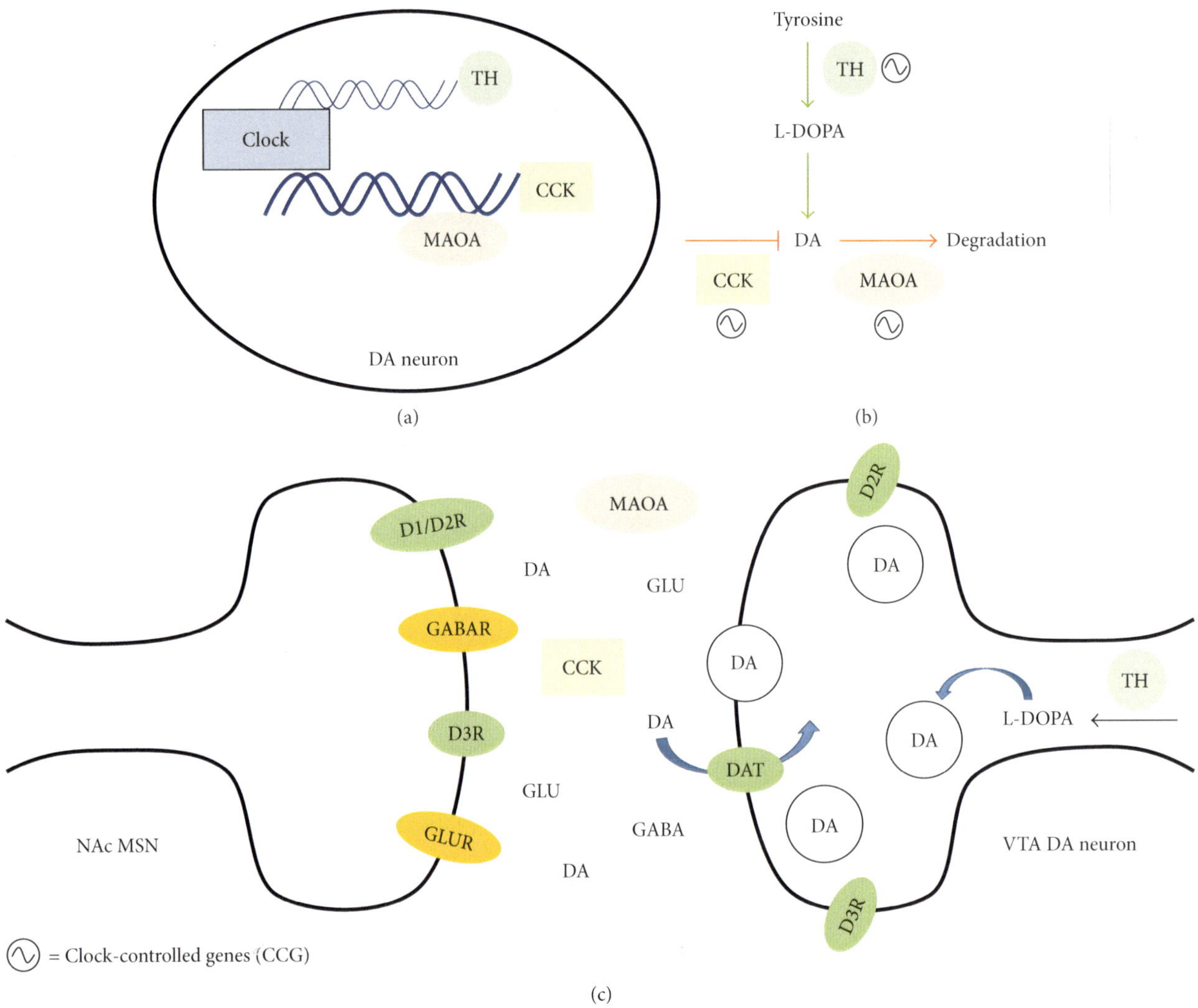

FIGURE 2: Potential mechanisms by which circadian rhythms impact reward. One of the primary mechanisms by which circadian rhythms might affect reward and reward-related behaviors is through monoaminergic signaling in the nucleus accumbens (NAc). In particular, circadian clock genes control regulatory processes involved in the synthesis, function, and degradation of dopamine (DA). Clock is thought to be a negative regulator of reward, since mutations in the *Clock* gene increase preference and drug taking. CLOCK and other related genes may be negatively regulating DA through their transcriptional actions. (a) Overall, dopaminergic signaling is reduced through CLOCK's actions (and increased in *ClockΔ19* mutant mice) because genes that increase dopaminergic signaling are negatively regulated by clock genes while genes that decrease dopaminergic signaling are positively regulated. (b) Tyrosine hydroxylase (TH), the rate-limiting enzyme in the synthesis of dopamine (DA), is negatively regulated, whereas monoamine oxidase A (MAOA), an enzyme which breaks down DA in the synapse and cholecystokinin (CCK), a regulatory peptide which negatively affects DA output is positively regulated by clock genes [114, 119]. (c) These changes in dopaminergic neurons in the VTA influence dopaminergic, and potentially glutamatergic, signaling in the NAc, which could mediate increases in reward seen in mice with mutations in clock genes. This could hold true in humans, with circadian disruptions or polymorphisms in circadian genes increasing dopaminergic signaling in the NAc, which leads to increased vulnerability to substance dependence.

hypothesized that this reduction in D2 signaling could be contributing to compulsive drug use.

Dopamine may also play a critical role in the relationship between reward and circadian rhythms (see Figure 2). Extracellular dopamine fluctuates rhythmically in the dorsal striatum, with its peak amplitude during the active phase [107]. Furthermore, D2R activity contributes to the rhythm of *Per2* expression in striatum [107], indicating that dopamine interacts with the circadian clock in reward-related brain regions. Therefore, drug-induced changes to the dopamine system may play a critical role in the disruption of circadian rhythms in addicts. For example, sleep disturbances are one of the key effects of chronic drug use in rodents [82, 87, 88] and in humans [7, 89, 90].

Sleep-wake disruptions may be regulated not only by circadian rhythms but also by ultradian rhythms, which are cycles that repeat every few hours in the body, such as alertness and appetite. The dopaminergic ultradian oscillator cycles with the circadian clock, but the two can become desynchronized when dopaminergic tone is elevated like in drug abuse [108]. This desynchronization can lead to aberrant arousal, similar to disturbed sleep-wake cycles seen across psychiatric disorders, including addiction. However, less is known about the mechanisms underlying ultradian rhythms compared to circadian rhythms. Future research should focus on dissecting the contributions of ultradian and circadian rhythm disturbances to drug addiction.

The relationship between circadian rhythms and addiction appears to be cyclical. Dopamine and drugs of abuse can disrupt rhythms, but sleep disturbances can also affect the dopaminergic system. Sleep deprivation decreases availability of D2 and D3R in the ventral striatum [109]. This finding seems to be a result of a downregulation of D2/D3 receptors in the ventral striatum, in lieu of dopamine increases, after sleep deprivation [110]. In this particularly translational study, a similar lack of change in dopamine levels in the ventral striatum was also seen in rats after one night of sleep deprivation [110]. Importantly, in cocaine abusers, sleep duration predicts D2/D3 availability [111]. This suggests that impaired sleep contributes to lower striatal D2/3 in cocaine abusers and that intervening with sleep patterns could improve treatment outcomes. However, it is again important to note that sleep disturbances might not necessarily correspond to changes in circadian rhythms.

Several studies have examined relationships between drugs of abuse, dopamine receptor type, the ventral striatum, and circadian genes. One study indicates that circadian genes might play a role in regulating dopamine receptor availability, possibly in the context of drug exposure. For example, striatal D2R levels are associated with the genotype of a novel variable number tandem repeat polymorphism in the *PER2* gene. Furthermore, genotype distribution is varied in cocaine abusers compared to controls [112].

Another study found that disturbing circadian rhythms with exposure to constant light increases expression of Per1, Per2, and D1R in the striatum could contribute to vulnerability to morphine consumption and preference in rats [113]. In mice, genetic manipulations of circadian clock genes impact cocaine preference as well as dopamine receptor expression (see Figure 2 for potential mechanisms). A dominant negative mutation in the *Clock* gene increases cocaine preference [114], whereas knocking out *NPAS2*, or knocking down NPAS2 in the ventral striatum, decreases cocaine preference [115]. *Clock*, and more so *Npas2*, is enriched in D1-containing neurons in the striatum, and ventral striatal NPAS2 knockdown disrupts the rhythmic expression of *Drd3* (dopamine receptor 3) [115]. Furthermore, chronic cocaine exposure disrupts diurnal rhythms in *Drd3* and *Drd1* [115].

Recently, a fair amount of research has investigated the role that circadian genes play in the effects of drugs of abuse on dopamine receptor availability and distribution in the ventral striatum. These studies emphasize the importance of circadian rhythms and circadian genes in one of the most prominent and well-studied mechanisms underlying addiction. Moving forward, we should continue to lay the groundwork for understanding how circadian rhythms and addiction are connected.

5. Summary

Taken together, these findings could help answer one of the most important questions facing the field of circadian rhythms and addiction today: do rhythms matter for treatment? Circadian rhythms appear to be important for drug taking and potentially for the transition to substance dependence and if rhythms matter for patient outcomes. It is critical to continue answering the questions posed in this review. Based on findings that sleep disturbances, whether induced by drugs of abuse or not, disrupt reward-related circuitry, it appears that treating sleep disturbances could be critically important. These treatments could occur preventively, for example, during development when sleep disruptions begin, or retrospectively, in the case of drug exposure where sleep disturbances are a symptom of use and withdrawal, which contribute to relapse. Moreover, determining the mechanisms by which drug taking is regulated by the circadian clock will lead to the development of novel therapies, including light therapy, and/or treatment approaches, such as phase-controlling treatment.

Fortunately, parallel findings studying circadian rhythms and/or sleep, and drug addiction are becoming more frequent in animal models. However, it is important to remember the shortcomings of mouse models. For example, the SCN appears to adapt much faster in rodents than it does in humans, which could lessen the severity or impact of sleep disruptions in rodent models. Therefore, care should be used when directly comparing circadian impairments and sleep disruptions across species.

Due to this additional factor, clinical research should take advantage of the mechanistic findings from animal models and try to create therapies for drug-induced impairments in circadian rhythm, but it is possible these mechanisms will be slightly different. Most of the animal literature is still building on a few, older human studies with very small sample size; therefore, updating and building on the existing human literature is imperative. In particular, studies aimed at manipulating circadian sleep and then investigating the effects on reward or vulnerability to drug use would be a crucial addition to the field.

Despite the difficulties, paralleling animal and human behavioral studies and manipulations will ensure the field progresses rapidly. Clinical research is critical, but we need to leverage those findings by using animal models to discover possible mechanisms and gain information about potential druggable targets. These results can be brought full circle into human studies in order to improve treatments options and approaches.

Conflicts of Interest

The authors declare that they have no conflicts of interest.

Acknowledgments

This study was supported by Grants DA039841, DA039865, DA042886, MH077159, and MH106460 (Colleen A. McClung) and Grants DA038654 and DA041872 (Ryan W. Logan).

References

[1] A. Wirz-Justice, "Biological rhythm disturbances in mood disorders," *International Clinical Psychopharmacology*, vol. 21, Supplement 1, pp. S11–S15, 2006.

[2] C. A. McClung, "Circadian genes, rhythms and the biology of mood disorders," *Pharmacology & Therapeutics*, vol. 114, pp. 222–232, 2007.

[3] E. M. Jones, D. Knutson, and D. Haines, "Common problems in patients recovering from chemical dependency," *American Family Physician*, vol. 68, pp. 1971–1978, 2003.

[4] P. T. Morgan, E. F. Pace-Schott, Z. H. Sahul, V. Coric, R. Stickgold, and R. T. Malison, "Sleep, sleep-dependent procedural learning and vigilance in chronic cocaine users: evidence for occult insomnia," *Drug and Alcohol Dependence*, vol. 82, pp. 238–249, 2006.

[5] D. A. Conroy, I. S. Hairston, J. T. Arnedt, R. F. Hoffmann, R. Armitage, and K. J. Brower, "Dim light melatonin onset in alcohol-dependent men and women compared with healthy controls," *Chronobiology International*, vol. 29, pp. 35–42, 2012.

[6] P. T. Morgan and R. T. Malison, "Cocaine and sleep: early abstinence," *The Scientific World Journal*, vol. 7, pp. 223–230, 2007.

[7] T. Schierenbeck, D. Riemann, M. Berger, and M. Hornyak, "Effect of illicit recreational drugs upon sleep: cocaine, ecstasy and marijuana," *Sleep Medicine Reviews*, vol. 12, pp. 381–389, 2008.

[8] D. A. A. Baranger, C. Ifrah, A. A. Prather et al., "PER1 rs3027172 genotype interacts with early life stress to predict problematic alcohol use, but not reward-related ventral striatum activity," *Frontiers in Psychology*, vol. 7, p. 464, 2016.

[9] J. Bi, J. Gelernter, J. Sun, and H. R. Kranzler, "Comparing the utility of homogeneous subtypes of cocaine use and related behaviors with DSM-IV cocaine dependence as traits for genetic association analysis," *American Journal of Medical Genetics Part B: Neuropsychiatric Genetics*, vol. 165, pp. 148–156, 2014.

[10] D. Blomeyer, A. F. Buchmann, J. Lascorz et al., "Association of PER2 genotype and stressful life events with alcohol drinking in young adults," *PLoS One*, vol. 8, article e59136, 2013.

[11] E. E. Forbes, R. E. Dahl, J. R. C. Almeida et al., "*PER2 rs2304672* polymorphism moderates circadian-relevant reward circuitry activity in adolescents," *Biological Psychiatry*, vol. 71, pp. 451–457, 2012.

[12] L. Kovanen, S. T. Saarikoski, J. Haukka et al., "Circadian clock gene polymorphisms in alcohol use disorders and alcohol consumption," *Alcohol and Alcoholism*, vol. 45, pp. 303–311, 2010.

[13] L. Dong, A. Bilbao, M. Laucht et al., "Effects of the circadian rhythm gene period 1 (*Per1*) on psychosocial stress-induced alcohol drinking," *The American Journal of Psychiatry*, vol. 168, pp. 1090–1098, 2011.

[14] J. J. Gamsby, E. L. Templeton, L. A. Bonvini et al., "The circadian *Per1* and *Per2* genes influence alcohol intake, reinforcement, and blood alcohol levels," *Behavioural Brain Research*, vol. 249, pp. 15–21, 2013.

[15] A. R. Ozburn, E. Falcon, S. Mukherjee et al., "The role of *Clock* in ethanol-related behaviors," *Neuropsychopharmacology*, vol. 38, pp. 2393–2400, 2013.

[16] A. R. Ozburn, E. B. Larson, D. W. Self, and C. A. McClung, "Cocaine self-administration behaviors in *Clock*Δ19 mice," *Psychopharmacology*, vol. 223, pp. 169–177, 2012.

[17] C. G. Jones, P. B. Yang, V. T. Wilcox, K. D. Burau, and N. Dafny, "Acute and chronic psychostimulant treatment modulates the diurnal rhythm activity pattern of WKY female adolescent rats," *Journal of Neural Transmission*, vol. 121, pp. 457–468, 2014.

[18] L. E. O'Dell, S. A. Chen, R. T. Smith et al., "Extended access to nicotine self-administration leads to dependence: circadian measures, withdrawal measures, and extinction behavior in rats," *Journal of Pharmacology and Experimental Therapeutics*, vol. 320, pp. 180–193, 2006.

[19] D. C. S. Roberts, K. Brebner, M. Vincler, and W. J. Lynch, "Patterns of cocaine self-administration in rats produced by various access conditions under a discrete trials procedure," *Drug and Alcohol Dependence*, vol. 67, pp. 291–299, 2002.

[20] W. J. Lynch, M. J. Girgenti, F. J. Breslin, S. S. Newton, and J. R. Taylor, "Gene profiling the response to repeated cocaine self-administration in dorsal striatum: a focus on circadian genes," *Brain Research*, vol. 1213, pp. 166–177, 2008.

[21] B. Chen, Y. Wang, X. Liu, Z. Liu, Y. Dong, and Y. H. Huang, "Sleep regulates incubation of cocaine craving," *The Journal of Neuroscience*, vol. 35, pp. 13300–13310, 2015.

[22] J. A. Cortes, G. Gomez, C. Ehnerd et al., "Altered activity-based sleep measures in rhesus monkeys following cocaine self-administration and abstinence," *Drug and Alcohol Dependence*, vol. 163, pp. 202–208, 2016.

[23] H. T. Jansen, A. Sergeeva, G. Stark, and B. A. Sorg, "Circadian discrimination of reward: evidence for simultaneous yet separable food- and drug-entrained rhythms in the rat," *Chronobiology International*, vol. 29, pp. 454–468, 2012.

[24] D. R. Keith, C. L. Hart, M. Robotham, M. Tariq, J. Le Sauter, and R. Silver, "Time of day influences the voluntary intake and behavioral response to methamphetamine and food reward," *Pharmacology Biochemistry and Behavior*, vol. 110, pp. 117–126, 2013.

[25] J. A. Mohawk, P. Pezuk, and M. Menaker, "Methamphetamine and dopamine receptor D1 regulate entrainment of murine circadian oscillators," *PLoS One*, vol. 8, article e62463, 2013.

[26] J. Mendoza, "Circadian clocks: setting time by food," *Journal of Neuroendocrinology*, vol. 19, pp. 127–137, 2007.

[27] A. A. van der Klaauw, E. A. H. von dem Hagen, J. M. Keogh et al., "Obesity-associated melanocortin-4 receptor mutations are associated with changes in the brain response to food cues," *The Journal of Clinical Endocrinology & Metabolism*, vol. 99, pp. E2101–E2106, 2014.

[28] N. D. Volkow, G.-J. Wang, D. Tomasi, and R. D. Baler, "Obesity and addiction: neurobiological overlaps," *Obesity Reviews*, vol. 14, pp. 2–18, 2013.

[29] Z. Liu, M. Huang, X. Wu et al., "PER1 phosphorylation specifies feeding rhythm in mice," *Cell Reports*, vol. 7, pp. 1509–1520, 2014.

[30] S. Yang, A. Liu, A. Weidenhammer et al., "The role of *mPer2* clock gene in glucocorticoid and feeding rhythms," *Endocrinology*, vol. 150, pp. 2153–2160, 2009.

[31] B. Guo, S. Chatterjee, L. Li et al., "The clock gene, brain and muscle Arnt-like 1, regulates adipogenesis *via* Wnt signaling pathway," *The FASEB Journal*, vol. 26, pp. 3453–3463, 2012.

[32] F. W. Turek, C. Joshu, A. Kohsaka et al., "Obesity and metabolic syndrome in circadian clock mutant mice," *Science*, vol. 308, pp. 1043–1045, 2005.

[33] D. M. Arble, J. Bass, A. D. Laposky, M. H. Vitaterna, and F. W. Turek, "Circadian timing of food intake contributes to weight gain," *Obesity*, vol. 17, pp. 2100–2102, 2009.

[34] R. Salgado-Delgado, M. Angeles-Castellanos, N. Saderi, R. M. Buijs, and C. Escobar, "Food intake during the normal activity phase prevents obesity and circadian desynchrony in a rat model of night work," *Endocrinology*, vol. 151, pp. 1019–1029, 2010.

[35] M. Hatori, C. Vollmers, A. Zarrinpar et al., "Time-restricted feeding without reducing caloric intake prevents metabolic diseases in mice fed a high-fat diet," *Cell Metabolism*, vol. 15, pp. 848–860, 2012.

[36] C. Escobar, R. Salgado, K. Rodriguez, A. S. Blancas Vázquez, M. Angeles-Castellanos, and R. M. Buijs, "Scheduled meals and scheduled palatable snacks synchronize circadian rhythms: consequences for ingestive behavior," *Physiology & Behavior*, vol. 104, pp. 555–561, 2011.

[37] V. van der Vinne, J. Akkerman, G. D. Lanting, S. J. Riede, and R. A. Hut, "Food reward without a timing component does not alter the timing of activity under positive energy balance," *Neuroscience*, vol. 304, pp. 260–265, 2015.

[38] F. Damiola, N. Le Minh, N. Preitner, B. Kornmann, F. Fleury-Olela, and U. Schibler, "Restricted feeding uncouples circadian oscillators in peripheral tissues from the central pacemaker in the suprachiasmatic nucleus," *Genes & Development*, vol. 14, pp. 2950–2961, 2000.

[39] R. A. Hut, V. Pilorz, A. S. Boerema, A. M. Strijkstra, and S. Daan, "Working for food shifts nocturnal mouse activity into the day," *PLoS One*, vol. 6, article e17527, 2011.

[40] V. van der Vinne, S. J. Riede, J. A. Gorter et al., "Cold and hunger induce diurnality in a nocturnal mammal," *Proceedings of the National Academy of Sciences of the United States of America*, vol. 111, pp. 15256–15260, 2014.

[41] M. Angeles-Castellanos, R. Salgado-Delgado, K. Rodríguez, R. M. Buijs, and C. Escobar, "Expectancy for food or expectancy for chocolate reveals timing systems for metabolism and reward," *Neuroscience*, vol. 155, pp. 297–307, 2008.

[42] A. Mitra, C. Lenglos, J. Martin, N. Mbende, A. Gagné, and E. Timofeeva, "Sucrose modifies *c-fos* mRNA expression in the brain of rats maintained on feeding schedules," *Neuroscience*, vol. 192, pp. 459–474, 2011.

[43] C. M. Gallardo, K. M. Gunapala, O. D. King, and A. D. Steele, "Daily scheduled high fat meals moderately entrain behavioral anticipatory activity, body temperature, and hypothalamic c-Fos activation," *PLoS One*, vol. 7, article e41161, 2012.

[44] S. W. Cain, C. H. Ko, J. A. Chalmers, and M. R. Ralph, "Time of day modulation of conditioned place preference in rats depends on the strain of rat used," *Neurobiology of Learning and Memory*, vol. 81, pp. 217–220, 2004.

[45] A. V. Monclaro, A. C. Sampaio, N. B. Ribeiro, and M. Barros, "Time-of-day effect on a food-induced conditioned place preference task in monkeys," *Behavioural Brain Research*, vol. 259, pp. 336–341, 2014.

[46] E. G. Marchant and R. E. Mistlberger, "Anticipation and entrainment to feeding time in intact and SCN-ablated C57BL/6j mice," *Brain Research*, vol. 765, pp. 273–282, 1997.

[47] Z. Boulos, A. M. Rosenwasser, and M. Terman, "Feeding schedules and the circadian organization of behavior in the rat," *Behavioural Brain Research*, vol. 1, pp. 39–65, 1980.

[48] F. K. Stephan, J. M. Swann, and C. L. Sisk, "Anticipation of 24-hr feeding schedules in rats with lesions of the suprachiasmatic nucleus," *Behavioral and Neural Biology*, vol. 25, pp. 346–363, 1979.

[49] C. Escobar, J. Y. Mendoza, A. Salazar-Juárez et al., "Rats made cirrhotic by chronic CCl4 treatment still exhibit anticipatory activity to a restricted feeding schedule," *Chronobiology International*, vol. 19, pp. 1073–1086, 2002.

[50] A.-M. Poulin and E. Timofeeva, "The dynamics of neuronal activation during food anticipation and feeding in the brain of food-entrained rats," *Brain Research*, vol. 1227, pp. 128–141, 2008.

[51] A. Blancas, S. D. González-García, K. Rodríguez, and C. Escobar, "Progressive anticipation in behavior and brain activation of rats exposed to scheduled daily palatable food," *Neuroscience*, vol. 281, pp. 44–53, 2014.

[52] J. Mendoza, M. Angeles-Castellanos, and C. Escobar, "Entrainment by a palatable meal induces food-anticipatory activity and c-Fos expression in reward-related areas of the brain," *Neuroscience*, vol. 133, pp. 293–303, 2005.

[53] A. M. Bao, R. Y. Liu, E. J. van Someren, M. A. Hofman, Y. X. Cao, and J. N. Zhou, "Diurnal rhythm of free estradiol during the menstrual cycle," *European Journal of Endocrinology*, vol. 148, pp. 227–232, 2003.

[54] M. Fatehi and Z. Fatehi-Hassanabad, "Effects of 17β-estradiol on neuronal cell excitability and neurotransmission in the suprachiasmatic nucleus of rat," *Neuropsychopharmacology*, vol. 33, pp. 1354–1364, 2008.

[55] J.-C. Dreher, P. J. Schmidt, P. Kohn, D. Furman, D. Rubinow, and K. F. Berman, "Menstrual cycle phase modulates reward-related neural function in women," *Proceedings of the National Academy of Sciences of the United States of America*, vol. 104, pp. 2465–2470, 2007.

[56] J. Thomas, E. Météreau, H. Déchaud, M. Pugeat, and J.-C. Dreher, "Hormonal treatment increases the response of the reward system at the menopause transition: a counterbalanced randomized placebo-controlled fMRI study," *Psychoneuroendocrinology*, vol. 50, pp. 167–180, 2014.

[57] Z. D. Cooper, R. W. Foltin, and S. M. Evans, "Effects of menstrual cycle phase on cocaine self-administration in rhesus macaques," *Hormones and Behavior*, vol. 63, pp. 105–113, 2013.

[58] H. Yang, W. Zhao, M. Hu, and J. B. Becker, "Interactions among ovarian hormones and time of testing on behavioral sensitization and cocaine self-administration," *Behavioural Brain Research*, vol. 184, pp. 174–184, 2007.

[59] L. R. Jackson, T. E. Robinson, and J. B. Becker, "Sex differences and hormonal influences on acquisition of cocaine self-administration in rats," *Neuropsychopharmacology*, vol. 31, pp. 129–138, 2005.

[60] M. Barrot, M. Marinelli, D. N. Abrous, F. Rougé-Pont, M. Le Moal, and P. V. Piazza, "The dopaminergic hyper-responsiveness of the shell of the nucleus accumbens is hormone-dependent," *The European Journal of Neuroscience*, vol. 12, pp. 973–979, 2000.

[61] M. Marinelli and P. V. Piazza, "Interaction between glucocorticoid hormones, stress and psychostimulant drugs," *The European Journal of Neuroscience*, vol. 16, pp. 387–394, 2002.

[62] E. R. Montoya, P. A. Bos, D. Terburg, L. A. Rosenberger, and J. van Honk, "Cortisol administration induces global down-regulation of the brain's reward circuitry," *Psychoneuroendocrinology*, vol. 47, pp. 31–42, 2014.

[63] A. J. Porcelli, A. H. Lewis, and M. R. Delgado, "Acute stress influences neural circuits of reward processing," *Frontiers in Neuroscience*, vol. 6, p. 157, 2012.

[64] R. J. DiLeone, J. R. Taylor, and M. R. Picciotto, "The drive to eat: comparisons and distinctions between mechanisms of food reward and drug addiction," *Nature Neuroscience*, vol. 15, pp. 1330–1335, 2012.

[65] A. Hajnal and R. Norgren, "Accumbens dopamine mechanisms in sucrose intake," *Brain Research*, vol. 904, pp. 76–84, 2001.

[66] G. P. Mark, D. S. Blander, and B. G. Hoebel, "A conditioned stimulus decreases extracellular dopamine in the nucleus accumbens after the development of a learned taste aversion," *Brain Research*, vol. 551, pp. 308–310, 1991.

[67] D. M. Small, M. Jones-Gotman, and A. Dagher, "Feeding-induced dopamine release in dorsal striatum correlates with meal pleasantness ratings in healthy human volunteers," *NeuroImage*, vol. 19, pp. 1709–1715, 2003.

[68] K. S. Burger and E. Stice, "Frequent ice cream consumption is associated with reduced striatal response to receipt of an ice cream-based milkshake," *The American Journal of Clinical Nutrition*, vol. 95, pp. 810–817, 2012.

[69] R. Gloria, L. Angelos, H. S. Schaefer et al., "An fMRI investigation of the impact of withdrawal on regional brain activity during nicotine anticipation," *Psychophysiology*, vol. 46, pp. 681–693, 2009.

[70] T. Tsurugizawa, A. Uematsu, H. Uneyama, and K. Torii, "Functional brain mapping of conscious rats during reward anticipation," *Journal of Neuroscience Methods*, vol. 206, pp. 132–137, 2012.

[71] D. M. Buffalari and R. E. See, "Amygdala mechanisms of pavlovian psychostimulant conditioning and relapse," *Current Topics in Behavioral Neurosciences*, vol. 3, pp. 73–99, 2010.

[72] R. Martin-Fardon, G. Cauvi, T. M. Kerr, and F. Weiss, "Differential role of hypothalamic orexin/hypocretin neurons in reward seeking motivated by cocaine versus palatable food," *Addiction Biology*, 2016.

[73] M. Lenoir, F. Serre, L. Cantin, and S. H. Ahmed, "Intense sweetness surpasses cocaine reward," *PLoS One*, vol. 2, article e698, 2007.

[74] D. N. Kearns, M. A. Gomez-Serrano, and B. J. Tunstall, "A review of preclinical research demonstrating that drug and non-drug reinforcers differentially affect behavior," *Current Drug Abuse Reviews*, vol. 4, pp. 261–269, 2011.

[75] C. Abarca, U. Albrecht, and R. Spanagel, "Cocaine sensitization and reward are under the influence of circadian genes and rhythm," *Proceedings of the National Academy of Sciences*, vol. 99, pp. 9026–9030, 2002.

[76] J. L. Trujillo, A. J. Roberts, and M. R. Gorman, "Circadian timing of ethanol exposure exerts enduring effects on subsequent ad libitum consumption in C57 mice," *Alcoholism, Clinical and Experimental Research*, vol. 33, pp. 1286–1293, 2009.

[77] I. C. Webb, "Circadian rhythms and substance abuse: chronobiological considerations for the treatment of addiction," *Current Psychiatry Reports*, vol. 19, p. 12, 2017.

[78] E. Falcon, A. Ozburn, S. Mukherjee, K. Roybal, and C. A. McClung, "Differential regulation of the period genes in striatal regions following cocaine exposure," *PLoS One*, vol. 8, article e66438, 2013.

[79] P. Zhou, J. H. Werner, D. Lee, A. D. Sheppard, S. Liangpunsakul, and G. E. Duffield, "Dissociation between diurnal cycles in locomotor activity, feeding behavior and hepatic PERIOD2 expression in chronic alcohol-fed mice," *Alcohol*, vol. 49, pp. 399–408, 2015.

[80] M. Eisenhardt, S. Leixner, R. Spanagel, and A. Bilbao, "Quantification of alcohol drinking patterns in mice," *Addiction Biology*, vol. 20, pp. 1001–1011, 2015.

[81] S. H. Ahmed and G. F. Koob, "Transition from moderate to excessive drug intake: change in hedonic set point," *Science*, vol. 282, pp. 298–300, 1998.

[82] E. S. Calipari, T. J. R. Beveridge, S. R. Jones, and L. J. Porrino, "Withdrawal from extended-access cocaine self-administration results in dysregulated functional activity and altered locomotor activity in rats," *The European Journal of Neuroscience*, vol. 38, pp. 3749–3757, 2013.

[83] G. Deneau, T. Yanagita, and M. H. Seevers, "Self-administration of psychoactive substances by the monkey," *Psychopharmacologia*, vol. 16, pp. 30–48, 1969.

[84] C. E. Johanson, R. L. Balster, and K. Bonese, "Self-administration of psychomotor stimulant drugs: the effects of unlimited access," *Pharmacology Biochemistry and Behavior*, vol. 4, pp. 45–51, 1976.

[85] T. J. Martin, W. Kahn, D. G. Cannon, and J. E. Smith, "Self-administration of heroin, cocaine and their combination under a discrete trial schedule of reinforcement in rats," *Drug and Alcohol Dependence*, vol. 82, pp. 282–286, 2006.

[86] J. Mantsch, V. Yuferov, A.-M. Mathieu-Kia, A. Ho, and M. Kreek, "Effects of extended access to high versus low cocaine doses on self-administration, cocaine-induced reinstatement and brain mRNA levels in rats," *Psychopharmacology*, vol. 175, pp. 26–36, 2004.

[87] M. A. Bozarth and R. A. Wise, "Toxicity associated with long-term intravenous heroin and cocaine self-administration in the rat," *JAMA*, vol. 254, pp. 81–83, 1985.

[88] L. M. Veatch, "Disruptions in sleep time and sleep architecture in a mouse model of repeated ethanol withdrawal," *Alcoholism: Clinical and Experimental Research*, vol. 30, pp. 1214–1222, 2006.

[89] K. J. Brower and J. M. Hall, "Effects of age and alcoholism on sleep: a controlled study," *Journal of Studies on Alcohol*, vol. 62, pp. 335–343, 2001.

[90] D. Mossberg, P. Liljeberg, and S. Borg, "Clinical conditions in alcoholics during long-term abstinence: a descriptive, longitudinal treatment study," *Alcohol*, vol. 2, pp. 551–553, 1985.

[91] R. A. Kowatch, S. S. Schnoll, J. S. Knisely, D. Green, and R. K. Elswick, "Electroencephalographic sleep and mood during cocaine withdrawal," *Journal of Addictive Diseases*, vol. 11, pp. 21–45, 1992.

[92] G. A. Angarita, S. V. Canavan, E. Forselius, A. Bessette, B. Pittman, and P. T. Morgan, "Abstinence-related changes in sleep during treatment for cocaine dependence," *Drug and Alcohol Dependence*, vol. 134, pp. 343–347, 2014.

[93] D. Matuskey, B. Pittman, E. Forselius, R. T. Malison, and P. T. Morgan, "A multistudy analysis of the effects of early cocaine abstinence on sleep," *Drug and Alcohol Dependence*, vol. 115, pp. 62–66, 2011.

[94] M. D. Puhl, M. Boisvert, Z. Guan, J. Fang, and P. S. Grigson, "A novel model of chronic sleep restriction reveals an increase in the perceived incentive reward value of cocaine in high drug-taking rats," *Pharmacology Biochemistry and Behavior*, vol. 109, pp. 8–15, 2013.

[95] R. F. Crossland, A. Balasa, R. Ramakrishnan, S. K. Mahadevan, M. L. Fiorotto, and I. B. Van den Veyver, "Chronic maternal low-protein diet in mice affects anxiety, night-time energy expenditure and sleep patterns, but not circadian rhythm in male offspring," *PLoS One*, vol. 12, article e0170127, 2017.

[96] A. M. Wells, E. Ridener, C. A. Bourbonais et al., "Effects of chronic social defeat stress on sleep and circadian rhythms are mitigated by kappa-opioid receptor antagonism," *The Journal of Neuroscience*, vol. 37, pp. 7656–7668, 2017.

[97] C. E. Bass, H. T. Jansen, and R. DCS, "Free-running rhythms of cocaine self-administration in rats held under constant lighting conditions," *Chronobiology International*, vol. 27, pp. 535–548, 2010.

[98] D. L. Graham, R. Hoppenot, A. Hendryx, and D. W. Self, "Differential ability of D1 and D2 dopamine receptor agonists to induce and modulate expression and reinstatement of cocaine place preference in rats," *Psychopharmacology*, vol. 191, pp. 719–730, 2007.

[99] M. K. Lobo, H. E. Covington, D. Chaudhury et al., "Cell type-specific loss of BDNF signaling mimics optogenetic control of cocaine reward," *Science*, vol. 330, pp. 385–390, 2010.

[100] M. Michaelides, P. K. Thanos, R. Kim et al., "PET imaging predicts future body weight and cocaine preference," *NeuroImage*, vol. 59, pp. 1508–1513, 2012.

[101] Z. Luo, N. D. Volkow, N. Heintz, Y. Pan, and C. Du, "Acute cocaine induces fast activation of D1 receptor and progressive deactivation of D2 receptor striatal neurons: *in vivo* optical microprobe $[Ca^{2+}]_i$ imaging," *The Journal of Neuroscience*, vol. 31, pp. 13180–13190, 2011.

[102] K. Park, N. D. Volkow, Y. Pan, and C. Du, "Chronic cocaine dampens dopamine signaling during cocaine intoxication and unbalances D_1 over D_2 receptor signaling," *The Journal of Neuroscience*, vol. 33, pp. 15827–15836, 2013.

[103] N. D. Volkow, D. Tomasi, G.-J. Wang et al., "Evidence that sleep deprivation downregulates dopamine D2R in ventral striatum in the human brain," *The Journal of Neuroscience*, vol. 32, pp. 6711–6717, 2012.

[104] D. Martinez, K. M. Carpenter, F. Liu et al., "Imaging dopamine transmission in cocaine dependence: link between neurochemistry and response to treatment," *The American Journal of Psychiatry*, vol. 168, pp. 634–641, 2011.

[105] N. D. Volkow, G.-J. Wang, J. S. Fowler et al., "Decreased striatal dopaminergic responsiveness in detoxified cocaine-dependent subjects," *Nature*, vol. 386, pp. 830–833, 1997.

[106] N. D. Volkow, D. Tomasi, G.-J. Wang et al., "Stimulant-induced dopamine increases are markedly blunted in active cocaine abusers," *Molecular Psychiatry*, vol. 19, pp. 1037–1043, 2014.

[107] S. Hood, P. Cassidy, M.-P. Cossette et al., "Endogenous dopamine regulates the rhythm of expression of the clock protein PER2 in the rat dorsal striatum via daily activation of D_2 dopamine receptors," *The Journal of Neuroscience*, vol. 30, pp. 14046–14058, 2010.

[108] I. D. Blum, L. Zhu, L. Moquin et al., "A highly tunable dopaminergic oscillator generates ultradian rhythms of behavioral arousal," *eLife*, vol. 3, 2014.

[109] N. D. Volkow, G.-J. Wang, F. Telang et al., "Sleep deprivation decreases binding of $[^{11}C]$raclopride to dopamine D_2/D_3 receptors in the human brain," *The Journal of Neuroscience*, vol. 28, pp. 8454–8461, 2008.

[110] N. D. Volkow, G.-J. Wang, J. S. Fowler, and D. Tomasi, "Addiction circuitry in the human brain," *Annual Review of Pharmacology and Toxicology*, vol. 52, pp. 321–336, 2012.

[111] C. E. Wiers, E. Shumay, E. Cabrera et al., "Reduced sleep duration mediates decreases in striatal D2/D3 receptor availability in cocaine abusers," *Translational Psychiatry*, vol. 6, article e752, 2016.

[112] E. Shumay, J. S. Fowler, G.-J. Wang et al., "Repeat variation in the human *PER2* gene as a new genetic marker associated with cocaine addiction and brain dopamine D2 receptor availability," *Translational Psychiatry*, vol. 2, article e86, 2012.

[113] B. Garmabi, N. Vousooghi, M. Vosough, A. Yoonessi, A. Bakhtazad, and M. R. Zarrindast, "Effect of circadian rhythm disturbance on morphine preference and addiction in male rats: involvement of period genes and dopamine D1 receptor," *Neuroscience*, vol. 322, pp. 104–114, 2016.

[114] C. A. McClung, K. Sidiropoulou, M. Vitaterna et al., "Regulation of dopaminergic transmission and cocaine reward by the clock gene," *Proceedings of the National Academy of Sciences*, vol. 102, pp. 9377–9381, 2005.

[115] A. R. Ozburn, E. Falcon, A. Twaddle et al., "Direct regulation of diurnal Drd3 expression and cocaine reward by NPAS2," *Biological Psychiatry*, vol. 77, pp. 425–433, 2015.

[116] A. Blancas-Velazquez, S. E. la Fleur, and J. Mendoza, "Effects of a free-choice high-fat high-sugar diet on brain PER2 and BMAL1 protein expression in mice," *Appetite*, vol. 117, pp. 263–269, 2017.

[117] C. Bainier, M. Mateo, M.-P. Felder-Schmittbuhl, and J. Mendoza, "Circadian rhythms of hedonic drinking behavior in mice," *Neuroscience*, vol. 349, pp. 229–238, 2017.

[118] L. J. Porrino, H. R. Smith, M. A. Nader, and T. J. R. Beveridge, "The effects of cocaine: a shifting target over the course of addiction," *Progress in Neuro-Psychopharmacology and Biological Psychiatry*, vol. 31, pp. 1593–1600, 2007.

[119] G. Hampp, J. A. Ripperger, T. Houben et al., "Regulation of monoamine oxidase a by circadian-clock components implies clock influence on mood," *Current Biology*, vol. 18, pp. 678–683, 2008.

10

Proteostasis and Mitochondrial Role on Psychiatric and Neurodegenerative Disorders: Current Perspectives

Pablo Olivero,[1,2] Carlo Lozano,[1,2,3] Ramón Sotomayor-Zárate,[4] Nicolás Meza-Concha,[1] Marcelo Arancibia,[1] Claudio Córdova,[1] Wilfredo González-Arriagada,[2,5] Ricardo Ramírez-Barrantes,[6] and Ivanny Marchant[1,2]

[1]*Laboratorio de Estructura y Función Celular, Escuela de Medicina, Facultad de Medicina, Universidad de Valparaíso, Hontaneda 2664, 2341386 Valparaíso, Chile*
[2]*Centro Interoperativo en Ciencias Odontológicas y Médicas, Universidad de Valparaíso, Valparaíso, Chile*
[3]*Servicio de Anatomía Patológica, Hospital Carlos van Buren, San Ignacio 725, Valparaíso, Chile*
[4]*Laboratorio de Neuroquímica y Neurofarmacología, Centro de Neurobiología y Fisiopatología Integrativa, Instituto de Fisiología, Facultad de Ciencias, Universidad de Valparaíso, Valparaíso, Chile*
[5]*Patología y Diagnóstico Oral, Facultad de Odontología, Universidad de Valparaíso, Valparaíso, Chile*
[6]*Escuela de Tecnologia Medica, Universidad Andres Bello, Quillota 980, 2531015 Viña del Mar, Chile*

Correspondence should be addressed to Ricardo Ramírez-Barrantes; ricardo.ramirez@unab.cl and Ivanny Marchant; ivanny.marchant@uv.cl

Academic Editor: Paola Bonsi

Proteostasis involves processes that are fundamental for neural viability. Thus, protein misfolding and the formation of toxic aggregates at neural level, secondary to dysregulation of the conservative mechanisms of proteostasis, are associated with several neuropsychiatric conditions. It has been observed that impaired mitochondrial function due to a dysregulated proteostasis control system, that is, ubiquitin-proteasome system and chaperones, could also have effects on neurodegenerative disorders. We aimed to critically analyze the available findings regarding the neurobiological implications of proteostasis on the development of neurodegenerative and psychiatric diseases, considering the mitochondrial role. Proteostasis alterations in the prefrontal cortex implicate proteome instability and accumulation of misfolded proteins. Altered mitochondrial dynamics, especially in proteostasis processes, could impede the normal compensatory mechanisms against cell damage. Thereby, altered mitochondrial functions on regulatory modulation of dendritic development, neuroinflammation, and respiratory function may underlie the development of some psychiatric conditions, such as schizophrenia, being influenced by a genetic background. It is expected that with the increasing evidence about proteostasis in neuropsychiatric disorders, new therapeutic alternatives will emerge.

1. Introduction

Ramón y Cajal, a pioneer in neuroscience, was the first to describe neurons as brain units that compose "cellular societies," from the point of view of functional morphology [1]. The story continues at the *Université de Paris*, where doctor Jean-Martin Charcot creates a chair on which all modern neurobiology develops. In fact, the autopsies performed by Charcot in illegitimate prostitutes' sons at the *Hôpital de la Salpêtrière* would change the vision of emerging neurobiology forever. Thanks to his contribution, it was possible to determine the existence of certain neuromuscular diseases and rudimentarily identify pathologies such as multiple sclerosis and Parkinson's disease. One hundred sixty years later, neuropathology could contribute to the study of neurodegenerative disorders through conventional techniques, for example, histopathology, histochemistry, or immunohistochemistry applied to the analysis of changes in normal distribution of various types of proteins in neurons and tissues. Then, in the 90s, the presence of the so-called inclusion bodies was demonstrated in prevalent neurodegenerative conditions like Alzheimer's disease (AD), Parkinson's disease (PD), Huntington's disease (HD), amyotrophic lateral sclerosis, polyglutamine diseases, and the Lewy body dementia. At the same time, immunohistochemistry revealed the role of the ubiquitin-proteasome system and molecular chaperones in the formation of inclusion bodies, particularly in AD and PD [2–7]. Nowadays, we know that besides neuronal involution and reactive gliosis, most neurodegenerative diseases are characterized by protein accumulation.

In protein biosynthesis, metabolic changes, mutations, and stress are frequent conditions that cause protein misfolding and hamper proper biological function. Being molecular machineries whose constituent elements are chaperones, the ubiquitin-proteasome system and the autophagy-lysosomal system [8, 9] constantly counteract these risks by avoiding the accumulation of nondegradable protein aggregates and the consequent cellular malfunction and death [10]. Preserving proteostasis, that is, stable conditions during processes such as biogenesis, folding, trafficking, or degradation of proteins, is crucial to guaranteeing cell functions and the ability to elaborate pertinent reactions to tissue-specific chronic and acute stressors [11]. Dysregulation of the conservative mechanisms of proteostasis involves processes that are fundamental for the viability of postmitotic cells such as neurons and has been associated with several neurodegenerative diseases, such as AD, PD, and HD, among others [12]. Thereby, with increasing knowledge about changes in the tissue protein distribution, new pathogenic mechanisms could be revealed as potential therapeutic targets, especially in the study of the ubiquitin-proteasome system and molecular chaperones [8, 13]. Besides, it has been observed that impaired mitochondrial function, which is influenced by the ubiquitin-proteasome system and chaperones, may also have effects on neurodegenerative disorders [14]. In the present work, we will review the main findings on the neurobiological implications of proteostasis, from a molecular perspective, in relation to the development of neurodegenerative and neuropsychiatric diseases. We discuss the genetic and molecular considerations of mitochondrial dysfunction, an important organelle in proteostasis, in schizophrenia. We conducted an exhaustive bibliographic search through the available articles on MEDLINE/PubMed database. Here, we present the main findings of the available literature, focusing on three main topics: (1) proteostasis in neurodegenerative disease, (2) TRPV1 and proteostasis, and (3) proteostasis and mitochondrial dysfunction in schizophrenia.

1.1. Proteostasis in Neurodegenerative Disease. The efficiency of the cellular physiological processes depends on proper protein localization and function. There is a molecular network that participates in the intricate mechanisms of synthesis, folding, trafficking, and degradation necessary to ensure the structure and function of proteins [15]. The maintenance of proteostasis thus involves the translational and folding machinery including their regulatory systems such as the unfolded protein response (UPR), as well as the large group of molecular chaperones such as HSP70, HSP90, DNAJ/HSP40, chaperonin/HSP60, and small HSP (sHSP) families [16, 17], which balance protein function and turnover. Chaperones' ATP-dependent function is impaired in cellular stress condition. Thus, poor physical recognition by chaperone networks and cellular metabolic stress condition may contribute to protein aggregation in aging and disease [18]. Proteins can be degraded individually or massively mainly in proteasomes by the ubiquitin-proteasome system (UPS) [15]. The UPS is part of the extensive system for protein quality control of neurons and other types of cells, regulating the degradation of misfolding or aberrant proteins to prevent detrimental aggregation. The proteins that will be degraded by the UPS are first ubiquitylated via a series of enzymatic reactions involving ubiquitin-activating (E1), conjugation (E2), and ligase (E3) enzymes [15]. Proteasomes include two subcomplexes, the core particle (CP, 20S) which is a barrel-shaped structure composed of four stacked rings, two identical outer α rings and two identical inner β rings, which carry the catalytic activity, and the regulatory particle (19S) which caps the extremities of the barrel and regulates the entry of ubiquitylated proteins into the catalytic center. The proteasomal network composition is highly dynamic; the levels of molecular chaperones and proteasome subunits can increase or decrease globally or specifically in some compartment, depending on factors such as environmental changes, genetic factors, and aging phenomena [19]. These changes lessen the ability of cells to regulate the accumulation of misfolded proteins, which can induce cell dysfunction and death [15]. The UPS in particular is able to modulate synaptic physiology both pre- and postsynaptically. UPS participation in the neuronal synapse implies regulating calcium channels and may have an impact on long-term memory [20].

Dysfunction of the proteostatic network decreases neuronal plasticity [21–23]. It has been reported that in response to LTP-inducing stimuli in the hippocampus, the activity of the proteasomes increases and also after activation of NMDAR [19]. The kinase CaMKIIα is activated by an entry of calcium via NMDAR which in turn phosphorylates and enhances the proteolytic activity of the proteasome, coupling the synaptic excitation with changes in proteostasis [19].

In mammalian neurons, proteasomal complexes attached to the plasma membrane have been described as nonconventional protein secretion systems. Once the proteins are degraded by these kinds of proteasomes, they are released into the extracellular space which in turn can stimulate postsynaptic neurons via NMDA-type receptors (involved in memory and learning). In addition, they are able to activate signals mediated by calcium [21]. Also, the application of proteasome inhibitors like MG132 induces a fast and several-fold increase in the frequency of spontaneous postsynaptic currents at excitatory and inhibitory synapses, which is independent of the accumulation of ubiquitylated proteins and specific by modulation of presynaptic neurons increasing the neurotransmitter release [24]. Furthermore, the inhibition of the proteasome system induces cell death in several cell types [22]. In neurons, the inhibition of proteasome has been shown to diminish the increase of cytosolic calcium that precedes programmed cell death, for example, before the activation of caspase-3 [22]. The progress of programmed cell death is very complex and depends on an orchestrated activation of proteins where calcium plays an important role. Experiments in primary cultures of neurons show that the activation of either a voltage-gated calcium channel or exchanger Na^+-Ca^{2+} in the plasma membrane during the initial steps in cell death attenuates the damage via increase of cytosolic Ca^{2+}. The inhibition of proteasome blocks this mechanism by reducing the increase of cytosolic calcium mediated by voltage-gated calcium channels [22]. Proteasome is also involved in other neural plasticity events like axonal growth, axonal guidance, and dendritic branching [23]. Failure of the proteostasis network may thus impede directly or indirectly the plasticity of neurons, by favoring the accumulation of aberrant proteins or modulating excitability, synapses, and growth.

Neurodegenerative diseases, which involve degradation of axons, loss of synapses, impairment of synaptic plasticity, and death of neurons, are one of the most enigmatic problems in medicine. Knowledge regarding these diseases has evolved from phenomenology description to mechanistic analysis, the hallmark being the aggregation and deposition of misfolded proteins [19]. AD, PD, and HD are today characterized by disrupted proteostasis, due to decreased function of the UPS, the accumulation of ubiquitylated proteins, and their aggregation, causing progressive neuronal dysfunction and death. Although ubiquitylated proteins can be localized in different brain areas, their high accumulation seems to be a common mechanism in all the diseases abovementioned and the UPS has been involved as primary or secondary cause. Mutations in genes encoding for UPS proteins [25] have also been associated with the development of hereditary forms of neurodegenerative diseases. Recent evidence shows that $A\beta$ peptides, α-synuclein, and mutant huntingtin protein, which are at the origin of the three most important neurodegenerative diseases, share a specific oligomeric conformation that impairs proteasome function. According to this study, the shared three-dimensional structure allows these oligomers to potently inhibit 20S and 26S proteasome gate opening, thus drastically reducing its function. This effect blocks the degradation of proteins favoring its abnormal accumulation [26]. In neurodegenerative disease, as previously described in prion diseases [27], the misfolding protein acts as a template and interacts directly with the native protein and converts the latter into a misfolded replicate. This is the process that aberrant proteins use to recruit and propagate intracellularly the misfolding protein [28]. This seeded aggregation mechanism is employed by $A\beta$ peptide, α-synuclein, and tau protein [28]. The accumulation of these proteins impairs the normal neuronal functions by altering the synaptic transmission [29] and causing cell death.

Besides neuronal dysfunction due to the accumulation of proteins, neurodegenerative disease could change the total protein expression. In particular in AD, a novel approach investigating postmortem the frontal cortex of sporadic AD patients using an integrated method of mass spectrometry-based quantitative proteomics revealed several clusters of modification of protein expression [30]. Using this method, the authors found 487 differentially expressed proteins with significantly altered levels. From this pool of proteins, 262 were upregulated while 225 were downregulated. In general terms, several functions in AD are altered which include proteostasis, RNA homeostasis, immune response, neuroinflammation, synaptic transmission, vesicular transport, cell signaling, cellular metabolism, lipid homeostasis, mitochondrial dynamics and function, cytoskeleton organization, and myelin-axon interactions. The identification of a wide spectrum of protein alterations strengthens the multifactorial and complex etiology of neurodegenerative disease and how the accumulation of altered proteins could alter completely the homeostasis of protein expression [30]. In the same line, AD proteomic applications indicate that the progression of the disease worsens several processes as energy production, signal transduction, synaptic plasticity, proteasome function, cellular morphology, and cell cycle [31].

In addition to protein misfolding and impaired proteostasis, neurodegenerative diseases are linked to imbalance of mitochondrial fission and fusion associated with an increase in oxidative stress. The association of mutant aberrant proteins with mitochondrial membrane has been reported to cause mitochondrial fragmentation, leading to mitochondrial dysfunction with concomitant production and liberation of reactive oxygen species. It is believed that this response would promote mitochondrial clearance by the cellular autophagic machinery via a process termed mitophagy [32], although the excess of activation of mitophagy could contribute to long-term neuronal degeneration [32]. This phenomenon is illustrated by PD where the abnormally degraded ubiquitylated proteins and α-synuclein often bind to mitochondrial membrane inducing mitochondrial dysfunction [33, 34].

Proteostasis is not limited to the cytoplasm only; it may occur in other cellular compartments. The most prominent are mitochondria and endoplasmic reticulum (ER), both organelles sharing multiple functions as calcium storage and lipid metabolism [35]. ER is considered the major site of cellular protein synthesis. One-third of the human proteome is synthesized in the ER, consisting in secreted proteins, integral membrane proteins, and functional proteins that connect the activity of ER and other organelles such as mitochondria [36].

C. elegans, *Drosophila*, and mammals, for instance, exhibit a mitochondrial unfolded protein response (mtUPR) against proteotoxic stress. This response could be activated by a wide range of noxious stimuli like depletion of mtDNA, impairment of mitochondrial chaperones or proteases, high concentration of ROS, or expression of misfolded proteins [37]. In general terms, this reaction consists in upregulating target genes that include organelle-specific chaperones and proteases to avoid the accumulation of toxic proteins [37]. Notably, this stress response is conserved in a cell culture model of HD, suggesting a general mechanism against stress [37].

Additional mechanisms may contribute to coordinated protein degradation between mitochondria and cytoplasm. The proteasome has been implied in the extraction and degradation of misfolded proteins of the mitochondrial outer membrane [38, 39]. In addition, it is possible that aggregates of cytosolic proteins can be sent to the mitochondria for their degradation by mitochondrial proteases [40]. Although this phenomenon remains incompletely understood, it is possible that the degradation system integrates the different cellular compartments to avoid protein aggregation not only in the cytoplasm but also in vital organelles such as endoplasmic reticulum and mitochondria, which can be altered by the aging process and neurodegenerative diseases. We present here below some examples of proteins involved in prevalent diseases and their particular role in neuron degeneration.

1.1.1. Tau Protein. Tau protein is abundant in the central nervous system, and its main physiological function is to stabilize the cytoskeleton through binding to microtubules [41, 42]. Recent information indicates that tau protein is involved in several other processes such as synaptic plasticity and memory. A knockout mouse model for tau ($Mapt^{-/-}$) evidenced aging-dependent short-term memory deficits, synaptic plasticity flaws, and impairment in long-term potentiation [43]. Some posttranslational modifications in tau protein such as phosphorylation, glycosylation, and ubiquitylation have been associated with neuropathologies. At the cellular level, Pick disease—a frontotemporal dementia that initiates with personality changes—is characterized by a large aggregation of hyperphosphorylated tau proteins that leads to production of Pick bodies [44, 45]. On the other hand, gliofibrillary tangles that characterize AD are composed of hyperphosphorylated tau proteins confined mainly to the entorhinal cortex [46, 47]. The accumulation of hyperphosphorylated tau is due to defective proteasomal degradation that may contribute to the build-up of tangles. In addition to phosphorylation, tau is also acetylated, and this modification impairs the proteasomal degradation and enhances the accumulation of tau. Together with Aβ-peptides, tau declines cognitive function, memory, and synaptic plasticity. These adverse effects produced by the combination of tau and Aβ can be prevented through the ablation of tau expression, leading to the hypothesis that tau is required for Aβ-induced synaptic dysfunction and memory deficits [43].

1.1.2. β-Amyloid. β-Amyloid is also involved in AD. This protein is formed from amyloid precursor protein, which is processed by α-, β-, and γ-secretase [48]. While the form $A\beta_{40}$ is the most common and soluble one, the more hydrophobic form $A\beta_{42}$ is considered the most amyloidogenic and, therefore, predominant component of senile plaques [49]. In fact, a great accumulation of senile plaques is associated with UPS dysfunction with consequent synaptic dysfunction and neuronal loss in cortical and subcortical regions, leading to cognitive impairment, memory loss, and motor disturbances [49].

1.1.3. α-Synuclein and PARK2. α-Synuclein is a soluble protein of 140 amino acids, which is abundant in neurons, and especially concentrated in presynaptic terminals [50]. This chaperone protein plays an important role in mediating protein-protein and protein-lipid interactions [51]. A mutated form of α-synuclein in patients with PD has been described [52], and again, the UPS is the main perturbed system favoring the accumulation of this protein. Selective inactivation of 26S proteasomes in substantia nigra dopaminergic neurons in a conditional knockout mouse model results in neurodegeneration and ubiquitin-positive aggregates resembling Lewy bodies (accumulation of α-synuclein). At a cognitive level, α-synuclein overexpression would induce a progressive loss of emotional memory secondary to mesolimbic dopaminergic dysfunction [53].

Parkin protein, now known as parkin RBR E3 ubiquitin-protein ligase (PARK2) [54], is part of the complex E3 ubiquitin ligase, necessary for the action of the ubiquitin-proteasome system. Parkin mutations have been associated with a familial form of early-onset PD [55, 56]. Interestingly, patients with PD with parkin mutations lack Lewy bodies, suggesting that parkin may be required for the formation and ubiquitination of these protein aggregates. Parkin has a role in neuroprotection by activating the PI3K-Akt pathway and also by cleansing dysfunctional mitochondria. Without the quality control of parkin, an increase in the number of dysfunctional mitochondria would lead to cell death. The dual-role context dependence of parkin should be better studied to understand neuronal physiology.

1.2. Coordinated Mitochondrial-Endoplasmic Reticulum Function Decline May Be Rescued by TRPV1 Control. The etiology of cognitive decline that occurs with aging is poorly understood; however, it is known that mitochondria are involved in this phenomenon [57]. Altered mitochondrial proteostasis and unfolded protein response could impede mitochondrial fusion and fission processes that normally reduce cell damage [14]. Disruptions of protein folding have also been associated to neurodegenerative disease with accumulation of misfolded proteins in the ER lumen, causing ER stress [35]. Several reports of increase in hyperphosphorylated tau protein in conjunction with stress markers in the ER in postmortem brain samples support this idea [58]. The "calcium hypothesis of brain aging and AD" intends to explain these findings. According to this hypothesis, Aβ would induce the ER to leach calcium that would be consequently taken by the mitochondria [59]. The calcium buffering mediated by mitochondria would induce overload of the ion in the mitochondrial matrix, reactive oxygen species production, and eventually, activation of programs of neuronal death [60, 61].

It should be noted that mammalian aging reduces pain perception associated with tissue damage by targeting the evolutionary conserved transient receptor potential cation channel subfamily V member 1 (TRPV1) that deploys a still unclear molecular mechanism for mitochondrial rescue [62]. TRPV1 mutations delay onset of age-related cognitive decline, maybe through SIRT1-dependent metabolic adaptation, which improves mitochondrial function and enhances several cellular antioxidant mechanisms [63]. The SIRT1 longevity factor is a deacetylase that plays a cytoprotective role in cellular response to stress. It is known that SIRT1 can modulate the heat shock response by deacetylation of the transcription factor HSF1, which triggers the production of molecular chaperones, promoting proteostasis and cellular viability [64]. In that sense, targeting mitochondrial proteostatic mechanisms, the natural TRPV1 agonist and antioxidant combined treatment synergistically would decrease glutamate toxicity, reactive oxygen species generation, and apoptotic neuronal death, offering a promising therapeutic approach to neurodegenerative disorders [65]. Activation of TRPV1 by capsaicin restores SIRT1 and suppresses NF-κB signaling recovering tissue damage generated by plaques of atheroma [66]. In addition, leptin is able to reduce brain infarct volume and improve functional outcome after stroke via increased expression of TRPV1 and SIRT-1, restoring mitochondrial function and avoiding apoptosis [67].

1.3. Targeting Mitochondrial Dysfunction in Neuropsychiatric Disorders: The Case of Schizophrenia. As stated above, mitochondria have a prominent role in proteostasis [14, 68]. Mitochondria by themselves are responsible for producing cellular energy through the oxidative phosphorylation system, managing calcium buffering, generating reactive oxygen species, and storing regulators related to apoptosis. These functions are physiologically relevant due to the energetically expensive neuronal activities that lead to successful synaptic plasticity or cell death [69]. Many findings point out that mitochondrial function abnormalities are essential components of the underlying neurobiology of a number of neuropsychiatric conditions, including schizophrenia.

1.4. The Role of DISC1. Disrupted in schizophrenia 1 (DISC1) is a scaffold protein involved in the regulation of neuronal proliferation, differentiation, migration, and cytoskeletal modulation [70] which has been extensively linked to schizophrenia and other major mental illnesses [71–73]. Although it is expressed most highly during fetal neurogenesis and in the adult hippocampus, DISC1 is expressed in different brain regions [74] and in other tissues as well [75]. DISC1 interactions with proteins of the dopaminergic system, such as fasciculation and elongation protein zeta 1, phosphodiesterase 4D9 and phosphodiesterase 4B, serine/threonine protein kinase Akt, and glycogen synthase kinase-3, have been studied due to their therapeutic potential [76, 77].

Unregulated expression of DISC1 and aberrant multimerization of DISC1-producing insoluble aggregates that are dysfunctional are associated with chronic neuropsychiatric diseases [75, 77]. Insoluble oligomers of DISC1 have indeed been found in postmortem brain samples of patients with schizophrenia [78]. The DISC1 mutant gene resulting from balanced translocation t(1;11)(q42;q14.3) was first identified in a Scottish lineage, and then it was found in other families, all of them with a history of schizophrenia among other mental disorders [79, 80]. In a recent systematic review, it was concluded that DISC1 would have a role in the regulation of dopaminergic function, installing dopaminergic dysregulation as a possible explanation for the higher rate of schizophrenia observed in patients with the DISC1 variant [77].

Inheritance of maternal mitochondrial DNA variants might be associated with the high prevalence of the disorder in relatives of schizophrenic patients [81]. Thus, Rollins et al. [82] verified that the synonymous base pair substitutions in the coding regions of the mitochondrial DNA genome in the dorsolateral prefrontal cortex of schizophrenics were increased by 22% compared to controls. Mostly found in mitochondria [83], DISC1 has been demonstrated to participate in neurite outgrowth, neurogenesis, neuronal migration, intracellular cAMP signaling, and many other neuronal processes [69]. Mitochondrial overexpressed truncated DISC1 isoforms may determine abnormal mitochondrial morphology, and depletion of DISC1 causes deficiencies in important mitochondrial enzyme activities and interferes mitochondrial trafficking throughout the axons [84]. Hence, the processes mediated by DISC1 in mitochondrial dynamics are necessary for neural development and dendritic branching [85]. Recent findings have shown that DISC1 plays a central role in mitochondrial function in association to mitofilin, a single-span mitochondrial inner membrane protein that is crucial for regulating mitochondrial cristae morphology and for preservation of mitochondrial DNA [69, 86]. DISC1 deficiencies are also linked with mitochondrial dysfunction such as decreased NADH dehydrogenase activity in the electron transport chain, reduced ATP contents, impaired mitochondrial calcium dynamics, and diminished activity of monoamine oxidase, which can be related to the loss of mitofilin stability as well as mitochondrial morphological abnormalities. Particularly, downregulation of monoamine oxidase activity is of utmost interest due to its link with the mesolimbic hyperdopaminergic tone, probably responsible for positive psychotic symptoms. Consequently, monoamine oxidase activity in DISC1-deficient neurons might indeed be a key element in hyperdopaminergic theory [69, 86].

In a critical and recent study of Park et al. [87], DISC1 deficiency is shown to elicit a hyperactivation in endoplasmic reticulum-mitochondrial Ca^{2+} transfer—through the mitochondrial associated endoplasmic reticulum membrane—triggered by oxidative stress and excessive glucocorticoids, causing abnormal mitochondrial Ca^{2+} storage. This process finally triggers an overproduction of ROS mediated by a disruption in mitochondrial membrane potential [87]. The authors concluded that DISC1 modulates neuronal stress response through ER-mitochondrial Ca^{2+} transfer. Thus, DISC1 association with cognitive and emotional deficits implies dysregulation of Ca^{2+} flux between ER and mitochondria through mitochondrion-associated membrane proteins and the consequent loss of proteostasis as a common mechanism shared by aging, as well as neurodegenerative and psychiatric diseases.

In other animal model explorations, DISC1 has been implicated in hypothalamic-pituitary-adrenal dysregulations [88, 89]. Specifically, in a mouse model it has been demonstrated that environmental stressors combined with an appropriate genetic risk can trigger, for example, neurochemical projections originating from the ventral tegmental area and behavioral changes induced by DISC1 expression [89]. Interestingly, these findings have allowed formulating the hypothesis that environmental stressors during childhood and adolescence could exert epigenetic control over the dopaminergic pathways and, therefore, set mental illnesses as schizophrenia.

1.4.1. Dendritic Spines and Mitochondrial Hypoplasia. Different studies indicate that the mitochondrial network displays important transcriptome alterations in layer III pyramidal cells in schizophrenics, supporting a molecular link between mitochondrial dysfunction and the important decrease in dendritic spine density observed in these neurons [90]. Mitochondria regulate dendritic spine morphogenesis and plasticity but are also involved in the negative regulation of dendritic branching during development. Overall, evidence intrinsically links mitochondrial copy number, localization, and function with dendritic spine morphology and synaptic transmission [91]. In this context, the most frequently found protein in postsynaptic density is PSD-95, a scaffolding protein which belongs to the kinase family. It is implied in excitatory synapses and plays a key role in synaptic plasticity through dendritic spine morphogenesis and long-term potentiation and long-term depression. Postmortem studies carried out in brains of schizophrenic patients have demonstrated a significant decrease in PSD-95 mRNA levels in specific areas as dorsolateral and dorsomedial prefrontal cortices [92]. This may be related to anomalous spine dynamics observed in neurodevelopmental and neuropsychiatric disorders, for example, schizophrenia and autism spectrum disorders [93]. Different explorations in patients with schizophrenia have found decreased numbers of mitochondria in presynaptic buttons in dopaminergic neurons of the substantia nigra [94]. Moreover, a reduction in the number of mitochondria in axons of drug-naïve schizophrenics has also been verified, but not in patients using antipsychotic drugs [95]. Findings also exhibit significant decreases in the mitochondrial density of oligodendroglial cells in the caudate nucleus and prefrontal areas in patients, particularly those with prominent negative symptoms [96].

1.4.2. Inflammation. Neuroprogression, a stage-related phenomenon of neurodegeneration and decline in neuronal plasticity and neurogenesis that has been employed as a research paradigm in schizophrenia, has demonstrated to be significantly influenced by neuroinflammation due to a synergistic effect with mitochondrial dysfunction and neuroprogressive immunoinflammatory, oxidative, and nitrosative stress pathways, activating a vicious cycle that conduces to neuronal death [97, 98]. Novel therapeutic strategies could focus on improving mitochondrial function, through promoting an endogenous antioxidant defense system and antioxidant treatment to compensate mitochondrial injury and increase the mitochondrial respiration rate [97].

Another potential therapeutic target regarding mitochondrial functioning is the translocator protein, located in the outer mitochondrial membrane of steroid-synthesizing nervous cells. It is involved in the permeability to water and small substances at the junction of the inner and outer membranes. Since it is linked with apoptosis and upregulated in some neurodegenerative diseases, this protein has been proposed as an inflammation biomarker and is currently being appraised in clinical trials of drug use [99].

1.4.3. Electron Transport Chain. Diverse neuroimaging studies have demonstrated an altered metabolism expressed as changes in ATP in different brain regions of schizophrenic patients [5]. The severity of negative symptoms and the neuropsychological performance would be correlated with ATP levels [100]. These results point out a dysfunction of brain mitochondrial oxidative phosphorylation, related intrinsically with processes as pre- and postsynaptic action potentials, neurotransmitter release, and postsynaptic currents [101, 102]. Specifically, the expression of multiple complex I subunits of the electron transport chain, such as NDUFV1, NDUFV2, and NDUFS1, is significantly altered in the prefrontal cortex, striatum, hippocampus, and parietooccipital cortex of schizophrenics [102, 103]. In fact, the NDUFV2 gene has been included as a high-risk gene for schizophrenia [104]. In this regard, a study conducted by Robicsek et al. [105] corroborated the impairments in maturation and differentiation into dopaminergic and glutamatergic neurons of schizophrenic-derived pluripotent stem cells, alongside a reduction in complex I-driven respiration, dissipation in mitochondrial membrane potential, altered mitochondrial network structure and connectivity, and aberrant expression degrees of NDUFV1, NDUFV2, and NDUFS1. Some interactions have also been proposed between oxidative phosphorylation and intramitochondrial calcium as complex I, complex II, and complex IV alterations are linked with abnormalities in calcium signaling [106].

With regards to pharmacotherapy, self-defeating findings indicate that typical and atypical antipsychotic drugs would inhibit complex I activity and complex I-driven respiration in isolated mitochondria and in intact neurons [102]. Comparable to these effects, dopamine also affects mitochondrial activity in neuronal cultures by diminishing complex I function and ATP synthesis. These findings could be related to the mitochondrial dopamine uptake, provoking a dose-dependent inhibition of complex I functioning [107]. Both antipsychotics and dopamine inhibit complex I activity, although they interact with the complex at different sites: dopamine interacts with the hydrophilic matrix-penetrating arm and antipsychotics with the hydrophobic inner membrane-embedded arm of the complex. While therapeutic effects of these drugs are due to their antagonism of the D2 receptor, side effects of antipsychotics might be explained by this drug-mitochondria interaction. Besides, dopamine and antipsychotic drugs may interact independently with mitochondria, participating in a compensatory phenomenon with the aim of overcoming mitochondrial dysfunction [102].

2. Conclusions

Our results show that a dysfunction of the proteostasis system is implicated in the etiology of a series of highly prevalent psychiatric and neurodegenerative processes such as PD, dementia, and schizophrenia, among others [12]. Indeed, proteostasis alterations in the prefrontal cortex implicate proteome instability and accumulation of misfolded proteins [45, 47, 49, 76] that could lead to detrimental behavioral and emotional functions in neuropsychiatric disorders [108]. Furthermore, altered mitochondrial dynamics, proteostasis, and mitochondrial unfolded protein response could impede mitochondrial fusion and fission, processes that normally reduce cell damage [14]. This may be related to the decline in prefrontal cortex performances observed during aging [109]. Mitochondrial alterations, specifically on its genetic bases [69, 86, 110], regulatory role in dendritic development [90, 91] and neuroinflammation [97, 98], could be the underlying phenomena of psychiatric disorders as schizophrenia. In the context of the neuronal relevance of mitochondrial functions [69], we hypothesize that it is possible to delay onset of age-related cognitive decline through metabolic SIRT1-dependent adaptation and improvement of mitochondrial function mediated by TRPV1 control. Thereby, TRPV1 modulation of the mitochondrial proteostasis mechanism could be used to design drug strategies against neural-dependent conditions, such as detrimental cognitive performance. Finally, we expect that with the increasing evidence about proteostasis in psychiatric and neurodegenerative disorders, new therapeutic alternatives will emerge.

Conflicts of Interest

The authors declare that they have no conflicts of interest.

Acknowledgments

The authors would like to thank Alvaro Cavieres for his precious comments on clinical concepts about neuropsychiatric disease development. This collaborative work was supported by *Fondo Nacional de Desarrollo Científico y Tecnológico*: Fondecyt 11100047 and Fondecyt 11110399.

References

[1] R. R. Llinás, "The contribution of Santiago Ramón y Cajal to functional neuroscience," *Nature Reviews Neuroscience*, vol. 4, no. 1, pp. 77–80, 2003.

[2] E. M. Hol, F. W. van Leeuwen, and D. F. Fischer, "The proteasome in Alzheimer's disease and Parkinson's disease: lessons from ubiquitin B^{+1}," *Trends in Molecular Medicine*, vol. 11, no. 11, pp. 488–495, 2005.

[3] C. P. Dohm, P. Kermer, and M. Bähr, "Aggregopathy in neurodegenerative diseases: mechanisms and therapeutic implication," *Neurodegenerative Diseases*, vol. 5, no. 6, pp. 321–338, 2008.

[4] A. B. Meriin and M. Y. Sherman, "Role of molecular chaperones in neurodegenerative disorders," *International Journal of Hyperthermia*, vol. 21, no. 5, pp. 403–419, 2005.

[5] F. Du, A. J. Cooper, T. Thida et al., "In vivo evidence for cerebral bioenergetic abnormalities in schizophrenia measured using 31P magnetization transfer spectroscopy," *JAMA Psychiatry*, vol. 71, no. 1, pp. 19–27, 2014.

[6] X. Gao and H. Hu, "Quality control of the proteins associated with neurodegenerative diseases," *Acta Biochimica et Biophysica Sinica*, vol. 40, no. 7, pp. 612–618, 2008.

[7] G. Luo and W. Le, "Collective roles of molecular chaperones in protein degradation pathways associated with neurodegenerative diseases," *Current Pharmaceutical Biotechnology*, vol. 11, no. 2, pp. 180–187, 2010.

[8] K. Gadhave, N. Bolshette, A. Ahire et al., "The ubiquitin proteasomal system: a potential target for the management of Alzheimer's disease," *Journal of Cellular and Molecular Medicine*, vol. 20, no. 7, pp. 1392–1407, 2016.

[9] Q. Zheng, T. Huang, L. Zhang et al., "Dysregulation of ubiquitin-proteasome system in neurodegenerative diseases," *Frontiers in Aging Neuroscience*, vol. 8, p. 303, 2016.

[10] M. Press, T. Jung, J. König, T. Grune, and A. Höhn, "Protein aggregates and proteostasis in aging: amylin and β-cell function," *Mechanisms of Ageing and Development*, 2018.

[11] J. A. Reisz, A. S. Barrett, T. Nemkov, K. C. Hansen, and A. D'Alessandro, "When nature's robots go rogue: exploring protein homeostasis dysfunction and the implications for understanding human aging disease pathologies," *Expert Review of Proteomics*, vol. 15, no. 4, pp. 293–309, 2018.

[12] C. Bobori, G. Theocharopoulou, and P. Vlamos, "Molecular chaperones in neurodegenerative diseases: a short review," *Advances in Experimental Medicine and Biology*, vol. 987, pp. 219–231, 2017.

[13] E. L. Friesen, M. L. De Snoo, L. Rajendran, L. V. Kalia, and S. K. Kalia, "Chaperone-based therapies for disease modification in Parkinson's disease," *Parkinson's Disease*, vol. 2017, Article ID 5015307, 11 pages, 2017.

[14] M. J. Baker, T. Tatsuta, and T. Langer, "Quality control of mitochondrial proteostasis," *Cold Spring Harbor Perspectives in Biology*, vol. 3, no. 7, 2011.

[15] J. Labbadia and R. I. Morimoto, "The biology of proteostasis in aging and disease," *Annual Review of Biochemistry*, vol. 84, no. 1, pp. 435–464, 2015.

[16] M. Haslbeck, T. Franzmann, D. Weinfurtner, and J. Buchner, "Some like it hot: the structure and function of small heat-shock proteins," *Nature Structural & Molecular Biology*, vol. 12, no. 10, pp. 842–846, 2005.

[17] Y. E. Kim, M. S. Hipp, A. Bracher, M. Hayer-Hartl, and F. Ulrich Hartl, "Molecular chaperone functions in protein folding and proteostasis," *Annual Review of Biochemistry*, vol. 82, no. 1, pp. 323–355, 2013.

[18] S.-A. Mok, C. Condello, R. Freilich et al., "Mapping interactions with the chaperone network reveals factors that protect against tau aggregation," *Nature Structural & Molecular Biology*, vol. 25, no. 5, pp. 384–393, 2018.

[19] B. Bingol and M. Sheng, "Deconstruction for reconstruction: the role of proteolysis in neural plasticity and disease," *Neuron*, vol. 69, no. 1, pp. 22–32, 2011.

[20] T. J. Jarome and F. J. Helmstetter, "The ubiquitin–proteasome system as a critical regulator of synaptic plasticity and long-term memory formation," *Neurobiology of Learning and Memory*, vol. 105, pp. 107–116, 2013.

[21] K. V. Ramachandran and S. S. Margolis, "A mammalian nervous-system-specific plasma membrane proteasome complex that modulates neuronal function," *Nature Structural & Molecular Biology*, vol. 24, no. 4, pp. 419–430, 2017.

[22] S. Wu, K. L. Hyrc, K. L. Moulder, Y. Lin, T. Warmke, and B. J. Snider, "Cellular calcium deficiency plays a role in neuronal death caused by proteasome inhibitors," *Journal of Neurochemistry*, vol. 109, no. 5, pp. 1225–1236, 2009.

[23] A. M. Hamilton and K. Zito, "Breaking it down: the ubiquitin proteasome system in neuronal morphogenesis," *Neural Plasticity*, vol. 2013, Article ID 196848, 10 pages, 2013.

[24] G. V. Rinetti and F. E. Schweizer, "Ubiquitination acutely regulates presynaptic neurotransmitter release in mammalian neurons," *The Journal of Neuroscience*, vol. 30, no. 9, pp. 3157–3166, 2010.

[25] H.-C. Tai and E. M. Schuman, "Ubiquitin, the proteasome and protein degradation in neuronal function and dysfunction," *Nature Reviews Neuroscience*, vol. 9, no. 11, pp. 826–838, 2008.

[26] T. A. Thibaudeau, R. T. Anderson, and D. M. Smith, "A common mechanism of proteasome impairment by neurodegenerative disease-associated oligomers," *Nature Communications*, vol. 9, no. 1, p. 1097, 2018.

[27] J. Rasmussen, M. Jucker, and L. C. Walker, "Aβ seeds and prions: how close the fit?," *Prion*, vol. 11, no. 4, pp. 215–225, 2017.

[28] J. Brettschneider, K. D. Tredici, V. M. Y. Lee, and J. Q. Trojanowski, "Spreading of pathology in neurodegenerative diseases: a focus on human studies," *Nature Reviews Neuroscience*, vol. 16, no. 2, pp. 109–120, 2015.

[29] E. A. André, P. A. Forcelli, and D. T. S. Pak, "What goes up must come down: homeostatic synaptic plasticity strategies in neurological disease," *Future Neurology*, vol. 13, no. 1, pp. 13–21, 2018.

[30] Q. Zhang, C. Ma, M. Gearing, P. G. Wang, L. S. Chin, and L. Li, "Integrated proteomics and network analysis identifies protein hubs and network alterations in Alzheimer's disease," *Acta Neuropathologica Communications*, vol. 6, no. 1, p. 19, 2018.

[31] A. M. Swomley, S. Förster, J. T. Keeney et al., "Abeta, oxidative stress in Alzheimer disease: evidence based on proteomics studies," *Biochimica et Biophysica Acta (BBA) - Molecular Basis of Disease*, vol. 1842, no. 8, pp. 1248–1257, 2014.

[32] S. Geisler, K. M. Holmström, D. Skujat et al., "PINK1/Parkin-mediated mitophagy is dependent on VDAC1 and p62/SQSTM1," *Nature Cell Biology*, vol. 12, no. 2, pp. 119–131, 2010.

[33] T. Ryan, V. V. Bamm, M. G. Stykel et al., "Cardiolipin exposure on the outer mitochondrial membrane modulates α-synuclein," *Nature Communications*, vol. 9, no. 1, p. 817, 2018.

[34] L. D. Osellame and M. R. Duchen, "Quality control gone wrong: mitochondria, lysosomal storage disorders and neurodegeneration," *British Journal of Pharmacology*, vol. 171, no. 8, pp. 1958–1972, 2014.

[35] D. Hughes and G. R. Mallucci, "The unfolded protein response in neurodegenerative disorders – therapeutic modulation of the PERK pathway," *The FEBS Journal*, 2018.

[36] C. Hetz and B. Mollereau, "Disturbance of endoplasmic reticulum proteostasis in neurodegenerative diseases," *Nature Reviews Neuroscience*, vol. 15, no. 4, pp. 233–249, 2014.

[37] E. A. Moehle, K. Shen, and A. Dillin, "Mitochondrial proteostasis in the context of cellular and organismal health and aging," *The Journal of Biological Chemistry*, 2018.

[38] S. R. Yoshii, C. Kishi, N. Ishihara, and N. Mizushima, "Parkin mediates proteasome-dependent protein degradation and rupture of the outer mitochondrial membrane," *The Journal of Biological Chemistry*, vol. 286, no. 22, pp. 19630–19640, 2011.

[39] P. Bragoszewski, M. Turek, and A. Chacinska, "Control of mitochondrial biogenesis and function by the ubiquitin–proteasome system," *Open Biology*, vol. 7, no. 4, article 170007, 2017.

[40] L. Ruan, C. Zhou, E. Jin et al., "Cytosolic proteostasis through importing of misfolded proteins into mitochondria," *Nature*, vol. 543, no. 7645, pp. 443–446, 2017.

[41] J. Avila, J. J. Lucas, M. Perez, and F. Hernandez, "Role of tau protein in both physiological and pathological conditions," *Physiological Reviews*, vol. 84, no. 2, pp. 361–384, 2004.

[42] G. V. W. Johnson and W. H. Stoothoff, "Tau phosphorylation in neuronal cell function and dysfunction," *Journal of Cell Science*, vol. 117, no. 24, pp. 5721–5729, 2004.

[43] F. Biundo, D. del Prete, H. Zhang, O. Arancio, and L. D'Adamio, "A role for tau in learning, memory and synaptic plasticity," *Scientific Reports*, vol. 8, no. 1, p. 3184, 2018.

[44] T. Uchihara, K. Ikeda, and K. Tsuchiya, "Pick body disease and Pick syndrome," *Neuropathology*, vol. 23, no. 4, pp. 318–326, 2003.

[45] K. Ando, K. Tomimura, V. Sazdovitch et al., "Level of PICALM, a key component of clathrin-mediated endocytosis, is correlated with levels of phosphotau and autophagy-related proteins and is associated with tau inclusions in AD, PSP and Pick disease," *Neurobiology of Disease*, vol. 94, pp. 32–43, 2016.

[46] G. W. Roberts, "Immunocytochemistry of neurofibrillary tangles in dementia pugilistica and Alzheimer's disease: evidence for common genesis," *The Lancet*, vol. 332, no. 8626-8627, pp. 1456–1458, 1988.

[47] S. S. Khan and G. S. Bloom, "Tau: the center of a signaling nexus in Alzheimer's disease," *Frontiers in Neuroscience*, vol. 10, no. 31, p. 31, 2016.

[48] D. K. V. Kumar, S. H. Choi, K. J. Washicosky et al., "Amyloid-β peptide protects against microbial infection in mouse and worm models of Alzheimer's disease," *Science Translational Medicine*, vol. 8, no. 340, article 340ra72, 2016.

[49] W. Cerpa, M. Dinamarca, and N. Inestrosa, "Structure-function implications in Alzheimer's disease: effect of Aβ oligomers at central synapses," *Current Alzheimer Research*, vol. 5, no. 3, pp. 233–243, 2008.

[50] K. Beyer, "α-synuclein structure, posttranslational modification and alternative splicing as aggregation enhancers," *Acta Neuropathologica*, vol. 112, no. 3, pp. 237–251, 2006.

[51] J. Diao, J. Burré, S. Vivona et al., "Native α-synuclein induces clustering of synaptic-vesicle mimics via binding to phospholipids and synaptobrevin-2/VAMP2," *eLife*, vol. 2, article e00592, 2013.

[52] C. W. Olanow and P. Brundin, "Parkinson's disease and alpha synuclein: is Parkinson's disease a prion-like disorder?," *Movement Disorders*, vol. 28, no. 1, pp. 31–40, 2013.

[53] A. Alvarsson, D. Caudal, A. Björklund, and P. Svenningsson, "Emotional memory impairments induced by AAV-mediated overexpression of human α-synuclein in dopaminergic neurons of the ventral tegmental area," *Behavioural Brain Research*, vol. 296, pp. 129–133, 2016.

[54] N. Hattori and Y. Mizuno, "Twenty years since the discovery of the parkin gene," *Journal of Neural Transmission*, vol. 124, no. 9, pp. 1037–1054, 2017.

[55] T. Kitada, S. Asakawa, N. Hattori et al., "Mutations in the parkin gene cause autosomal recessive juvenile parkinsonism," *Nature*, vol. 392, no. 6676, pp. 605–608, 1998.

[56] K. M. Doherty, L. Silveira-Moriyama, L. Parkkinen et al., "Parkin disease: a clinicopathologic entity?," *JAMA Neurology*, vol. 70, no. 5, pp. 571–579, 2013.

[57] F. Gonzalez-Lima, B. R. Barksdale, and J. C. Rojas, "Mitochondrial respiration as a target for neuroprotection and cognitive enhancement," *Biochemical Pharmacology*, vol. 88, no. 4, pp. 584–593, 2014.

[58] W. Scheper and J. J. M. Hoozemans, "The unfolded protein response in neurodegenerative diseases: a neuropathological perspective," *Acta Neuropathologica*, vol. 130, no. 3, pp. 315–331, 2015.

[59] V. H. Cornejo and C. Hetz, "The unfolded protein response in Alzheimer's disease," *Seminars in Immunopathology*, vol. 35, no. 3, pp. 277–292, 2013.

[60] A. C. R. G. Fonseca, E. Ferreiro, C. R. Oliveira, S. M. Cardoso, and C. F. Pereira, "Activation of the endoplasmic reticulum stress response by the amyloid-beta 1–40 peptide in brain endothelial cells," *Biochimica et Biophysica Acta (BBA) - Molecular Basis of Disease*, vol. 1832, no. 12, pp. 2191–2203, 2013.

[61] C. Supnet and I. Bezprozvanny, "The dysregulation of intracellular calcium in Alzheimer disease," *Cell Calcium*, vol. 47, no. 2, pp. 183–189, 2010.

[62] C. E. Riera and A. Dillin, "Tipping the metabolic scales towards increased longevity in mammals," *Nature Cell Biology*, vol. 17, no. 3, pp. 196–203, 2015.

[63] C. Cantó, L. Q. Jiang, A. S. Deshmukh et al., "Interdependence of AMPK and SIRT1 for metabolic adaptation to fasting and exercise in skeletal muscle," *Cell Metabolism*, vol. 11, no. 3, pp. 213–219, 2010.

[64] R. Raynes, J. Brunquell, and S. D. Westerheide, "Stress inducibility of SIRT1 and its role in cytoprotection and cancer," *Genes & Cancer*, vol. 4, no. 3-4, pp. 172–182, 2013.

[65] J.-G. Lee, J. M. Yon, C. Lin, A. Y. Jung, K. Y. Jung, and S. Y. Nam, "Combined treatment with capsaicin and resveratrol enhances neuroprotection against glutamate-induced toxicity in mouse cerebral cortical neurons," *Food and Chemical Toxicology*, vol. 50, no. 11, pp. 3877–3885, 2012.

[66] M. J. Zhang, Y. Zhou, L. Chen et al., "Impaired SIRT1 promotes the migration of vascular smooth muscle cell-derived foam cells," *Histochemistry and Cell Biology*, vol. 146, no. 1, pp. 33–43, 2016.

[67] Y. Avraham, N. Davidi, M. Porat et al., "Leptin reduces infarct size in association with enhanced expression of CB2, TRPV1, SIRT-1 and leptin receptor," *Current Neurovascular Research*, vol. 7, no. 2, pp. 136–143, 2010.

[68] L. MacPherson and K. Tokatlidis, "Protein trafficking in the mitochondrial intermembrane space: mechanisms and links to human disease," *The Biochemical Journal*, vol. 474, no. 15, pp. 2533–2545, 2017.

[69] C. Park and S. K. Park, "Molecular links between mitochondrial dysfunctions and schizophrenia," *Molecules and Cells*, vol. 33, no. 2, pp. 105–110, 2012.

[70] N. J. Gamo, A. Duque, C. D. Paspalas et al., "Role of disrupted in schizophrenia 1 (DISC1) in stress-induced prefrontal cognitive dysfunction," *Translational Psychiatry*, vol. 3, no. 12, article e328, 2013.

[71] Y. Xu, J. Ren, and H. Ye, "Association between variations in the *disrupted in schizophrenia 1* gene and schizophrenia: a meta-analysis," *Gene*, vol. 651, pp. 94–99, 2018.

[72] M. Niwa, T. Cash-Padgett, K. I. Kubo et al., "DISC1 a key molecular lead in psychiatry and neurodevelopment: No-More *Disrupted-in-Schizophrenia 1*," *Molecular Psychiatry*, vol. 21, no. 11, pp. 1488-1489, 2016.

[73] J. K. Millar, J. C. Wilson-Annan, S. Anderson et al., "Disruption of two novel genes by a translocation co-segregating with schizophrenia," *Human Molecular Genetics*, vol. 9, no. 9, pp. 1415–1423, 2000.

[74] S. Miyata, T. Hattori, S. Shimizu, A. Ito, and M. Tohyama, "Disturbance of oligodendrocyte function plays a key role in the pathogenesis of schizophrenia and major depressive disorder," *BioMed Research International*, vol. 2015, Article ID 492367, 26 pages, 2015.

[75] D. J. Porteous, J. K. Millar, N. J. Brandon, and A. Sawa, "DISC1 at 10: connecting psychiatric genetics and neuroscience," *Trends in Molecular Medicine*, vol. 17, no. 12, pp. 699–706, 2011.

[76] T. Dahoun, S. V. Trossbach, N. J. Brandon, C. Korth, and O. D. Howes, "The impact of *Disrupted-in-Schizophrenia 1 (DISC1)* on the dopaminergic system: a systematic review," *Translational Psychiatry*, vol. 7, no. 1, article e1015, 2017.

[77] N. J. Brandon, J. K. Millar, C. Korth, H. Sive, K. K. Singh, and A. Sawa, "Understanding the role of DISC1 in psychiatric disease and during normal development," *The Journal of Neuroscience*, vol. 29, no. 41, pp. 12768–12775, 2009.

[78] W. Ratta-apha, A. Hishimoto, K. Mouri et al., "Association analysis of the DISC1 gene with schizophrenia in the Japanese population and DISC1 immunoreactivity in the postmortem brain," *Neuroscience Research*, vol. 77, no. 4, pp. 222–227, 2013.

[79] D. St Clair, D. Blackwood, W. Muir et al., "Association within a family of a balanced autosomal translocation with major mental illness," *The Lancet*, vol. 336, no. 8706, pp. 13–16, 1990.

[80] N. A. Sachs, A. Sawa, S. E. Holmes, C. A. Ross, L. E. DeLisi, and R. L. Margolis, "A frameshift mutation in Disrupted in Schizophrenia 1 in an American family with schizophrenia and schizoaffective disorder," *Molecular Psychiatry*, vol. 10, no. 8, pp. 758–764, 2005.

[81] N. Doi, Y. Hoshi, M. Itokawa, C. Usui, T. Yoshikawa, and H. Tachikawa, "Persistence criteria for susceptibility genes for schizophrenia: a discussion from an evolutionary viewpoint," *PLoS One*, vol. 4, no. 11, article e7799, 2009.

[82] B. Rollins, M. V. Martin, P. A. Sequeira et al., "Mitochondrial variants in schizophrenia, bipolar disorder, and major depressive disorder," *PLoS One*, vol. 4, no. 3, article e4913, 2009.

[83] R. James, R. R. Adams, S. Christie, S. R. Buchanan, D. J. Porteous, and J. K. Millar, "Disrupted in schizophrenia 1 (DISC1) is a multicompartmentalized protein that predominantly localizes to mitochondria," *Molecular and Cellular Neurosciences*, vol. 26, no. 1, pp. 112–122, 2004.

[84] E. Piñero-Martos, B. Ortega-Vila, J. Pol-Fuster et al., "Disrupted in Schizophrenia 1 (DISC1) is a constituent of the mammalian Mitochondrial contact site and Cristae Organizing System (MICOS) complex, and is essential for oxidative phosphorylation," *Human Molecular Genetics*, vol. 25, no. 19, pp. 4157–4169, 2016.

[85] R. Norkett, S. Modi, N. Birsa et al., "DISC1-dependent regulation of mitochondrial dynamics controls the morphogenesis of complex neuronal dendrites," *The Journal of Biological Chemistry*, vol. 291, no. 2, pp. 613–629, 2016.

[86] Y. U. Park, J. Jeong, H. Lee et al., "*Disrupted-in-schizophrenia 1* (DISC1) plays essential roles in mitochondria in collaboration with Mitofilin," *Proceedings of the National Academy of Sciences of the United States of America*, vol. 107, no. 41, pp. 17785–17790, 2010.

[87] S. J. Park, S. B. Lee, Y. Suh et al., "DISC1 modulates neuronal stress responses by gate-keeping ER-mitochondria Ca^{2+}

transfer through the MAM," *Cell Reports*, vol. 21, no. 10, pp. 2748–2759, 2017.

[88] H. Eachus, C. Bright, V. T. Cunliffe, M. Placzek, J. D. Wood, and P. J. Watt, "*Disrupted-in-Schizophrenia-1* is essential for normal hypothalamic-pituitary-interrenal (HPI) axis function," *Human Molecular Genetics*, vol. 26, no. 11, pp. 1992–2005, 2017.

[89] M. Niwa, H. Jaaro-Peled, S. Tankou et al., "Adolescent stress-induced epigenetic control of dopaminergic neurons via glucocorticoids," *Science*, vol. 339, no. 6117, pp. 335–339, 2013.

[90] D. Arion, J. P. Corradi, S. Tang et al., "Distinctive transcriptome alterations of prefrontal pyramidal neurons in schizophrenia and schizoaffective disorder," *Molecular Psychiatry*, vol. 20, no. 11, pp. 1397–1405, 2015.

[91] B. E. Hjelm, B. Rollins, F. Mamdani et al., "Evidence of mitochondrial dysfunction within the complex genetic etiology of schizophrenia," *Molecular Neuropsychiatry*, vol. 1, no. 4, pp. 201–219, 2015.

[92] V. S. Catts, D. S. Derminio, C.-G. Hahn, and C. S. Weickert, "Postsynaptic density levels of the NMDA receptor NR1 subunit and PSD-95 protein in prefrontal cortex from people with schizophrenia," *npj Schizophrenia*, vol. 1, no. 1, article 15037, 2015.

[93] A. A. Coley and W.-J. Gao, "PSD95: a synaptic protein implicated in schizophrenia or autism?," *Progress in Neuro-Psychopharmacology and Biological Psychiatry*, vol. 82, pp. 187–194, 2018.

[94] N. S. Kolomeets and N. A. Uranova, "Synaptic contacts in schizophrenia: studies using immunocytochemical identification of dopaminergic neurons," *Neuroscience and Behavioral Physiology*, vol. 29, no. 2, pp. 217–221, 1999.

[95] L. Kung and R. C. Roberts, "Mitochondrial pathology in human schizophrenic striatum: a postmortem ultrastructural study," *Synapse*, vol. 31, no. 1, pp. 67–75, 1999.

[96] N. A. Uranova, D. D. Orlovskaia, O. V. Vikhreva, I. S. Zimina, and V. I. Rakhmanova, "Morphometric study of ultrastructural changes in oligodendroglial cells in the postmortem brain in endogenous psychoses," *Vestnik Rossiĭskoĭ Akademii Meditsinskikh Nauk*, no. 7, pp. 42–48, 2001.

[97] A. Rajasekaran, G. Venkatasubramanian, M. Berk, and M. Debnath, "Mitochondrial dysfunction in schizophrenia: pathways, mechanisms and implications," *Neuroscience & Biobehavioral Reviews*, vol. 48, pp. 10–21, 2015.

[98] G. Anderson, M. Maes, and M. Berk, "Schizophrenia is primed for an increased expression of depression through activation of immuno-inflammatory, oxidative and nitrosative stress, and tryptophan catabolite pathways," *Progress in Neuro-Psychopharmacology and Biological Psychiatry*, vol. 42, pp. 101–114, 2013.

[99] M. D. Filiou, R. B. Banati, and M. B. Graeber, "The 18-kDa translocator protein as a CNS drug target: finding our way through the neuroinflammation fog," *CNS & Neurological Disorders - Drug Targets*, vol. 16, no. 9, pp. 990–999, 2018.

[100] H. P. Volz, R. Rzanny, G. Röger et al., "Decreased energy demanding processes in the frontal lobes of schizophrenics due to neuroleptics? A ^{31}P-magneto-resonance spectroscopic study," *Psychiatry Research: Neuroimaging*, vol. 76, no. 2-3, pp. 123–129, 1997.

[101] C. N. Hall, M. C. Klein-Flugge, C. Howarth, and D. Attwell, "Oxidative phosphorylation, not glycolysis, powers presynaptic and postsynaptic mechanisms underlying brain information processing," *The Journal of Neuroscience*, vol. 32, no. 26, pp. 8940–8951, 2012.

[102] O. Bergman and D. Ben-Shachar, "Mitochondrial oxidative phosphorylation system (OXPHOS) deficits in schizophrenia: possible interactions with cellular processes," *Canadian Journal of Psychiatry*, vol. 61, no. 8, pp. 457–469, 2016.

[103] S. Akarsu, D. Torun, A. Bolu et al., "Mitochondrial complex I and III gene mRNA levels in schizophrenia, and their relationship with clinical features," *Journal of Molecular Psychiatry*, vol. 2, no. 1, p. 6, 2014.

[104] M. Ayalew, H. le-Niculescu, D. F. Levey et al., "Convergent functional genomics of schizophrenia: from comprehensive understanding to genetic risk prediction," *Molecular Psychiatry*, vol. 17, no. 9, pp. 887–905, 2012.

[105] O. Robicsek, R. Karry, I. Petit et al., "Abnormal neuronal differentiation and mitochondrial dysfunction in hair follicle-derived induced pluripotent stem cells of schizophrenia patients," *Molecular Psychiatry*, vol. 18, no. 10, pp. 1067–1076, 2013.

[106] P. H. G. M. Willems, J. A. M. Smeitink, and W. J. H. Koopman, "Mitochondrial dynamics in human NADH:ubiquinone oxidoreductase deficiency," *The International Journal of Biochemistry & Cell Biology*, vol. 41, no. 10, pp. 1773–1782, 2009.

[107] H. Brenner-Lavie, E. Klein, R. Zuk, H. Gazawi, P. Ljubuncic, and D. Ben-Shachar, "Dopamine modulates mitochondrial function in viable SH-SY5Y cells possibly via its interaction with complex I: relevance to dopamine pathology in schizophrenia," *Biochimica et Biophysica Acta (BBA) - Bioenergetics*, vol. 1777, no. 2, pp. 173–185, 2008.

[108] A. Bechara, H. Damasio, and A. R. Damasio, "Emotion, decision making and the orbitofrontal cortex," *Cerebral Cortex*, vol. 10, no. 3, pp. 295–307, 2000.

[109] Y. Ouchi and M. Kikuchi, "A review of the default mode network in aging and dementia based on molecular imaging," *Reviews in the Neurosciences*, vol. 23, no. 3, pp. 263–268, 2012.

[110] J. E. Eykelenboom, G. J. Briggs, N. J. Bradshaw et al., "A t(1;11) translocation linked to schizophrenia and affective disorders gives rise to aberrant chimeric *DISC1* transcripts that encode structurally altered, deleterious mitochondrial proteins," *Human Molecular Genetics*, vol. 21, no. 15, pp. 3374–3386, 2012.

11

Operant Up-Conditioning of the Tibialis Anterior Motor-Evoked Potential in Multiple Sclerosis: Feasibility Case Studies

Aiko K. Thompson[1] **Briana M. Favale,**[2] **Jacqueline Velez,**[2] **and Patricia Falivena**[2]

[1]*Department of Health Sciences and Research, College of Health Professions, Medical University of South Carolina, Charleston, SC 29425, USA*
[2]*Helen Hayes Hospital, New York State Department of Health, West Haverstraw, New York City, NY 10993, USA*

Correspondence should be addressed to Aiko K. Thompson; thompsai@musc.edu

Academic Editor: J. Michael Wyss

Damage to the corticospinal pathway often results in weak dorsiflexion of the ankle, thereby limiting the mobility of people with multiple sclerosis (MS). Thus, strengthening corticospinal connectivity may improve locomotion. Here, we investigated the feasibility of tibialis anterior (TA) motor-evoked potential (MEP) operant conditioning and whether it can enhance corticospinal excitability and alleviate locomotor problems in people with chronic stable MS. The protocol consisted of 6 baseline and 24 up-conditioning sessions over 10 weeks. In all sessions, TA MEPs were elicited at 10% above active threshold while the sitting subject provided 30–35% maximum voluntary contraction (MVC) level of TA background EMG. During baseline sessions, MEPs were simply measured. During conditioning trials of the conditioning sessions, the subject was encouraged to increase MEP and was given immediate feedback indicating whether MEP size was above a criterion. In 3/4 subjects, TA MEP increased 32–75%, MVC increased 28–52%, locomotor EMG modulation improved in multiple leg muscles, and foot drop became less severe. In one of them, MEP and MVC increases were maintained throughout 3 years of extensive follow-up sessions. These initial results support a therapeutic possibility of MEP operant conditioning for improving locomotion in people with MS or other CNS disorders, such as spinal cord injury and stroke.

1. Introduction

Transcranial magnetic stimulation (TMS) and its motor-evoked potential (MEP) have been widely used to study corticospinal excitability and connectivity noninvasively [1]. Generally, for a given intensity of stimulation, the larger the response size, the stronger the corticospinal connectivity and/or excitability [1–3]. Corticospinal activity is essential in human motor control, including walking [1, 3–6], and its restoration is important for regaining motor skills after CNS lesions [7–11]. In fact, CNS lesions that damage descending connections from the brain, such as spinal cord injury and multiple sclerosis (MS), reduce MEP size [6, 12–16], reflecting diminished corticospinal function in these populations. In people with MS, particularly, MEP measurements have been found useful in detecting and predicting the progression of disability and recovery [14, 15, 17–21]. Importantly, people with MS can display corticospinal plasticity [22, 23], which plays a key role in motor function recovery [7, 8, 24–28]. Thus, new methods for strengthening corticospinal connectivity and enhancing corticospinal function may improve motor function in people with MS. In the present case studies, we explored the possibility that enhancing the excitability and connectivity of corticospinal pathways to the ankle dorsiflexors through MEP operant conditioning can improve impaired locomotion due to moderately severe secondary progressive MS.

Operant conditioning is a powerful method for modifying a behavior based on its consequences. The past 35 years of spinal reflex operant conditioning studies in monkeys, rats, mice, and humans show that even a simple spinal reflex behavior can be gradually changed through learning and practice [29–31]. Animal studies have revealed that a hierarchy of spinal and supraspinal plasticity (from the cerebellum to sensorimotor cortex to corticospinal tract to spinal cord) is involved in inducing and maintaining the operant conditioning-induced change in the evoked response [31, 32]. Thus, operant conditioning of an EMG-evoked response that induces spinal and supraspinal plasticity may be used as a gateway to encouraging the production of specific patterns of CNS activity that are potentially linked to better motor function recovery after CNS damage [33–36]. In the present studies, an operant up-conditioning protocol was applied to the tibialis anterior (TA) MEP of people with MS who suffer from foot drop. The subjects were trained to strengthen the pathway specifically responsible for generating the TA MEP, so as to improve locomotion that also needs this pathway.

The purpose of this study was to investigate the feasibility and a therapeutic possibility of MEP operant conditioning for improving locomotion in people with chronic stable MS.

2. Materials and Methods

2.1. MEP Operant Conditioning Protocol. The MEP operant conditioning protocol used in this study is a modified version of the conditioning protocols developed and used in human subjects with and without spinal cord injury [34, 37, 38]. The study protocol was approved by the Institutional Review Board of Helen Hayes Hospital, New York State Department of Health, and all subjects gave written consent prior to participation.

At the beginning of the study, the subject was familiarized with the protocol and TMS in several preliminary sessions. Then, each subject completed 6 baseline sessions and 24 up-conditioning sessions that occurred at a pace of 3 times per week (Figure 1(a)). In one of the subjects, follow-up sessions occurred over the following 3 years at varying intervals (1 week to several months). To avoid variability due to possible diurnal variation in response size [39, 40], a subject's sessions always occurred at the same time of day (i.e., within the same 3 hr time window). In all sessions, TA MEPs were measured while the sitting subject provided a preset level (typically 30–35% maximum voluntary contraction (MVC) level, determined during preliminary sessions) of TA background EMG with ankle, knee, and hip joint angles fixed at $\approx 100^\circ$, $\approx 120^\circ$, and $\approx 110^\circ$, respectively.

At the beginning of each session, self-adhesive surface Ag-AgCl electrodes (2.2 × 3.5 cm, Vermed Inc., Bellows Falls, VT) were placed over the muscle bellies of TA and soleus for EMG recording [13, 41]. EMG signal was amplified, band-pass filtered (10–1000 Hz), and sampled at 5000 Hz. Absolute TA EMG during MVC was measured in two 3 s maximum isometric dorsiflexion trials, while the subject sat in a chair with hip, knee, and ankle joints fixed in a custom-made apparatus (Figure 1(c)). Then, the common peroneal nerve was stimulated at the neck of fibula, using surface electrodes (2.2 × 2.2 cm for cathode, 2.2 × 3.5 cm for anode, Vermed Inc.) and 0.5 ms wide single square pulses delivered from Grass S88 stimulator with an SIU-5 stimulation isolation unit and a CCU1 constant current unit (Astro-Med Inc., West Warwick, RI), while the subject sat at rest. Four EMG responses were averaged at each of 10 stimulus intensities varied from below M-wave threshold to just above the maximum M-wave (M_{max}) [42]. This TA M_{max} measurement was followed by control MEP trials (Figure 1(b)). In all trials of baseline sessions and the first 20 trials of conditioning sessions, the subject received no feedback as to MEP size (i.e., control MEPs). The subject simply needed to maintain the preset level of TA EMG activity. In contrast, in 225 conditioning trials of each conditioning session (i.e., conditioning MEPs), the subject was encouraged to increase TA MEP size and received immediate feedback as to whether MEP size was above a criterion (i.e., whether the trial was a success, Figure 1(d)). The criterion was based on the average MEP size for the previous block of trials. In each conditioning session, the criterion value for the first block of 75 conditioning trials was determined based on the immediately preceding block of 20 control trials, and the criterion values for the second and third conditioning blocks were based on the immediately preceding block of 75 conditioning trials. The criterion was selected so that if MEP values for the new block were similar to those for the previous block, 50–60% of the trials would be successful [34, 37]. For each block, the subject earned a modest extra monetary reward if the success rate exceeded 50% (see [37] for full details of the protocol.). For all trials, TMS at 10% above threshold was used to evoke the MEP. The same absolute TMS intensity (expressed as % maximum output of the stimulator) was used throughout the study. TA and soleus background EMG levels were kept stable throughout data collection. In order to minimize the session-to-session variability in nerve stimulation and EMG recording, the positions of all electrodes were measured in relation to landmarks on the skin (e.g., scars or moles) during the first preliminary session, and the same measures were used to place the electrodes in all subsequent sessions.

2.2. Subjects. Four women (age: 47–56 years) with chronic foot drop due to secondary progressive MS participated. Inclusion criteria were (1) neurologically stable for >6 months; (2) medical clearance to participate (with the expectation that current medication and therapy schedule would be maintained without change for at least 4 months)*; (3) ability to ambulate with or without an assistive device (i.e., Expanded Disability Status Scale (EDSS) 2 to 6 [43]); and (4) clinical signs of weak dorsiflexion of the ankle at least unilaterally. Exclusion criteria were (1) lower motor neuron damage; (2) known cardiac condition; (3) medical instability; (4) cognitive impairment; (5) a history of epileptic seizures; (6) metal implants in the head; and (7) implanted biomedical device in or above the chest. *Except for subject A, who had been taking 4-aminopyridine (Ampyra®) for 5 years at the time of enrollment, none were on neuromodulatory medication (e.g., baclofen). These subjects maintained their long-term MS medication, such as beta interferons (e.g., Avonex®), rituximab (Rituxan®), and dimethyl fumarate (Tecfidera®), throughout the 10 weeks of main study period.

The subject profiles are summarized in Table 1. In subject B, the MEP could be elicited only in one leg, and therefore that leg was studied. In subjects A, C, and D, the MEP could be elicited in both legs, and the more severely affected leg was studied (i.e., more severe foot drop). Before and after the 24

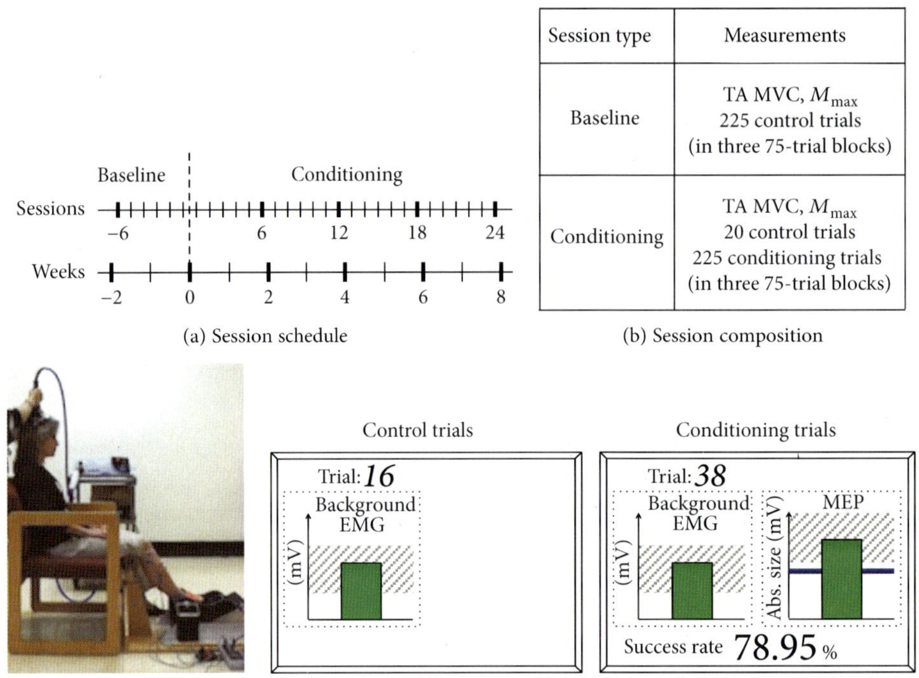

(a) Session schedule

(b) Session composition

(c) Setup view

(d) Visual feedback screens

FIGURE 1: (a) Session schedule. Six baseline sessions are followed by 24 conditioning sessions. (b) Composition of baseline and conditioning sessions. (c) Setup view. The subject sits in a chair with hip, knee, and ankle angles fixed at ≈100°, ≈120°, and ≈110°, respectively, in a custom-made apparatus. (d) Visual feedback screens for control and conditioning trials. In all trials, the number of the current trial within its block is displayed, and the background EMG panel shows the correct range (shaded) and the current value (green vertical bar, updated every 200 ms). If TA EMG activity stays in the correct range for at least 2 s and at least 5.5 s has passed since the last trial, an MEP is elicited. In control trials (left), the MEP panel is not shown. In conditioning trials (right), the shading in the MEP panel indicates the rewarded MEP range for up-conditioning. The dark horizontal line is the average MEP size of the baseline sessions, and the vertical bar is the MEP size (i.e., the average rectified EMG in the MEP interval (e.g., 45–75 ms after TMS)) for the most recent trial (it appears 200 ms after TMS). If that MEP size reaches into the shaded area, the bar is green and the trial is a success. If it falls below the shaded area, the bar is red and the trial is a not a success. The running success rate for the current block is shown at the bottom.

TABLE 1

Subj.	Age	Yrs	EDSS	ROM		Strength		FIM		25 ft time (s)	
				Pre	Post	Pre	Post	Pre	Post	Pre	Post
A	56	27	4.0	N (WNL)	WNL (WNL)	3− (5)	5 (5)	6	6	13.46	10.54
B	57	35	5.0	WNL (N)	N (10)	1 (0)	3 (1−)	6	6	26.45	19.51
C	47	26	5.0	WNL (WNL)	WNL (WNL)	2 (2)	3 (3)	6	6	27.51	36.80*
D	54	30	5.5	WNL (WNL)	WNL (WNL)	4+ (5)	5− (5)	2	2	39.84	33.80

Yrs: years since the original diagnosis of MS; EDSS: Expanded Disability Status Scale; ROM: passive ankle dorsiflexion range of motion (WNL: within normal limits; N: to neutral); Strength: manual muscle strength testing score for dorsiflexion, graded from 0 to 5 (0: no contractions felt in the muscle; 5: normal). ROM and Strength were measured bilaterally. The first row in each subject is for the conditioned leg and the second row (assessments indicated in ()) is for the contralateral leg. *In subject C, the post functional assessment was performed one month after the completion of 24 conditioning sessions.

conditioning sessions, Dr. Falivena and Ms. Velez, who were blinded to the subjects' conditioning results, assessed the clinical and functional states of disability: EDSS [43], evaluation of ankle joint passive range of motion, extent of voluntary movement control with manual muscle testing, and presence of movement abnormalities. 25 ft walking time was measured [44], and a functional independence measure (FIM) motor score was obtained.

2.3. Transcranial Magnetic Stimulation. TMS was performed using Magstim 200^2 and a custom-made double-cone coil (in subjects B, C, and D) or a bat-wing coil (in subject A) with radii of 9 cm (Jali Medical Inc., Woburn, MA), held over the scalp such that the induced current flowed in the posterior–anterior direction in the brain. When the absolute TA EMG level was maintained within the preset range (determined as 30–35% MVC level during preliminary sessions, and not changed throughout the entire study [34, 37]), an MEP was elicited by TMS, with a minimum interval of >5.5 s between stimuli. In preliminary sessions, the optimal TMS location at which the lowest stimulus intensity elicited the TA MEP was determined by moving the coil over the scalp. At the optimal location, the input-output curve of the corticospinal pathway was measured by increasing the TMS intensity, represented as a percentage of the maximum current that can be discharged into the coil, in steps of 5% until the MEP reached its plateau. Four MEPs were collected at each intensity, and the peak-to-peak and mean rectified amplitudes were plotted against the stimulus intensity [13, 45–47]. From the input-output curve measurement in several preliminary sessions, a stimulus intensity that was ≈10% above threshold was determined for each subject, and the same absolute TMS intensity was used throughout all the baseline and conditioning sessions.

Along with control and conditioned MEP size measurements, we also measured the silent period (SP) as the period from the end of the MEP to the recovery of background EMG activity in 50% of the responses [13, 45, 46, 48].

2.4. Locomotor EMG Measurement. Overground locomotor EMG activity was measured before and after the 24 conditioning sessions. Subject B, who wore an ankle foot orthosis on her unconditioned leg, was asked to remove it for this measurement. Surface EMG was recorded from the TA, soleus, biceps femoris, and vastus lateralis bilaterally. To detect foot contact for each leg, foot-switch cells were inserted between the subject's shoes and feet. For analysis, the foot-contact signal was used to define the beginning of the step cycle. Rectified EMG signals from individual steps were normalized to the mean step cycle time and averaged together to obtain the locomotor EMG activity over the step cycle [34, 49, 50]. Fifty or more steps were averaged. For quantitative analysis, the step cycle was divided into 12 equal bins and EMG activity was averaged for each bin. Then, each bin's average EMG amplitude was expressed in percent of the amplitude in the bin with the highest amplitude [38]. To determine for each muscle the extent of EMG modulation over the step cycle, a modulation index (MI) was calculated in percent as 100 × [(highest bin amplitude − lowest bin amplitude)/highest bin amplitude] [34, 38]. In each muscle, the MIs across the 12 bins were compared before and after conditioning.

2.5. Data Analysis. For each session of each subject, we calculated average MEP sizes for the 20 within-session control trials and for all three 75-trial blocks together. For these calculations, MEP size was defined as average absolute EMG in the MEP interval minus average background EMG. Changes in these MEP sizes across sessions were quantified in percent of their average values for the 6 baseline sessions. We also determined for each subject the final effects of conditioning on the conditioned MEP by averaging the MEPs for the 75-trial conditioning blocks of conditioning sessions 22–24 and expressing the result in % of the average MEP for the 75-trial blocks of the 6 baseline sessions. (Thus, a value of 100% indicates no change in the MEP.) The final effect on the control MEP was calculated by averaging the MEPs for the 20 within-session control trials of conditioning sessions 22–24 and expressing the result in % of the average MEP for the first 20 trials of the 6 baseline sessions (see [37]).

To determine for each subject whether MEP up-conditioning was successful, the average conditioned MEPs of the final 6 conditioning sessions were compared to the average MEPs of the 6 baseline sessions by unpaired *t*-test (two-tailed) [34, 37]. To evaluate in each subject the stability of the M_{max} and background EMG levels over all sessions and assess changes in MVC and SP, a factorial ANOVA was used across successive 6-session blocks (i.e., baseline sessions 1–6 and conditioning sessions 1–6, 7–12, 13–18, and 19–24) [37]. TA M_{max} and TA and soleus background EMG levels in control and conditioning trials remained stable throughout the study ($p > 0.07$ for all parameters by one-way factorial ANOVA in each of the subjects). Typically, TA M_{max} remained within ±15% to the mean across all the sessions, TA background EMG remained within ±5%, and soleus background EMG remained under 5 μV (i.e., resting EMG level) throughout the study.

3. Results

In 3 of the 4 subjects, TA MEP increased significantly, together with the TA MVC; and at the end of conditioning, all three spontaneously reported better leg movement in their daily walking. Here, we describe each subject's results individually.

3.1. Subject A. Over the course of conditioning, her left TA MEP increased progressively. Her final conditioned MEP size was 175% of the baseline value (Figure 2(a)). This increase consisted of a 33% increase in the control MEP (reflecting long-term across-session change) and a 42% within-session increase (i.e., task-dependent change) (not shown in figures, see [34, 35, 37] for discussion of them). TA MVC also increased gradually; the final MVC was 128% of the baseline value (Figure 2(b)), while the SP duration decreased steadily from 205 ms in baseline sessions to 98 ms in the conditioning sessions 22–24 (Figure 2(c)).

There were several noteworthy observations over the course of study. First, this subject had no visible voluntary ankle dorsiflexion at the beginning and needed a cane to compensate for the limited motion in the left leg. After 24 conditioning sessions, she was able to flex the left ankle even against resistance (Table 1); and at the post conditioning clinical evaluation, she surprised Dr. Falivena by saying that she forgot to bring a cane. She commented that her cane usage had decreased over the course of study. After conditioning, 25 ft walking time was decreased, indicating a 28% increase in walking speed (Table 1). Figure 2(d) shows the changes in locomotor EMG activity after conditioning. The conditioned leg's TA burst during the swing phase is clearly

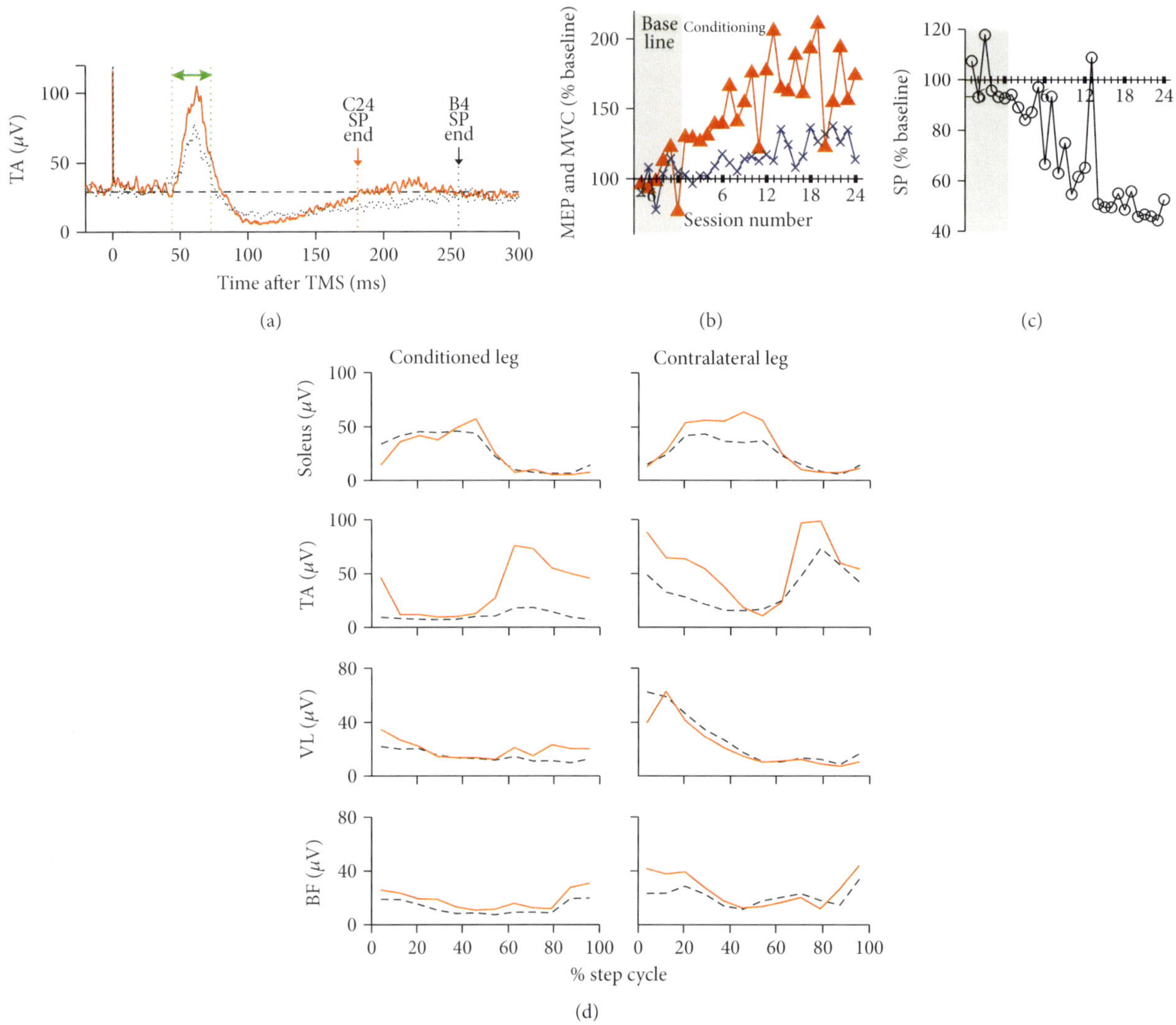

Figure 2: Changes in tibialis anterior (TA) motor-evoked potential (MEP), maximum voluntary contraction (MVC), and silent period (SP) over the course of study, and bilateral locomotor EMG activity in subject A. (a) Rectified EMG signals from the fourth baseline session (dashed black) and the last (i.e., 24th) conditioning session (solid red). Two hundred twenty-five responses were averaged together for each sweep. A pair of dashed vertical lines (green) indicates the time window for this subject's MEP size calculation. The horizontal line at 30 μV indicates the background EMG level. (b) Mean MEP size (i.e., the mean of 225 control (in baseline sessions) or 225 conditioned (in conditioning sessions) MEP trials) (filled triangle) and MVC (cross) in 6 baseline (shaded part of the panel) and 24 conditioning sessions. (c) Mean SP duration (i.e., as marked in panel (a)). (d) Rectified locomotor EMG activity in soleus, TA, vastus lateralis (VL), and biceps femoris (BF) muscles of both legs before (dashed black) and after (solid red) conditioning. The step cycle is divided into 12 equal bins, starting from foot contact. Generally, bins 1–7 (i.e., up to 60% of the step cycle) are for the stance phase and bins 8–12 (i.e., 60–100% of the step cycle) are for the swing phase. After successful MEP up-conditioning, EMG modulation over the step cycle becomes greater in the muscles of both legs.

increased, enabling ankle dorsiflexion during the swing phase and heel contact at the beginning of the stance phase. Thus, after conditioning, this subject no longer suffered from foot drop. As Figure 2(d) also shows, the swing phase burst was increased in the contralateral TA as well. Locomotor EMG MI was increased in 6 of 8 leg muscles, indicating an overall improvement of EMG modulation during locomotion.

In this subject, 66 follow-up sessions were performed over 161 weeks (3 years) after the last conditioning session (Figure 3). During this period, her official diagnosis changed from secondary progressive MS to relapsing-remitting MS, and the medication changed accordingly. Also, on week 70, we repeated cortical mapping of the TA MEP. At that point, we found that the MEP size at the vertex was similar to that elicited at the original optimum location (i.e., 2.5 cm lateral and 1.5 cm anterior to the vertex). Thus, from week 71 on, TMS was applied at the vertex, not at the original optimum location. Also, the TMS intensity and coil were changed from 80% of stimulator's maximum output with a bat-wing coil to 70% with a double-cone coil, which generated control MEPs comparable to those generated by 80% with the bat-wing coil. Larger conditioned MEP size observed from week 71 on may be partially due to less-focused wider-spread stimulation with the double-cone coil. Most importantly, over this

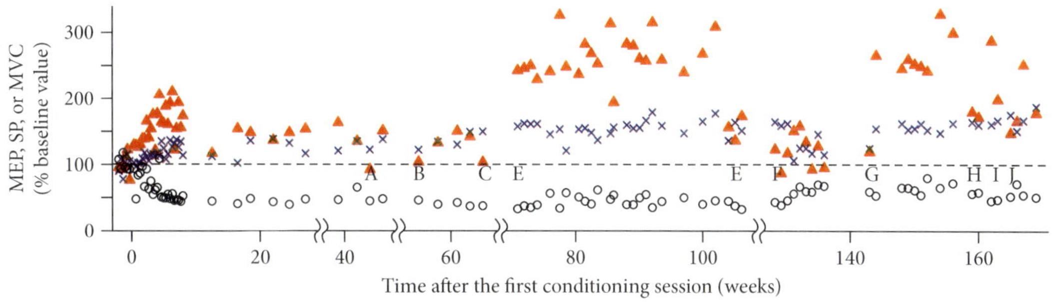

FIGURE 3: TA MEP (filled triangle), MVC (cross), and SP (circle) over 3.3 years of study including baseline to conditioning to follow-up periods in subject A. During the follow-up period (i.e., after 8 weeks of conditioning), her official diagnosis changed (from secondary progressive MS to relapsing-remitting MS) and so did her medication. Notable events in her life and neurological/medical history during the study period are indicated as A–J. (A) A few days after the first rituximab injection. (B) Feeling tired due to personal life issue. (C) Going through divorce. (D) Cortical mapping had been redone. TMS location was changed from "2.5 cm lateral and 1.5 cm anterior to the vertex". (E) Kidney infection. (F) MS relapse diagnosed; started taking dimethyl fumarate (tecfidera); her gait had worsened. No visible ankle dorsiflexion. (*Visible dorsiflexion returned several weeks later.) (G) Frequent urinary tract infection for the past several weeks. (H) Started taking ropinirole hydrochloride (requip). Also started on tamsulosin and oxybutynin for UTI treatment/prevention. (I) Her mother just had a stroke. (J) Started taking interferon beta Ia (avonex). Throughout this lengthy follow-up and many life events, the MEP and MVC increases and the SP decrease associated with MEP up-conditioning persisted.

extensive follow-up, her MVC increase was well maintained (M_{max} remained around 3.8 mV for the entire 172 weeks of her study). An increased MEP and decreased SP duration were also present in most of the follow-up sessions. At the study conclusion (i.e., 3 years after conditioning), voluntary ankle dorsiflexion remained visible and improved.

3.2. Subject B. The TA MEP increased over the course of study (Figure 4(a)). Her final conditioned MEP size was 132% of the baseline value; this came from within-session increase. There was no long-term change in the control MEP. TA MVC increase paralleled MEP change; the final MVC was 142% of the baseline value (Figure 4(a)). SP duration did not change (from 277 ms in baseline sessions to 265 ms in the conditioning sessions 22–24, Figure 4(b)).

After conditioning, the conditioned leg's TA burst in the late swing phase of walking and soleus burst during the stance phase were clearly increased (Figure 4(c)). Locomotor EMG MI was increased in 7 of 8 muscles measured, indicating overall improvement in EMG modulation. These improvements in the locomotor EMG activity, together with improved dorsiflexion strength (Table 1), were associated with a 36% increase in walking speed (Table 1).

3.3. Subject C. Her final conditioned MEP size was 172% of the baseline value (Figure 4(d)), which consisted of 45% increase in the control MEP (i.e., long-term increase) and a 27% within-session task-dependent increase (not shown in figures). MVC increase paralleled MEP change; the final MVC was 152% of the baseline value (Figure 4(d)). We were unable to determine the SP duration, as she was unable to maintain the background EMG level after TMS in many of the trials of the baseline sessions.

The TA burst in the swing phase of locomotion increased after conditioning in both the conditioned and the contralateral legs (Figure 4(e)). Locomotor EMG MI was increased in 6 of 8 muscles measured, indicating overall improvement in EMG modulation. However, soon after the last conditioning session, the neurologist noted that her MS resumed to progress; at the post functional assessment that was performed one month after the last conditioning session (this delay of assessment was caused by her physical condition and scheduling conflicts), the walking speed was decreased (Table 1).

3.4. Subject D. MEP up-conditioning did not increase her MEP (Figure 4(f)). Her final conditioned MEP size was 106% of the baseline value, which consisted of 9% within-session increase and 3% across-session control MEP decrease. TA MVC did not increase either; the final MVC was 101% of the baseline value (Figure 4(f)). SP duration also did not change over the course of conditioning (234 ms in baseline sessions and 231 ms in the conditioning sessions 22–24, Figure 4(g)). No clear changes were observed in her locomotor EMG activity after conditioning (Figure 4(f)). Locomotor EMG MI was increased in 3 of 8 muscles while unchanged or decreased in 5 of 8 muscles measured, suggesting no overall improvement in EMG modulation. However, her 25 ft walking time was reduced after conditioning by 15% (Table 1). This speed improvement may be a nonspecific (psychological) effect of the procedures (see also [34]). Altogether, the results show that unsuccessful conditioning in this subject was unlikely due to her MS status and did not worsen her gait.

4. Discussion

4.1. Effects of Up-Conditioning on MEP and SP in People with MS. In three of 4 subjects with MS, up-conditioning successfully increased MEP over the course of 24 conditioning sessions, supporting the possibility and feasibility of MEP operant conditioning in people with chronic stable MS.

In two of the 3 successfully conditioned subjects, the conditioned MEP increase consisted of within-session task-dependent adaptation and cumulative long-term change, similar to previous studies of H-reflex operant conditioning [34, 37, 38]. Since the long-term change represents the

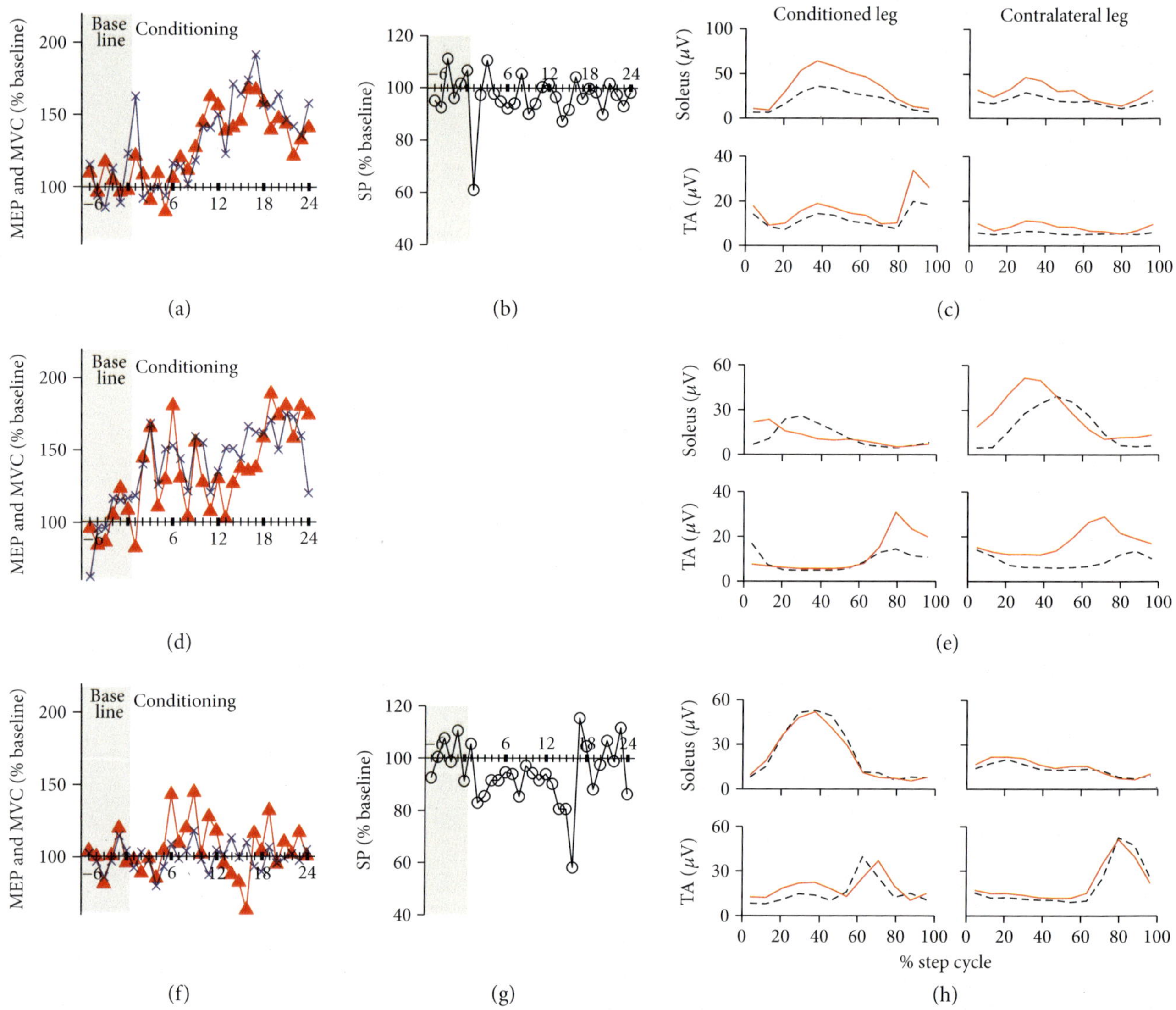

FIGURE 4: Changes in the TA MEP, MVC, and SP over the course of study and bilateral locomotor EMG in subjects B, C, and D. (a, b, c) Subject B. (a) Mean MEP size (filled triangle) and MVC (cross) in 6 baseline (shaded part of the panel) and 24 conditioning sessions. (b) Mean SP duration. (c) Rectified locomotor EMG activity in soleus and TA of both legs before (black) and after (red) conditioning. After successful MEP up-conditioning, locomotor EMG modulation increases in TA and soleus of both legs; not only the conditioned TA but also the soleus burst amplitude increased. (d, e) Subject C. (d) Mean MEP size and MVC in 6 baseline and 24 conditioning sessions. (e) Rectified locomotor EMG activity in soleus and TA bilaterally, before and after conditioning. After successful MEP up-conditioning, TA EMG burst amplitude increased in both legs. SP duration could not be measured in this subject. (f, g, h) Subject D. (f) Mean MEP size and MVC in 6 baseline and 24 conditioning sessions. (g) Mean SP duration. (h) Rectified locomotor EMG activity in soleus and TA bilaterally, before and after conditioning. In this subject, unlike subjects A–C, MEP up-conditioning had no significant effect.

plasticity that persists outside of the conditioning paradigm [34, 38, 42], we expected that functional improvement (i.e., in locomotion and MVC) would be linked to the presence and extent of long-term increase in MEP size. However, increased MVC, improved locomotor EMG, and increased walking speed were present even in the subject with little long-term MEP increase (Figures 4(a)–4(c), Table 1). Thus, it is possible that the relationship between the long-term change and functional impact may differ between the pathways targeted by different operant conditioning protocols. Different from reflex conditioning, functional impact of MEP conditioning may be better estimated with the total conditioning-induced change (i.e., the sum of long-term and task-dependent changes) or the task-dependent change of corticospinal excitability. Since corticospinal drive is directly involved in the activation of TA during the swing phase of locomotion [4, 5], after successful MEP up-conditioning, the corticospinal pathways that were trained to increase their connectivity during conditioning trials would also do so during walking.

In all of these subjects with MS, we noticed that the SP duration was very long (i.e., >200 ms) during the baseline sessions. Since baclofen, a common antispastic medication for people with MS, spinal cord injury, and cerebral palsy

[51–53], is a $GABA_B$ receptor agonist and known to prolong the SP duration [54, 55], one might suspect that the observed long SP would be due to medication. However, that would not be the case here; none of the present subjects had been taking baclofen or any other known antispastic medication (e.g., diazepam). Therefore, it is likely that their long SP reflects their underlying physiology, not GABAergic medication effects. The later part of long SP (e.g., >100 ms) originates from $GABA_B$-mediated intracortical inhibition [56–58]. The prolonged SP observed in the present subjects with MS could, thus, be due to enhanced intracortical inhibition [54] that may be linked to their motor impairments [59]. In subject A, the SP duration progressively decreased over the course of study (Figures 2(a) and 2(c)), suggesting a decrease in intracortical inhibition. We have observed similar decreases in SP duration with MEP up-conditioning in neurologically normal subjects, in whom baseline SP duration was not quite long (≈100 ms, [60]). Considering this clear difference in the baseline SP duration between normal subjects and subjects with MS and the fact that SP duration did not decrease in subject B, further studies are needed to investigate the consistency and mechanisms of SP decrease with MEP up-conditioning.

4.2. Functional Implications. In 3 of the 4 subjects, operant up-conditioning of TA MEP was successful and was accompanied by increased MVC, increased TA burst during the swing-phase of locomotion, and improved EMG modulation during locomotion. In 2 of the 3 subjects, the ankle dorsiflexor strength and walking speed also improved; in the third subject, disease progression near the end of the study may have prevented walking speed improvement despite significant increases in MEP, MVC, and locomotor EMG modulation. The increased corticospinal drive to the conditioned TA may explain increases in TA MEP, TA MVC, and TA burst amplitude during the swing phase of walking [4, 5, 26], but it cannot explain widespread improvements in locomotor EMG activity; locomotor EMG modulation improved in the ankle extensors, knee flexors, and knee extensors of both legs. This wide effect of MEP up-conditioning is very similar to the locomotor improvements produced by H-reflex down-conditioning in people with SCI [34]. As discussed in detail elsewhere [34, 35], bilateral locomotor EMG improvements in proximal and distal leg muscles probably occurred through additional plasticity in other spinal pathways that are involved in locomotion. The acquisition of a new behavior (e.g., increasing corticospinal excitability for the TA) through 8 weeks of operant conditioning probably triggered a widespread adaptive plasticity in many CNS pathways that resulted in better locomotion [32, 33, 35]. These widespread effects are explainable in terms of the negotiated equilibrium hypothesis [32].

One of the cases presented here (subject A) has an important implication for future therapeutic applications. Over 3 years of follow-up sessions, her TA MEP, MVC, and SP improvements and the voluntary ankle dorsiflexion that she had not had before conditioning were essentially maintained (Figure 3), despite changes in diagnosis, medication, and personal life. This case supports the possibility of long-term maintenance of improvement with periodic follow-up sessions, after completion of initial intense conditioning. The intervals between follow-up sessions varied from a week to months in this subject; the minimum effective follow-up interval needs to be determined through thorough systematic studies.

4.2.1. Limitations. The present study investigated the feasibility of MEP operant conditioning in a small number of individuals with MS. Thus, while the initial results support a therapeutic possibility of this approach for improving locomotion in people with MS (and potentially other CNS disorders), its wider applicability is yet to be confirmed through future clinical studies of larger scales.

Disclosure

Part of this work has been presented in an abstract form at Neuroscience 2014 (Society for Neuroscience 44th Annual Meeting, Program no. 537.05) in Washington, D.C., in 2014.

Conflicts of Interest

The authors declare that there is no conflict of interest regarding the publication of this paper.

Acknowledgments

The authors thank Dr. Jonathan R. Wolpaw for helpful comments on the manuscript, Ms. Gina Fiorenza and Mr. Alex J. Amsterdam for assistance in data analysis, and Ms. Laura Tenteromano for study coordination. This work was supported in part by the National Institute of Neurological Disorders and Stroke (NS069551 to Aiko K. Thompson), the Helen Hayes Hospital Foundation (to Aiko K. Thompson), and the National Institute of General Medical Sciences (GM104941, Institutional Development Award (IDeA) to Binder-MacLeod).

References

[1] A. Pascual-Leone, N. J. Davey, J. Rothwell, E. M. Wassermann, and B. K. Puri, *Handbook of Transcranial Magnetic Stimulation*, A. Pascual-Leone, N. J. Davey, J. Rothwell, E. M. Wassermann, and B. K. Puri, Eds., Arnold, a member of the Hodder headline Group, London, UK, 2002.

[2] M. Hallett, "Transcranial magnetic stimulation and the human brain," *Nature*, vol. 406, no. 6792, pp. 147–150, 2000.

[3] M. C. Ridding and J. C. Rothwell, "Stimulus/response curves as a method of measuring motor cortical excitability in man," *Electroencephalography and Clinical Neurophysiology/Electromyography and Motor Control*, vol. 105, no. 5, pp. 340–344, 1997.

[4] C. Capaday, B. A. Lavoie, H. Barbeau, C. Schneider, and M. Bonnard, "Studies on the corticospinal control of human walking. I. Responses to focal transcranial magnetic stimulation of the motor cortex," *Journal of Neurophysiology*, vol. 81, no. 1, pp. 129–139, 1999.

[5] N. T. Petersen, J. E. Butler, V. Marchand-Pauvert et al., "Suppression of EMG activity by transcranial magnetic stimulation

in human subjects during walking," *The Journal of Physiology*, vol. 537, no. 2, pp. 651–656, 2001.

[6] D. Barthélemy, M. Willerslev-Olsen, H. Lundell et al., "Impaired transmission in the corticospinal tract and gait disability in spinal cord injured persons," *Journal of Neurophysiology*, vol. 104, no. 2, pp. 1167–1176, 2010.

[7] J. Liepert, H. Bauder, H. R. Wolfgang, W. H. Miltner, E. Taub, and C. Weiller, "Treatment-induced cortical reorganization after stroke in humans," *Stroke*, vol. 31, no. 6, pp. 1210–1216, 2000.

[8] R. J. Nudo, "Adaptive plasticity in motor cortex: implications for rehabilitation after brain injury," *Journal of Rehabilitation Medicine*, vol. 35, no. 0, pp. 7–10, 2003.

[9] U. Ziemann, T. V. Ilić, C. Pauli, F. Meintzschel, and D. Ruge, "Learning modifies subsequent induction of long-term potentiation-like and long-term depression-like plasticity in human motor cortex," *Journal of Neuroscience*, vol. 24, no. 7, pp. 1666–1672, 2004.

[10] D. Ramanathan, J. M. Conner, and M. H. Tuszynski, "A form of motor cortical plasticity that correlates with recovery of function after brain injury," *Proceedings of the National Academy of Sciences of the United States of America*, vol. 103, no. 30, pp. 11370–11375, 2006.

[11] K. L. Bunday and M. A. Perez, "Motor recovery after spinal cord injury enhanced by strengthening corticospinal synaptic transmission," *Current Biology*, vol. 22, no. 24, pp. 2355–2361, 2012.

[12] N. J. Davey, H. C. Smith, G. Savic, D. W. Maskill, P. H. Ellaway, and H. L. Frankel, "Comparison of input-output patterns in the corticospinal system of normal subjects and incomplete spinal cord injured patients," *Experimental Brain Research*, vol. 127, no. 4, pp. 382–390, 1999.

[13] A. K. Thompson, B. Lapallo, M. Duffield, B. M. Abel, and F. Pomerantz, "Repetitive common peroneal nerve stimulation increases ankle dorsiflexor motor evoked potentials in incomplete spinal cord lesions," *Experimental Brain Research*, vol. 210, no. 1, pp. 143–152, 2011.

[14] N. Kale, J. Agaoglu, G. onder, and O. Tanik, "Correlation between disability and transcranial magnetic stimulation abnormalities in patients with multiple sclerosis," *Journal of Clinical Neuroscience*, vol. 16, no. 11, pp. 1439–1442, 2009.

[15] A. Gagliardo, F. Galli, A. Grippo et al., "Motor evoked potentials in multiple sclerosis patients without walking limitation: amplitude vs. conduction time abnormalities," *Journal of Neurology*, vol. 254, no. 2, pp. 220–227, 2007.

[16] A. Conte, D. Lenzi, V. Frasca et al., "Intracortical excitability in patients with relapsing–remitting and secondary progressive multiple sclerosis," *Journal of Neurology*, vol. 256, no. 6, pp. 933–938, 2009.

[17] F. Mori, H. Kusayanagi, C. G. Nicoletti, S. Weiss, M. G. Marciani, and D. Centonze, "Cortical plasticity predicts recovery from relapse in multiple sclerosis," *Multiple Sclerosis Journal*, vol. 20, no. 4, pp. 451–457, 2013.

[18] R. Schlaeger, M. D'Souza, C. Schindler et al., "Prediction of long-term disability in multiple sclerosis," *Multiple Sclerosis*, vol. 18, no. 1, pp. 31–38, 2012.

[19] K. Schmierer, K. Irlbacher, P. Grosse, S. Roricht, and B. U. Meyer, "Correlates of disability in multiple sclerosis detected by transcranial magnetic stimulation," *Neurology*, vol. 59, no. 8, pp. 1218–1224, 2002.

[20] P. Fuhr and L. Kappos, "Evoked potentials for evaluation of multiple sclerosis," *Clinical Neurophysiology*, vol. 112, no. 12, pp. 2185–2189, 2001.

[21] P. Fuhr, A. Borggrefe-Chappuis, C. Schindler, and L. Kappos, "Visual and motor evoked potentials in the course of multiple sclerosis," *Brain*, vol. 124, no. 11, pp. 2162–2168, 2001.

[22] D. Zeller, K. aufm Kampe, A. Biller et al., "Rapid-onset central motor plasticity in multiple sclerosis," *Neurology*, vol. 74, no. 9, pp. 728–735, 2010.

[23] R. B. Stein, D. G. Everaert, F. D. Roy, S. Chong, and M. Soleimani, "Facilitation of corticospinal connections in able-bodied people and people with central nervous system disorders using eight interventions," *Journal of Clinical Neurophysiology*, vol. 30, no. 1, pp. 66–78, 2013.

[24] S. L. Thomas and M. A. Gorassini, "Increases in corticospinal tract function by treadmill training after incomplete spinal cord injury," *Journal of Neurophysiology*, vol. 94, no. 4, pp. 2844–2855, 2005.

[25] R. B. Stein, S. L. Chong, D. G. Everaert et al., "A multicenter trial of a footdrop stimulator controlled by a tilt sensor," *Neurorehabilitation and Neural Repair*, vol. 20, no. 3, pp. 371–379, 2006.

[26] D. G. Everaert, A. K. Thompson, Su Ling Chong, and R. B. Stein, "Does functional electrical stimulation for foot drop strengthen corticospinal connections?," *Neurorehabilitation and Neural Repair*, vol. 24, no. 2, pp. 168–177, 2010.

[27] R. J. Nudo, "Postinfarct cortical plasticity and behavioral recovery," *Stroke*, vol. 38, no. 2, pp. 840–845, 2007.

[28] V. Tomassini, P. M. Matthews, A. J. Thompson et al., "Neuroplasticity and functional recovery in multiple sclerosis," *Nature Reviews Neurology*, vol. 8, no. 11, pp. 635–646, 2012.

[29] J. R. Wolpaw and A. M. Tennissen, "Activity-dependent spinal cord plasticity in health and disease," *Annual Review of Neuroscience*, vol. 24, no. 1, pp. 807–843, 2001.

[30] J. R. Wolpaw, "Spinal cord plasticity in acquisition and maintenance of motor skills," *Acta Physiologica*, vol. 189, no. 2, pp. 155–169, 2007.

[31] A. K. Thompson and J. R. Wolpaw, "Operant conditioning of spinal reflexes: from basic science to clinical therapy," *Frontiers in Integrative Neuroscience*, vol. 8, p. 25, 2014.

[32] J. R. Wolpaw, "What can the spinal cord teach us about learning and memory?," *The Neuroscientist*, vol. 16, no. 5, pp. 532–549, 2010.

[33] A. K. Thompson and J. R. Wolpaw, "Chapter 7 - targeted neuroplasticity for rehabilitation," *Progress in Brain Research*, vol. 218, pp. 157–172, 2015.

[34] A. K. Thompson, F. R. Pomerantz, and J. R. Wolpaw, "Operant conditioning of a spinal reflex can improve locomotion after spinal cord injury in humans," *Journal of Neuroscience*, vol. 33, no. 6, pp. 2365–2375, 2013.

[35] A. K. Thompson and J. R. Wolpaw, "Restoring walking after spinal cord injury: operant conditioning of spinal reflexes can help," *The Neuroscientist*, vol. 21, no. 2, pp. 203–215, 2014.

[36] A. K. Thompson and J. R. Wolpaw, "The simplest motor skill: mechanisms and applications of reflex operant conditioning," *Exercise and Sport Sciences Reviews*, vol. 42, no. 2, pp. 82–90, 2014.

[37] A. K. Thompson, X. Y. Chen, and J. R. Wolpaw, "Acquisition of a simple motor skill: task-dependent adaptation plus long-term change in the human soleus H-reflex," *Journal of Neuroscience*, vol. 29, no. 18, pp. 5784–5792, 2009.

[38] Y. Makihara, R. L. Segal, J. R. Wolpaw, and A. K. Thompson, "Operant conditioning of the soleus H-reflex does not induce long-term changes in the gastrocnemius H-reflexes and does not disturb normal locomotion in humans," *Journal of Neurophysiology*, vol. 112, no. 6, pp. 1439–1446, 2014.

[39] O. Lagerquist, E. P. Zehr, E. R. L. Baldwin, P. M. Klakowicz, and D. F. Collins, "Diurnal changes in the amplitude of the Hoffmann reflex in the human soleus but not in the flexor carpi radialis muscle," *Experimental Brain Research*, vol. 170, no. 1, pp. 1–6, 2006.

[40] A. S. Tamm, O. Lagerquist, A. L. Ley, and D. F. Collins, "Chronotype influences diurnal variations in the excitability of the human motor cortex and the ability to generate torque during a maximum voluntary contraction," *Journal of Biological Rhythms*, vol. 24, no. 3, pp. 211–224, 2009.

[41] A. K. Thompson, K. L. Estabrooks, S. L. Chong, and R. B. Stein, "Spinal reflexes in ankle flexor and extensor muscles after chronic central nervous system lesions and functional electrical stimulation," *Neurorehabilitation and Neural Repair*, vol. 23, no. 2, pp. 133–142, 2008.

[42] A. K. Thompson, X. Yang Chen, and J. R. Wolpaw, "Soleus H-reflex operant conditioning changes the H-reflex recruitment curve," *Muscle & Nerve*, vol. 47, no. 4, pp. 539–544, 2013.

[43] J. F. Kurtzke, "Rating neurologic impairment in multiple sclerosis: an expanded disability status scale (EDSS)," *Neurology*, vol. 33, no. 11, pp. 1444–1452, 1983.

[44] A. D. Goodman, T. R. Brown, L. B. Krupp et al., "Sustained-release oral fampridine in multiple sclerosis: a randomised, double-blind, controlled trial," *The Lancet*, vol. 373, no. 9665, pp. 732–738, 2009.

[45] M. E. Knash, A. Kido, M. Gorassini, K. M. Chan, and R. B. Stein, "Electrical stimulation of the human common peroneal nerve elicits lasting facilitation of cortical motor-evoked potentials," *Experimental Brain Research*, vol. 153, no. 3, pp. 366–377, 2003.

[46] A. Kido Thompson and R. B. Stein, "Short-term effects of functional electrical stimulation on motor-evoked potentials in ankle flexor and extensor muscles," *Experimental Brain Research*, vol. 159, no. 4, pp. 491–500, 2004.

[47] A. K. Thompson, B. Doran, and R. B. Stein, "Short-term effects of functional electrical stimulation on spinal excitatory and inhibitory reflexes in ankle extensor and flexor muscles," *Experimental Brain Research*, vol. 170, no. 2, pp. 216–226, 2006.

[48] M. A. Garvey, U. Ziemann, D. A. Becker, C. A. Barker, and J. J. Bartko, "New graphical method to measure silent periods evoked by transcranial magnetic stimulation," *Clinical Neurophysiology*, vol. 112, no. 8, pp. 1451–1460, 2001.

[49] A. Kido, N. Tanaka, and R. B. Stein, "Spinal reciprocal inhibition in human locomotion," *Journal of Applied Physiology*, vol. 96, no. 5, pp. 1969–1977, 2004.

[50] Y. Makihara, R. L. Segal, J. R. Wolpaw, and A. K. Thompson, "H-reflex modulation in the human medial and lateral gastrocnemii during standing and walking," *Muscle & Nerve*, vol. 45, no. 1, pp. 116–125, 2012.

[51] M. Kita and D. E. Goodkin, "Drugs used to treat spasticity," *Drugs*, vol. 59, no. 3, pp. 487–495, 2000.

[52] I. Stetkarova, K. Brabec, P. Vasko, and L. Mencl, "Intrathecal baclofen in spinal spasticity: frequency and severity of withdrawal syndrome," *Pain Physician*, vol. 18, no. 4, pp. E633–E641, 2015.

[53] M. P. Barnes, R. M. Kent, J. K. Semlyen, and K. M. McMullen, "Spasticity in multiple sclerosis," *Neurorehabilitation and Neural Repair*, vol. 17, no. 1, pp. 66–70, 2003.

[54] H. R. Siebner, J. Dressnandt, C. Auer, and B. Conrad, "Continuous intrathecal baclofen infusions induced a marked increase of the transcranially evoked silent period in a patient with generalized dystonia," *Muscle & Nerve*, vol. 21, no. 9, pp. 1209–1212, 1998.

[55] I. Stetkarova and M. Kofler, "Differential effect of baclofen on cortical and spinal inhibitory circuits," *Clinical Neurophysiology*, vol. 124, no. 2, pp. 339–345, 2013.

[56] R. Chen, A. M. Lozano, and P. Ashby, "Mechanism of the silent period following transcranial magnetic stimulation. Evidence from epidural recordings," *Experimental Brain Research*, vol. 128, no. 4, pp. 539–542, 1999.

[57] M. N. McDonnell, Y. Orekhov, and U. Ziemann, "The role of $GABA_B$ receptors in intracortical inhibition in the human motor cortex," *Experimental Brain Research*, vol. 173, no. 1, pp. 86–93, 2006.

[58] K. J. Werhahn, E. Kunesch, S. Noachtar, R. Benecke, and J. Classen, "Differential effects on motorcortical inhibition induced by blockade of GABA uptake in humans," *The Journal of Physiology*, vol. 517, no. 2, pp. 591–597, 1999.

[59] J. Classen, "The motor syndrome associated with exaggerated inhibition within the primary motor cortex of patients with hemiparetic," *Brain*, vol. 120, no. 4, pp. 605–619, 1997.

[60] A. K. Thompson, R. H. Cote, and C. R. Thompson, "Operant conditioning of the tibialis anterior motor evoked potential to transcranial magnetic stimulation," *Converging Clinical and Engineering Research on Neurorehabilitation: Proceedings of the 3rd International Conference on NeuroRehabilitation (ICNR2016)*, Springer, Segovia, Spain, 2016.

12

Thrombin Inhibition Reduces the Expression of Brain Inflammation Markers upon Systemic LPS Treatment

Efrat Shavit Stein,[1] Marina Ben Shimon,[1,2] Avital Artan Furman,[1] Valery Golderman,[1,2] Joab Chapman,[1,2] and Nicola Maggio[1,2,3,4]

[1]*Department of Neurology, The Chaim Sheba Medical Center at Tel HaShomer, 52621 Ramat Gan, Israel*
[2]*Department of Neurology and Neurosurgery, Sackler Faculty of Medicine, Tel Aviv University, 6997801 Tel Aviv, Israel*
[3]*Talpiot Medical Leadership Program, The Chaim Sheba Medical Center at Tel HaShomer, 52621 Ramat Gan, Israel*
[4]*Sagol School of Neuroscience, Tel Aviv University, 6997801 Tel Aviv, Israel*

Correspondence should be addressed to Nicola Maggio; nicola.maggio@sheba.health.gov.il

Academic Editor: Carlo Cavaliere

Systemic inflammation and brain pathologies are known to be linked. In the periphery, the inflammation and coagulation systems are simultaneously activated upon diseases and infections. Whether this well-established interrelation also counts for neuroinflammation and coagulation factor expression in the brain is still an open question. Our aim was to study whether the interrelationship between coagulation and inflammation factors may occur in the brain in the setting of systemic inflammation. The results indicate that systemic injections of lipopolysaccharide (LPS) upregulate the expression of both inflammatory and coagulation factors in the brain. The activity of the central coagulation factor thrombin was tested by a fluorescent method and found to be significantly elevated in the hippocampus following systemic LPS injection (0.5 ± 0.15 mU/mg versus 0.2 ± 0.03 mU/mg in the control). A panel of coagulation factors and effectors (such as thrombin, FX, PAR1, EPCR, and PC) was tested in the hippocampus, isolated microglia, and N9 microglia cell by Western blot and real-time PCR and found to be modulated by LPS. One central finding is a significant increase in FX expression level following LPS induction both in vivo in the hippocampus and in vitro in N9 microglia cell line (5.5 ± 0.6- and 2.3 ± 0.1-fold of increase, resp.). Surprisingly, inhibition of thrombin activity (by a specific inhibitor NAPAP) immediately after LPS injection results in a reduction of both the inflammatory (TNFα, CXL9, and CCL1; $p < 0.006$) and coagulation responses (FX and PAR1; $p < 0.004$) in the brain. We believe that these results may have a profound clinical impact as they might indicate that reducing coagulation activity in the setting of neurological diseases involving neuroinflammation may improve disease outcome and survival.

1. Introduction

A growing body of evidence links systemic inflammation and disease pathogenesis in the brain [1–3]. Upon stimulation by endogenous (e.g., injury, stroke, and autoimmune processes) or exogenous challenges (e.g., pathogens or severe psychological stressors), the immune system upregulates the expression of several cytokines in the brain [4–10]. This results in microglia alteration and ultimately disruption of the delicate neuroglial interactive balance causing alteration of cognition and behavior [11, 12]. Brain inflammation has as well been linked to neuronal damage and neurodegeneration [2, 13, 14].

In the periphery, systemic inflammation has been shown to alter the expression of blood coagulation factors [15]. Indeed, in either autoimmune and/or severe infections (i.e., sepsis), inflammation and coagulation systems are simultaneously activated [16]. A crosstalk among them amplifies and maintains their activation with profound local and systemic implications [17]. Thrombin, the main coagulation factor, has pronounced proinflammatory effects [18]. Acting via specific cell membrane receptors, the protease-activated receptors (PARs), which are abundantly expressed in all arterial vessel wall constituents, thrombin has the potential to exert proatherogenic actions, such as leukocyte migration, cellular proliferation, regulation of vascular permeability and tone, platelet activation, and edema formation [19–23].

Thrombin and its inactive precursor prothrombin have been also detected in the brain [24, 25]. Although the precise cellular source of thrombin in the brain and the molecular mechanisms responsible for its formation and release warrant further investigation, experimental evidence has been provided that neural prothrombin expression and thrombin activity are highly regulated under physiological and pathological conditions [24, 26].

While several evidences point out at an interrelation between systemic inflammation and coagulation, to date, there are no proofs on whether neuroinflammation could interact with the expression of coagulation factors in the brain.

In this manuscript, we investigated whether an interrelationship between coagulation and inflammation factors may occur in the brain in the setting of systemic inflammation [2, 13, 14, 27]. Our data show that systemic injections of lipopolysaccharide (LPS, a component of the bacterial wall) upregulate the expression of both inflammatory and coagulation factors in the brain. Surprisingly, inhibition of thrombin activity prior to LPS injection results in a reduction of both the inflammatory and coagulation responses in the brain. We believe that these results may have a profound clinical impact as they might indicate that reducing coagulation activity in the setting of neurological diseases involving neuroinflammation may improve disease outcome and survival.

2. Materials and Methods

2.1. Experimental Setting. The experiments were approved by the Institutional Animal Care and Use Committee of the Sheba Medical Center which obeys to the national- and NIH-approved rules (1000/15). The minimal number of animals was used, and all efforts were made to minimize suffering. The study was carried out in 8-week-old male C57BL/6 mice, purchased from Envigo Laboratories, Israel. Mice were injected IP (intraperitoneal) with LPS (*Escherichia coli* 0111:B4, Sigma L4130, 1 mg/kg, diluted in saline) only, LPS and NAPAP (Sigma Pefabloc 76308, 0.75 mg/kg), NAPAP or 150 μl saline only ($n = 6$ for each group). 24 hrs following the injection, mice were anesthetized with pentobarbital (0.8 mg/kg) and the brains were removed for hippocampus dissection.

2.2. Cell Cultures. The microglial cell model murine microglial cell line N9 was used [28]. Cells were a generous gift from Professor Dan Frenkel of Tel Aviv University. Cells were grown in RPMI 1640, supplemented with 10% fetal bovine serum, 1% glutamine, and 1% Pen.-Strep. Cells were kept at 37°C with 5% CO_2 and 95% relative humidity. For experiments, N9 cells were seeded into 6-well plates at a density of 10^4 cells per well. The medium was supplemented with 0.1 μg/ml LPS for 24 hrs, then the cells were harvested for protein and mRNA analysis ($n = 3$).

2.3. Quantitative PCR. Prior to the harvest, the animals were anesthetized with pentobarbital. The brains were removed and the hippocampi were dissected. The RNA tissue was extracted using the TRIzol (Thermo Fisher 15596026) solubilization method followed by phase separation with chloroform. Samples were placed in 1 ml TRIzol and homogenized with bullet blender homogenizer (Next Advance) at a maximum speed for 1 minute. RNA phase cleaning was performed using Bio-Rad Aurum 732-6820 (Bio-Rad Laboratories, Hercules, CA, USA). N9 cell mRNA was extracted by lysis buffer addition to the cells accordingly the Bio-Rad Aurum 732-6820 kit. Two micrograms of total RNA was used for reverse transcription using high-capacity cDNA reverse transcription kit (Applied Biosystems). Quantitative real-time polymerase chain reaction was performed on the StepOne™ Real-Time PCR System (Applied Biosystems, Rhenium, Israel) using Fast SYBR Green Master (ROX) (Applied Biosystems). Hypoxanthine guanine phosphoribosyltransferase (HPRT) served as a reference gene in this analysis (primer list). A standard amplification program was used (1 cycle of 95°C for 20 seconds (s) and 40 cycles of 95°C for 3 s and 60°C for 30 s. The primers used in this analysis are listed in Table 1. The results were normalized to reference gene expression within the same cDNA sample and calculated using the ΔCt method with results reported as fold changes relative to control brains of sham animals and reported as mean ± SE.

2.4. Western Blot. N9 cell line samples ($n = 3$) were lysed in RIPA buffer (containing in mM: 50 TRIS HCl pH 8, 150 NaCl, 1% NP-40, 0.5% sodium deoxycholate, and 0.1% SDS) and a protease inhibitor cocktail (Merck Millipore 539134). The homogenates were centrifuged (13,000g × 5 min) at 4°C. The supernatants were collected, and protein concentration was determined through a bicinchoninic acid (BCA) assay. 20 μg from each sample was separated by SDS-polyacrylamide gel electrophoresis. The proteins were transferred onto nitrocellulose membranes. Membranes were incubated with rabbit anti-FX (1 : 1000, BS-77622, Bioss), thrombin (1 : 400, BS-19142, Bioss), PAR1 (1 : 500, BS-0828R, Bioss), EPCR (1 : 500, NBP2-21578 Novous Biologicals), protein C (1 : 400, 251142 Abbiotec), and TNFα (1 : 500, gtx-110520) over night at 4°C and washed with tris-buffered saline and 0.1% Tween 20 (TBST). Membranes were then incubated at room temperature with horseradish peroxidase-conjugated goat anti-rabbit antibody (1 : 10,000, Jackson Immunoresearch Laboratories). Protein bands were detected by a peroxidase-based ECL method. Upon detection, the membranes were stripped and reincubated with a mouse anti-HSC70 antibody (1 : 10,000, sc-7298) and redetected by ECL. Analysis of the protein band density was performed with ImageJ software.

2.5. Thrombin Activity. Thrombin enzymatic activity was measured using a fluorometric assay based on the cleavage rate of the synthetic substrate Boc-Asp(OBzl)-ProArg-AMC (I-1560; Bachem, Bubendorf, Switzerland) and defined by the linear slope of the fluorescence intensity versus time, as previously described [29, 30]. 24 hrs following LPS injection, mice ($n = 6$) were anesthetized with pentobarbital and brains were removed for hippocampus dissection. The dorsal part of

Table 1

Gene	Forward	Reverse
HPRT	GATTAGCGATGATGAACCAGGTT	CCTCCCATCTCCTTCATGA CA
PT (prothrombin)	CCGAAAGGGCAACCTAGAGC	GGCCCAGAACACGTCTGTG
FX (factor X)	GTGGCCGGGAATGCAA	AACCCTTCATTGTCTTCGTTAATGA
PAR1	TGAACCCCCGCTC ATTCTTTC	TGAACCCCCGCTC ATTCTTTC
EPCR	ATGTGGCCGTGAATGGAAGCGC	CCATCAGGATGCCCAGGACC
TNFα	GACCCTCACACTCAGATCATCTTCT	CCTCCACTTGGTGGTTTGCT
IL1β	CTGGTGTGTGACGTTCCCATTA	CCGACAGCACGAGGCTTT
CCL2	CCGGCTGGAGCATCCACGTGT	TGGGGTCAGCACAGACCTCTCTCT
CXL9	TCCTTTTGGGCATCATCTTCC	TTTGTAGTGGATCGTGCCTCG
CCL1	CACAGGGGCGCCTATCGCCAA	CAAGGCAAGCCTCGCGACCAT

the hippocampus was collected for thrombin-like activity assay. The hippocampal tissue was then placed into 96-well black microplate (Nunc, Roskilde, Denmark) containing the substrate buffer. Measurements were carried out using a microplate reader (Tecan; Infinite 200; Switzerland) with excitation and emission filters of 360 ± 35 and 460 ± 35 nm, respectively. Reported values are normalized to protein concentration of each sample (±SEM).

2.6. Microglia Cell Separation. Microglia cells were isolated from hippocampus homogenates. Mice were anesthetized with ketamine/xylazine solution (100 mg/kg and 18.6 mg/kg, resp.) and perfused with cold PBS. The brains were removed and the hippocampi from two mice were pooled. The pooled samples ($n = 3$–8) per tested target gene were triturated using mechanical homogenization by syringe, in Hank's Balanced Salt Solution (HBSS), pH 7.4. Resulting homogenates were passed through a 70 μm nylon cell strainer and centrifuged at 975g, 4°C for 5 min. Supernatants were removed and cell pellets were resuspended in 40% isotonic Percoll (Sigma, p1644) at room temperature. The gradient was centrifuged for 15 min at 975g, and the supernatant was discarded. Cells were washed in staining buffer (at 375g for 6 min) and then stained with FITC anti-mouse CD11b (BioLegend, 101205), APC anti-mouse CD45 (BioLegend, 103111), and Pacific blue anti-mouse Ly-6G (BioLegend, 127611). The number of viable cells was determined using a hemocytometer and 0.1% trypan blue staining. Positive microglia cells were collected according to the gating definition: Ly-6G$^-$/CD11b$^+$/CD45^{low}. The positive cells were collected in RNA lysis buffer and RNA was purified immediately (Qiagen RNeasy Plus Micro Kit 74034).

2.7. Statistical Analysis. Statistical analysis was performed using the GraphPad Prism 7 software. The statistical comparisons between groups were performed using a Student t-test and ANOVA followed by Tukey's multiple comparison test. p values ≤ 0.05 were considered significant between means. All results present as mean ± SE of the mean.

3. Results

3.1. Systemic Injection of LPS Activates the Inflammation and Coagulation Response in Microglia. Systemic injections of LPS activate the inflammatory response in the periphery and in the brain [31]. Microglia, the brain resident macrophage cells, are the first and main form of active immune defense in the central nervous system. Upon 24 hours from i.p. LPS injections, TNFα gene expression level in microglia increased significantly (7.9 ± 0.4-fold, $p = 0.0006$, $n = 4$) as well as those of the cytokine IL1β (1.8 ± 0.3-fold, $n = 8$, Figure 1(a)). Chemockine (C-C motif) ligand 2 (CCL2), a gene encoding for a factor recruiting inflammatory cells during the inflammatory response [32], was upregulated (2.1 ± 0.6-fold, $n = 4$) in microglia cells from LPS-treated animals (Figure 1(a)). Interestingly, LPS was able to activate the expression of factor X, a coagulation factor, which increased by 7.5-fold ($n = 4$) in microglia of LPS-treated animals compared to control (Figure 1(a)).

Treating microglia cell lines (N9) with LPS resulted in a similar upregulation of inflammation-related gene expression (Figure 1(b)). In this setting, the expression levels of TNFα, IL1β, and CCL2β were increased (13.8 ± 0.47-, 129 ± 8.5-, and 13.6 ± 0.33-fold, resp., $p < 0.0001$) (Figure 1(b)). TNFα protein levels likely raised significantly compared to control (1.5 ± 0.187, $p = 0.03$) following LPS treatment (Figure 1(c)). Interestingly, the coagulation factors were equally affected following LPS treatment in microglia cells (Figures 1(a)–1(c)). The expression of genes for factor X, prothrombin, and EPCR reached levels of 2.34 ± 0.2, 1.9 ± 0.4, and 1.8 ± 0.2 ($p \leq 0.01$) compared to their corresponding controls, respectively (Figure 1(b)). Coagulation factor protein levels as well increased following LPS treatment of microglia cell lines. Specifically, thrombin, PAR1, EPCR, and PC reached the highest levels of expressions compared to their respective controls (1.6 ± 0.03, 1.6 ± 0.1, 3.6 ± 0.1, and 2.2 ± 0.16, $p \leq 0.04$) while factor X was lightly upregulated with its value not reaching statistical significance (Figure 1(c)).

All in all, these data indicate that upon LPS challenge, inflammation and coagulation factors are upregulated in microglia both in an *in vivo* setting and an *in vitro* setting.

3.2. Blockade of Thrombin Activity Reduces the Expression of Inflammation and Coagulation Markers in the Hippocampus. The activity of the central coagulation factor thrombin was found to be significantly elevated in the hippocampus following systemic LPS injection (0.5 ± 0.15 mU/mg versus

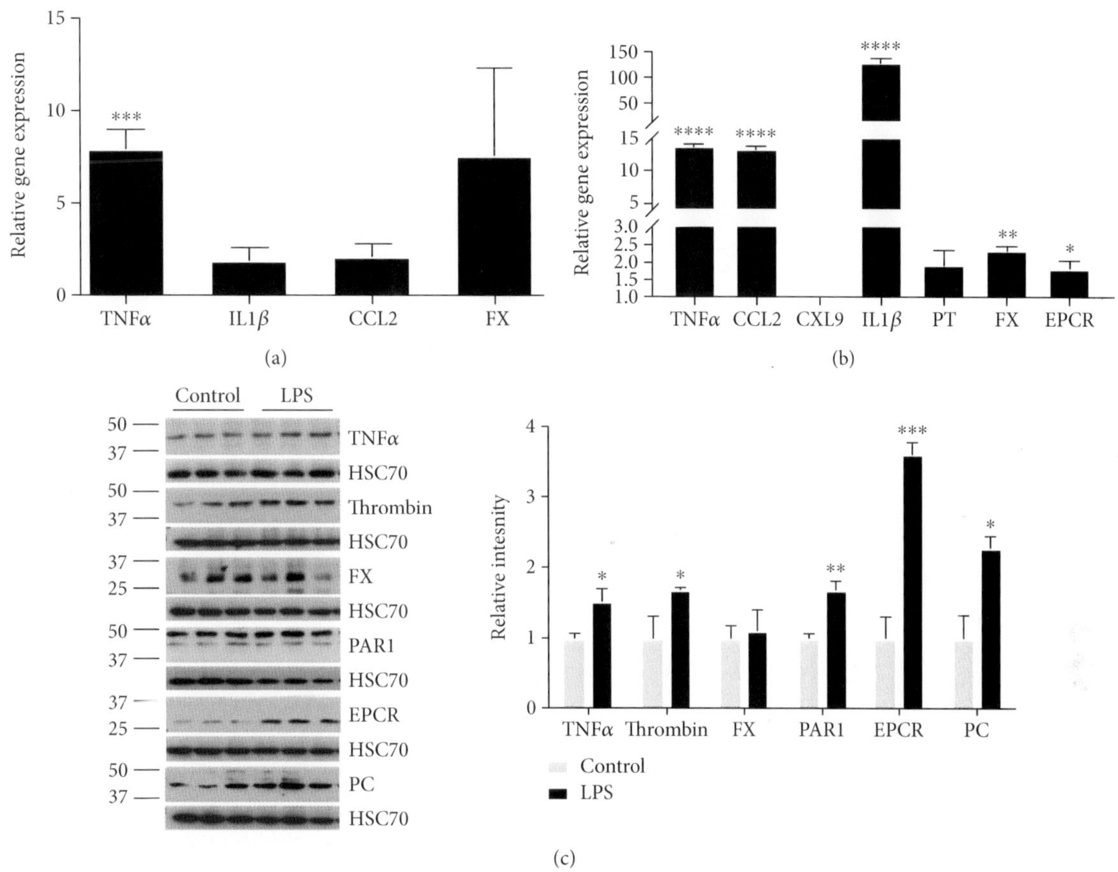

FIGURE 1: LPS induces inflammation in microglia cells *in vivo* and *in vitro*. Gene expression in mouse hippocampal isolated microglia cells 24 hrs following systemic LPS injection (a). Inflammation and coagulation gene expression in N9 microglial cell line, 24 hrs following LPS treatment (b). Protein expression of coagulation and inflammation factors in N9 microglial cell line. Representative blots are presented on the left panel; each protein of interest normalized to HSC70 protein. The graph represents relative intensities that reported as fold change relative to control samples (c). Results are presented as mean ± SEM. $^{*}p \leq 0.05$, $^{**}p \leq 0.01$, $^{***}p \leq 0.001$, and $^{****}p \leq 0.0001$.

0.2 ± 0.03 mU/mg in the control, $p \leq 0.03$, Figure 2(a)). Such result raised the question whether the upregulation of inflammatory cytokines and coagulation factors in the LPS-challenged microglia cells may mirror a situation occurring in the brain. We decided to check the gene expression of those factors in the whole hippocampus. Upon 24 hours from LPS injection, TNFα, IL1β, CCL2, CXL9, and CCL1 reached levels of 12.2 ± 0.8, 8 ± 1.8, 12.5 ± 2.2, 4.58 ± 1, and 27.3 ± 3.8 ($p \leq 0.01$), respectively, compared to their respective controls (Figure 2(b)). Factor X and PAR1 gene expression were as well upregulated to 5.5 ± 0.6 and 1.6 ± 0.1, ($p \leq 0.0001$), respectively, compared to control (Figure 2(b)).

In the periphery, inflammation and coagulation are strictly interconnected [15]; therefore, we decided to evaluate whether blocking thrombin activity may affect the expression of both the inflammatory and coagulation markers. In this experiment, immediately after LPS challenge, mice received NAPAP, an irreversible blocker of thrombin activity. In this setting, NAPAP was able to significantly reduce the expression of both inflammatory and coagulation markers (Figure 2(b)). Indeed, in animals treated with NAPAP and LPS, the expression of TNFα, CXL9, and CCL1 dropped to levels of 5.8 ± 1.7, 1 ± 0.3, and 9 ± 3.5 ($p \leq 0.005$), compared to their respective LPS-injected control (Figure 2(b)). IL1β and CCL2 decreased in a nonsignificant manner to 4.6 ± 1.7 and 6 ± 3 compared to their respective LPS-injected control (Figure 2(b)). Factor X and PAR1 gene expression were downregulated to 2.2 ± 0.5 and 1.2 ± 0.05, $p \leq 0.003$, respectively, compared to LPS-injected control (Figure 2(b)).

Overall, the gene expression profile in the hippocampus (Figure 2(b)) shares a similar pattern to the one obtained in the cells (Figures 1(a)-1(b)), that is, TNFα. Nevertheless, a difference was noted with respect to the levels of expression in the different settings. This may possibly be due to the cellular composition of the tested preparations, with the hippocampus containing a wide range of cells (i.e., neurons, etc.) rather than only glia.

4. Discussion

In this manuscript, we report that an LPS challenge upregulated the expression of both inflammatory and coagulation factors in microglia and in the hippocampus. Strikingly, inhibiting thrombin activity resulted in a downregulation of inflammatory and coagulation factors in the brain.

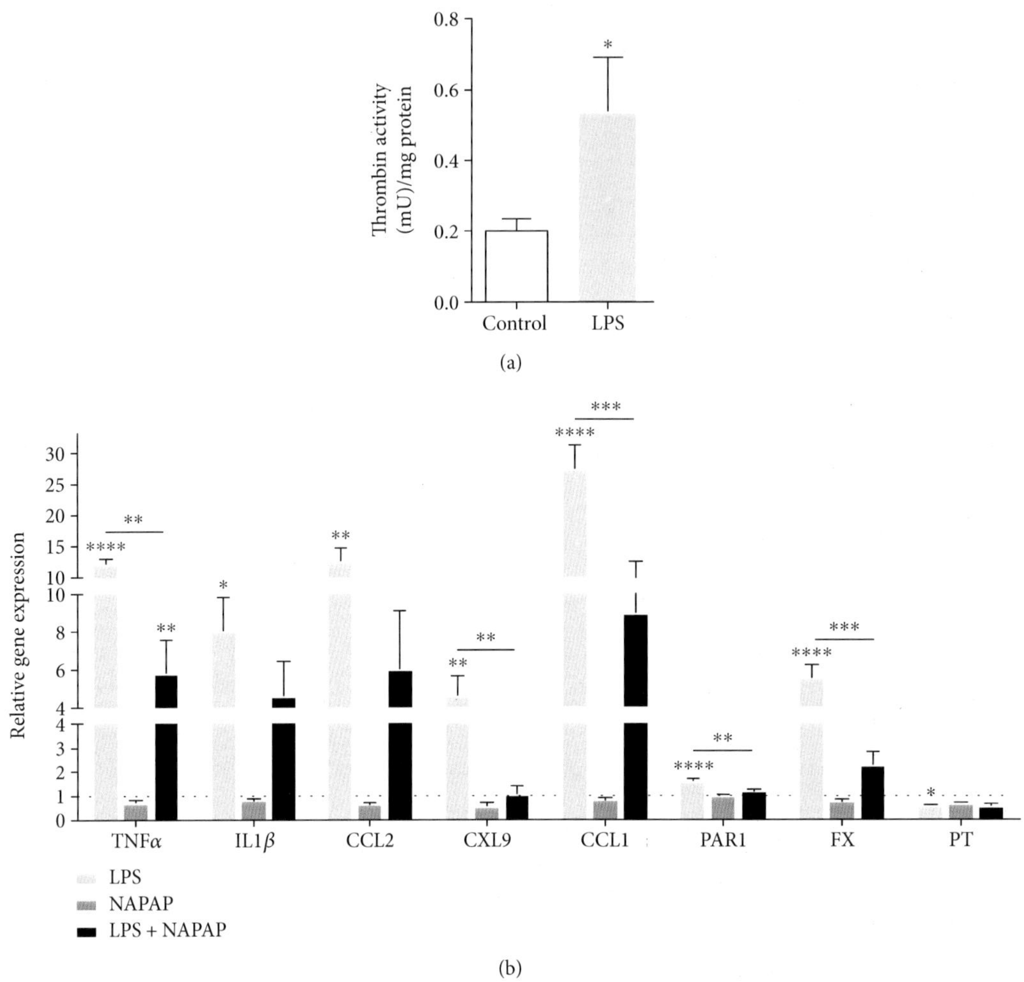

FIGURE 2: NAPAP treatment modifies hippocampal gene expression following LPS activation. Thrombin activity measured in the hippocampus (mU) and normalized to mg protein (a). $n = 6$, t-test. Gene expression analysis of the hippocampus from mice treated with NAPAP and LPS (b). $n = 6$, one-way ANOVA. $^{*}p \le 0.05$, $^{**}p \le 0.01$, $^{***}p \le 0.001$, and $^{****}p \le 0.0001$

LPS has been shown to activate coagulation and inflammation in the periphery [31]. Here, we show that a systemic LPS inflammatory drives the gene expression of inflammation and coagulation factors and their protein synthesis in the brain as well. Microglia seem to be directly involved in this process. It is tempting to speculate about the mechanisms in charge of this phenomenon. A possibility could be that upon LPS exposure, activated macrophages in the periphery may cross the blood-brain barrier (BBB) [31], change their conformation into microglia, and orchestrate the inflammatory response [31, 33]. Alternatively, LPS may break the BBB [34, 35], get into the brain, and activate the resident microglia. More experiments addressing the time scale of microglia activation following a systemic LPS treatment may help in elucidating these mechanisms.

In the periphery, systemic inflammation and coagulation are directly linked [15, 16]. Inflammation initiates clotting while decreasing the activity of natural anticoagulant mechanisms and impairing the fibrinolytic system [15, 22]. Inflammatory cytokines are the major mediators involved in the activation of coagulation [4, 10, 15]. The natural anticoagulants function to dampen the elevation of cytokine levels [15, 36]. Furthermore, components of the natural anticoagulant cascades, like thrombomodulin, minimize endothelial cell dysfunction by rendering the cells less responsive to inflammatory mediators [37], facilitate the neutralization of some inflammatory mediators, and decrease the loss of endothelial barrier function [36, 38, 39]. Hence, downregulation of anticoagulant pathways not only promotes thrombosis but also amplifies the inflammatory process [40, 41]. When the inflammation-coagulation interactions overwhelm the natural defense systems, catastrophic events occur, such as in severe sepsis or in autoimmune diseases [15, 16].

Our data suggest that a crosstalk between inflammation and coagulation may occur in the brain as well. However, the implications for such interactions are far less clear. On the one side, neuroinflammation has profound physiological implications in protecting the brain from internal and/or external injuries [42, 43]. On the other side, amplification of the neuroinflammatory response has been linked to the pathophysiology of stroke and several neurodegenerative diseases [44]. The role of coagulation factors in the brain has only started to be unrevealed. Thrombin in the brain is implicated in synaptic plasticity and learning and memory [45–49], yet upregulation of thrombin in the brain has been linked to seizures [46, 47, 50], maladaptive synaptic plasticity [49, 51], and brain death [52]. How neuroinflammation and brain coagulation interact among themselves is currently unknown. Several data have reported that in neurological diseases, both inflammation and coagulation are upregulated in the brain [7, 27, 53]. In ischemic and hemorrhagic stroke, microglia are recruited to the site of injury where they mediate neuronal death [54] and contribute to brain recovery [44]. In these settings, the upregulated brain concentrations of thrombin have been linked to neuronal damage [26, 29, 30, 55, 56]. In Alzheimer's disease and in vascular dementia, high levels of thrombin and other coagulation factors have been detected in the brain aside with the recruitment of microglia and additional inflammatory components [57–59].

The evidence that the bidirectional relationship between coagulation and inflammation plays a pivotal role in the mechanisms leading to organ failure in patients with severe infection or sepsis has promoted the theory that a pharmacological restoration of the anticoagulant mechanisms may be a logical action in the treatment of septic patients with coagulation abnormalities [60]. Our experiments show that, in the brain, blockade of thrombin activity (i.e., and consequently of the coagulation system) may reduce neuroinflammation and possibly limit the neuronal damage associated to it. If several experimental and initial clinical studies have been started to better address the interaction between inflammation and coagulation in the periphery, similarly, additional studies in the brain are needed. Better investigating the cross-talk between neuroinflammation and coagulation in the brain may result in the development of novel therapeutic strategies for brain disorders.

Disclosure

This work was performed in partial fulfillment of the requirements for a Ph.D. degree of Marina Ben Shimon.

Conflicts of Interest

The authors have no conflict of interest to declare.

Authors' Contributions

Efrat Shavit Stein and Marina Ben Shimon contributed equally to this work.

Acknowledgments

This work was supported by a Kamin research program grant (no. 56338) from the Israeli Ministry of Economy and Industry to Nicola Maggio. Nicola Maggio is a recipient of a Talpiot Medical Leadership Program Fellowship from the Chaim Sheba Medical Center.

References

[1] C. A. Thomson, A. McColl, J. Cavanagh, and G. J. Graham, "Peripheral inflammation is associated with remote global gene expression changes in the brain," *Journal of Neuroinflammation*, vol. 11, no. 1, p. 73, 2014.

[2] R. Sankowski, S. Mader, and S. Iván Valdés-Ferrer, "Systemic inflammation and the brain: novel roles of genetic, molecular, and environmental cues as drivers of neurodegeneration," *Frontiers in Cellular Neuroscience*, vol. 9, p. 28, 2015.

[3] N. Maggio, E. Shavit-Stein, A. Dori, I. Blatt, and J. Chapman, "Prolonged systemic inflammation persistently modifies synaptic plasticity in the hippocampus: modulation by the stress hormones," *Frontiers in Molecular Neuroscience*, vol. 6, p. 46, 2013.

[4] A. Al Mamun, A. Chauhan, H. Yu, Y. Xu, R. Sharmeen, and F. Liu, "Interferon regulatory factor 4/5 signaling impacts on microglial activation after ischemic stroke in mice," *European Journal of Neuroscience*, vol. 47, no. 2, pp. 140–149, 2018.

[5] M. Gelderblom, M. Gallizioli, P. Ludewig et al., "IL-23 (interleukin-23)–producing conventional dendritic cells control the detrimental IL-17 (interleukin-17) response in stroke," *Stroke*, vol. 49, no. 1, pp. 155–164, 2017.

[6] S. Gyoneva and R. M. Ransohoff, "Inflammatory reaction after traumatic brain injury: therapeutic potential of targeting cell–cell communication by chemokines," *Trends in Pharmacological Sciences*, vol. 36, no. 7, pp. 471–480, 2015.

[7] L. E. Collins-Praino, A. Arulsamy, V. Katharesan, and F. Corrigan, "The effect of an acute systemic inflammatory insult on the chronic effects of a single mild traumatic brain injury," *Behavioural Brain Research*, vol. 336, pp. 22–31, 2018.

[8] Y.-F. Lin, T.-T. Liu, C.-H. Hu, C. C. Chen, and J. Y. Wang, "Expressions of chemokines and their receptors in the brain after heat stroke-induced cortical damage," *Journal of Neuroimmunology*, vol. 318, pp. 15–20, 2018.

[9] A. Mizuma and M. A. Yenari, "Anti-inflammatory targets for the treatment of reperfusion injury in stroke," *Frontiers in Neurology*, vol. 8, 2017.

[10] T. Rodney, N. Osier, and J. Gill, "Pro- and anti-inflammatory biomarkers and traumatic brain injury outcomes: a review," *Cytokine*, 2018.

[11] J. Czerniawski and J. F. Guzowski, "Acute neuroinflammation impairs context discrimination memory and disrupts pattern separation processes in hippocampus," *The Journal of Neuroscience*, vol. 34, no. 37, pp. 12470–12480, 2014.

[12] J. Czerniawski, T. Miyashita, G. Lewandowski, and J. F. Guzowski, "Systemic lipopolysaccharide administration impairs retrieval of context–object discrimination, but not spatial, memory: evidence for selective disruption of specific hippocampus-dependent memory functions during acute neuroinflammation," *Brain, Behavior, and Immunity*, vol. 44, pp. 159–166, 2015.

[13] S. Rossi, R. Furlan, V. de Chiara et al., "Interleukin-1β causes synaptic hyperexcitability in multiple sclerosis," *Annals of Neurology*, vol. 71, no. 1, pp. 76–83, 2012.

[14] S. Rossi, C. Motta, V. Studer et al., "Tumor necrosis factor is elevated in progressive multiple sclerosis and causes excitotoxic neurodegeneration," *Multiple Sclerosis Journal*, vol. 20, no. 3, pp. 304–312, 2014.

[15] M. Levi and T. van der Poll, "Coagulation and sepsis," *Thrombosis Research*, vol. 149, pp. 38–44, 2017.

[16] T. Iba and J. H. Levy, "Inflammation and thrombosis: roles of neutrophils, platelets and endothelial cells and their interactions in thrombus formation during sepsis," *Journal of Thrombosis and Haemostasis*, vol. 16, no. 2, pp. 231–241, 2018.

[17] C. T. Esmon, K. Fukudome, T. Mather et al., "Inflammation, sepsis, and coagulation," *Haematologica*, vol. 84, no. 3, pp. 254–259, 1999.

[18] C. T. Esmon, "Targeting factor Xa and thrombin: impact on coagulation and beyond," *Thrombosis and Haemostasis*, vol. 111, no. 4, pp. 625–633, 2014.

[19] R. Reiter, U. Derhaschnig, A. Spiel et al., "Regulation of protease-activated receptor 1 (PAR1) on platelets and responsiveness to thrombin receptor activating peptide (TRAP) during systemic inflammation in humans," *Thrombosis and Haemostasis*, vol. 90, pp. 898–903, 2003.

[20] R. A. Schuepbach and M. Riewald, "Coagulation factor Xa cleaves protease-activated receptor-1 and mediates signaling dependent on binding to the endothelial protein C receptor," *Journal of Thrombosis and Haemostasis*, vol. 8, no. 2, pp. 379–388, 2010.

[21] D. CHEN and A. DORLING, "Critical roles for thrombin in acute and chronic inflammation," *Journal of Thrombosis and Haemostasis*, vol. 7, pp. 122–126, 2009.

[22] G. R. Sambrano, E. J. Weiss, Y. W. Zheng, W. Huang, and S. R. Coughlin, "Role of thrombin signalling in platelets in haemostasis and thrombosis," *Nature*, vol. 413, no. 6851, pp. 74–78, 2001.

[23] S. R. Coughlin, "Protease-activated receptors in vascular biology," *Thrombosis and Haemostasis*, vol. 86, no. 1, pp. 298–307, 2001.

[24] Y. Hua, J. Wu, R. F. Keep, J. T. Hoff, and G. Xi, "Thrombin exacerbates brain edema in focal cerebral ischemia," *Acta Neurochirurgica. Supplement*, vol. 86, pp. 163–166, 2003.

[25] M. Dihanich, M. Kaser, E. Reinhard, D. Cunningham, and D. Monard, "Prothrombin mRNA is expressed by cells of the nervous system," *Neuron*, vol. 6, no. 4, pp. 575–581, 1991.

[26] E. S. Stein, Z. Itsekson-Hayosh, A. Aronovich et al., "Thrombin induces ischemic LTP (iLTP): implications for synaptic plasticity in the acute phase of ischemic stroke," *Scientific Reports*, vol. 5, no. 1, p. 7912, 2015.

[27] J. Chapman, "Coagulation in inflammatory diseases of the central nervous system," *Seminars in Thrombosis and Hemostasis*, vol. 39, no. 8, pp. 876–880, 2013.

[28] B. Stansley, J. Post, and K. Hensley, "A comparative review of cell culture systems for the study of microglial biology in Alzheimer's disease," *Journal of Neuroinflammation*, vol. 9, no. 1, 2012.

[29] D. Bushi, M. Ben Shimon, E. Shavit Stein, J. Chapman, N. Maggio, and D. Tanne, "Increased thrombin activity following reperfusion after ischemic stroke alters synaptic transmission in the hippocampus," *Journal of Neurochemistry*, vol. 135, no. 6, pp. 1140–1148, 2015.

[30] D. Bushi, J. Chapman, A. Katzav et al., "Quantitative detection of thrombin activity in an ischemic stroke model," *Journal of Molecular Neuroscience*, vol. 51, no. 3, pp. 844–850, 2013.

[31] I. C. M. Hoogland, C. Houbolt, D. J. van Westerloo, W. A. van Gool, and D. van de Beek, "Systemic inflammation and microglial activation: systematic review of animal experiments," *Journal of Neuroinflammation*, vol. 12, no. 1, p. 114, 2015.

[32] M. C. Lebre, T. Burwell, P. L. Vieira et al., "Differential expression of inflammatory chemokines by Th1- and Th2-cell promoting dendritic cells: a role for different mature dendritic cell populations in attracting appropriate effector cells to peripheral sites of inflammation," *Immunology and Cell Biology*, vol. 83, no. 5, pp. 525–535, 2005.

[33] C. Cunningham, "Microglia and neurodegeneration: the role of systemic inflammation," *Glia*, vol. 61, no. 1, pp. 71–90, 2013.

[34] B. Wispelwey, A. J. Lesse, E. J. Hansen, and W. M. Scheld, "Haemophilus influenzae lipopolysaccharide-induced blood brain barrier permeability during experimental meningitis in the rat," *The Journal of Clinical Investigation*, vol. 82, no. 4, pp. 1339–1346, 1988.

[35] W. A. Banks and M. A. Erickson, "The blood–brain barrier and immune function and dysfunction," *Neurobiology of Disease*, vol. 37, no. 1, pp. 26–32, 2010.

[36] C. T. Esmon, "The interactions between inflammation and coagulation," *British Journal of Haematology*, vol. 131, no. 4, pp. 417–430, 2005.

[37] Y. Xu, X. Xu, H. Jin, X. Yang, Q. Gu, and K. Liu, "Effects of a thrombomodulin-derived peptide on monocyte adhesion and intercellular adhesion molecule-1 expression in lipopolysaccharide-induced endothelial cells," *Molecular Vision*, vol. 19, pp. 203–212, 2013.

[38] J. Wenzel, J. C. Assmann, and M. Schwaninger, "Thrombomodulin–a new target for treating stroke at the crossroad of coagulation and inflammation," *Current Medicinal Chemistry*, vol. 21, no. 18, pp. 2025–2034, 2014.

[39] C. Esmon, "Inflammation and the activated protein C anticoagulant pathway," *Seminars in Thrombosis and Hemostasis*, vol. 32, pp. 049–060, 2006.

[40] S. Gando, "Role of fibrinolysis in sepsis," *Seminars in Thrombosis and Hemostasis*, vol. 39, no. 4, pp. 392–399, 2013.

[41] C. T. Esmon, "Crosstalk between inflammation and thrombosis," *Maturitas*, vol. 47, no. 4, pp. 305–314, 2004.

[42] T. Taib, C. Leconte, J. van Steenwinckel et al., "Neuroinflammation, myelin and behavior: temporal patterns following mild traumatic brain injury in mice," *PLoS One*, vol. 12, no. 9, article e0184811, 2017.

[43] N. Kim, J. Y. Kim, and M. A. Yenari, "Anti-inflammatory properties and pharmacological induction of Hsp70 after brain injury," *Inflammopharmacology*, vol. 20, no. 3, pp. 177–185, 2012.

[44] S. Wang, H. Zhang, and Y. Xu, "Crosstalk between microglia and T cells contributes to brain damage and recovery after ischemic stroke," *Neurological Research*, vol. 38, no. 6, pp. 495–503, 2016.

[45] H. Wang, J. Sun, and H. Goldstein, "Human immunodeficiency virus type 1 infection increases the in vivo capacity of peripheral monocytes to cross the blood-brain barrier into the brain and the in vivo sensitivity of the blood-brain barrier to disruption by lipopolysaccharide," *Journal of Virology*, vol. 82, no. 15, pp. 7591–7600, 2008.

[46] N. Maggio, E. Shavit, J. Chapman, and M. Segal, "Thrombin induces long-term potentiation of reactivity to afferent stimulation and facilitates epileptic seizures in rat hippocampal slices: toward understanding the functional consequences of cerebrovascular insults," *The Journal of Neuroscience*, vol. 28, no. 3, pp. 732–736, 2008.

[47] N. Maggio, C. Cavaliere, M. Papa, I. Blatt, J. Chapman, and M. Segal, "Thrombin regulation of synaptic transmission:

implications for seizure onset," *Neurobiology of Disease*, vol. 50, pp. 171–178, 2013.

[48] N. Maggio, Z. Itsekson, D. Dominissini et al., "Thrombin regulation of synaptic plasticity: implications for physiology and pathology," *Experimental Neurology*, vol. 247, pp. 595–604, 2013.

[49] M. Ben Shimon, M. Lenz, B. Ikenberg et al., "Thrombin regulation of synaptic transmission and plasticity: implications for health and disease," *Frontiers in Cellular Neuroscience*, vol. 9, p. 151, 2015.

[50] N. Maggio, I. Blatt, A. Vlachos, D. Tanne, J. Chapman, and M. Segal, "Treating seizures and epilepsy with anticoagulants?," *Frontiers in Cellular Neuroscience*, vol. 7, p. 19, 2013.

[51] A. Strehl, M. Lenz, Z. Itsekson-Hayosh et al., "Systemic inflammation is associated with a reduction in synaptopodin expression in the mouse hippocampus," *Experimental Neurology*, vol. 261, pp. 230–235, 2014.

[52] L. M. Willems, N. Zahn, N. Ferreirós et al., "Sphingosine-1-phosphate receptor inhibition prevents denervation-induced dendritic atrophy," *Acta Neuropathologica Communications*, vol. 4, no. 1, p. 28, 2016.

[53] C. De Luca, A. Virtuoso, N. Maggio, and M. Papa, "Neuro-coagulopathy: blood coagulation factors in central nervous system diseases," *International Journal of Molecular Sciences*, vol. 18, no. 10, p. 2128, 2017.

[54] A. Tuttolomondo, D. di Raimondo, R. di Sciacca, A. Pinto, and G. Licata, "Inflammatory cytokines in acute ischemic stroke," *Current Pharmaceutical Design*, vol. 14, no. 33, pp. 3574–3589, 2008.

[55] D. Bushi, E. S. Stein, V. Golderman et al., "A linear temporal increase in thrombin activity and loss of its receptor in mouse brain following ischemic stroke," *Frontiers in Neurology*, vol. 8, p. 138, 2017.

[56] O. Gera, E. Shavit-Stein, D. Bushi et al., "Thrombin and protein C pathway in peripheral nerve Schwann cells," *Neuroscience*, vol. 339, pp. 587–598, 2016.

[57] P. L. MCGeer, A. Klegeris, D. G. Walker, O. Yasuhara, and E. G. MCGeer, "Pathological proteins in senile plaques," *The Tohoku Journal of Experimental Medicine*, vol. 174, no. 3, pp. 269–277, 1994.

[58] S. Thameem Dheen, C. Kaur, and E. A. Ling, "Microglial activation and its implications in the brain diseases," *Current Medicinal Chemistry*, vol. 14, no. 11, pp. 1189–1197, 2007.

[59] P. Grammas and J. M. Martinez, "Targeting thrombin: an inflammatory neurotoxin in Alzheimer's disease," *Journal of Alzheimer's Disease*, vol. 42, Supplement 4, pp. S537–S544, 2014.

[60] J. Chapman, "Thrombin in inflammatory brain diseases," *Autoimmunity Reviews*, vol. 5, no. 8, pp. 528–531, 2006.

Intraspinal Grafting of Serotonergic Neurons Modifies Expression of Genes Important for Functional Recovery in Paraplegic Rats

Krzysztof Miazga,[1] Hanna Fabczak,[1] Ewa Joachimiak,[1] Małgorzata Zawadzka,[1] Łucja Krzemień-Ojak,[1] Marek Bekisz,[1] Anna Bejrowska,[1] Larry M. Jordan,[2] and Urszula Sławińska[1]

[1]*Nencki Institute of Experimental Biology, Polish Academy of Sciences, Warsaw, Poland*
[2]*Department of Physiology and Phatophysiology, University of Manitoba, Winnipeg, MB, Canada*

Correspondence should be addressed to Urszula Sławińska; u.slawinska@nencki.gov.pl

Academic Editor: Junichi Ushiba

Serotonin (5-hydroxytryptamine; 5-HT) plays an important role in control of locomotion, partly through direct effects on motoneurons. Spinal cord complete transection (SCI) results in changes in 5-HT receptors on motoneurons that influence functional recovery. Activation of 5-HT$_{2A}$ and 5-HT$_7$ receptors improves locomotor hindlimb movements in paraplegic rats. Here, we analyzed the mRNA of 5-HT$_{2A}$ and 5-HT$_7$ receptors (encoded by *Htr2a* and *Htr7* genes, resp.) in motoneurons innervating tibialis anterior (TA) and gastrocnemius lateralis (GM) hindlimb muscles and the tail extensor caudae medialis (ECM) muscle in intact as well as spinal rats. Moreover, the effect of intraspinal grafting of serotonergic neurons on *Htr2a* and *Htr7* gene expression was examined to test the possibility that the graft origin 5-HT innervation in the spinal cord of paraplegic rats could reverse changes in gene expression induced by SCI. Our results indicate that SCI at the thoracic level leads to changes in *Htr2a* and *Htr7* gene expression, whereas transplantation of embryonic serotonergic neurons modifies these changes in motoneurons innervating hindlimb muscles but not those innervating tail muscles. This suggests that the upregulation of genes critical for locomotor recovery, resulting in limb motoneuron plasticity, might account for the improved locomotion in grafted animals.

1. Introduction

Motoneurons (MNs) respond to 5-HT with an increase in excitability [1–3]. We and others have previously argued that 5-HT$_{2A}$ and 5-HT$_7$ receptors are important in the initiation and control of locomotion [3–12], and that these receptors mediate hindlimb locomotor recovery produced in paraplegic animals after replacement of 5-HT neurons into the sublesional spinal cord by grafts of fetal brainstem [10, 13]. One of the effects of spinal cord transection, which interrupts the 5-HT pathway from the brainstem to the spinal cord, is plasticity in 5-HT receptors of spinal MNs [14, 15]. The 5-HT$_7$ receptors have been implicated in control of MNs or reflexes involved in respiration, jaw movement, micturition, and locomotion [16–21] as well as in the control of pain after spinal cord injury [22, 23], while the 5-HT$_{2A}$ receptor has been implicated in the control of respiration, development of spasticity in tail and hindlimb digit MNs, and the recovery of locomotor capability after spinal cord injury [24–27]. Intraspinal grafting of serotonergic neurons leads to functional recovery and involves activation of 5-HT$_{2A}$ and 5-HT$_7$ receptors [10]. We asked whether the facilitation of locomotion by our grafts might be mediated by plasticity in these key receptors that are necessary for locomotor recovery.

The 5-HT$_7$ receptor protein is found in MNs of the spinal cord [28], with some MN populations (e.g., Onuf's nucleus) more intensely labeled than others. MNs in the L4 spinal cord, where MNs to hindlimb muscles are located, displayed a relatively low level of labeling. These receptors have been shown to have excitatory effects on some MNs, including phrenic MNs [29] and trigeminal MNs [19], but not hypoglossal respiratory MNs [30, 31].

The afterhyperpolarization (AHP) in many types of neurons is reduced by 5-HT, and this effect may be mediated by 5-HT_7 receptors [19, 32]. MNs of limb muscles have reduced AHPs during locomotion [33, 34], and lamprey MNs have reduced AHP due to 5-HT [35, 36]. This effect serves as a means of increasing MN spiking.

The 5-HT_{2A} receptor is abundant in ventral horn MNs [37, 38], with variable expression levels depending upon the functional role of the cell. For example, 5-HT_{2A} receptors are differentially distributed on MNs to the physiological extensor soleus muscle and extensor digitorum longus, a physiological flexor muscle [39]. Plasticity in the 5-HT_{2A} receptor protein has been examined after sacral spinal cord injury, where the changes have been suggested to underlie the development of tail spasticity (reviewed in [14, 15]). Contusive spinal cord injury at the thoracic level resulted in upregulation of 5-HT_{2A} receptor protein in MNs of the rostral dorsolateral nucleus innervating the plantar muscles of the foot, with an associated increase in the H-reflex recorded from the plantar muscles of the hindpaw [40]. Cervical spinal cord hemisections give rise to increased 5-HT_{2A} receptor protein in phrenic MNs and their subsequent increased excitability [27].

Chopek et al. [41] demonstrated that the extensor monosynaptic reflex in hindlimb MNs of passively cycled spinal rats responded to quipazine (a 5-HT_2 agonist). This plasticity could be related to changes in 5-HT receptors in MNs; 5-HT_{2A} receptor mRNA increased after injury and increased further after passive cycling [42]. An increase in 5-HT_{2A} mRNA after sacral SCI was observed in tail MNs [43]. Chopek et al. [42] found no change in 5-HT_7 receptor gene expression in lumbar MNs 3 months after spinal cord transection, but passive cycling increased 5-HT_7 receptor mRNA. Giroux et al. [44] found spinal 5-HT receptors increased at 15 and 30 days after spinal cord injury, but returned to baseline levels after 60 days or more. They used [3H]8-OH-DPAT to label 5-HT receptors, a ligand that can bind to 5-HT_7 receptors.

There is increasing evidence that activation of specific serotonin receptors in the spinal cord is effective for enhancing locomotor recovery in spinal rats [11, 45, 46]. Out of many serotonergic receptors present in the spinal cord, the 5-HT_{2A} and 5-HT_7 receptors are the major ones implicated in the control of locomotion [3, 6, 7, 12, 25, 47–49]. The most commonly used agonists that are effective in enhancing the locomotor hindlimb movements when applied systemically are quipazine, which has high affinity for both 5-HT_{2A} and 5-HT_{2C} receptors and 8-hydroxy-2-(di-n-propylamino)-tetralin (8-OH-DPAT), which binds selectively to 5-HT_7 and 5-HT_{1A} receptors [46, 47, 50]. We previously demonstrated that intraspinal grafting of embryonic brainstem tissue containing serotonergic neurons below a thoracic total transection enhances recovery of hindlimb locomotor movements [10, 13, 51]. We also demonstrated that graft-related recovery is mediated in part by 5-HT_{2A} and 5-HT_7 receptors because application of their antagonists diminished the restored hindlimb locomotor movements [10, 13]. Constitutive activity in 5-HT_2 receptors is implicated in the recovery of locomotion after SCI [25, 52], and intrathecal application of a selective 5-HT_7 receptor antagonist during unrestrained locomotion in intact adult rats [4] blocks voluntary locomotion. Similar effects were obtained with 5-HT_2 antagonists [53].

Here, we hypothesize that the plastic changes in these receptors that occur after spinal cord injury might be affected by the restoration of 5-HT innervation from grafted 5-HT neurons so as to reverse or normalize these changes. This hypothesis is consistent with the findings that the presence of 5-HT or other ligands for these receptors can downregulate, upregulate, or desensitize these 5-HT receptors [54, 55]. We tested this hypothesis on identified MNs of the lumbar enlargement that innervate muscles with known actions during locomotion (ankle flexor (TA), extensor (GM), and tail elevator (ECM)), and we attempted to induce plasticity in the receptors on these MNs using thoracic spinal cord transection. We monitored the changes in receptor mRNA expression produced in these identified lumbar MNs at 1 month and 4 months after spinal cord transection, and we determined whether intraspinal grafting of embryonic serotonergic neurons in spinal rats reverses the effects of spinal total transection on expression of these genes. We show, for the first time, that intraspinal grafting of embryonic serotonergic neurons reverses injury-evoked changes in 5-HT_{2A} and 5-HT_7 receptor gene expression in the MN populations supplying hindlimb but not tail muscles. We propose that these changes may account for the effects of the grafts on neural plasticity responsible for locomotor recovery achieved by intraspinal grafting of embryonic raphe nuclei in paraplegic rats. A preliminary report of these findings has been published [56].

2. Materials and Methods

Experiments were performed on WAG (Wistar Albino Glaxo) 3-month-old female rats ($n = 35$) at the time of spinal cord injury. All procedures were conducted with care to minimize pain and suffering of animals with the approval of the First Local Ethics Committee in Poland, according to the principles of experimental conditions and laboratory animal care of European Union and the Polish Law on Animal Protection.

2.1. Spinal Cord Transection. Complete spinal cord transection (SCI) was performed ($n = 23$) at the Th9/10 level under deep anesthesia (isoflurane: 5% to induce and then maintained with 2% in oxygen 0.2–0.3 l/min and Butomidor: 0.05 mg/kg b.w.) as previously described [10]. To prevent the possibility of axonal regrowth through the cavity of the lesion, 1-2 mm of spinal cord tissue was aspirated using a glass pipette. Then, the muscles and fascia overlying the paravertebral muscles were closed in layers using sterile sutures, and the skin was closed with stainless steel surgical clips. After surgery, the animals received a nonsteroidal anti-inflammatory and analgesic treatment (s.c., Tolfedine

4 mg/kg b.w.) and antibiotics (s.c., Baytril 5 mg/kg b.w.; gentamicin 2 mg/kg b.w.) for the following 5–7 days. The bladder was emptied manually twice a day until the voiding reflex was reestablished.

2.2. Grafting of Embryonic 5-HT Cells. One month after SCI, nine out of 23 spinal rats were selected randomly for intraspinal grafting of embryonic serotonergic cells (SCI_{TR}). Fourteen-day-old embryos (E14; E0—the day after mating) from time-pregnant female WAG rats were removed by Caesarean section and transferred to Hanks' buffered solution containing 0.5% glucose. A small piece of the embryonic caudal brainstem area containing the B1, B2, and B3 serotonergic regions was dissected under a microscope (for more details, see [10, 57]).

At the same time, the spinal cord of a recipient rat (isoflurane anesthesia, 5% to induce and then maintained with 2% in oxygen 0.2–0.3 l/min) was exposed by a small laminectomy at the Th11/12 vertebrae level (at least one segment below the total spinal cord transection), and a solid piece of embryonic tissue (approximately 2 μl) was injected by pressure into the spinal cord 1 mm below the pial surface through a sharpened micropipette attached to the Hamilton syringe. The micropipette was then slowly withdrawn to avoid graft movement. Control spinal rats ($n = 11$) were subjected to a sham grafting procedure where the operation was identical to that described above, but no tissue was injected into the spinal cord [10, 13, 51].

2.3. Behavioral Assessment of Locomotor Ability in Spinal Rats. Before starting the procedure of collecting data for qRT-PCR analysis, two months after grafting (3 months after complete spinal cord transection), all the rats were subjected to behavioral testing to confirm the quality of their hindlimb plantar stepping. This was established in rats suspended above a treadmill with their forelimbs and thorax placed on a platform and with their hindlimbs touching the treadmill belt. To elicit hindlimb movements, a tail pinch was used. Stimulation of tail has been used for eliciting locomotion in many cases of complete spinal cord transection [46, 58] and has been used in all prior attempts to reveal locomotor recovery after brainstem neuron grafting [10, 13, 57, 59, 60]. The tail stimulus was adjusted by the experimenter to maximize the quality of plantar stepping. All the spinal grafted rats considered for the further investigation of gene expression in defined MNs or for immunohistochemistry of the spinal cord presented good plantar walking performance and were not different from those described in our previous paper [10, 13, 51, 57].

2.4. Implantation of EMG Electrodes. To evaluate the quality of hindlimb movements, we routinely use electromyography (EMG). In rats from the SCI_{4m} group (three months after total transection) and in the rats from the SCI_{TR} group (two months after intraspinal grafting), bipolar electrodes for EMG recordings were implanted under isoflurane anesthesia (5% to induce and then maintained with 2% in oxygen 0.2–0.3 l/min) in Sol muscle (physiological extensor active during the stance phase of the step cycle) and TA muscle (physiological flexor active during the swing phase of the step cycle) of both hindlimbs. The electrodes were made of Teflon-coated stainless steel wire (0.24 mm in diameter; AS633, CoonerWire Co., Chatsworth, CA, USA). The tips of the electrodes with 1–1.5 mm of the insulation removed were pulled through a cutaneous incision on the back of the animal, and each of the hook electrodes was inserted into the appropriate muscle and secured by a suture [10, 51, 57]. The distance between the electrode tips in the muscle was 1-2 mm. The ground electrode was placed under the skin on the back of the animal in some distance from the hindlimb muscles. The connector with the other ends of the wires fixed to it, covered with dental cement (Spofa Dental, Prague, Czech Republic) and silicone (3140 RTV, Dow Corning), was secured to the back of the animal. After surgery, the animals received antibiotic treatment (Baytril, 5 mg/kg s.c.).

2.5. Tissue Preparation and Immunohistochemistry: Morphological Verification of Spinal Reactive Gliosis in Spinal Rats with and without the Graft. After testing the quality of locomotor hindlimb movements, three grafted rats and three spinal control rats without the graft were subjected to perfusion to prepare the spinal cord tissue for histological investigation of the graft condition and presence of inflammatory responses at the spinal level in which the MNs were collected.

For immunochemistry, the spinal cords were collected from the animals deeply anesthetized with pentobarbital and transcardially perfused with cold 0.1 M phosphate-buffered saline (PBS), pH 7.2, for 2-3 min and subsequently with cold 4% paraformaldehyde in PBS for 15 min. The spinal cords were postfixed and then cryoprotected gradually up to 30% sucrose in PBS, embedded in OCT, frozen on dry ice, and sectioned in a cryotome (12 μm). The collected cross sections were immobilized on poly-L-lysine-covered glass slides and stored at −20°C.

The primary antibodies that were used in the immunohistochemistry were mouse antiglial fibrillary acidic protein (GFAP, 1 : 1000, BD Pharmingen) for astrocytes and mouse neuronal nuclear protein antibody (NeuN, 1 : 100 Millipore) for neuronal labeling. Isolectin B4 (FITC-conjugated, 20 μg/ml, Sigma-Aldrich) was used for activated microglia detection. To identify 5-HT-positive fibers, rabbit anti-5-HT antibody (1 : 1000, ImmunoStar) was used. The Alexa Fluor secondary antibodies were used: 488-conjugated donkey antibody against mouse IgG, 647-conjugated goat antibody against mouse IgG, and 555-conjugated donkey antibody against rabbit IgG, (1 : 1000 Invitrogen). Nuclei were stained with DAPI dye (1 μg/ml in H_2O, Sigma-Aldrich).

For the immunostaining, frozen cross sections, after several rinses in PBS, were blocked in 10% normal donkey or donkey/goat serum with 0.5% Triton X-100 in PBS at RT for 2 h and then incubated overnight at 4°C with primary antibodies followed by incubation with fluorophore-conjugated secondary antibodies for 2 h at room temperature. The specimens were coverslipped in fluorescence mounting medium (Dako) after several washes in PBS and examined

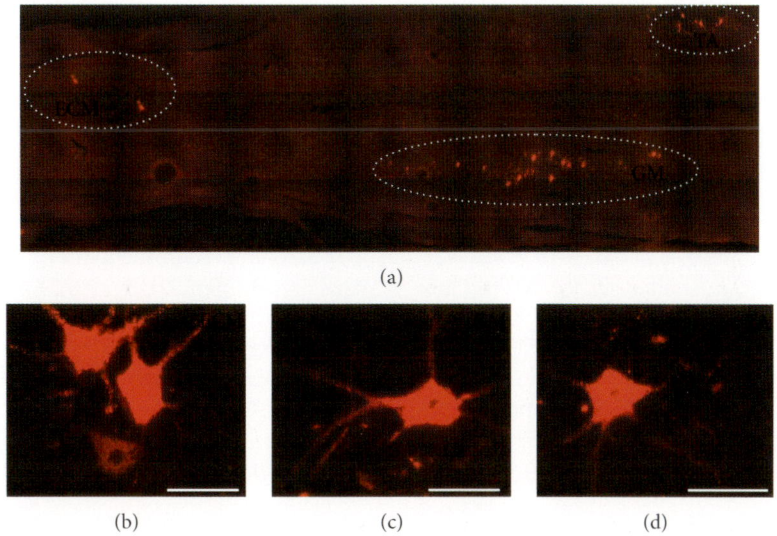

FIGURE 1: (a) Examples of labeled motoneurons (cholera toxin subunit B coupled with Alexa Fluor 555) innervating selected muscles: extensor caudae medialis (ECM) of the right side (b), gastrocnemius lateralis (GM) in the left hindlimb (c), and tibialis anterior (TA) in the right hindlimb (d). Scale bar: 50 μm.

on either a Zeiss Fluorescence Microscope Axio Imager.M2 or a Leica SP5 Laser Scanning Confocal Microscope.

2.6. Motoneuron Labeling. One week before the animal euthanasia, populations of MNs innervate the following muscles: TA of the right hindlimb, GM of the left hindlimb, and ECM of the right side of the tail were labeled by intramuscular injection by cholera toxin subunit B (CTB) coupled with Alexa Fluor 555 dye (see examples of CTB-labeled MNs innervating TA, GM, and ECM muscles in Figure 1). The TA and GM muscles were selected on the left and right sides to provide easy differentiation between the two MN pools innervating these two muscles when the same type of labeling was used in both of them. Also, the left ECM pool MN labeling (the most caudally localized) is a marker of the left side helping in identification of the GM MN pool. At the same time, the ECM and TA MN pools are separated with the most rostrocaudal distance. The ECM muscle was also selected because it plays a role in elevation of the tail, an indicator of functional recovery after spinal cord injury, according to the BBB score [61]. Animals were anesthetized using isoflurane (5% to induce and then maintained with 2% in oxygen 0.2–0.3 l/min), and proper muscles were exposed by small skin incisions enabling injection with 0.5% CTB using Hamilton syringe (TA and GM muscles $3 \times 15\,\mu$l of CTB and ECM muscle $2 \times 20\,\mu$l of CTB). The CTB injection was performed over a period of 2 minutes, the needle was slowly (2 min) withdrawn, and the skin incision was closed.

2.7. Htr2a and Htr7 Gene Expression Analysis

2.7.1. Experiment Scheme. In order to examine the *Htr2a* and *Htr7* gene expression in MNs innervating selected hindlimb and tail muscles, we performed experiments on 29 WAG female rats, in which specific motoneuron pools were labeled by injection of retrograde tracer molecules into a target muscle. Our investigations were performed on rats from four experimental groups: INT: intact ($n = 12$); SCI_{TR}: spinal cord injury followed by intraspinal transplantation of embryonic brainstem tissue containing serotonergic neurons ($n = 6$); SCI_{1m}: 1 month after spinal cord injury ($n = 5$); SCI_{4m}: 4 months after spinal cord injury ($n = 6$)-the time matched with the time of euthanasia of rats from the SCI_{TR} group.

Animals from the SCI_{1m} and SCI_{4m} groups were subjected to a spinal cord total transection procedure performed at the thoracic level. Animals from the INT group were the control animals that were not subjected to any procedure. Animals from the SCI_{TR} group received an intraspinal graft of 14-day-old rat embryonic brainstem one month after spinal cord total transection. Three months after intraspinal grafting in SCI_{TR} group and four months after complete transection in rats of both groups, SCI_{TR} and SCI_{4m} (seven days after motoneuron tracer injection with cholera toxin subunit B coupled with Alexa Fluor 555) rats were transcardially perfused with PBS solution to remove any bloodborne 5-HT receptors, and the spinal cord was dissected and prepared for further analysis (animals from the SCI_{4m} and SCI_{TR} groups were euthanized 4 months after spinal cord total transection).

2.7.2. Laser Capture Microdissection (LCM) of Selected Motoneurons. Spinal cord tissue was collected from animals that were deeply anesthetized and transcardially perfused with PBS solution. Then, the spinal cords were immediately dissected and frozen by fast immersion in isopentane (−80°C) and stored at −80°C until future processing. Horizontal sections (20 μm) of the lumbar-sacral spinal cord fragment were cut on the cryostat in −20°C and mounted on PEN Membrane Frame Slides (Applied Biosystems). Slides were stored at −80°C until future use.

Slides were dehydrated by immersion in increasing concentrations (70%, 90%, and 100%) of ethyl alcohol (ETOH) followed by immersion in xylene. Motoneuron collection was performed using an Arcturus Laser

Table 1: Description of assays used in real-time PCR.

Gene symbol	Reference number	Gene name	Assay ID	Amplicon length
Ppia	NM_017101.1	Cyclophilin A	Rn00690933_m1	149
Htr2a	NM_017254.1	Receptor 5-HT_{2A}	Rn00568473_m1	71
Htr7	NM_022938.2	Receptor 5-HT_7	Rn00576048_m1	85

Microdissection System (Applied Biosystems). Tissue sections were photographed using a filter set for Alexa Fluor 555 to identify CTB-labeled MNs. Individual MNs were dissected using UV laser and collected on *Cap Sure Macro LCM Caps* (Applied Biosystems). After incubation in lysis buffer (*Arcturus Pico Pure RNA Isolation Kit*, Applied Biosystems) for 30 minutes, the samples were stored at −80°C until future processing.

2.7.3. RNA Isolation. RNA was isolated using an *Arcturus Pico Pure RNA Isolation Kit* (Applied Biosystems) according to the manufacturer's instructions. Any residual genomic DNA was removed using supplementary DNAse I (*RQ1 RNase-Free DNase*, Promega) treatment. Three independent measurements of RNA concentration were obtained using NanoDrop (Thermo Scientific). RNA samples were pooled by mixing the same RNA amount isolated from one motoneuron population from all rats in a particular experimental group (i.e., equal amounts of RNA collected from the particular selected motoneuron populations in different rats in the same experimental group were pooled). RNA samples were stored at −80°C.

2.7.4. Reverse Transcription PCR and cDNA Preamplification. Reverse transcription PCR (RT-PCR) was performed in a *MJ Mini Personal Thermal Cycler* (Bio-Rad) using a *High Capacity cDNA Reverse Transcription Kit* (Applied Biosystems) according to the manufacturer's instructions (10 min, 25°C; 120 min, 37°C; 5 min, 85°C; storage 4°C) with use of 31 ng of purified RNA as a sample. Synthesized cDNA was stored at −20°C for future use.

Preamplification was performed to increase the number of cDNA copies to the level necessary for accurate detection in the real-time PCR reaction. cDNA was preamplified in *MJ Mini Personal Thermal Cycler* (Bio-Rad) using *TaqMan PreAmp Master Mix Kit* (Applied Biosystems). Reactions were conducted in standard conditions according to the preamplification kit manufacturer's instructions: 95°C for 10 min; then 14 cycles: 95°C for 15 s; 60°C for 4 min.

2.7.5. Real-Time PCR. Expression of the *Htr2a and Htr7* genes (encoding the 5-HT_{2A} and 5-HT_7 receptors, resp.) in the selected MN populations was measured by semiquantitative real-time PCR (qRT-PCR) using a *Step One Plus* (Applied Biosystems) thermocycler and TaqMan gene-specific FAM/MGB assays (Applied Biosystems). *Ppia* gene encoding cyclophilin A was used as the housekeeping gene. The description of TaqMan assays used in the qRT-PCR reaction is shown in Table 1.

Reactions were run in triplicate for each sample and for each assay in 20 μl reaction mix prepared in accordance with *TaqMan Gene Expression Master Mix* (Applied Biosystems) manufacturer recommendations. Reactions were run in standard, recommended by *TaqMan Gene Expression Master Mix* manufacturer conditions (2 min, 50°C; 10 min, 95°C; then 40 cycles: 15 s, 95°C; 1 min, 60°C). Relative expression levels of analyzed genes were then calculated using the comparative CT method.

2.8. Statistical Analysis. For comparison of results from two experimental groups, Student's t-test analysis was used after normal distribution was confirmed using Shapiro-Wilk test (Prism, GraphPad Software, La Jolla, CA). For statistical analysis of the results collected from qRT-PCR of more than two experimental groups that were expressed in relation to those established in INT rats, the nonparametric Kruskal-Wallis test for multiple independent sample comparison followed by Conover post hoc (further adjusted by the Holm family-wise error rate (FWER) method and in one case the method of Benjamini-Hochberg false discovery rate (FDR) when the FWER method just approached significance) was used (http://astatsa.com/KruskalWallisTest/).

3. Results

3.1. Locomotor Ability in Spinal Rats. As we published before, the SCI rats (SCI_{1m} and SCI_{4m}) presented very limited hindlimb movements [10, 11, 13, 46, 51]. Usually, their hindlimbs were outstretched passively behind the hindquarters without any spontaneous hindlimb movement present and there was hardly any EMG activity recorded in the hindlimb flexor (TA) and extensor (Sol) muscles (Figure 2(a)). In contrast, the hindlimbs of the SCI_{TR} rats moving in the home cage were abducted with partial flexion in the ankle joint or flexed at all joints with the foot plantar surface touching the ground, but without noticeable body weight support in spite presence of some EMG activity in hindlimb Sol and TA muscles (Figure 2(c)). Tail pinching in SCI rats suspended over a treadmill induced only irregular, limited hindlimb movements characterized by obvious lack of body weight support with no plantar stepping. EMG activity of hindlimb flexor and extensor muscles was irregular with lack of the long burst of Sol EMG activity related to the stance phase of the step cycle that is observed in normal locomotor activity of intact rats (Figure 2(b)). In SCI_{TR} rats suspended over the treadmill, tail pinch was effective to induce regular plantar hindlimb walking with nice regular EMG muscle activity with typical alternating pattern of EMG Sol versus TA bursts of activity and long burst of Sol related to the stance phase of step cycle in both hindlimbs (Figure 2(d)).

3.2. Morphological Verification of Reactive Gliosis in Spinal Rats with and without the Graft. As we published before

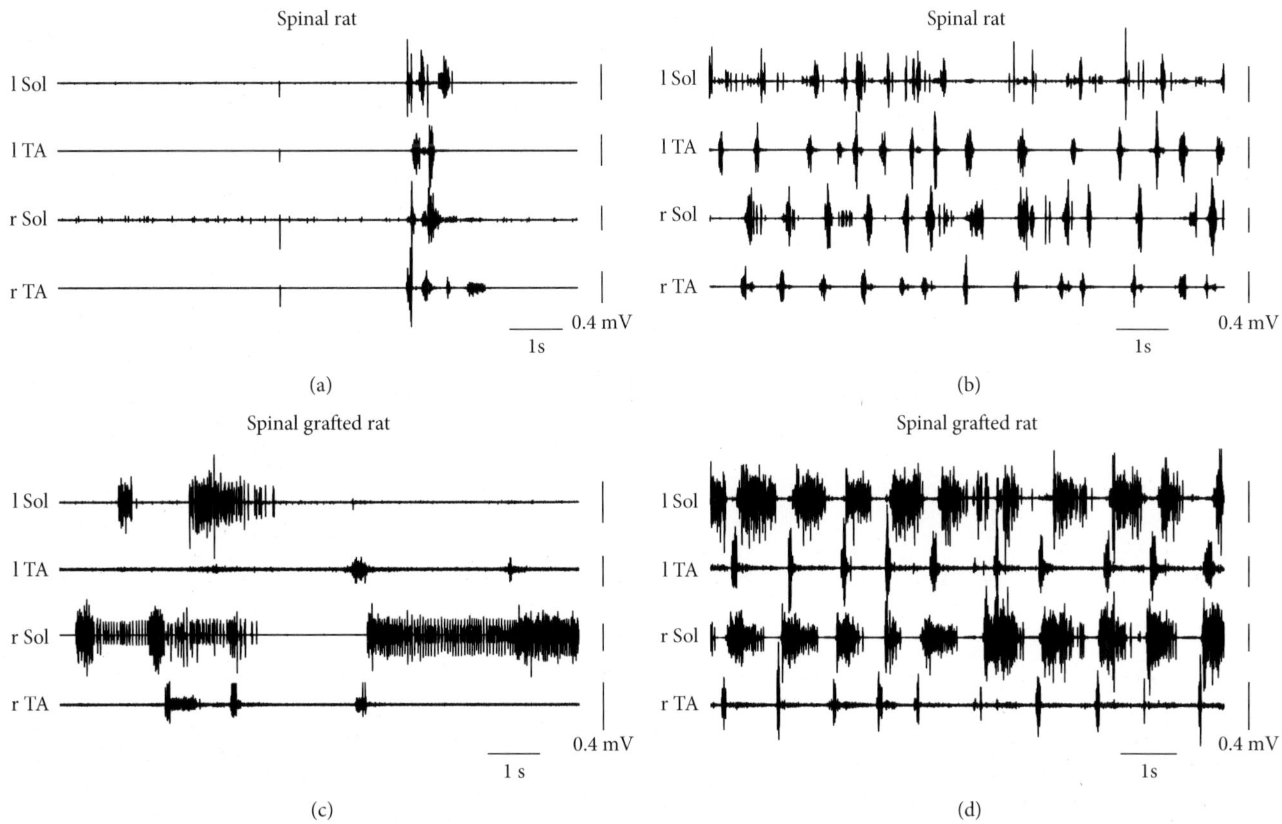

FIGURE 2: Examples of EMG recordings from hindlimb muscles of the spinal rats (a) and (b) and spinal grafted rat (c) and (d) during exploratory behavior in the home cage (a) and (c) and during locomotor-like hindlimb movements on a treadmill induced by tail pinching (b and d). Note that in spinal control rats during spontaneous movement in the home cage, the hindlimb muscles were usually silent but a brief episode of EMG activity could be induced by a sudden touch of the rat tail (a), while in the spinal grafted rats, the spontaneous EMG activity of Sol and TA muscles could be obtained without any external intervention (c) (for more details, see [10, 13, 51, 57]. Sol: soleus muscle; TA: tibialis anterior muscle; l/r: left/right.

[10, 51, 57], intraspinally grafted 5-HT neurons survive the grafting procedure and their axons grow into the distal part of the host spinal cord, spreading caudally for a considerable distance below the total transection. Figure 3(b) shows a representative example of fetal grafted tissue located in the spinal cord one/two segments below the total transection of the spinal grafted rat. The sham-operated spinal SCI_{4m} rats do not possess any 5-HT innervation in the spinal cord below the total transection (Figure 3(a)). Here, we also verified the presence of activated microglia and astrocytes in the spinal cord below transection in spinal rats with (SCI_{TR}) and without the graft (SCI_{4m}) long after the injury (4 months). While there was moderate microglia activation detectable within white matter and virtually no activation in grey matter at Th13/L1 (the level of a real or sham grafting), we were not able to detect any sign of inflammation at L4/L5 in any of the animals, regardless of whether they were sham or grafted ones (Figure 3 left and middle panels). Moreover, while we identified a slightly increased number of astrocytes in ventral horns at the grafting level compared to control, the same numbers of astrocytes were observed at L4/L5 in both SCI_{4m} and SCI_{TR} rats. However, none of the detected astrocytes showed the morphology of reactive cells (Figure 3, right panel). Thus, we assumed that 4 months after transplantation of embryonic tissue, there is no inflammatory reaction in the ventral horn at and below of L4/L5 spinal cord levels, where our samples were taken. This finding demonstrates that a role for inflammation in changes in 5-HT receptors such as previously suggested after sacral spinal cord injury [43] does not apply in our case.

3.3. Htr2a and Htr7 Gene Expression in MNs of Intact Adult Rats. The relative abundance of the distinct mRNAs was established by the minimal number of amplification cycles necessary to detect a given mRNA and was presented at graph as 1/ΔCt value. In all analyzed populations of MNs innervating the TA, GM, and ECM muscles, expression of *Htr2a* and *Htr7* genes (encoding $5\text{-}HT_{2A}$ and $5\text{-}HT_7$ receptors, resp.) was detectable and expression of *Htr2a* gene in all analyzed motoneurons was significantly higher (Student's t-test $p < 0.0001$) than expression of gene encoding $5\text{-}HT_7$ serotonin receptor (Figure 4).

3.4. Htr2a Gene Expression in MNs. In comparison to INT rats, in SCI_{1m} rats, the *Htr2a* gene expression was reduced by ~60% in TA MNs (nonparametric Kruskal-Wallis test (df: 3, $p = 0.015$) with Conover post hoc test $p < 0.001$) and by ~50% in the GM MNs (nonparametric Kruskal-Wallis test

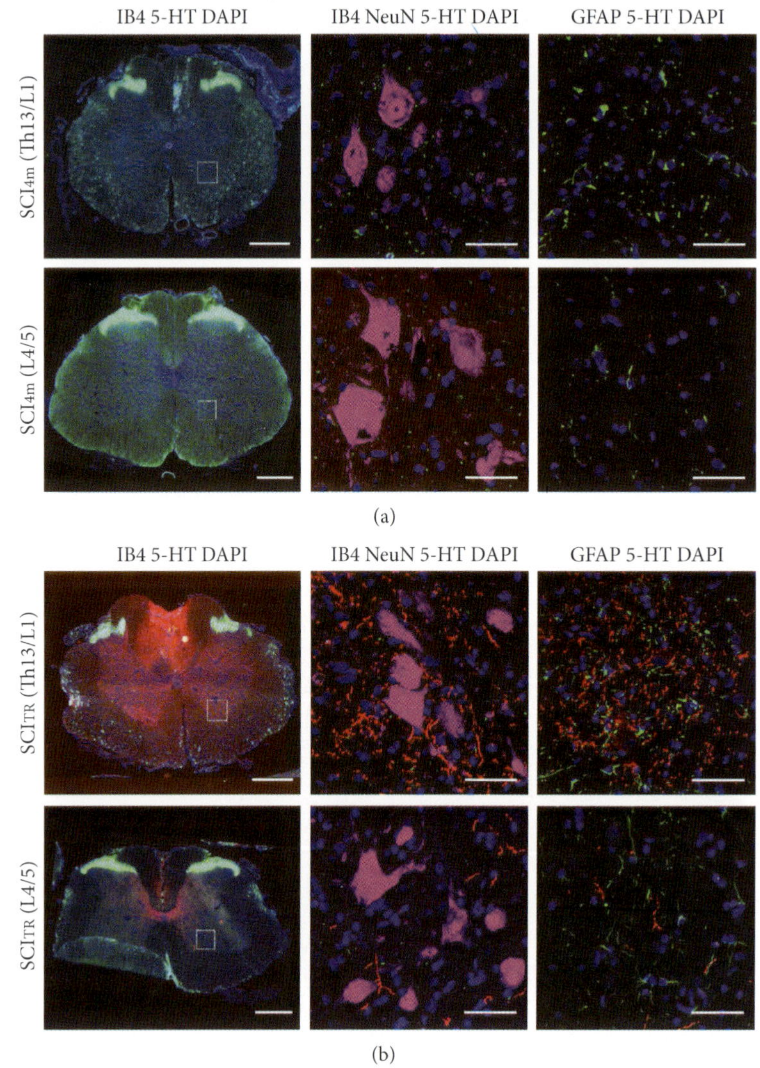

FIGURE 3: Immunofluorescent detection of inflammatory response in control SCI_{4m} (a) and transplanted SCI_{TR} (b) rats at 4 months after total spinal transection and 3 months after transplantation (sham grafting in SCI_{4m}). The first panel shows general view of spinal cord cross section labeled with isolectin B4 (IB4) to visualize activated microglia in low power; the next two panels show boxed area labeled with IB4 (green; left and middle panel) for microglia and GFAP (green; right panel) for astrocytes, reimaged using confocal microscope. Note grafted tissue at Th13/L1 and serotonin-positive fibers (5-HT, red) located closely to ventral horn motoneurons (NeuN; purple) at L4/L5. Representative images: scale bar: 500 μm and 50 μm in low- and high-power images, respectively.

(df: 3, $p = 0.019$) with Conover post hoc test $p < 0.01$) and increased by 103% in ECM MNs (nonparametric Kruskal-Wallis test (df: 3, $p = 0.015$) with Conover post hoc $p < 0.0001$) when normalized to the *Htr2a* gene expression in MNs of INT animals (Figure 5).

In SCI_{4m} rats, the *Htr2a* gene expression was also lower than in INT rats (~45% of INT) in TA MNs (Conover post hoc test $p < 0.001$) and GM MNs (Conover post hoc test $p < 0.05$). There was also a small difference in gene expression in SCI_{4m} rats in comparison to SCI_{1m} rats (Conover post hoc test $p < 0.05$) in MNs of both TA and GM muscles. In SCI_{4m}, the *Htr2a* gene expression in the ECM MNs decreased by ~44% (Conover post hoc $p < 0.001$) in comparison to the gene expression level measured in SCI_{1m} rats. Expression of the *Htr2a* gene in TA and GM MNs of SCI_{4m} rats was still much lower than expression of this gene in INT rats (Figure 5).

Intraspinal grafting of embryonic brainstem serotonergic neurons reversed to some extent changes in the *Htr2a* gene expression observed in the TA and GM MNs of SCI_{1m} rats (Figure 5). Expression of the *Htr2a* gene in TA and in GM MNs in SCI_{TR} rats was significantly higher by 112% and 110%, respectively, than that in SCI_{1m} (Conover post hoc test $p < 0.001$ for both MN populations) and by 52% and 93%, respectively, than that in SCI_{4m} (Conover post hoc test $p < 0.05$ and $p < 0.01$, resp., for both MN populations). However, *Htr2a* gene expression remained ~14% lower in comparison to MNs of INT TA (Conover post hoc test $p < 0.05$) but in the GM MNs was restored to the level of INT (Conover post hoc test $p > 0.05$). The expression of the *Htr2a* gene in ECM MNs of SCI_{TR} rats remained increased by ~25% in comparison to that in MNs of INT rats (Conover post hoc test $p < 0.001$).

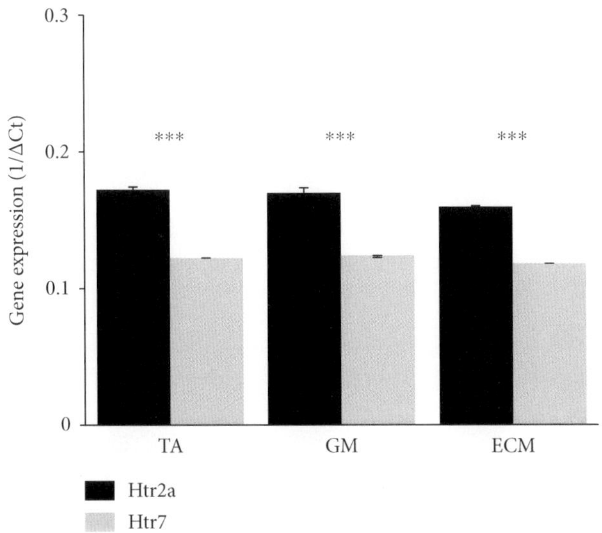

FIGURE 4: Expression level of *Htr2a* and *Htr7* genes (encoding 5-HT_{2A} and 5-HT_7 receptors, resp.) in motoneuron populations innervating TA, GM, and ECM muscles in intact adult rats. Expression levels of *Htr2a* and *Htr7* genes were normalized to the expression level of the constitutively active *Ppia* (cyclophyline A) gene and was presented as the 1/ΔCt value of the analyzed genes. Student's *t*-test $^{***}p < 0.0001$. Data are presented as mean ± standard deviation (mean ± SD). TA: tibialis anterior muscle; GM: gastrocnemius muscle; ECM: extensor caudae medialis muscle.

3.5. Htr7 Gene Expression in MNs. In SCI_{1m} rats, the *Htr7* gene expression was reduced by ~22% in TA MNs (nonparametric Kruskal-Wallis test (df: 3, $p = 0.015$) with Conover post hoc test $p < 0.001$), by ~50% in GM MNs (nonparametric Kruskal-Wallis test (df: 3, $p = 0.022$) with Conover post hoc test $p < 0.05$), and by ~20% in ECM MNs (nonparametric Kruskal-Wallis test (df: 3, $p = 0.025$) with Conover post hoc test $p < 0.001$) when normalized to the *Htr7* gene expression in MNs of INT animals (Figure 6).

In SCI_{4m} rats, the *Htr7* gene expression was also lower than in INT rats in TA MNs (Conover post hoc test $p < 0.05$) and in GM MNs (Conover post hoc test $p < 0.01$). There was also a small increase in gene expression in SCI_{4m} rats in comparison to SCI_{1m} rats (Conover post hoc test $p < 0.05$) in TA MNs but remained significantly lower in comparison to that of INT ($p < 0.01$). In MNs of GM muscle, *Htr7* gene expression was unchanged (Conover post hoc test $p > 0.05$) in comparison to that of SCI_{1m} rats but remained lower in comparison to that of INT (Conover post hoc test $p < 0.01$). In SCI_{4m}, the *Htr7* gene expression in the ECM MNs increased by ~12% (Conover post hoc test $p < 0.05$) in comparison to the gene expression level measured in SCI_{1m} rats (Figure 6).

Intraspinal grafting of embryonic brainstem serotonergic neurons reversed changes in the *Htr7* gene expression observed in the TA and GM MNs of SCI_{1m} rats (Figure 6). Expression of the *Htr7* gene in the TA MNs (nonparametric Kruskal-Wallis test (df: 3, $p = 0.015$) with post hoc Conover method for multiple comparisons $p < 0.001$) and in the GM MNs (nonparametric Kruskal-Wallis test $p = 0.022$ and Conover post hoc adjusted with FDR method for multiple comparisons $p < 0.05$) in SCI_{TR} rats was higher than that in the INT rats. Expression of the *Htr7* gene in SCI_{TR} significantly increased by ~109% (Conover post hoc $p < 0.01$) and ~215% (Conover post hoc test $p < 0.001$) in the TA and GM MNs, respectively, in comparison to the *Htr7* gene expression in the SCI_{1m} and by ~86% (Conover post hoc $p < 0.001$) and ~215% (Conover post hoc test $p < 0.001$) in the TA and GM MNs, respectively, in comparison to the *Htr7* gene expression in SCI_{4m} rats. On the other hand, in the ECM MNs, expression of the *Htr7* gene in the SCI_{TR} rats was not different in comparison to the *Htr7* expression in the SCI_{4m} rats (nonparametric Kruskal-Wallis (df: 3, $p = 0.025$ with Conover post hoc $p = 0.81$)).

4. Discussion

In our previous papers, we demonstrated that intraspinal grafting of embryonic neurons destined to form the descending 5-HT system of the rat brain stem effectively restores coordinated plantar stepping in adult spinal rats [10, 13, 51, 57]. We also demonstrated that such recovery is mediated by 5-HT_{2A} and 5-HT_7 serotonergic receptors [10, 13].

In the present paper, we confirmed expression of the *Htr2a* and *Htr7* genes in MN populations of intact and paraplegic rats. We showed for the first time that intraspinal transplantation of rat E14 embryo brainstem containing serotonergic neurons increases expression of these genes in the TA and GM hindlimb MNs in comparison to ungrafted spinal animals. We found that 5-HT_7 receptor mRNA was decreased at 1 month and 4 months after spinal cord injury in all 3 types of MNs. In the presence of the grafts, 5-HT_7 mRNA levels increased above those at 1 and 4 months and were significantly different from the intact condition in TA, GM, and ECM MNs. The graft tended to reverse the decrease in 5-HT_7 receptor mRNA in TA and GM MNs, with a sustained increase after 4 months in the grafted rats. The grafts did not have such an effect in ECM (tail) MNs. One month after SCI, 5-HT_{2A} receptor mRNA decreased in flexor and extensor MNs, while it increased in tail MNs. Flexor and extensor MNs had decreased 5-HT_{2A} mRNA after 4 months, while 5-HT_{2A} mRNA in the tail MNs decreased in comparison to that observed one month after SCI but remained slightly higher than that in INT. Grafting resulted in 5-HT_{2A} mRNA levels that did not differ from the intact condition in GM MNs, but 5-HT_{2A} mRNA expression continued to be slightly downregulated in TA MNs and upregulated in ECM MNs. It is possible to conclude that the presence of the grafts tended to normalize the levels of 5-HT receptor mRNA in limb muscle MNs, as predicted by our hypothesis, but not in MNs of tail muscle. A possible mechanism for the effect of the grafts might be that increased *Htr2a* gene expression may be a consequence of the increased presence of 5-HT derived from the graft, which can occur in some cells [62]. The mechanism for regulation of *Htr2a* gene expression in MNs of different types may vary. This is a suitable topic for further research.

Our data showing 5-HT_{2A} mRNA upregulation in ECM is similar to findings on receptor protein upregulation in

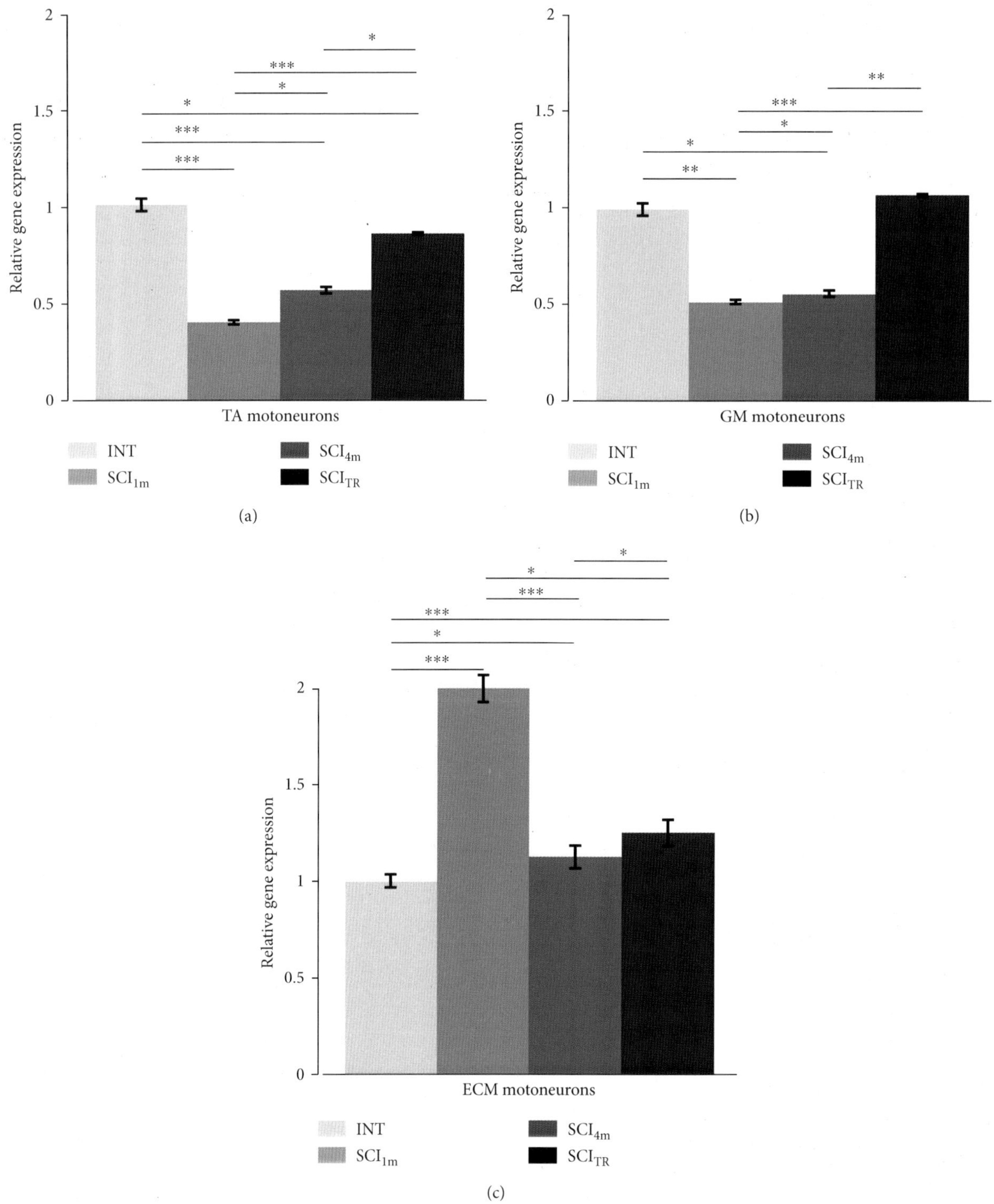

FIGURE 5: Changes in the *Htr2a* gene expression in MNs innervating the TA (a), GM (b), and ECM (c) muscles in rats one and four months after total spinal cord transection and in spinal rats with a graft of 14-day-old rat embryonic brainstem tissue containing serotonergic neurons. INT: intact rats; SCI_{1m}: rats 1 month after spinal cord transection; SCI_{4m}: rats 4 months after spinal cord transection; SCI_{TR}: rats 4 months after spinal cord transection with a graft; TA: tibialis anterior muscle; GM: gastrocnemius muscle; ECM: extensor caudae medialis muscle. Data normalized to the expression of *Htr2a* gene in MNs of INT rats are presented as mean ± SD (standard deviation). Nonparametric Kruskal-Wallis test with Conover post hoc method for multiple comparison ($^*p < 0.05$; $^{**}p < 0.01$; $^{***}p < 0.001$).

more distal tail muscle MNs [63–65]. In MNs innervating hindlimb muscles, $5\text{-}HT_{2A}$ receptor protein levels have been observed to be upregulated 4–6 weeks after contusive SCI [66, 67]. Protein levels for this receptor have not been examined at later time points after injury. Absence of an increase in *Htr2a* gene expression after total transection observed here is consistent with in situ hybridization data obtained by Ung and colleagues showing a clear tendency

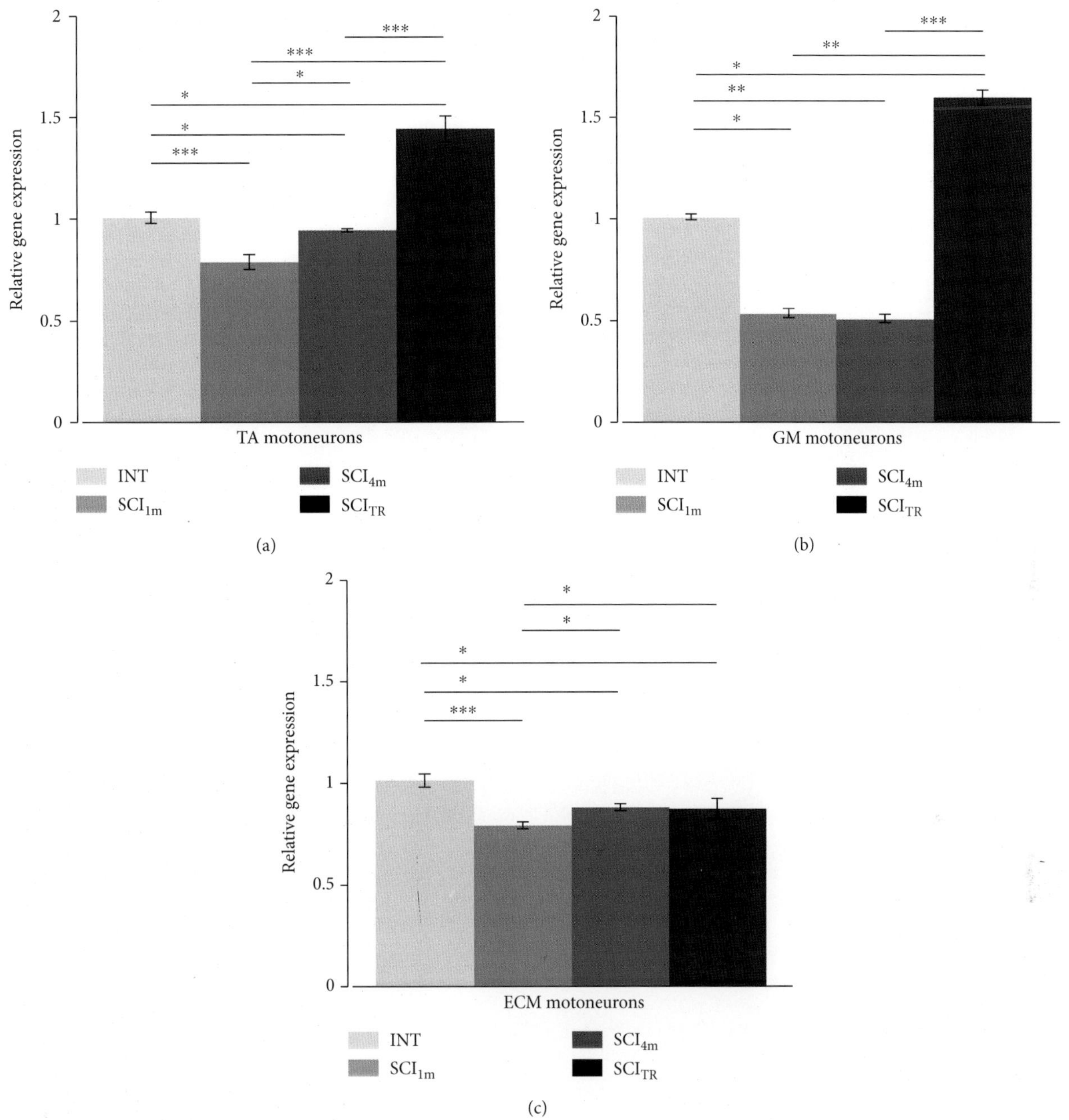

FIGURE 6: Changes in the *Htr7* gene expression in MNs innervating TA (a), GM (b), and ECM (c) muscles in rats one and four months after total spinal cord transection and in spinal rats with a graft of 14-day-old rat embryonic brainstem tissue containing serotonergic neurons. INT: intact rats; SCI_{1m}: rats 1 month after spinal cord transection; SCI_{4m}: rats 4 months after spinal cord transection; SCI_{TR}: rats 4 months after spinal cord transection with a graft; TA: tibialis anterior muscle; GM: gastrocnemius muscle; ECM: extensor caudae medialis muscle. Data normalized to the expression of *Htr7* gene in MNs of INT rats are presented as mean ± SD (standard deviation). Nonparametric Kruskal-Wallis test with Conover post hoc method for multiple comparison ($^{*}p < 0.05$; $^{**}p < 0.01$; $^{***}p < 0.001$).

of 5-HT_{2A} mRNA to decrease in the ventral horn of lumbar segments 28 days after spinal cord transection in adult mice [68]. Our data on 5-HT_{2A} receptor mRNA are not predictive of the increase in 5-HT_{2A} receptor protein. Maier et al. [69] reviewed the common observation that mRNA and protein expression can be uncorrelated. They conclude that the major posttranslational factor influencing mRNA-protein correlation is the individual half-life of proteins. Our observation of a decrease in mRNA expression at times when increases in protein expression occur [66, 67] can be explained by the relative half-life of the mRNA and the 5-HT_{2A} receptor protein. In situ hybridization results [68] are consistent with a decrease in *Htr2a* gene expression after spinal cord injury in the ventral horn (28 days in their case and one month and 4 months in our case). In the paper by Chopek et al. [42], the samples were taken 3 months after injury. Since mRNA expression is not maintained in a steady state [69], some fluctuation in mRNA expression over time is to be expected. For example, in laser-captured phrenic motoneurons [70], mRNA for 5-HT_{2A} receptors was upregulated 14 days after cervical hemisection, but had returned to normal or below at 21 days. Fuller et al. [27], in contrast, found upregulation of 5-HT_{2A} protein after 7–14 days in the same preparation (cervical hemisection). The decrease in *Htr2a* gene expression may be an autoregulatory response to increased receptor density [71].

Chopek and others [42] found significant increases in *Htr2a* gene expression in motoneurons innervating hindlimb flexor and extensor muscles after spinal cord transection. This is not surprising given the frequent absence of correlation between gene and protein expression after injury. What might account for the differences between our findings and those of Chopek et al? They might be an effect of different selection of motoneurons for analysis. We compared MNs innervating TA with those innervating GM based upon the fact that these muscles have comparable composition of the three types of motor units, but they are different in function (extensor versus flexor). Chopek and others collected MNs innervating both soleus and gastrocnemius lateralis muscles to the extensor pool and MNs innervating extensor digitorum longus and tibialis anterior muscles to the flexor pool. Soleus is a typical slow muscle, and extensor digitorum longus is a typical fast muscle, so including these MNs in their extensor and flexor pools, respectively, may have influenced the results. MNs of different sizes may express 5-HT_{2A} receptors differently, and they react differently to spinal cord injury [72]. Moreover, Chopek and others [42] use *SDHA* as the reference gene for qPCR analysis, which may have influenced the results, because expression of this gene may be altered by spinal cord injury. This is the case after disuse in microgravity, and it appears to induce changes in *SDHA* expression differently in motoneurons of different sizes [73, 74]. We selected the *Ppia* gene after Navarrett and others [75], who verified it as suitable for use in spinal cord tissue after injury. We also eliminated any effects of 5-HT receptors in blood [76] by perfusing the rat with PBS before dissecting the spinal cord and further preparation for laser capture of the motoneurons, whereas this was not done by others who observed an increase in 5-HT_{2A} mRNA [42, 43]. In the Di Narzo et al. [43] study, the sample was taken from the sacral cord and was not limited to motoneurons. Another possible explanation for the differences between our observations on 5-HT_{2A} mRNA levels after injury and those of Chopek et al. [42] and Di Narzo et al. [43] is that they used Sprague-Dawley rats, while WAG (Wistar Albino Glaxo) rats were used in our study.

Di Narzo et al. [43] described recently that in rat spinal cord, the mRNA expression of *Htr2c* gene is influenced by inflammation caused by total transection at the sacral level (0.6 mm below and above the SCI). Our analysis of the inflammatory responses in the spinal cord of spinal rats with and without a graft revealed that in the ventral horn of the lumbar segments (6 mm below the graft site—the shortest distance below the graft that MNs of TA and GM muscles were collected), there was no increased level of astrocytes and no presence of activated microglia. Thus, inflammation induced by intraspinal grafting is not likely to be responsible for the observed changes in *Htr2a* and *Htr7* gene expression.

There is good evidence for constitutive activity in 5-HT_2 receptors in sacral MNs after S2 spinal cord injury (reviewed in [14]), but the evidence that this is true in MNs innervating limb muscles is less complete. The degree of constitutive activity of 5-HT_{2A} receptors is thought to be dependent upon mRNA expression [75]. The reduction in mRNA after SCI may be interpreted as an indication of decreased constitutive activity in both 5-HT_{2A} and 5-HT_7 receptors. Our finding that limb motoneuron 5-HT_{2A} and 5-HT_7 mRNA expression is increased by the grafts could therefore reflect an increase in constitutive activity in these receptors. Whether this can account for the efficacy of the grafts for improving locomotor recovery in paraplegic rats will require further investigation. These results suggest that the mechanisms regulating 5-HT receptor mRNA expression in limb and tail MNs after SCI might be different.

Our results showing 5-HT_7 receptor mRNA upregulation after grafting provides support for the suggestion that the graft improves locomotion by increasing the role of this receptor in these MNs. Both 5-HT_{2A} and 5-HT_7 receptors are expressed in phrenic MNs, and both receptors facilitate spinal motor plasticity [77, 78]. Their coexistence results in mutual crosstalk inhibition (Fuller and Mitchell respiratory neuroplasticity) due to the downstream effects induced by Gq (5-HT_{2A}) and Gs (5-HT_7) activation. The details of this crosstalk inhibition are not well defined, but this factor needs to be taken into account if the function of neurons expressing both these G protein receptors is to be understood. In the case of limb motoneurons, it is possible that such crosstalk inhibition could result in mutual downregulation of receptor expression. Further investigations of the effects of 5-HT_7 receptors on limb motoneurons are warranted. A description of the mechanisms involved in the increased expression of RNAs for both receptors induced by the grafts will require further investigation.

5-HT_7 receptors appear to be expressed in limb MNs, but their role in controlling motoneuron function has not been established. Zhang [79] found that a 5-HT_7 receptor agonist produced depolarization when applied iontophoretically onto lumbar MNs in cat spinal cord. MN excitability might be increased if 5-HT_7 receptors mediated a reduction in the afterhyperpolarization in limb MNs, which appears to be the case in trigeminal MNs [19]. Limb MN AHPs are reduced by iontophoretically applied 5-HT [80], but the receptor responsible for this effect has not been determined. These issues need to be investigated, along with the possibility of inhibitory crosstalk between 5-HT_{2A} and 5-HT_7 receptors which occurs in phrenic motoneurons [77, 78], when both receptors are present in the same cell.

5. Conclusion

Our results indicate that thoracic spinal cord transection leads to changes in *Htr2a* and *Htr7* gene expression, whereas transplantation of embryonic serotonergic neurons reverses these changes in MNs innervating hindlimb muscles but not those innervating the tail muscle. These differences in *Htr2a* and *Htr7* gene expression between MNs innervating hindlimb and tail muscles can be a result of the distance from the graft to the motoneurons. The fibers of grafted 5-HT neurons do not extend farther than to the level of L4-L5 lumbar segments [10, 57], so motoneurons innervating the ECM muscle may not be supplied by serotonergic innervation of graft origin. Alternatively, it may be that motoneurons that innervate tail muscles have unique adaptations to spinal injury and the effects of intraspinal grafts of 5-HT neurons, such as reliance on constitutive activity of 5-HT_2 receptors after spinal cord injury. Increased *Htr2a* and *Htr7* gene expression induced by the graft could restore motoneuron excitability and lead to improved motor function, such as we observed in the grafted rats [10, 57]. Here, we show for the first time that changes in gene expression induced by the graft may account for this recovery.

Conflicts of Interest

The authors declare that there is no conflict of interest regarding the publication of this paper.

Acknowledgments

This work was supported by grants from the Polish National Science Centre (UMO-2013/09/B/NZ4/02885) to Urszula Sławińska and the Operational Programme Human Capital - Priority 8.2.2, engaged in the innovative scientific research in areas considered particularly important for the development of Masovian Voivodeship for Krzysztof Miazga. Research subject was carried out with the use of CePT infrastructure (the Arcturus Laser Microdissection System, Laboratory of Molecular Neurobiology, headed by Professor B. Kamińska) financed by the European Union - the European Regional Development Fund within the Operational Programme "Innovative Economy" for 2007–2013.

References

[1] J. Hounsgaard, "Motor neurons," *Comprehensive Physiology*, vol. 7, no. 2, pp. 463–484, 2017.

[2] J. F. Perrier and F. Cotel, "Serotonergic modulation of spinal motor control," *Current Opinion in Neurobiology*, vol. 33, pp. 1–7, 2015.

[3] B. J. Schmidt and L. M. Jordan, "The role of serotonin in reflex modulation and locomotor rhythm production in the mammalian spinal cord," *Brain Research Bulletin*, vol. 53, no. 5, pp. 689–710, 2000.

[4] A. M. Cabaj, H. Majczyński, E. Couto et al., "Serotonin controls initiation of locomotion and afferent modulation of coordination via 5-HT7 receptors in adult rats," *The Journal of Physiology*, vol. 595, no. 1, pp. 301–320, 2017.

[5] F. Gackiere and L. Vinay, "Serotonergic modulation of post-synaptic inhibition and locomotor alternating pattern in the spinal cord," *Frontiers in Neural Circuits*, vol. 8, 2014.

[6] J. Liu and L. M. Jordan, "Stimulation of the parapyramidal region of the neonatal rat brain stem produces locomotor-like activity involving spinal 5-HT7 and 5-HT2A receptors," *Journal of Neurophysiology*, vol. 94, no. 2, pp. 1392–1404, 2005.

[7] J. Liu, T. Akay, P. B. Hedlund, K. G. Pearson, and L. M. Jordan, "Spinal 5-HT7 receptors are critical for alternating activity during locomotion: in vitro neonatal and in vivo adult studies using 5-HT7 receptor knockout mice," *Journal of Neurophysiology*, vol. 102, no. 1, pp. 337–348, 2009.

[8] M. A. Madriaga, L. C. McPhee, T. Chersa, K. J. Christie, and P. J. Whelan, "Modulation of locomotor activity by multiple 5-HT and dopaminergic receptor subtypes in the neonatal mouse spinal cord," *Journal of Neurophysiology*, vol. 92, no. 3, pp. 1566–1576, 2004.

[9] E. Pearlstein, F. Ben Mabrouk, J. F. Pflieger, and L. Vinay, "Serotonin refines the locomotor-related alternations in the in vitro neonatal rat spinal cord," *European Journal of Neuroscience*, vol. 21, no. 5, pp. 1338–1346, 2005.

[10] U. Sławińska, K. Miazga, A. M. Cabaj et al., "Grafting of fetal brainstem 5-HT neurons into the sublesional spinal cord of paraplegic rats restores coordinated hindlimb locomotion," *Experimental Neurology*, vol. 247, pp. 572–581, 2013.

[11] U. Sławińska, K. Miazga, and L. M. Jordan, "5-HT2 and 5-HT7 receptor agonists facilitate plantar stepping in chronic spinal rats through actions on different populations of spinal neurons," *Frontiers in Neural Circuits*, vol. 8, 2014.

[12] S. Hochman, S. M. Garraway, D. W. Machacek, and B. L. Shay, "5-HT receptors and the neuromodualatory control of spinal cord function," in *Motor Neurobiology of the Spinal Cord*, T. C. Cope, Ed., pp. 48–87, CRC Press, New York, 2001.

[13] H. Majczyński, K. Maleszak, A. Cabaj, and U. Sławińska, "Serotonin-related enhancement of recovery of hind limb motor functions in spinal rats after grafting of embryonic raphe nuclei," *Journal of Neurotrauma*, vol. 22, no. 5, pp. 590–604, 2005.

[14] J. M. D'Amico, E. G. Condliffe, K. J. B. Martins, D. J. Bennett, and M. A. Gorassini, "Recovery of neuronal and network excitability after spinal cord injury and implications for spasticity," *Frontiers in Integrative Neuroscience*, vol. 8, 2014.

[15] M. Zhang, "Normal distribution and plasticity of serotonin receptors after spinal cord injury and their impacts on motor outputs," in *Recovery of Motor Function Following Spinal Cord Injury*, H. Fuller and M. Gates, Eds., InTech, 2016.

[16] M. S. Hoffman and G. S. Mitchell, "Spinal 5-HT7 receptors and protein kinase A constrain intermittent hypoxia-induced phrenic long-term facilitation," *Neuroscience*, vol. 250, pp. 632–643, 2013.

[17] M. S. Hoffman and G. S. Mitchell, "Spinal 5-HT7 receptor activation induces long-lasting phrenic motor facilitation," *The Journal of Physiology*, vol. 589, no. 6, pp. 1397–1407, 2011.

[18] W. Gang, T. Hongjian, C. Jasheng et al., "The effect of the 5-HT7 serotonin receptor agonist, LP44, on micturition in rats with chronic spinal cord injury," *Neurourology and Urodynamics*, vol. 33, no. 7, pp. 1165–1170, 2014.

[19] T. Inoue, S. Itoh, S. Wakisaka, S. Ogawa, M. Saito, and T. Morimoto, "Involvement of 5-HT7 receptors in serotonergic effects on spike afterpotentials in presumed jaw-closing motoneurons of rats," *Brain Research*, vol. 954, no. 2, pp. 202–211, 2002.

[20] K. Matsumoto-Miyai, M. Yoshizumi, and M. Kawatani, "Regulatory effects of 5-hydroxytryptamine receptors on voiding

function," *Advances in Therapy*, vol. 32, Supplement 1, pp. 3–15, 2015.

[21] J. Ogilvie, M. Wigglesworth, L. Appleby, T. O. W. Kingston, and R. W. Clarke, "On the role of 5-HT1B/1D receptors in modulating transmission in a spinal reflex pathway in the decerebrated rabbit," *British Journal of Pharmacology*, vol. 128, no. 3, pp. 781–787, 1999.

[22] A. Dogrul, M. Seyrek, E. O. Akgul, T. Cayci, S. Kahraman, and H. Bolay, "Systemic paracetamol-induced analgesic and antihyperalgesic effects through activation of descending serotonergic pathways involving spinal 5-HT7 receptors," *European Journal of Pharmacology*, vol. 677, no. 1-3, pp. 93–101, 2012.

[23] F. Viguier, B. Michot, M. Hamon, and S. Bourgoin, "Multiple roles of serotonin in pain control mechanisms—implications of 5-HT7 and other 5-HT receptor types," *European Journal of Pharmacology*, vol. 716, no. 1-3, pp. 8–16, 2013.

[24] N. Cao, J. Ni, X. Wang et al., "Chronic spinal cord injury causes upregulation of serotonin (5-HT)2A and 5-HT2C receptors in lumbosacral cord motoneurons," *BJU International*, vol. 121, no. 1, pp. 145–154, 2018.

[25] K. Fouad, M. M. Rank, R. Vavrek, K. C. Murray, L. Sanelli, and D. J. Bennett, "Locomotion after spinal cord injury depends on constitutive activity in serotonin receptors," *Journal of Neurophysiology*, vol. 104, no. 6, pp. 2975–2984, 2010.

[26] P. J. Harvey, X. Li, Y. Li, and D. J. Bennett, "5-HT2 receptor activation facilitates a persistent sodium current and repetitive firing in spinal motoneurons of rats with and without chronic spinal cord injury," *Journal of Neurophysiology*, vol. 96, no. 3, pp. 1158–1170, 2006.

[27] D. D. Fuller, T. L. Baker-Herman, F. J. Golder, N. J. Doperalski, J. J. Watters, and G. S. Mitchell, "Cervical spinal cord injury upregulates ventral spinal 5-HT2A receptors," *Journal of Neurotrauma*, vol. 22, no. 2, pp. 203–213, 2005.

[28] S. Doly, J. Fischer, M. J. Brisorgueil, D. Verge, and M. Conrath, "Pre- and postsynaptic localization of the 5-HT7 receptor in rat dorsal spinal cord: immunocytochemical evidence," *The Journal of Comparative Neurology*, vol. 490, no. 3, pp. 256–269, 2005.

[29] D. P. Fields, S. R. Springborn, and G. S. Mitchell, "Spinal 5-HT7 receptors induce phrenic motor facilitation via EPAC-mTORC1 signaling," *Journal of Neurophysiology*, vol. 114, no. 3, pp. 2015–2022, 2015.

[30] P. Fenik and S. C. Veasey, "Pharmacological characterization of serotonergic receptor activity in the hypoglossal nucleus," *American Journal of Respiratory and Critical Care Medicine*, vol. 167, no. 4, pp. 563–569, 2003.

[31] S. Okabe, M. Mackiewicz, and L. Kubin, "Serotonin receptor mRNA expression in the hypoglossal motor nucleus," *Respiration Physiology*, vol. 110, no. 2-3, pp. 151–160, 1997.

[32] C. H. Gill, E. M. Soffin, J. J. Hagan, and C. H. Davies, "5-HT7 receptors modulate synchronized network activity in rat hippocampus," *Neuropharmacology*, vol. 42, no. 1, pp. 82–92, 2002.

[33] R. M. Brownstone, L. M. Jordan, D. J. Kriellaars, B. R. Noga, and S. J. Shefchyk, "On the regulation of repetitive firing in lumbar motoneurones during fictive locomotion in the cat," *Experimental Brain Research*, vol. 90, no. 3, pp. 441–455, 1992.

[34] B. J. Schmidt, "Afterhyperpolarization modulation in lumbar motoneurons during locomotor-like rhythmic activity in the neonatal rat spinal cord in vitro," *Experimental Brain Research*, vol. 99, no. 2, pp. 214–222, 1994.

[35] P. A. M. ban Dongen, S. Grillner, and T. Hökfelt, "5-Hydroxytryptamine (serotonin) causes a reduction in the afterhyperpolarization following the action potential in lamprey motoneurons and premotor interneurons," *Brain Research*, vol. 366, no. 1-2, pp. 320–325, 1986.

[36] P. Wallén, J. Christenson, L. Brodin, R. Hill, A. Lansner, and S. Grillner, "Chapter 26 Mechanisms underlying the serotonergic modulation of the spinal circuitry for locomotion in lamprey," *Progress in Brain Research*, vol. 80, pp. 321–327, 1989.

[37] S. Doly, A. Madeira, J. Fischer et al., "The 5-HT2A receptor is widely distributed in the rat spinal cord and mainly localized at the plasma membrane of postsynaptic neurons," *The Journal of Comparative Neurology*, vol. 472, no. 4, pp. 496–511, 2004.

[38] V. Cornea-Hebert, M. Riad, C. Wu, S. K. Singh, and L. Descarries, "Cellular and subcellular distribution of the serotonin 5-HT2A receptor in the central nervous system of adult rat," *The Journal of Comparative Neurology*, vol. 409, no. 2, pp. 187–209, 1999.

[39] F. Vult von Steyern and T. Lomo, "Postnatal appearance of 5-HT2A receptors on fast flexor and slow extensor rat motor neurons," *Neuroscience*, vol. 136, no. 1, pp. 87–93, 2005.

[40] J. K. Lee, C. S. Johnson, and J. R. Wrathall, "Up-regulation of 5-HT2 receptors is involved in the increased H-reflex amplitude after contusive spinal cord injury," *Experimental Neurology*, vol. 203, no. 2, pp. 502–511, 2007.

[41] J. W. Chopek, C. W. MacDonell, K. Gardiner, and P. F. Gardiner, "Daily passive cycling attenuates the hyperexcitability and restores the responsiveness of the extensor monosynaptic reflex to quipazine in the chronic spinally transected rat," *Journal of Neurotrauma*, vol. 31, no. 12, pp. 1083–1087, 2014.

[42] J. W. Chopek, P. C. Sheppard, K. Gardiner, and P. F. Gardiner, "Serotonin receptor and KCC2 gene expression in lumbar flexor and extensor motoneurons posttransection with and without passive cycling," *Journal of Neurophysiology*, vol. 113, no. 5, pp. 1369–1376, 2015.

[43] A. F. Di Narzo, A. Kozlenkov, Y. Ge et al., "Decrease of mRNA editing after spinal cord injury is caused by down-regulation of ADAR2 that is triggered by inflammatory response," *Scientific Reports*, vol. 5, no. 1, article 12615, 2015.

[44] I. Giroux, E. M. Kurowska, and K. K. Carroll, "Role of dietary lysine, methionine, and arginine in the regulation of hypercholesterolemia in rabbits," *The Journal of Nutritional Biochemistry*, vol. 10, no. 3, pp. 166–171, 1999.

[45] M. Antri, J. Y. Barthe, C. Mouffle, and D. Orsal, "Long-lasting recovery of locomotor function in chronic spinal rat following chronic combined pharmacological stimulation of serotonergic receptors with 8-OHDPAT and quipazine," *Neuroscience Letters*, vol. 384, no. 1-2, pp. 162–167, 2005.

[46] U. Sławińska, H. Majczyński, Y. Dai, and L. M. Jordan, "The upright posture improves plantar stepping and alters responses to serotonergic drugs in spinal rats," *The Journal of Physiology*, vol. 590, no. 7, pp. 1721–1736, 2012.

[47] E. S. Landry, N. P. Lapointe, C. Rouillard, D. Levesque, P. B. Hedlund, and P. A. Guertin, "Contribution of spinal 5-HT1A and 5-HT7 receptors to locomotor-like movement induced by 8-OH-DPAT in spinal cord-transected mice," *The European Journal of Neuroscience*, vol. 24, no. 2, pp. 535–546, 2006.

[48] R. Bos, K. Sadlaoud, P. Boulenguez et al., "Activation of 5-HT2A receptors upregulates the function of the neuronal K-Cl cotransporter KCC2," *Proceedings of the National

Academy of Sciences of the United States of America, vol. 110, no. 1, pp. 348–353, 2013.

[49] M. J. Dunbar, M. A. Tran, and P. J. Whelan, "Endogenous extracellular serotonin modulates the spinal locomotor network of the neonatal mouse," *The Journal of Physiology*, vol. 588, no. 1, pp. 139–156, 2010.

[50] M. Antri, C. Mouffle, D. Orsal, and J. Y. Barthe, "5-HT1A receptors are involved in short- and long-term processes responsible for 5-HT-induced locomotor function recovery in chronic spinal rat," *The European Journal of Neuroscience*, vol. 18, no. 7, pp. 1963–1972, 2003.

[51] U. Sławińska, H. Majczyński, and R. Djavadian, "Recovery of hindlimb motor functions after spinal cord transection is enhanced by grafts of the embryonic raphe nuclei," *Experimental Brain Research*, vol. 132, no. 1, pp. 27–38, 2000.

[52] K. C. Murray, A. Nakae, M. J. Stephens et al., "Recovery of motoneuron and locomotor function after spinal cord injury depends on constitutive activity in 5-HT2C receptors," *Nature Medicine*, vol. 16, no. 6, pp. 694–700, 2010.

[53] U. Sławińska, L. M. Jordan, B. Burger, H. Fabczak, and H. Majczyński, "Locomotion of intact adult rats is controlled by 5-HT2A and 5-HT7 but not 5-HT2C receptors; 2012," in *Society of Neuroscience*, Neuroscience Meeting Planner, New Orleans, LA, USA, 2012, Program No. 85.09.

[54] K. L. Wohlpart and P. B. Molinoff, "Regulation of levels of 5-HT2A receptor mRNA," *Annals of the New York Academy of Sciences*, vol. 861, no. 1 ADVANCES IN S, pp. 128–135, 1998.

[55] D. Van Oekelen, W. H. M. L. Luyten, and J. E. Leysen, "5-HT2A and 5-HT2C receptors and their atypical regulation properties," *Life Sciences*, vol. 72, no. 22, pp. 2429–2449, 2003.

[56] K. Miazga, E. Joachimiak, H. Fabczak, and U. Sławińska, "Grafted serotonergic neurons can reverse changes in gene expression in motoneurons produced by spinal cord injury in rats.; 2015. Programm: P9.6," in *12th International Congress of the Polish Neuroscience Society*, Gdańsk, Poland, September 2015.

[57] U. Sławińska, K. Miazga, and L. M. Jordan, "The role of serotonin in the control of locomotor movements and strategies for restoring locomotion after spinal cord injury," *Acta Neurobiologiae Experimentalis*, vol. 74, no. 2, pp. 172–187, 2014.

[58] A. Lev-Tov, A. Etlin, and D. Blivis, "Sensory-induced activation of pattern generators in the absence of supraspinal control," *Annals of the New York Academy of Sciences*, vol. 1198, no. 1, pp. 54–62, 2010.

[59] D. Feraboli-Lohnherr, D. Orsal, A. Yakovleff, M. Gimenez y Ribotta, and A. Privat, "Recovery of locomotor activity in the adult chronic spinal rat after sublesional transplantation of embryonic nervous cells: specific role of serotonergic neurons," *Experimental Brain Research*, vol. 113, no. 3, pp. 443–454, 1997.

[60] M. G. y Ribotta, J. Provencher, D. Feraboli-Lohnherr, S. Rossignol, A. Privat, and D. Orsal, "Activation of locomotion in adult chronic spinal rats is achieved by transplantation of embryonic raphe cells reinnervating a precise lumbar level," *The Journal of Neuroscience*, vol. 20, no. 13, pp. 5144–5152, 2000.

[61] D. M. Basso, M. S. Beattie, and J. C. Bresnahan, "Graded histological and locomotor outcomes after spinal cord contusion using the NYU weight-drop device versus transection," *Experimental Neurology*, vol. 139, no. 2, pp. 244–256, 1996.

[62] R. C. Ferry, C. D. Unsworth, R. P. Artymyshyn, and P. B. Molinoff, "Regulation of mRNA encoding 5-HT2A receptors in P11 cells through a post-transcriptional mechanism requiring activation of protein kinase C," *The Journal of Biological Chemistry*, vol. 269, no. 50, pp. 31850–31857, 1994.

[63] X. Y. Kong, J. Wienecke, M. Chen, H. Hultborn, and M. Zhang, "The time course of serotonin 2a receptor expression after spinal transection of rats: an immunohistochemical study," *Neuroscience*, vol. 177, pp. 114–126, 2011.

[64] X.-Y. Kong, J. Wienecke, H. Hultborn, and M. Zhang, "Robust upregulation of serotonin 2A receptors after chronic spinal transection of rats: an immunohistochemical study," *Brain Research*, vol. 1320, pp. 60–68, 2010.

[65] Y. Zhang, R. X. Zhang, M. Zhang et al., "Electroacupuncture inhibition of hyperalgesia in an inflammatory pain rat model: involvement of distinct spinal serotonin and norepinephrine receptor subtypes," *British Journal of Anaesthesia*, vol. 109, no. 2, pp. 245–252, 2012.

[66] Y. Ryu, T. Ogata, M. Nagao et al., "The swimming test is effective for evaluating spasticity after contusive spinal cord injury," *PLoS One*, vol. 12, no. 2, article e0171937, 2017.

[67] Y. Ryu, T. Ogata, M. Nagao, Y. Sawada, R. Nishimura, and N. Fujita, "Effects of treadmill training combined with serotonergic interventions on spasticity after contusive spinal cord injury," *Journal of Neurotrauma*, vol. 35, no. 12, pp. 1358–1366, 2018.

[68] R. V. Ung, E. S. Landry, P. Rouleau, N. P. Lapointe, C. Rouillard, and P. A. Guertin, "Role of spinal 5-HT2 receptor subtypes in quipazine-induced hindlimb movements after a low-thoracic spinal cord transection," *European Journal of Neuroscience*, vol. 28, no. 11, pp. 2231–2242, 2008.

[69] T. Maier, M. Guell, and L. Serrano, "Correlation of mRNA and protein in complex biological samples," *FEBS Letters*, vol. 583, no. 24, pp. 3966–3973, 2009.

[70] C. B. Mantilla, J. P. Bailey, W. Z. Zhan, and G. C. Sieck, "Phrenic motoneuron expression of serotonergic and glutamatergic receptors following upper cervical spinal cord injury," *Experimental Neurology*, vol. 234, no. 1, pp. 191–199, 2012.

[71] M. Zaniewska, N. Alenina, K. Wydra et al., "Discovering the mechanisms underlying serotonin (5-HT)2A and 5-HT2C receptor regulation following nicotine withdrawal in rats," *Journal of Neurochemistry*, vol. 134, no. 4, pp. 704–716, 2015.

[72] J. Celichowski, W. Mrówczyński, P. Krutki, T. Górska, H. Majczyński, and U. Sławińska, "Changes in contractile properties of motor units of the rat medial gastrocnemius muscle after spinal cord transection," *Experimental Physiology*, vol. 91, no. 5, pp. 887–895, 2006.

[73] A. Ishihara, F. Nagatomo, H. Fujino, H. Kondo, and Y. Ohira, "Decreased succinate dehydrogenase activity of gamma and alpha motoneurons in mouse spinal cords following 13 weeks of exposure to microgravity," *Neurochemical Research*, vol. 38, no. 10, pp. 2160–2167, 2013.

[74] A. Ishihara, R. R. Roy, and V. R. Edgerton, "Succinate dehydrogenase activity and soma size of motoneurons innervating different portions of the rat tibialis anterior," *Neuroscience*, vol. 68, no. 3, pp. 813–822, 1995.

[75] S. Navarrett, L. Collier, C. Cardozo, and S. Dracheva, "Alterations of serotonin 2C and 2A receptors in response to T10 spinal cord transection in rats," *Neuroscience Letters*, vol. 506, no. 1, pp. 74–78, 2012.

[76] N. Herr, C. Bode, and D. Duerschmied, "The effects of serotonin in immune cells," *Frontiers in Cardiovascular Medicine*, vol. 4, p. 48, 2017.

[77] D. P. Fields and G. S. Mitchell, "Divergent cAMP signaling differentially regulates serotonin-induced spinal motor plasticity," *Neuropharmacology*, vol. 113, no. Part A, pp. 82–88, 2017.

[78] D. D. Fuller and G. S. Mitchell, "Respiratory neuroplasticity – overview, significance and future directions," *Experimental Neurology*, vol. 287, Part 2, pp. 144–152, 2017.

[79] L. Zhang, "Effects of 5-hydroxytryptamine on cat spinal motoneurons," *Canadian Journal of Physiology and Pharmacology*, vol. 69, no. 2, pp. 154–163, 1991.

[80] S. R. White and S. J. Fung, "Serotonin depolarizes cat spinal motoneurons in situ and decreases motoneuron afterhyperpolarizing potentials," *Brain Research*, vol. 502, no. 2, pp. 205–213, 1989.

14

The Activation of the Mirror Neuron System during Action Observation and Action Execution with Mirror Visual Feedback in Stroke

Jack J. Q. Zhang,[1] Kenneth N. K. Fong,[1] Nandana Welage,[2] and Karen P. Y. Liu[2]

[1]*Department of Rehabilitation Sciences, The Hong Kong Polytechnic University, Kowloon, Hong Kong*
[2]*School of Science and Health, Western Sydney University, Penrith, NSW, Australia*

Correspondence should be addressed to Kenneth N. K. Fong; rsnkfong@polyu.edu.hk

Academic Editor: Ambra Bisio

Objective. To evaluate the concurrent and training effects of action observation (AO) and action execution with mirror visual feedback (MVF) on the activation of the mirror neuron system (MNS) and its relationship with the activation of the motor cortex in stroke individuals. *Methods.* A literature search using CINAHL, PubMed, PsycINFO, Medline, Web of Science, and SCOPUS to find relevant studies was performed. *Results.* A total of 19 articles were included. Two functional magnetic resonance imaging (fMRI) studies reported that MVF could activate the ipsilesional primary motor cortex as well as the MNS in stroke individuals, whereas two other fMRI studies found that the MNS was not activated by MVF in stroke individuals. Two clinical trials reported that long-term action execution with MVF induced a shift of activation toward the ipsilesional hemisphere. Five fMRI studies showed that AO activated the MNS, of which, three found the activation of movement-related areas. Five electroencephalography (EEG) studies demonstrated that AO or MVF enhanced mu suppression over the sensorimotor cortex. *Conclusions.* MVF may contribute to stroke recovery by revising the interhemispheric imbalance caused by stroke due to the activation of the MNS. AO may also promote motor relearning in stroke individuals by activating the MNS and motor cortex.

1. Introduction

Stroke is one of the leading causes of adult disability. Patients commonly suffer lasting motor impairments and functional disability following a stroke [1]. A substantial number of advanced rehabilitation strategies have been applied in upper limb stroke rehabilitation, such as robot-assisted therapy [2], constraint-induced movement training (CIMT) [3], and virtual reality- (VR-) based rehabilitation [4], which are aimed at helping stroke survivors relearn motor skills through intensive training. These rehabilitation strategies have been reported to improve patients' motor functions by inducing experience-dependent neuroplasticity in their damaged hemispheres [5–7]. However, the neuroplasticity resulting from intensive-based interventions may be limited if the residual motor functions of the patients are also extremely limited. It is crucial to find an adjunct therapy, on top of limb training, to enhance the recovery of the ipsilesional motor cortex of patients with severe hemiplegia, in order to overcome the learned nonuse phenomenon in such patient populations [8].

There is evidence to support the theory that cortical areas involved in motor execution can be activated by observing actions performed by others, which is attributed to the function of the mirror neuron system (MNS). The MNS is a class of neural substrates that discharges during action observation (AO) and action execution [9, 10]. The MNS is also associated with various human functions, such as motor preparation [11], motion imitation [12, 13], language [14], and emotion recognition [15, 16]. In humans, the core MNS is understood to be located in the inferior frontal gyrus (IFG), including the ventral premotor cortex (PMv), the inferior parietal lobule (IPL), and the intraparietal sulcus (IPS) [9, 17]. An extended MNS involves additional brain regions, such as the primary motor cortex, the primary somatosensory cortex, and the middle frontal cortex [18]. A bilaterally distributed parietofrontal network with mirror neuron (MN) properties (i.e., parietofrontal MNS) has been proposed, which serves as a neural substrate to achieve the transformation of visual information into cortical areas for motor execution (i.e., visuomotor transformation) [19].

Based on this theory, researchers believe that the motor cortex could be primed by activating the MNS, thus boosting the efficacy of standardized rehabilitation for patients after strokes [17, 20]. Subsequently, various rehabilitative strategies, aimed at facilitating the motor cortex through activating the MNS, have been applied in stroke rehabilitation, including action observation training (AOT) [21, 22] and action execution with MVF [23]. AOT usually consists of a session of AO followed by a session of imitating the observed action [22]. Some clinical trials have supported the efficacy of AO as a motor priming tool in stroke rehabilitation [24–28]. Previous neuroimaging studies have identified a bilateral AO network over the frontal, parietal, temporal, and occipital areas in the brain, which encompass the core MNS [29, 30]. Action execution with MVF, including mirror therapy (MT) [23], mirror box therapy [31], and VR-based MT [32], is already a commonly employed regimen in stroke rehabilitation. By virtue of MVF, patients receive a visual illusion showing that their hemiplegic upper limbs are moving normally when they move their nonparetic upper limbs simultaneously [23]. MVF could boost the effects of the conventional upper limb rehabilitation of stroke [33]. It has been proposed that the training-induced effects of MVF arise from the activation of the ipsilesional primary motor cortex by enriching the visual and proprioceptive inputs to the MNS [10, 19, 34], but this hypothesis has not been duly confirmed in human studies [35].

It is feasible nowadays for researchers to objectively measure the brain's activities before and after interventions using advanced functional neuroimaging and electrophysiological techniques [36]. An increasing number of studies regarding the effects of these two promising motor priming techniques (AO and MVF) on brain activation in stroke individuals have been published. However, there is a lack of focused reviews investigating the effects of AO or action execution with MVF on the activation of MNS and its subsequent effects on the activation of the motor cortex in patients who have had a stroke. We conducted this systematic review to evaluate the concurrent and training effects of AO and action execution with MVF on the activation of the MNS in stroke individuals, by reviewing available experimental studies as well as clinical trials with functional neuroimaging or electrophysiological examinations. In order to understand the role of the MNS in upper limb stroke rehabilitation, we have summarized the following information in this review: (1) MNS activation and (2) MNS activation and its relationship with the activation of the motor cortex.

2. Methods

2.1. Literature Search. A literature search for relevant studies was conducted using CINAHL (the Cumulative Index to Nursing and Allied Health Literature), PubMed, PsycINFO, Medline, SCIE (Science Citation Index Expanded), and SCOPUS. Two of the authors of this review independently identified the relevant studies. Keywords used during the search were "stroke" OR "hemiplegia"; "action observation" OR "action observation training" OR "mirror visual feedback" OR "mirror neuron" OR "mirror therapy" OR "mirror box therapy"; and "functional imaging" OR "functional magnetic resonance imaging" OR "fMRI" OR "electroencephalography" OR "EEG" OR "near-infrared spectrometry" OR "NIRS" OR "magnetoencephalography" OR "MEG" OR "positron emission tomography" OR "PET". The date of publication was limited to 10 years, from January 2007 to November 2017. The reference lists of the retrieved articles were manually searched to identify any further relevant articles.

2.2. Selection Criteria. We used the PICOS method to formulate our selection criteria. Studies that satisfied all the following criteria were considered for this review.

Population (P): studies recruiting adult patients diagnosed with having had strokes; *intervention (I)*: interventions or experimental paradigms using AO or MVF in regard to upper limb actions; *comparison (C)*: control conditions without AO or MVF or using sham AO or MVF; *outcomes (O)*: studies providing anatomical evidence of brain activation induced by AO or action execution with MVF, as represented by signal changes in PET, fMRI, or fNIRS; or using previously validated electrophysiological indices of MN activities, such as event-related desynchronization (ERD) of the mu band (i.e., mu suppression) [37] or the ERD of the beta band (i.e., beta suppression) [38]; or employing an advance analysis to explore the neural network related to AO or MVF, including but not limited to dynamic casual modelling (DCM) in regard to fMRI or a coherence analysis of EEG; and *study design (S)*: clinical trials investigating the training effects or experimental studies investigating the concurrent effects of the relevant experimental condition.

Studies were excluded if (1) they only recruited healthy subjects or patients with other primary diagnoses (e.g., Parkinson's disease); (2) they only focused on the lower limb or trunk actions; (3) the final analyzed sample size was less than five; (4) they were published as conference proceedings, dissertations, or in books; and (5) they were not published in English language.

2.3. Data Extraction. After identifying relevant studies, two authors independently extracted the following information from each article: (1) the characteristics of participants; (2) the protocol of the intervention or experiment; (3) the modalities of the functional neuroimaging or electrophysiological techniques used in the study; and (4) the main results of the studies. Any disagreement was settled by discussion with the third author.

2.4. Quality Assessment. We assessed the quality of the randomized controlled trials (RCTs) in regard to the training effects of AOT or action execution with MVF in patients who have had strokes, based on the Physiotherapy Evidence Database (PEDro) scale. Both independent reviewers evaluated each article. The PEDro scale consists of 11 items. The first criterion, item eligibility, is not scored, as it is used as a component of external validity. The other criteria included random allocation, concealment of allocation, baseline equivalence, blinding procedure, intention to treat analysis, adequate follow-up, between-group statistical analysis, measurement of data variability, and point estimates. Any scoring discrepancies were resolved.

3. Results

3.1. Identification Process for the Selection of the Studies. The initial search yielded 332 results. After removing duplicates, a total of 191 records were screened, of which, 138 citations were excluded for the following reasons: the studies were reviews or meta-analyses ($n = 18$); the studies' protocols ($n = 6$); the studies focused on infants, children, or adolescents ($n = 4$); the studies enrolled only healthy participants or patients with neurological diseases other than strokes ($n = 58$); or the studies were irrelevant ($n = 52$). The remaining 53 articles were subjected to full-text reading, of which 34 articles were removed for the following reasons: the studies did not use functional neuroimaging or electrophysiological techniques for stroke participants ($n = 17$); the final analyzed sample sizes of the studies were less than five ($n = 8$); studies of motion observation with a brain-computer interface ($n = 2$); the visual feedback was based on the lower limbs or trunk actions, rather than upper limb actions ($n = 4$) [39–42]; or the studies used EEG spectrum analysis alone ($n = 1$) [43]. One study focused on the functional neuroplasticity induced by observing the skills of tool use, which was hard to compare with other protocols of AO. Another study enrolled both patients who have had strokes and brain tumors, and the data of stroke participants could not be separated; these studies were hence excluded [16, 44]. Finally, 19 articles satisfied our inclusion criteria and were included in the present review [13, 22, 28, 34, 45–59]. Figure 1 shows the identification process for the selection of studies.

3.2. Clinical Trials regarding the Training Effects of Long-Term Intervention. Among the included studies, six studies focused on the training effects of long-term therapeutic programs [22, 28, 45, 46, 52, 59]. Four of these were RCTs [22, 28, 45, 52], and the other two were interventional studies with pre-post comparisons [46, 59]. Three studies investigated the training effects of bimanual training with MVF (four- to eight-week interventions) [45, 46, 52]. Of these, two identified a shift of activation toward the ipsilesional hemisphere [46, 52], evidenced by fMRI. Cortical areas activated by MVF mainly included the primary motor cortex [46, 52] and the premotor cortex (PMC) [46]. A study with EEG reported that mu suppression over sensorimotor cortex (SMC) was higher in the group with MVF [45]. Sun et al., who also used mu suppression as an index, reported additional benefits of AO on the basis of motor imagery (MI) in regard to enhancing mu suppression over the ipsilesional SMC, compared with the control group (MI alone) [28]. A fNIRS study measured the difference in brain activity of participants before and after four weeks of MT in addition to conventional rehabilitation; however, the difference in the activation pattern over the primary motor cortex and the precuneus was insignificant over time [59].

An RCT investigating the training effects of AO found that the four-week AOT (AO followed by imitation) induced more evident activation over bilateral PMv, bilateral superior temporal gyrus (STG), supplementary motor area (SMA) over the contralesional hemisphere, and supramarginal gyrus (SMG) over the ipsilesional hemisphere, relative to the control group watching nonbiological videos followed by action execution [22]. Characteristics of these studies are summarized in Table 1.

3.3. Experimental Studies with fMRI Findings. Eight articles explored the concurrent effects of AO or action execution with MVF on brain activation, evidenced by fMRI [34, 47, 48, 50, 53, 55–57]. In studies regarding MVF, Michielsen et al. found that bimanual movement with MVF led to significant activation of the precuneus and the posterior cingulate cortex (PCC), rather than the MNS [53]. However, Saleh et al. [34, 55] reported that the ipsilesional primary motor cortex was activated by MVF, and connectivity between the ipsilesional primary somatosensory cortex and the primary motor cortex was stronger, relative to the control group without MVF [55]. The source of the ipsilesional primary motor cortex activation was further found by the DCM to be the contralesional intraparietal sulcus (IPS) [34]. Wang et al. reported that lateralized activation toward the affected hemisphere was in favor of virtual MVF, as reflected by the peak T value of the precuneus in the majority of their samples [57].

For studies concerning AO, Szameitat et al. found that AO of wrist movement activated the PMC and IPL; however, the pattern of neural activation in action execution more resembled MI, rather than AO [56]. Garrison et al. reported that left IFG, SMG, and bilateral precentral gyrus were activated during right-hand (paretic side) observation of reach and grasp actions. Lateralized activation toward the ipsilesional hemisphere was also noted [50]. During left-hand AO (nonparetic side), the bilateral activation was relatively symmetrical in stroke individuals. Brunner et al. [47] devised a protocol to observe bimanual action; they reported that stroke individuals (within one-to-two weeks after the stroke) showed activation in inferior and superior parietal lobes, IFG, and the primary motor cortex during AO. In the second fMRI exam (three months after the stroke), the neural response to AO was extended to more movement-related areas, including the PMC, primary motor cortex, and the SMA. The neural response to AO was increased from one or two weeks to three months after the individual suffered a stroke. Dettmers et al. compared the brain activities during AO and MI of patients with left or right subcortical strokes and reported that patients with left subcortical strokes presented higher levels of activity than those with right subcortical strokes [48]. The brain activation induced by AO or MVF shown by fMRI are summarized in Table 2.

3.4. Experimental Studies with EEG or MEG. Four experiments measured the concurrent effects of AO on mu rhythm

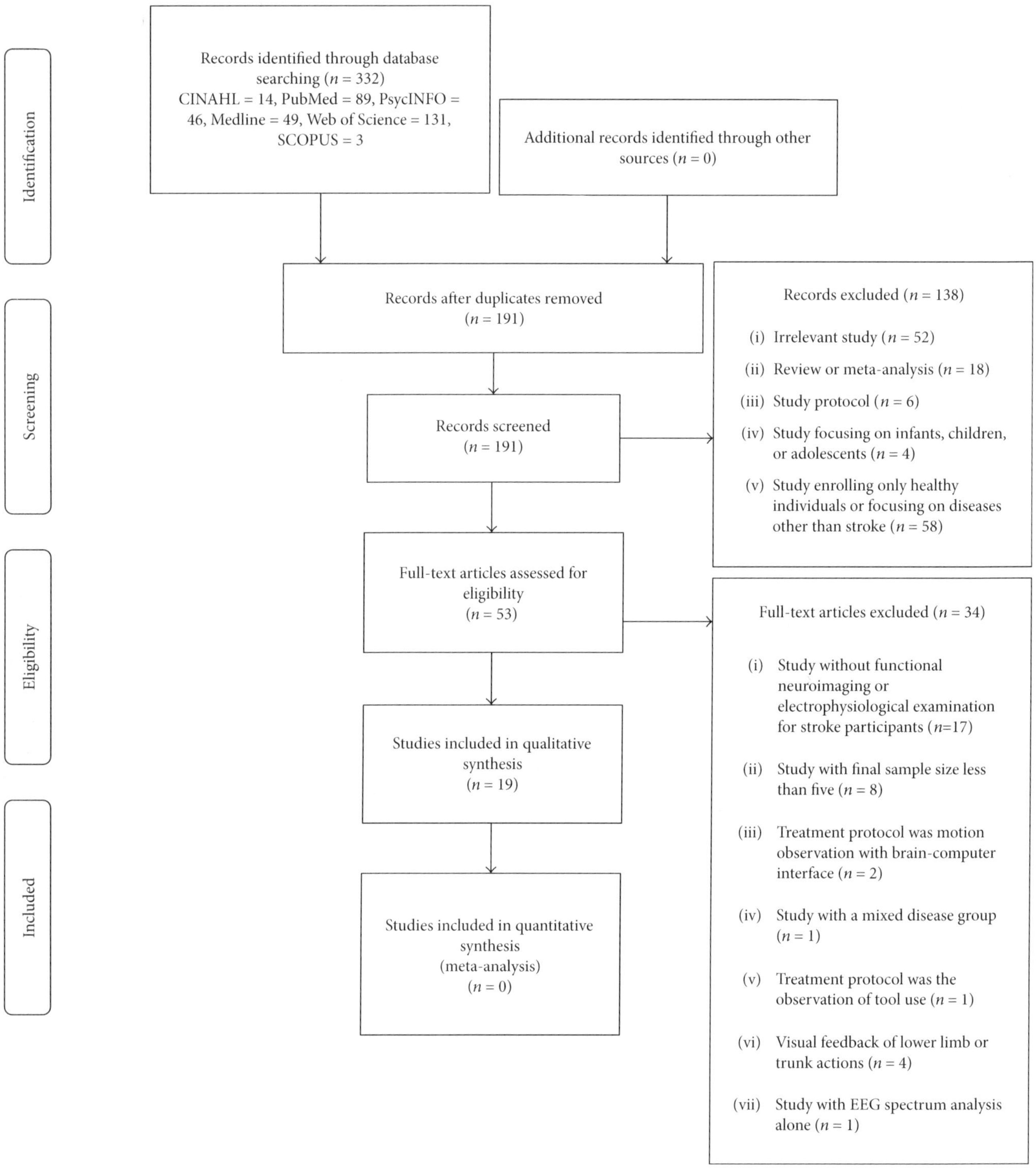

Figure 1: Flowchart of literature search.

using EEG [13, 49, 51, 58]. Another study used MEG to measure the difference in beta suppression during bimanual movement with and without MVF [54]. Kuk et al. reported the whole brain topography based on mu rhythm before and after AO and found that the middle frontal gyrus (MFG) was less active after a total of five sessions of AO [51]. Frenkel-Toledo et al. reported that observations of the reach-and-grasp hand action could induce mu suppression over the SMC, but the magnitude of mu suppression was significantly lower in the affected hemisphere, relative to the unaffected hemisphere. Mu suppression over the unaffected side was attenuated in patients with lesions over the right IPL [13, 49]. Tani et al. also showed that AO of the open-and-close action by the paretic hand induced stronger

TABLE 1: Characteristics of studies regarding the effects of long-term training on brain activation in stroke patients.

Study	Characteristics of stroke participants	Severity of hemiplegia	Intervention protocol	Intervention protocol	Imaging modality	Main results	
						Neuroimaging findings	Behavioral improvements
Ertelt et al. [22]	15 chronic stroke patients (>six months after stroke), aged 38–69.	Moderate arm paralysis (FAT: 0 to 5; WMFT (time): 2.41 to 41.29 seconds).	EG ($n = 7$): AOT (videos of upper limb actions followed by practice of observed actions, using the paretic upper limb); CG ($n = 8$): control (nonbiological videos followed by practice of the same actions, using the paretic upper limb).	Four-week intervention (90 minutes/ session, 18 sessions in total).	fMRI (EG = 7 and CG = 6).	More evident activation of PMv, SMA, insula, and STG over the nonaffected hemisphere and PMv, SMG, and STG over the affected hemisphere in EG than CG.	FAT posttreatment (EG > CG) WMFT-posttreatment (−) SIS-posttreatment (EG > CG). No significant difference between posttreatment and follow-up in three assessments.
Michielsen et al. [52]	40 chronic stroke patients (>one year after stroke), aged 55.3 ± 12.0 (MT)/58.7 ± 13.5 (CG).	Brunnstrom stage for the upper extremity III-V.	MT ($n = 20$): bimanual exercise with MVF of the unaffected hand; CG ($n = 20$): bimanual exercise with direct view of both hands.	Six-week intervention (one hour/ session, five sessions/week).	fMRI (MT = 9 and CG = 7).	A shift of activation toward the M1 over the affected hemisphere in MT.	FMA posttreatment (MT > CG); FMA 6-month follow-up (−) Jamar handheld dynamometer (−) Tardieu scale (−) ARAT (−) Stroke-ULAM (−) EQ-5D (−).
Bhasin et al. [46]	20 stroke patients (three 14 months after stroke), aged 45.45 ± 6.6.	Brunnstrom stage of the hand II-IV.	Bilateral hand exercise with virtual MVF of the nonparetic hand.	Eight-week intervention (five days/week, 60–90 minutes/ session).	fMRI.	LI of BA 4 and BA 6 was increased at eight weeks.	FM scale (posttreatment and 24-week follow-up > pretreatment) MBI (posttreatment and 24-week follow-up > pretreatment) MRC grade scale (−) Brunnstrom stage (−).
Bae et al. [45]	20 stroke patients (<six months after stroke), aged 55.2 ± 8.5 (MT)/52.6 ± 11.2 (CG).	Brunnstrom stage of the hand II–IV.	MT ($n = 10$): bilateral upper limb exercise with MVF; CG ($n = 10$): paretic arm exercise only.	Four-week intervention (30 minutes/ session, five times/week).	EEG.	Mu suppression at C3, Cz, and C4 was higher in MT than CG.	MFT posttreatment (MT > CG).
Sun et al. [28]	10 stroke patients (<two months after stroke), aged 59.4 ± 4.94.	Severe arm paralysis (FMA: 10 to 25).	On top of the CR, patients received the training: EG ($n = 5$): AO (paretic upper limb actions) with MI; CG ($n = 5$): MI alone.	Four-week intervention.	EEG.	AO with MI increased to higher mu suppression over C3 than MI at week 2, 3 and 4.	FMA week 2, 3 and 4; (EG > CG) PST week 3 and 4 (EG > CG).

Table 1: Continued.

Study	Characteristics of stroke participants	Severity of hemiplegia	Intervention protocol	Intervention protocol	Imaging modality	Main results	
						Neuroimaging findings	Behavioral improvements
Brunetti et al. [59]	11 stroke patients (15–92 days after stroke), aged 49–74.	Severe hand paralysis (a wrist extension of less than 20 degrees and metacarpophalangeal joint extension of less than 10 degrees).	On top of the CR, patients performed a bilateral exercise with MVF of nonparetic side.	Four-week intervention (30 minutes/ session, five sessions/week).	fNIRS.	The activation pattern of M1 and precuneus was stable over time.	Six of eleven patients showed improvement (gain scores from one to eight) in FMA-finger.

FAT: Frenchay arm test; WMFT: Wolf motor function test; EG: experimental group; CG: control group; AOT: action observation training; fMRI: functional magnetic resonance image; PMv: ventral premotor cortex; SMA: supplementary motor area; STG: superior temporal gyrus; SMG: supramarginal gyrus; SIS: stroke impact scale; MVF: mirror visual feedback; MT: mirror therapy; M1: primary motor cortex; FMA: Fugl-Meyer assessment; ARAT: action research arm test; Stroke-ULAM: stroke upper limb activity monitor; EQ-5D: EuroQOL five-dimension questionnaire; LI: laterality index; BA: Broadman area; MBI: modified Barthel index; MRC: Medical Research Council; EEG: electroencephalography; BA: Broadman area; MFT: manual function test; PT: physical training; CR: conventional rehabilitation; AO: action observation; MI: motor imagery; ERD: event-related desynchronization; PST: pinch strength test; fNIRS: functional near-infrared spectroscopy.

Table 2: Brain activation or lateralization of brain activation measured by fMRI.

Brain areas	Concurrent effect of MVF versus the control without MVF during a motor task	Long-term rehabilitation with MVF versus the control without MVF	Concurrent effect of AO versus the control	Long-term rehabilitation with AO versus the control without AO
Frontal lobes				
Primary motor cortex	Ipsilesional activation [34, 55]	Ipsilesional lateralization [46, 52]	Bilateral activation [47]; ipsilesional lateralization [50]	
Premotor cortex		Ipsilesional lateralization [46]	Bilateral activation [47]; ipsilesional activation [56]	Bilateral activation [22]
Supplementary motor area			Bilateral activation [47]	Contralesional activation [22]
Superior frontal gyrus			Ipsilesional activation [48]	
Inferior frontal gyrus			Bilateral activation [47]; ipsilesional lateralization [48, 50]	
Prefrontal gyrus			Ipsilesional activation [48]	
Parietal lobes				
Primary somatosensory cortex	Bilateral activation [34, 55]			
Superior parietal gyrus			Bilateral activation [47]; ipsilesional activation [48]	
Precuneus	Bilateral activation [34, 53, 55]; ipsilesional lateralization [57]			
Inferior parietal gyrus			Ipsilesional activation [56]; bilateral activation [47]	
Supramarginal gyrus	Contralesional activation [34, 55]		Ipsilesional lateralization [50]	Ipsilesional activation [22]
Intraparietal sulcus	Contralesional activation [34, 55]			
Posterior cingular cortex	Contralesional activation [53]			
Temporal lobes				
Superior temporal gyrus				Bilateral activation [22]
Inferior temporal gyrus			Bilateral activation [47]	
Occipital lobes				
Occipital gyrus			Bilateral activation [47]	

Notes: MVF: mirror visual feedback; AO: action observation. Garrison et al. [50]: results of AO of the paretic hand movement were used; Bhasin et al [46]: the result of within-group difference was used, because the study did not have a control group.

mu suppression than the MI of the same action in stroke individuals [58]. Interhemispheric imbalance of movement-related beta suppression was noted in stroke participants in the study by Rossiter et al. when performing the bimanual open-and-close action. The initial asymmetricity was partially attenuated by MVF [54]. Characteristics of the experimental studies are summarized in Table 3, and brain activation induced by AO or MVF, measured by fMRI, is summarized in Table 2.

3.5. Methodological Quality of Included Randomized Controlled Trials. Four RCTs were included in this review [22, 28, 45, 52]. The results of the assessment of methodological quality are summarized in Table 4.

4. Discussion

The present study is aimed at systematically evaluating the evidence of MNS activation induced by AO or MVF and its potential effects on the activation of the motor cortex in patients who have had strokes. The main findings of the present review are (1) the ipsilesional primary motor cortex can be facilitated by MVF [46, 52], which may be achieved by recruiting the MNS [34, 55]; (2) long-term action execution

Table 3: Characteristics of studies regarding the concurrent effects of single-session or multiple-session experiments on brain activation in stroke patients.

Study	Characteristics of stroke participants	Severity of hemiplegia	Experiment conditions	Imaging modality	Main results
Garrison et al. [50]	12 chronic stroke patients (two to 17 years after stroke), aged 39 to 85.	Moderate to severe arm paresis (FMA-UE: 13 to 48).	AO (reach to grasp objects by the right or left hand) and fixation.	fMRI.	Right-hand (paretic side) AO resulted in lateralization toward the left hemisphere, including IFG pars opercularis, IFG pars triangularis, SMG, and precentral gyrus.
Michielsen et al. [53]	18 chronic stroke patients (>one year after stroke), aged 54.7 ± 9.9.	Brunnstrom stage for the upper extremity III-V.	Unimanual exercise (open-and-close action by the unaffected hand) with MVF; unimanual exercise without MVF; bimanual exercise (bilateral open-and-close actions) with MVF; bimanual exercise without MVF.	fMRI.	Bimanual exercise with MVF significantly increased the activity in precuneus and PCC, more than other conditions.
Szameitat et al. [56]	Five chronic right-hemispheric stroke patients (>one year after stroke), aged 57 to 67.	Unclear.	Action execution (left wrist flexion and extension), MI (MI of the same wrist movement), AO (watching a video showing the same action), passive movement and baseline.	fMRI.	AO activated right lateral medial anterior PMC and a small focus of right IPL than baseline result.
Wang et al. [57]	Five stroke patients (29 to 93 days after stroke), aged 53 to 72.	Severe arm paresis (a wrist extension ability of less than 20 degrees and metacarpophalangeal joint extension ability of less than 10 degrees).	Unilateral index finger-thumb opposition (by nonparetic hands) with virtual normal visual feedback or virtual MVF.	fMRI.	Four out of five patients displayed the lateralized activation toward the affected hemisphere (reflected by peak *T* values within the precuneus), evoked by virtual MVF.
Brunner et al. [47]	18 stroke patients, aged 41 to 79; first scan: 8.9 ± 4.1 days after stroke; second scan: 89.3 ± 8.3 days after stroke.	NHPT < 0.5 (pegs per second).	AO (a video of bimanual twisting of a cylindrical device) and its resting condition (a still image of the device being held); action execution (bimanual twisting of a cylindrical device) and its resting condition (hold the device without twisting).	fMRI.	AO (first scan): involvement of the occipital and temporal visual areas bilaterally with activation maxima in the MTG and ITG and occipital lobe. Patients also showed activation in the parietal and frontal areas and the IPL, SPL, IFG, and M1 were involved; AO (second scan): most activated clusters were observed in ITG and the ventral anterior of the thalamus, also in premotor areas, SMA and M1.
Dettmers et al. [48]	18 subcortical stroke patients (nine left stroke patients, aged 59.2 ± 7.1, 28.2 ± 40.9 months after stroke and nine right stroke patients aged 63 ± 10.3, 47.1 ± 89.5 months after stroke).	With the ability to grip a small object and release it by the paretic hand.	AO (static pictures) of object-related hand action by the paretic side, AO (movies) of object-related hand action by the paretic side, AO (same movies) with imagery (performing the shown action) and fixation.	fMRI.	AO (movies) elicited activation in visual cortex, SPL, prefrontal cortex, and superior and inferior frontal cortexes in both patient groups. AO (movies) with imagery revealed a very similar network as during AO (movies) alone.
Saleh et al. [55]	15 chronic stroke patients (>six months after stroke), aged 54 ± 12.	CMA: four to seven; CMH: three to seven.	Nonparetic hand action (finger flexion) with veridical feedback or MVF and the control (nonanthropomorphic objects).	fMRI (14 data).	MVF induced significant activation of the ipsilesional postcentral gyrus, M1, precuneus, contralesional postcentral gyrus, superior bank of the intraparietal

Table 3: Continued.

Study	Characteristics of stroke participants	Severity of hemiplegia	Experiment conditions	Imaging modality	Main results
					sulcus and precuneus, and SMG. Connectivity between BA 1 and M1 and between BA 1 and S1 was significantly stronger after MVF.
Saleh et al. [34]	15 chronic stroke patients (>six months after stroke), aged 54 ± 12.	CMA: four to seven; CMH: three to seven.	Nonparetic hand action (finger flexion) with veridical feedback or MVF and the control (nonanthropomorphic objects).	fMRI (12 data).	MVF-induced activation of the ipsilesional primary motor cortex arose from the contralesional parietal cortex, in a region along the IPS.
Frenkel-Toledo et al. [49]	33 stroke patients aged 24 to 76, 23 to 132 days after stroke.	FMA zero to 66.	AO (reach and grasp action by left or right hands), observation of nonbiological videos and the eye close condition.	EEG.	AO induced mu suppression over SMC rather than observation of nonbiological videos; mu suppression was significantly diminished in the ipsilesional SMC (C3 or C4), compared with the contralesional SMC (C3 or C4); right IPL damage lowered mu suppression over the unaffected hemisphere.
Rossiter et al. [54]	10 stroke patients aged 56 ± 12, one to 114 months after stroke.	ARAT zero to 57.	Bilateral open-and-close hand action with MVF of nonparetic hand and bilateral open-and-close hand movement while viewing the paretic hand.	MEG.	Movement-related beta desynchronization was greater in contralesional compared to ipsilesional hemisphere. The asymmetry in movement-related beta desynchronization was more symmetrical in the condition with MVF.
Frenkel-Toledo et al. [13]	36 stroke patients aged 24 to 81 years, 23 to 132 days after stroke.	FMA zero to 66.	AO (reach and grasp action by left or right hands), observation of nonbiological videos, and the eye close condition.	EEG.	Failure to imitate correlated with diminished mu suppression in patients with IPL or IFG pars opercularis damage.
Kuk et al. [51]	20 chronic stroke patients (>six months after stroke); EG ($n = 10$): stroke patients aged 60.0 ± 9.36; CG ($n = 10$): stroke patients aged 59.70 ± 6.58.	With the ability to grasp a small cube (2.5 cm^3) by the paretic hand.	EG: AO (watching videos of the actions of BBT performed by both hands), followed by performing the same task; CG: observation of nonbiological videos, followed by performing the same task.	EEG ($n = 10$, only for EG).	MTG was not activated after five sessions of AO, compared with pretraining.
Tani et al. [58]	11 stroke patients (18 to 1919 days after stroke), aged 64.1 ± 7.8.	Brunnstrom stage of the hand III–V.	AO (open-and-grasp action by the paretic hand), MI (the same actions by the paretic hand), and fixation.	EEG.	AO induced stronger mu suppression over the ipsilesional SMC (C3 or C4) than MI.

EG: experimental group; CG: control group; FMA-UE: Fugl-Meyer assessment upper extremity; AO: action observation; IFG: inferior frontal gyrus; SMG: supramarginal gyrus; fMRI: functional magnetic resonance imaging; MVF: mirror visual feedback; PCC: posterior cingular cortex; MI: motor imagery; PMC: premotor cortex; SMC: sensorimotor cortex; S1: primary somatosensory cortex; M1: primary motor cortex; NHPT: nine-hole peg test; MTG: middle temporal gyrus; ITG: inferior temporal gyrus; SPL: superior parietal lobe; IPL: inferior parietal lobe; PMd: dorsal premotor cortex; SMC: sensorimotor cortex; CMA: Chedokee-McMaster motor assessment arm scale; CMH: Chedokee-McMaster motor assessment hand scale; BA: Broadman area; EEG: electroencephalography; IPS: intraparietal sulcus; ARAT: action research arm test; MEG: magnetoencephalography; BBT: box and block test; ERD: event-related desynchronization.

TABLE 4: Methodological assessment of included studies using the PEDro scale*.

Criterion	Ertelt et al. [22]	Michielsen et al. [52]	Bae et al. [45]	Sun et al. [28]
Eligibility criteria	Yes	Yes	No	Yes
Random allocation	1	1	1	1
Concealed allocation	0	1	0	0
Baseline comparability	1	1	1	1
Blind subjects	0	0	0	0
Blind therapists	0	0	0	0
Blind assessors	0	1	0	1
Adequate follow-up	1	1	0	1
Intention-to-treat analysis	0	1	0	1
Between group comparisons	1	1	1	1
Point estimates and variability	1	1	1	1
Total scores	5	8	4	7

*The PEDro scores were taken from the PEDro website, except Ertelt et al. [22] and Sun et al. [28], which were rated by our team.

with MVF resulted in a shifted activation toward the ipsilesional hemispheres in patients who have had strokes; hence, a more symmetrical state between the two hemispheres may be achieved [46, 52]; (3) AO induced broader brain activation in the frontal, parietal, temporal, and occipital areas in patients who have had strokes, which encompassed the MNS, as well as cortical areas of motor execution, including the primary motor cortex, PMC, and SMA [22, 47, 48, 50]; (4) mu suppression can be induced by AO in patients who have had strokes; however, mu suppression over the affected hemisphere is relatively diminished [13, 49, 58]; and (5) MVF [45] or AO [28] embedded in long-term rehabilitation could bring about additional neurophysiological effects in patients after they have had strokes, reflected by more evident mu suppression, which may indicate that MN activities can be increased by this training.

A classical pathological change following stroke involves the activities of the affected hemispheres being suppressed, while those of less affected hemispheres are heightened, due to interhemispheric competition rivalry [60]; hence, successful motor recovery in patients who have had strokes could be achieved by normalizing the interhemispheric asymmetricity and promoting the neuroplasticity of the ipsilesional motor cortex [61, 62]. As the present review has shown, long-term MVF can contribute to a shift in activation toward the affected hemisphere [46, 52]. Furthermore, MVF transiently attenuates the asymmetric activities of movement-related beta suppression [54]. These findings can partially explain the beneficial effects of MT, which induces more symmetrical activities between the two hemispheres in patients who have had strokes. This is in line with previous findings regarding the effects of MVF on the healthy brain [35]. However, evidence to support the way in which AO can induce a shift of activation toward the affected hemisphere is relatively limited [50].

The difference between the activation patterns of MVF and AO can be identified. MVF mainly activates the ipsilesional primary motor cortex [34, 40, 46, 52, 55], the PMC [46], the primary somatosensory cortex [34, 40, 55], and the IPL [34, 55]. Two articles (one study) using effective connectivity and DCM have proposed that MVF could increase the connectivity between the ipsilesional primary somatosensory and primary motor cortex [55]. This study also suggests that the activation of the ipsilesional primary motor cortex may arise from contralesional IPS [34], which is a part of the MNS. These results are in line with the assumed functions of the MNS: visuomotor transformation. However, this conclusion should be interpreted with caution, since some studies have not identified the MNS activation by MVF in either patients who have had strokes [53] or healthy subjects [35]. The studies by Saleh et al. did not choose another frontal MNS (e.g., PMC) as the node in the DCM [34, 55]. As the first fMRI study with DCM that supports the activation of the MNS induced by MVF and its subsequent effects on the activation of the primary motor cortex [34], it is worthwhile to further explore the neural network underlying the MVF, in order to explain the role of the MNS in the network.

For AO, the activated brain regions were much broader, including IFG [47, 50], the PMC [22, 47, 48], the IPL [47], the primary motor cortex [47, 50], and temporal and occipital structures, which encompass the parietofrontal MNS as well as the cortical areas for motor execution (e.g., the primary motor cortex, PMC, and SMA). Small et al. proposed a model of brain repair after a stroke, which hypothesized that the MNS activation induced by AO may promote the reorganization of the cortical motor loop (i.e., the primary motor cortex, PMC, and SMA), thereby improving the motor functions of stroke survivors [63]. Our findings provide anatomical evidence to support this model. Observations of the bimanual action elicited a similar activation pattern as the execution of the same action in one study [47], whereas another study showed that AO (of a simple wrist movement) activated a part of the PMC and IPL, which did not resemble the activation pattern of action execution to such a great extent [56]. This difference may be attributed to different experimental paradigms of AO. The AO network, which may be involved in the understanding of motor intention, may have a stronger response to an object-directed or goal-directed action [64, 65], relative to a single action without meaning, although this is still inconclusive [66]. All in all, the results are still consistent with previously defined bilateral AO networks in healthy human brains [29, 30]. The neural network underlying the AO remains unclear.

The activation patterns of MVF and AO are obviously different. AO elicited broader activation of the frontal, parietal, temporal, and occipital areas, while the activated regions of MVF mainly covered the frontal and parietal structures. The difference between these two regimens is that the participants were required to perform bilateral or unilateral movement themselves when observing the visual feedback in the

MVF experiments, while this was not required in the AO experiments. Previous studies have assumed that there are different neural networks in response to AO and MVF [35, 67], and this opinion was confirmed by the present review in the stroke cohorts. Even though the underlying neural network cannot be fully understood at this stage, MNS activation seems to play a key role in both AO- and MVF-induced functional plasticities. There have been several TMS studies that have provided indirect evidence of the activation of the primary motor cortex by AO or MVF [27, 68]. Therefore, these two modalities can be viewed as optional motor priming tools for stroke rehabilitation. However, there is still a lack of studies directly comparing the clinical improvements and the pattern of neuroplasticity induced by MVF and AO [69] and whether or not the activation pattern is congruent with the clinical improvements in patients with stroke.

Brain waveforms recorded by EEG are altered by AO, reflected by lower alpha power and higher beta power over the frontal, central, and occipital electrodes [41, 42]. Some studies have also shown that the electrophysiological responses to AO may decrease after repetitive stimulations [43, 51]. These changes may be related to the changes in cognitive activities related to the understanding of motor intention after receiving visual feedback [70]. However, pure spectrum analysis is less likely than detailed EEG analyses, for example, time-frequency analysis, to reflect MN activity and stroke recovery [71, 72]. A recent meta-analysis indicated that both AO and action execution could induce the suppression of mu rhythm with a significant effect size [73]. This property of dual activation makes the mu suppression a signature of human mirror neuron activity [37, 74]. Regarding the studies included in the present review, two articles investigated AO-induced mu suppression in stroke individuals and its relationship with brain lesions [13, 49]. They found that the magnitude of mu suppression was reduced in the affected hemisphere, relative to the unaffected hemisphere, which was also identified by another study [58]. Two RCTs demonstrated that AO- or MI-induced mu suppression can be enhanced after long-term AOT [28] or training with MVF [45], which implies enhanced MN activities after the AO or MI training. Lesion analysis also showed that the damage over IPL or IFG was correlated with the diminished mu suppression, which indicates that mu suppression may be a specific index of MN activities [13, 16, 49].

One study demonstrated that behavioral improvement is correlated with the neural response to AO (measured by fMRI) in stroke individuals, which indicates that the AO-induced neural response is likely to be an indicator that can evaluate the arm motor recovery of patients who have had strokes within the first three months [47]. As the MNS is correlated with motion imitation [75], its activation may be a neurobiomarker that can measure the potential of motor learning in patients who have had strokes [47], which could also be measured by mu suppression. The predictive value of mu suppression and its relationship with motor improvement remain speculative. Other frequency bands related to action execution and AO, such as the beta band, might also be suitable candidates in regard to measuring MN activities [38, 76], although evidence of this in the stroke population is fairly limited [54]. As EEG is a relatively low-cost technique, further studies are encouraged to longitudinally explore the role of the ERD of different frequency ranges over various brain regions in patients who have had strokes. This neurobiomarker may also serve as a useful reference of the patients' motor recovery trajectory and motor relearning potential, promoted by MNS activation in stroke individuals.

There are some limitations in the present review. First, the heterogeneous protocols of AO and MVF and different experimental designs in regard to implementing neuroimaging hindered us from giving a firm and precise conclusion. Second, potentially confounding factors cannot be fully explained, based on currently available evidence, such as the dominance of handedness [48] and the nature of stroke lesions [48], which may result in different responses to AO and MVF. Further studies are warranted to answer these questions. Finally, restricting our review to English publications may have resulted in language bias.

5. Conclusions

MVF may contribute to stroke recovery by revising the interhemispheric imbalance, and MNS recruitment may be one of the potential neural mechanisms in this process. AO is associated with the activation of the MNS and motor cortex, which may promote motor relearning in stroke individuals. More rigorous studies with functional neuroimaging or electrophysiological techniques should be performed to further explain the different functional neural networks underlying AO or MVF and to explore the relationship between MN activities and clinical recovery in patients who have had strokes.

Abbreviations

AO: Action observation
MVF: Mirror visual feedback
MNS: Mirror neuron system
fMRI: Functional magnetic resonance imaging
EEG: Electroencephalography
CIMT: Constraint-induced movement training
VR: Virtual reality
IFG: Inferior frontal gyrus
PMv: Ventral premotor cortex
IPL: Inferior parietal lobule
IPS: Intraparietal sulcus
MT: Mirror therapy
MEG: Magnetoencephalography
PET: Positron emission tomography
NIRS: Near-infrared spectrometry
ERD: Event-related desynchronization
DCM: Dynamic casual modelling
PMC: Premotor cortex
SMC: Sensorimotor cortex
MI: Motor imagery
STG: Superior temporal gyrus
SMA: Supplementary motor area
SMG: Supramarginal gyrus
PCC: Posterior cingulate cortex
MFG: Middle frontal gyrus.

Conflicts of Interest

The authors declare that they have no conflicts of interest.

Acknowledgments

This work was partially funded by a grant from the General Research Fund (GRF) (Grant no. 151039/15M), Research Grants Council, University Grants Committee, Hong Kong, to Kenneth N. K. Fong.

References

[1] B. H. Dobkin, "Rehabilitation after stroke," *New England Journal of Medicine*, vol. 352, no. 16, pp. 1677–1684, 2005.

[2] A. C. Lo, P. D. Guarino, L. G. Richards et al., "Robot-assisted therapy for long-term upper-limb impairment after stroke," *New England Journal of Medicine*, vol. 362, no. 19, pp. 1772–1783, 2010.

[3] G. Kwakkel, J. M. Veerbeek, E. E. H. van Wegen, and S. L. Wolf, "Constraint-induced movement therapy after stroke," *The Lancet Neurology*, vol. 14, no. 2, pp. 224–234, 2015.

[4] K. E. Laver, S. George, S. Thomas, J. E. Deutsch, and M. Crotty, "Virtual reality for stroke rehabilitation," *Cochrane Database of Systematic Reviews*, no. 2, article CD008349, 2015.

[5] Y. T. Fan, K. C. Lin, H. L. Liu, C. Y. Wu, Y. Y. Wai, and T. H. Lee, "Neural correlates of motor recovery after robot-assisted stroke rehabilitation: a case series study," *Neurocase*, vol. 22, no. 5, pp. 416–425, 2016.

[6] J. Liepert, W. H. R. Miltner, H. Bauder et al., "Motor cortex plasticity during constraint-induced movement therapy in stroke patients," *Neuroscience Letters*, vol. 250, no. 1, pp. 5–8, 1998.

[7] S. Saleh, G. Fluet, Q. Qiu, A. Merians, S. V. Adamovich, and E. Tunik, "Neural patterns of reorganization after intensive robot-assisted virtual reality therapy and repetitive task practice in patients with chronic stroke," *Frontiers in Neurology*, vol. 8, no. 452, p. 452, 2017.

[8] V. Ramachandran, "Plasticity and functional recovery in neurology," *Clinical Medicine*, vol. 5, no. 4, pp. 368–373, 2005.

[9] G. Rizzolatti and L. Craighero, "The mirror-neuron system," *Annual Review of Neuroscience*, vol. 27, no. 1, pp. 169–192, 2004.

[10] G. Rizzolatti and G. Luppino, "The cortical motor system," *Neuron*, vol. 31, no. 6, pp. 889–901, 2001.

[11] L. Fadiga, L. Fogassi, G. Pavesi, and G. Rizzolatti, "Motor facilitation during action observation: a magnetic stimulation study," *Journal of Neurophysiology*, vol. 73, no. 6, pp. 2608–2611, 1995.

[12] G. Buccino, S. Vogt, A. Ritzl et al., "Neural circuits underlying imitation learning of hand actions: an event-related fMRI study," *Neuron*, vol. 42, no. 2, pp. 323–334, 2004.

[13] S. Frenkel-Toledo, D. G. Liebermann, S. Bentin, and N. Soroker, "Dysfunction of the human mirror neuron system in ideomotor apraxia: evidence from mu suppression," *Journal of Cognitive Neuroscience*, vol. 28, no. 6, pp. 775–791, 2016.

[14] W. Chen, Q. Ye, X. Ji et al., "Mirror neuron system based therapy for aphasia rehabilitation," *Frontiers in Psychology*, vol. 6, p. 1665, 2015.

[15] T. F. Yuan and R. Hoff, "Mirror neuron system based therapy for emotional disorders," *Medical Hypotheses*, vol. 71, no. 5, pp. 722–726, 2008.

[16] A. Perry, S. N. Saunders, J. Stiso et al., "Effects of prefrontal cortex damage on emotion understanding: EEG and behavioural evidence," *Brain*, vol. 140, no. 4, pp. 1086–1099, 2017.

[17] K. A. Garrison, C. J. Winstein, and L. Aziz-Zadeh, "The mirror neuron system: a neural substrate for methods in stroke rehabilitation," *Neurorehabilitation and Neural Repair*, vol. 24, no. 5, pp. 404–412, 2010.

[18] J. A. Pineda, "Sensorimotor cortex as a critical component of an 'extended' mirror neuron system: does it solve the development, correspondence, and control problems in mirroring?," *Behavioral and Brain Functions*, vol. 4, no. 1, p. 47, 2008.

[19] G. Rizzolatti and C. Sinigaglia, "The functional role of the parieto-frontal mirror circuit: interpretations and misinterpretations," *Nature Reviews Neuroscience*, vol. 11, no. 4, pp. 264–274, 2010.

[20] T. F. Yuan, W. Chen, C. Shan et al., "Activity-dependent neurorehabilitation beyond physical trainings: "mental exercise" through mirror neuron activation," *CNS & Neurological Disorders - Drug Targets*, vol. 14, no. 10, pp. 1267–1271, 2015.

[21] E. Sarasso, M. Gemma, F. Agosta, M. Filippi, and R. Gatti, "Action observation training to improve motor function recovery: a systematic review," *Archives of Physiotherapy*, vol. 5, no. 1, p. 14, 2015.

[22] D. Ertelt, S. Small, A. Solodkin et al., "Action observation has a positive impact on rehabilitation of motor deficits after stroke," *NeuroImage*, vol. 36, pp. T164–T173, 2007.

[23] E. L. Altschuler, S. B. Wisdom, L. Stone et al., "Rehabilitation of hemiparesis after stroke with a mirror," *The Lancet*, vol. 353, no. 9169, pp. 2035-2036, 1999.

[24] K. Sugg, S. Müller, C. Winstein, D. Hathorn, and A. Dempsey, "Does action observation training with immediate physical practice improve hemiparetic upper-limb function in chronic stroke?," *Neurorehabilitation and Neural Repair*, vol. 29, no. 9, pp. 807–817, 2015.

[25] M. Franceschini, M. G. Ceravolo, M. Agosti et al., "Clinical relevance of action observation in upper-limb stroke rehabilitation: a possible role in recovery of functional dexterity. A randomized clinical trial," *Neurorehabilitation and Neural Repair*, vol. 26, no. 5, pp. 456–462, 2012.

[26] T. Cowles, A. Clark, K. Mares, G. Peryer, R. Stuck, and V. Pomeroy, "Observation-to-imitate plus practice could add little to physical therapy benefits within 31 days of stroke: translational randomized controlled trial," *Neurorehabilitation and Neural Repair*, vol. 27, no. 2, pp. 173–182, 2013.

[27] J. Fu, M. Zeng, F. Shen et al., "Effects of action observation therapy on upper extremity function, daily activities and motion evoked potential in cerebral infarction patients," *Medicine*, vol. 96, no. 42, article e8080, 2017.

[28] Y. Sun, W. Wei, Z. Luo, H. Gan, and X. Hu, "Improving motor imagery practice with synchronous action observation in stroke patients," *Topics in Stroke Rehabilitation*, vol. 23, no. 4, pp. 245–253, 2016.

[29] S. Caspers, K. Zilles, A. R. Laird, and S. B. Eickhoff, "ALE meta-analysis of action observation and imitation in the human brain," *NeuroImage*, vol. 50, no. 3, pp. 1148–1167, 2010.

[30] V. M. Pomeroy, C. A. Clark, J. S. G. Miller, J. C. Baron, H. S. Markus, and R. C. Tallis, "The potential for utilizing the "mirror neurone system" to enhance recovery of the severely

affected upper limb early after stroke: a review and hypothesis," *Neurorehabilitation and Neural Repair*, vol. 19, no. 1, pp. 4–13, 2005.

[31] V. S. Ramachandran and E. L. Altschuler, "The use of visual feedback, in particular mirror visual feedback, in restoring brain function," *Brain*, vol. 132, no. 7, pp. 1693–1710, 2009.

[32] K. Eng, E. Siekierka, P. Pyk et al., "Interactive visuo-motor therapy system for stroke rehabilitation," *Medical & Biological Engineering & Computing*, vol. 45, no. 9, pp. 901–907, 2007.

[33] S. F. M. Toh and K. N. K. Fong, "Systematic review on the effectiveness of mirror therapy in training upper limb hemiparesis after stroke," *Hong Kong Journal of Occupational Therapy*, vol. 22, no. 2, pp. 84–95, 2012.

[34] S. Saleh, M. Yarossi, T. Manuweera, S. Adamovich, and E. Tunik, "Network interactions underlying mirror feedback in stroke: a dynamic causal modeling study," *NeuroImage: Clinical*, vol. 13, pp. 46–54, 2017.

[35] F. J. A. Deconinck, A. R. P. Smorenburg, A. Benham, A. Ledebt, M. G. Feltham, and G. J. P. Savelsbergh, "Reflections on mirror therapy: a systematic review of the effect of mirror visual feedback on the brain," *Neurorehabilitation and Neural Repair*, vol. 29, no. 4, pp. 349–361, 2015.

[36] A. M. Auriat, J. L. Neva, S. Peters, J. K. Ferris, and L. A. Boyd, "A review of transcranial magnetic stimulation and multimodal neuroimaging to characterize post-stroke neuroplasticity," *Frontiers in Neurology*, vol. 6, p. 226, 2015.

[37] H. M. Hobson and D. V. M. Bishop, "Mu suppression – a good measure of the human mirror neuron system?," *Cortex*, vol. 82, pp. 290–310, 2016.

[38] S. D. Muthukumaraswamy and K. D. Singh, "Modulation of the human mirror neuron system during cognitive activity," *Psychophysiology*, vol. 45, no. 6, pp. 896–905, 2008.

[39] R. S. Calabrò, A. Naro, M. Russo et al., "The role of virtual reality in improving motor performance as revealed by EEG: a randomized clinical trial," *Journal of NeuroEngineering and Rehabilitation*, vol. 14, no. 1, p. 53, 2017.

[40] F. Guo, Q. Xu, H. M. Abo Salem, Y. Yao, J. Lou, and X. Huang, "The neuronal correlates of mirror therapy: a functional magnetic resonance imaging study on mirror-induced visual illusions of ankle movements," *Brain Research*, vol. 1639, pp. 186–193, 2016.

[41] J. Kim, B. Lee, H. S. Lee, K. H. Shin, M. J. Kim, and E. Son, "Differences in brain waves of normal persons and stroke patients during action observation and motor imagery," *Journal of Physical Therapy Science*, vol. 26, no. 2, pp. 215–218, 2014.

[42] J. H. Kim and B. H. Lee, "Action observation training for functional activities after stroke: a pilot randomized controlled trial," *NeuroRehabilitation*, vol. 33, no. 4, pp. 565–574, 2013.

[43] M. Y. Chang, H. H. Kim, K. M. Kim, J. S. Oh, C. Jang, and T. H. Yoon, "Effects of observation of hand movements reflected in a mirror on cortical activation in patients with stroke," *Journal of Physical Therapy Science*, vol. 29, no. 1, pp. 38–42, 2017.

[44] M. Martin, K. Nitschke, L. Beume et al., "Brain activity underlying tool-related and imitative skills after major left hemisphere stroke," *Brain*, vol. 139, no. 5, pp. 1497–1516, 2016.

[45] S. H. Bae, W. S. Jeong, and K. Y. Kim, "Effects of mirror therapy on subacute stroke patients' brain waves and upper extremity functions," *Journal of Physical Therapy Science*, vol. 24, no. 11, pp. 1119–1122, 2012.

[46] A. Bhasin, R. Bhatia, S. S. Kumaran, S. Mohanty, and M. V. Padma Srivastava, "Neural interface of mirror therapy in chronic stroke patients: a functional magnetic resonance imaging study," *Neurology India*, vol. 60, no. 6, pp. 570–576, 2012.

[47] I. C. Brunner, J. S. Skouen, L. Ersland, and R. Gruner, "Plasticity and response to action observation: a longitudinal fMRI study of potential mirror neurons in patients with subacute stroke," *Neurorehabilitation and Neural Repair*, vol. 28, no. 9, pp. 874–884, 2014.

[48] C. Dettmers, V. Nedelko, and M. Ariel Schoenfeld, "Impact of left versus right hemisphere subcortical stroke on the neural processing of action observation and imagery," *Restorative Neurology and Neuroscience*, vol. 33, no. 5, pp. 701–712, 2015.

[49] S. Frenkel-Toledo, S. Bentin, A. Perry, D. G. Liebermann, and N. Soroker, "Mirror-neuron system recruitment by action observation: effects of focal brain damage on mu suppression," *NeuroImage*, vol. 87, pp. 127–137, 2014.

[50] K. A. Garrison, L. Aziz-Zadeh, S. W. Wong, S. L. Liew, and C. J. Winstein, "Modulating the motor system by action observation after stroke," *Stroke*, vol. 44, no. 8, pp. 2247–2253, 2013.

[51] E. J. Kuk, J. M. Kim, D. W. Oh, and H. J. Hwang, "Effects of action observation therapy on hand dexterity and EEG-based cortical activation patterns in patients with post-stroke hemiparesis," *Topics in Stroke Rehabilitation*, vol. 23, no. 5, pp. 318–325, 2016.

[52] M. E. Michielsen, R. W. Selles, J. N. van der Geest et al., "Motor recovery and cortical reorganization after mirror therapy in chronic stroke patients: a phase II randomized controlled trial," *Neurorehabilitation and Neural Repair*, vol. 25, no. 3, pp. 223–233, 2011.

[53] M. E. Michielsen, M. Smits, G. M. Ribbers et al., "The neuronal correlates of mirror therapy: an fMRI study on mirror induced visual illusions in patients with stroke," *Journal of Neurology, Neurosurgery & Psychiatry*, vol. 82, no. 4, pp. 393–398, 2011.

[54] H. E. Rossiter, M. R. Borrelli, R. J. Borchert, D. Bradbury, and N. S. Ward, "Cortical mechanisms of mirror therapy after stroke," *Neurorehabilitation and Neural Repair*, vol. 29, no. 5, pp. 444–452, 2015.

[55] S. Saleh, S. V. Adamovich, and E. Tunik, "Mirrored feedback in chronic stroke: recruitment and effective connectivity of ipsilesional sensorimotor networks," *Neurorehabilitation and Neural Repair*, vol. 28, no. 4, pp. 344–354, 2014.

[56] A. J. Szameitat, S. Shen, A. Conforto, and A. Sterr, "Cortical activation during executed, imagined, observed, and passive wrist movements in healthy volunteers and stroke patients," *NeuroImage*, vol. 62, no. 1, pp. 266–280, 2012.

[57] J. Wang, C. Fritzsch, J. Bernarding et al., "Cerebral activation evoked by the mirror illusion of the hand in stroke patients compared to normal subjects," *NeuroRehabilitation*, vol. 33, no. 4, pp. 593–603, 2013.

[58] M. Tani, Y. Ono, M. Matsubara et al., "Action observation facilitates motor cortical activity in patients with stroke and hemiplegia," *Neuroscience Research*, 2017.

[59] M. Brunetti, N. Morkisch, C. Fritzsch et al., "Potential determinants of efficacy of mirror therapy in stroke patients – a pilot study," *Restorative Neurology and Neuroscience*, vol. 33, no. 4, pp. 421–434, 2015.

[60] P. Marque, D. Gasq, E. Castel-Lacanal, X. De Boissezon, and I. Loubinoux, "Post-stroke hemiplegia rehabilitation: evolution of the concepts," *Annals of Physical and Rehabilitation Medicine*, vol. 57, no. 8, pp. 520–529, 2014.

[61] T. Askim, B. Indredavik, T. Vangberg, and A. Haberg, "Motor network changes associated with successful motor skill relearning after acute ischemic stroke: a longitudinal functional magnetic resonance imaging study," *Neurorehabilitation and Neural Repair*, vol. 23, no. 3, pp. 295–304, 2009.

[62] D. A. Nowak, C. Grefkes, M. Ameli, and G. R. Fink, "Interhemispheric competition after stroke: brain stimulation to enhance recovery of function of the affected hand," *Neurorehabilitation and Neural Repair*, vol. 23, no. 7, pp. 641–656, 2009.

[63] S. L. Small, G. Buccino, and A. Solodkin, "Brain repair after stroke—a novel neurological model," *Nature Reviews Neurology*, vol. 9, no. 12, pp. 698–707, 2013.

[64] L. Koski, A. Wohlschläger, H. Bekkering et al., "Modulation of motor and premotor activity during imitation of target-directed actions," *Cerebral Cortex*, vol. 12, no. 8, pp. 847–855, 2002.

[65] S. L. Liew, K. A. Garrison, J. Werner, and L. Aziz-Zadeh, "The mirror neuron system: innovations and implications for occupational therapy," *OTJR: Occupation, Participation and Health*, vol. 32, no. 3, pp. 79–86, 2012.

[66] R. Newman-Norlund, H. T. van Schie, M. E. C. van Hoek, R. H. Cuijpers, and H. Bekkering, "The role of inferior frontal and parietal areas in differentiating meaningful and meaningless object-directed actions," *Brain Research*, vol. 1315, pp. 63–74, 2010.

[67] F. Hamzei, C. H. Lappchen, V. Glauche, I. Mader, M. Rijntjes, and C. Weiller, "Functional plasticity induced by mirror training: the mirror as the element connecting both hands to one hemisphere," *Neurorehabilitation and Neural Repair*, vol. 26, no. 5, pp. 484–496, 2012.

[68] Y. Kang, H. Park, H. Kim et al., "Upper extremity rehabilitation of stroke: facilitation of corticospinal excitability using virtual mirror paradigm," *Journal of NeuroEngineering and Rehabilitation*, vol. 9, no. 1, p. 71, 2012.

[69] T. Y. Shih, C. Y. Wu, K. C. Lin et al., "Effects of action observation therapy and mirror therapy after stroke on rehabilitation outcomes and neural mechanisms by MEG: study protocol for a randomized controlled trial," *Trials*, vol. 18, no. 1, p. 459, 2017.

[70] L. Fogassi, P. F. Ferrari, B. Gesierich, S. Rozzi, F. Chersi, and G. Rizzolatti, "Parietal lobe: from action organization to intention understanding," *Science*, vol. 308, no. 5722, pp. 662–667, 2005.

[71] S. Giaquinto, A. Cobianchi, F. Macera, and G. Nolfe, "EEG recordings in the course of recovery from stroke," *Stroke*, vol. 25, no. 11, pp. 2204–2209, 1994.

[72] C. Neuper, M. Wortz, and G. Pfurtscheller, "ERD/ERS patterns reflecting sensorimotor activation and deactivation," *Progress in Brain Research*, vol. 159, pp. 211–222, 2006.

[73] N. A. Fox, M. J. Bakermans-Kranenburg, K. H. Yoo et al., "Assessing human mirror activity with EEG mu rhythm: a meta-analysis," *Psychological Bulletin*, vol. 142, no. 3, pp. 291–313, 2016.

[74] H. M. Hobson and D. V. M. Bishop, "The interpretation of mu suppression as an index of mirror neuron activity: past, present and future," *Royal Society Open Science*, vol. 4, no. 3, article 160662, 2017.

[75] G. Rizzolatti, L. Cattaneo, M. Fabbri-Destro, and S. Rozzi, "Cortical mechanisms underlying the organization of goal-directed actions and mirror neuron-based action understanding," *Physiological Reviews*, vol. 94, no. 2, pp. 655–706, 2014.

[76] C. Babiloni, C. del Percio, F. Vecchio et al., "Alpha, beta and gamma electrocorticographic rhythms in somatosensory, motor, premotor and prefrontal cortical areas differ in movement execution and observation in humans," *Clinical Neurophysiology*, vol. 127, no. 1, pp. 641–654, 2016.

15

Newly Generated Cells in the Dentate Gyrus Differentially Respond to Brief Spatial Exploration and Forced Swim in Adult Female Balb/C Mice

Gerardo Bernabé Ramírez-Rodríguez, María del Ángel Ocaña-Fernández, and Leonardo Ortiz-López

Laboratory of Neurogenesis, Division of Clinical Research, National Institute of Psychiatry "Ramón de la Fuente Muñiz", Calzada México-Xochimilco 101, 14370 Mexico City, Mexico

Correspondence should be addressed to Gerardo Bernabé Ramírez-Rodríguez; gbernabe@imp.edu.mx

Academic Editor: Michele Fornaro

Neurogenesis in the hippocampus is influenced by several factors including external stimuli. In addition to their involvement in learning and memory processes, newborn neurons of the dentate gyrus (DG) buffer against the effects of stress. Although the response of these cells to environmental stimuli has been shown, the age of the cells that respond to a brief spatial exploration or a stressful situation produced by forced-swim stress in adult female Balb/C mice is still unknown. Here, we investigated the activation of newborn neurons after three (IdU) or six weeks (CldU) postlabelling with the expression of Arc in the same mice but exposed to different environmental stimuli. Mice housed in standard conditions showed an increase in the activation of CldU-labelled cells after two exposures to a brief spatial exploration but no increase in the activation of IdU-labelled cells compared with the control group. Additionally, we analysed neuronal activation in the DG of mice housed in standard conditions and further exposed to forced-swim stress. We found a decreased activation of IdU-labelled cells in mice exposed to forced-swim stress with increase number of CldU-labelled cells. Our results suggest that based on their time postlabelling, newly generated hippocampal neurons show a different response to several environmental stimuli.

1. Introduction

The generation of newborn neurons in the DG of the hippocampus during adulthood is regulated by several external stimuli (i.e., [1–4]). Among them, voluntary physical activity and environmental enrichment have proven to have beneficial effects on neuroplasticity in, but not limited to, the hippocampus (i.e., [1–4]). Additionally, hippocampal neurogenesis is negatively regulated by stressful paradigms such as acute stress, psychosocial stress, or unpredictable chronic mild stress (i.e., [4, 5]).

Interestingly, newly generated hippocampal neurons play an important role in the processing of information related to spatial memory (i.e., [6–8]). Additionally, the presence of more neurons in the DG is indicative for their participation in the adaptation to complex environments, particularly because newborn neurons can help buffer the effects of stress (i.e., [9, 10]).

The enrolment of newly generated neurons in information processing has been studied by examining the expression of immediate early gene (IEG) products such as c-Fos, zif268, and activity-regulated cytoskeletal-associated protein (Arc) (i.e., [11–19]). The IEGs are transiently and rapidly induced in response to several stimuli. These genes and their products have relevant roles in several processes including brain development, learning, and long-term synaptic plasticity (for review, see [20]).

Additionally, depending on the age of the newborn neurons, they have been suggested to be able to be involved not only in processing specific information such as spatial learning, spatial memory retrieval, contextual memory, and spatial exploration but also in processing a stressful experience in rodents (i.e., [11–21]).

In this sense, hippocampal newly generated cells of ages ranging between 28 and 42 days old in C57Bl6 mice previously exposed to voluntary physical activity show a decrease in activation after exposure to a cold forced-swim stress [17]. Moreover, no difference was found in cells 7 and 84 days old after forced-swim exposure in mice preexposed to ENR conditions [22].

Despite the information related to the activation of newborn cells in the DG, there is still a discrepancy, from our point of view, in the age of newborn hippocampal cells that are activated in response to different environmental stimuli. Thus, we hypothesized that depending on their age, newborn neurons will differentially respond to environmental stimuli. Then, we determined the age and the environmental stimuli to which newly generated cells in the DG respond in adult female Balb/C mice, a strain of mice with low baseline adult neurogenesis [23] but with the capability to reflect the regulation of adult hippocampal neurogenesis (i.e., [24–26]). We exposed standard housed mice to different configurations of spatial exploration or to forced-swim stress as was previously reported for rats and mice [11] to explore the response of newly generated cells, at 3 or 6 weeks postlabelling, to the environmental stimuli.

2. Materials and Methods

2.1. Animals. Thirty Balb/C female mice were used in this study. They were held in standard laboratory cages with 12 h light/12 h dark cycles at a temperature of $23 \pm 1^{\circ}$C in the animal facilities of the National Institute of Psychiatry Ramón de la Fuente Muñiz. Mice had access to food and water ad libitum and were left to acclimate to their environment until animals reached ten weeks of age. All institutional and legal regulations regarding animal ethics and handling were followed for in vivo experiments (IACUC: CEI/C/009/2013).

2.2. CldU and IdU Labelling. All animals were injected intraperitoneally (ip) with two analogues of thymidine: 5-chloro-2′-deoxyuridine (CldU) and 5-iodo-2′-deoxyuridine (IdU) (MP Biomedicals, Santa Ana, CA, USA). On the first day of housing, all mice received a single injection of CldU (42.5 mg/kg), and on the twenty-first day of housing, all mice received one single IdU injection (57.5 mg/kg) [27]. Six weeks later, after the beginning of the housing protocol, mice experienced a behavioural task. With this procedure, we identified newborn cells at 21 days postlabelling (IdU) or 42 days postlabelling (CldU).

2.3. Experiments

2.3.1. Experiment 1. Mice were maintained in standard housing conditions, and on day 42, animals experienced a behavioural task. Animals were distributed into four groups: (1) mice decapitated directly from their cages (control, CTL); (2) mice that explored environment A once (A); (3) mice that explored environment A twice, each separated by 20 min (A + A); or (4) mice that explored two different environments, A and B, each separated by 20 min (A + B). The exploration time in each environment was 5 min. Mice were adapted to handling and transportation procedures for 3 minutes each day for seven consecutive days before the behavioural task. The day before environmental explorations, animals were left undisturbed.

Environment A was a square open box (30 × 30 cm) with 8.5 cm high walls, two of which were covered with black foamy paper. The box was divided into nine squares; two of them were covered by brown corrugated paper. Environment A was placed in a rectangular room (2 × 1.5 m) with spatial stimuli on the walls.

Environment B was a rectangular open box (25 × 35 cm) with 8.5 cm high walls; two of which were covered with blue foamy paper. The box was divided in 8 rectangular sections; three of which were covered with green corrugated paper. Exposure to environment B was done in another room of similar size but with different spatial stimuli on the walls. Both environments, A and B, were different; however, they had a similar level of complexity [11]. In each exploration session, mice were lifted and randomly placed in the centre of the grids of the corresponding explored environment for 15 seconds for a total period of five minutes [11, 21]. Fifty-five minutes after the first environmental exposure, mice were sacrificed.

2.3.2. Experiment 2. To test the effect of stress on Arc protein expression in newly generated cells, mice were exposed or not exposed to forced-swim stress on day 42. Mice were maintained in standard housing conditions for six weeks. Mice were divided into two groups: (1) mice housed in standard conditions and sacrificed directly from their cages (No-FS) or (2) mice housed in standard conditions followed by exposure to forced-swim stress (FS).

The forced-swim stress paradigm, also known as Porsolt's test, is a test that measures an animal's response to a stressful situation in which they are forced to swim in a cylinder from which there is no opportunity for escape. Mice were gently placed in a cylinder (18 cm in diameter) filled with water maintained at room temperature to a depth of approximately 15 cm. Each mouse was tested for 6 min; the first 2 min served as a habituation period. The time spent immobile during the last 4 min was recorded. Immobility was assessed when a mouse was floating in the water without struggling and only making movements necessary to keep its head above water. After testing, each mouse was gently dried and returned to their cage covered by an absorbent paper towel [28, 29]. Fifty-four minutes later, mice were sacrificed by transcardial perfusion [30].

2.4. Tissue Preparation. Brains were immersed in 4% *p*-formaldehyde and kept for 7 days. Then, brains were cryoprotected before they were cut into 40 μm coronal sections on a sliding microtome (Leica, Buffalo Grove, IL, USA). The sections were stored at 4°C in cryoprotective solution containing 25% ethylene glycol and 25% glycerol in 0.05 M phosphate buffer [30].

2.5. Immunohistochemistry and Immunofluorescence. Sections were stained following the free-floating immunohistochemistry method [30]. To visualize the expression of Arc protein, IdU, and CldU, we used the peroxidase method, as previously described [30]. For IdU and CldU immunodetection, brain slices were pretreated with 2 N HCl for 30 min at 37°C followed by 2 washes in 0.1 M borate buffer (pH 8.5) for 10 min each. The antibodies used were the rat anti-BrdU (CldU; 1:500; Accurate), mouse anti-BrdU (IdU; 1:500; BD Pharmingen), and rabbit anti-Arc antibody (1:5000; Synaptic Systems) to measure neuronal activation in the DG. Secondary antibodies were biotinylated and added for 2 additional hours of incubation at room temperature. All secondary antibodies were from Jackson ImmunoResearch Laboratories (West Grove, PA, USA). Finally, the cells that were positive for the different markers were visualized using the ABC-DAB system (Vector Labs; Burlingame, CA, USA). Sections were clarified and mounted with Neo-Mount medium (Merck Millipore; Naucalpan, Estado de México, México).

Identification of newly formed cells in the DG of adult mice that expressed the Arc protein was performed by double immunofluorescence (CldU/Arc or IdU/Arc). The primary antibodies were mouse anti-IdU, rat anti-CldU, and rabbit anti-Arc. The fluorophore coupled secondary antibodies were anti-rat FITC, anti-mouse FITC, and anti-rabbit TRITC. All secondary antibodies were raised in donkey and diluted 1:200 [31]. Sections were mounted in polyvinyl alcohol with diazabicyclo-octane as an antifading agent (PVA-DABCO).

2.6. Cellular Quantification and Neuronal Activation Colabelling. The number of IdU-, CldU-, and Arc-labelled cells was determined in series of every 6th section from all animals. Positive cells were counted using a 40x objective throughout the rostrocaudal extent of the granular cell layer on a light microscope (Leica) (Bregma −1.34 to −3.20). Counting was done as previously described with a modified optical fractionator method. The cells appearing in the uppermost focal plane were not counted [30]. The estimate of the total number of cells was calculated from the resulting numbers through multiplication by 6.

Analysis of newly formed cells activated in the DG was performed in a one-in-twelve series of sections from all animals. The number of IdU- and CldU-labelled cells coexpressing the Arc protein was quantified by confocal microscopy (TCS SP2, Leica, and on a Zeiss LSM 510 Meta, Zeiss, Ciudad de México, México) in a sequential scanning mode to avoid cross-bleeding between channels. Double labelling was confirmed by three-dimensional reconstructions of z-series covering the entire nucleus or cell in question. IdU-Arc or CldU-Arc cells were calculated from the percentages of the respective labelled cells and the total number of IdU- or CldU-labelled cells [25, 29, 30].

2.7. Statistical Analysis. Analysis was performed using SigmaStat 3.1 software (Systat Software Inc., Chicago, IL, USA). The results are presented as the mean ± standard error of the mean; SEM. Mean differences between two groups were analysed using unpaired Student's t-test. Mean differences among groups were analysed using a one-way ANOVA followed by Student-Newman-Keuls post hoc test. Differences were considered statistically significant at $p \leq 0.05$.

3. Results

3.1. Newborn Cells Generated in the Dentate Gyrus during Housing Conditions. To visualize IdU or CldU newborn cells in the same animals housed in standard conditions, we injected two analogues of thymidine (Figure 1(a)); we quantified IdU- and CldU-labelled cells in the DG (Figure 1(b)) of mice exposed to brief spatial exploration (CTL, A, A + A, or A + B) or in mice of the second experiment exposed to forced-swim stress. Mice of the first experiment did not show significant differences in the number of IdU- (CTL = 445 ± 63, A = 498 ± 60, A + A = 441 ± 41, and A + B = 451 ± 39; $F_{3,19} = 0.25$; $p = 0.85$) or CldU-labelled cells (CTL = 367 ± 43, A = 408 ± 104, A + A = 336 ± 82, and A + B = 367 ± 38; $F_{3,19} = 0.16$; $p = 0.91$) (Figure 1(c)). Moreover, mice of the second experiment exposed to forced-swim stress (FS) did not show significant differences in the number of IdU- or CldU-labelled cells compared with the not-exposed-to-FS group (No-FS) (IdU: No − FS = 339 ± 33, FS = 439 ± 54, $p = 0.16$; CldU: No − FS = 523 ± 59, FS = 414 ± 158, $p = 0.54$). Thus, these results showed newborn cells at 3 or 6 weeks after administration of different analogues of thymidine in the same mice.

3.2. Distribution of Arc in Cells of the Granular Cell Layer of the Dentate Gyrus. First, we studied Arc distribution in cells of the granular cell layer of the DG (Figures 2(a) and 2(b)). Arc cells showed a well-stained nucleus within oval or round somas. Also, some Arc-positive cells exhibited a short dendrite. Moreover, some Arc-positive cells showed one primary dendrite with one branching point or a well-defined dendrite projecting to the direction of and reaching the molecular layer. Similar distribution of Arc was observed by immunofluorescence (Figure 2(c)). In accordance with the images, we confirmed that Arc distribution was not limited to the nucleus of immunoreactive cells of the GCL of the DG.

3.3. Arc Expression Increased in the Dentate Gyrus after Spatial Exploration or Forced-Swim Stress. On day 42, mice experienced a brief spatial exploration task or were exposed to the forced-swim stress (Figures 3(a) and 4(a)). To assess the activation of granule cells in the DG in response to each task, we identified the cells labelled with Arc.

Analysis of experiment 1 showed significant differences among the groups ($F_{3,19} = 15.53$, $p < 0.001$; Figures 3(b) and 3(c)). The post hoc test did not show a difference between the *CTL* group (1106 ± 130 cells) and mice exposed to environment A a single time (1379 ± 63 cells; $p = 0.709$). However, there was a significant increase in the number of Arc-labelled cells in mice exposed to environment A twice *(2624 ± 231 cells)* compared with that in the control group ($p = 0.001$) or with that in mice exposed to environment A once ($p = 0.006$). Similarly, we found significant differences between group A + B (2780 ± 335 cells) and the control group ($p = 0.001$) and group A ($p = 0.002$). However, there was no significant difference between the mice in the A + A and A + B groups ($p = 0.961$).

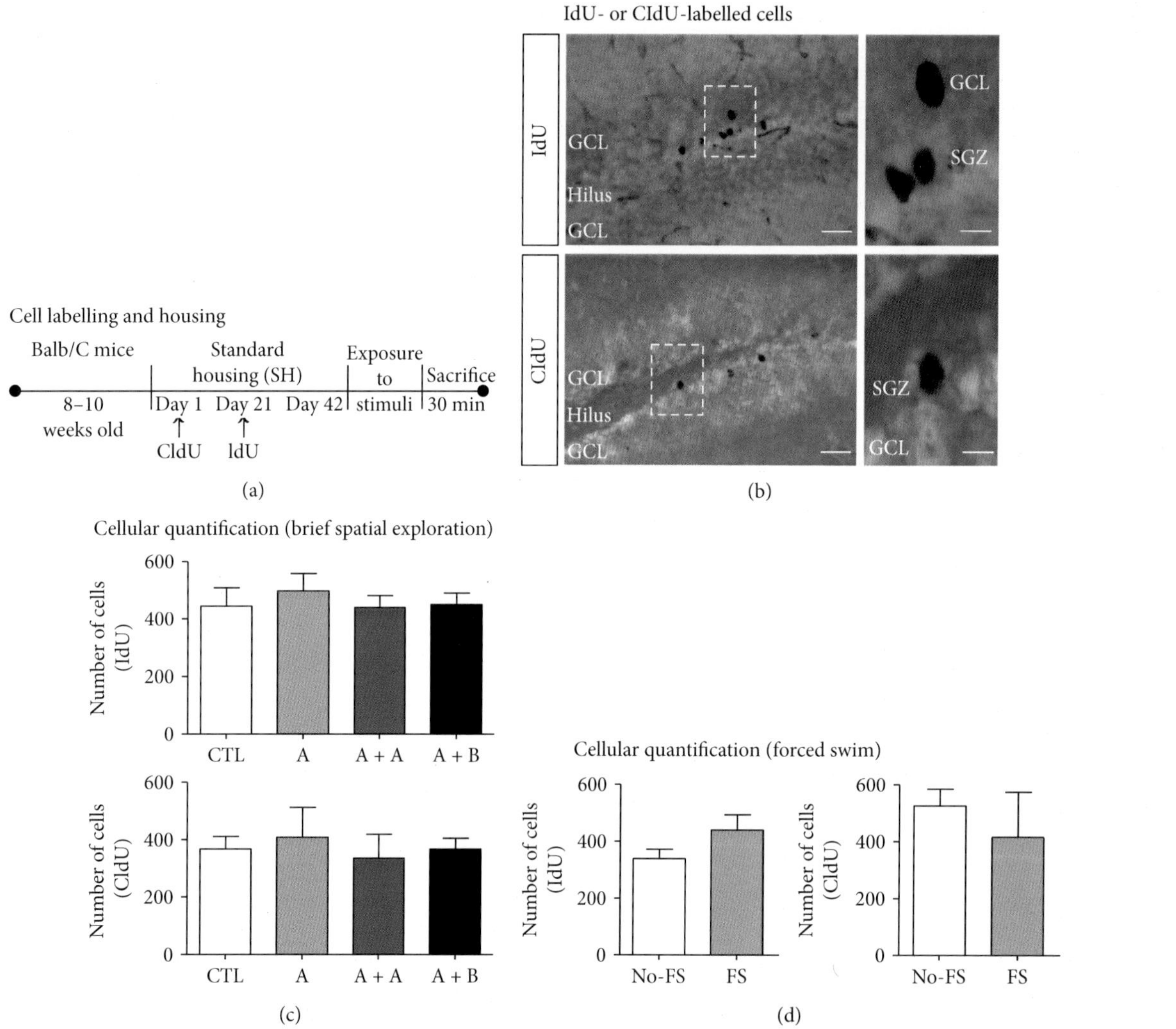

Figure 1: The experimental design to visualize newborn cells in the dentate gyrus of adult mice. (a) Female Balb/C mice were kept under standard housing (SH) conditions. Mice received one single injection of CldU (day 1) and another injection of IdU at day 21. Then, mice were housed for an additional 22 days in SH conditions. (b) Representative micrographs of IdU- or CldU-labelled cells in the SH group. High-power images exhibit the presence of IdU- or CldU-labelled cells. Labels identify granule cell layer (GCL), subgranular zone (SGZ), and the hilus. Scale bars are equal to 40 and 10 μm. (c) Quantification of IdU- and CldU-labelled cells was done in mice decapitated directly from their cages (control, CTL), mice that explored environment A once (a), mice that explored environment A twice, each separated by 20 min (A-A), or 4) mice that explored two different environments, (a) and (b), each separated by 20 min (A–B). $n = 5$ per group. Data are expressed as the mean ± SEM of the absolute number of Arc-cells, and comparisons in (c) were performed with a one-way ANOVA followed by Student-Newman-Keuls post hoc test. Also in the second experiment, cellular quantification was done in mice housed in standard conditions and sacrificed directly from their cages and not exposed to forced swim (No-FS) or mice housed in standard conditions followed by exposure to forced-swim stress (FS). $n = 5$ per group. Data are expressed as the mean ± SEM of the absolute number of Arc cells, and comparisons in (d) were performed with an unpaired Student t-test.

Moreover, analysis of Arc-labelled cells in experiment 2 (Figure 4(a)), in which mice were kept in standard conditions for 42 days followed by forced-swim exposure, revealed that the forced-swim condition showed a statistically significant effect on the expression of the Arc protein in the granule cells of the DG (Figures 4(b) and 4(c); No − FS = 948 ± 129 cells, FS = 1658 ± 186 cells; $p = 0.035$).

3.4. IdU-Labelled Cells Were Not Affected but CldU-Labelled Cells Increased Their Coexpressing Arc after Spatial Exploration. To obtain information about the activation of IdU- and CldU-labelled cells after behaviour, we analysed cells coexpressing the Arc protein as indicative of neuronal activation in the DG (Figure 5(a)). Analysis of IdU/Arc-labelled cells in the mice from experiment 1 reflected that the number of newborn cells at three weeks post-IdU labelling was not significantly increased in the DG of mice exposed once (125 ± 13 cells) or twice to environment A (131 ± 8 cells) compared to the cells found in mice of the control group (97 ± 11 cells). Moreover, no differences were found in mice exposed to environments A and B (83 ± 8 cells) when compared with the control mice. The one-way ANOVA yielded the following values: $F_{3,19} = 4.59$; $p = 0.016$; Figure 5(b)).

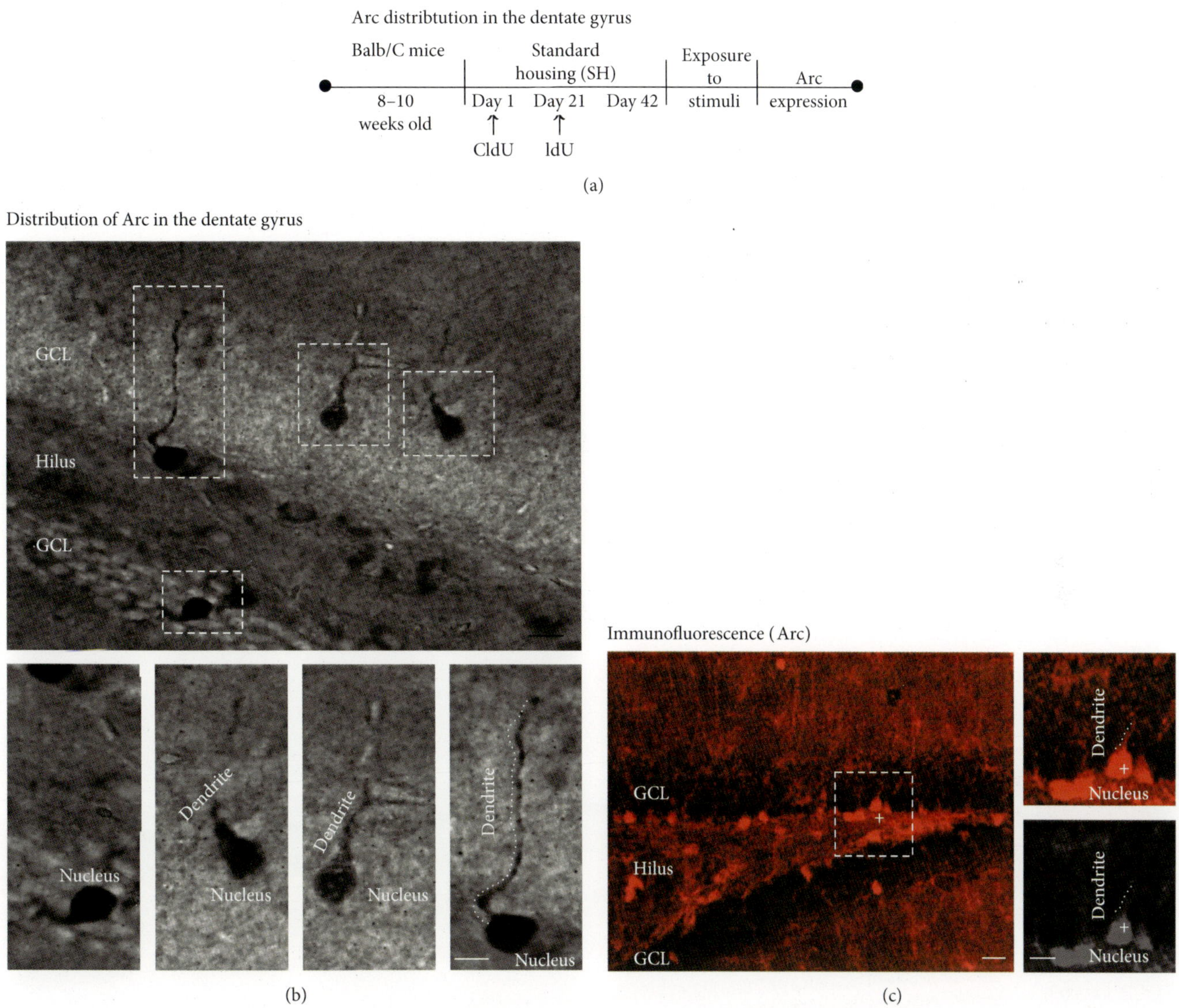

FIGURE 2: Arc expression in the dentate gyrus of adult mice. (a) Experimental design. (b) Arc-positive cells are present in the dentate gyrus. Bright field also shows the granule cell layer (GCL), hilus (H), and molecular layer (ML). High-power images exhibit the presence of Arc in the nucleus, and Arc labelling is present in the dendrites projecting to the ML. The scale bar in (b) is equal to 10 μm (c) Also, the distribution of Arc is shown by immunofluorescence. Scale bars in (c) are equal to 20 and 10 μm.

In addition, the analysis of CldU/Arc protein-labelled cells revealed that mice exposed once to environment A (75 ± 7 cells) showed a trend toward an increase in the number of CldU/Arc-labelled cells compared to control mice (38 ± 9 cells). However, mice exposed to environment A twice (106 ± 20 cells) or mice exposed to environment A followed by environment B (133 ± 9 cells) showed activation at six weeks post-CldU labelling of cells in the DG compared with the control group ($p = 0.03$ and $p = 0.001$, respectively; Figure 5(c)). Additionally, we found more CldU/Arc cells in mice exposed to environment A followed by environment B than in mice exposed once to environment A ($p = 0.03$), but no differences were found between groups A + A and A + B. The one-way ANOVA yielded the following values: $F3, 19 = 7.082$; $p = 0.0046$.

3.5. The Coexpressing Arc of IdU-Labelled Cells Decreased but That of CldU-Labelled Cells Increased after Forced-Swim Stress. The analysis of experiment 2 showed differences in the number of IdU/Arc-labelled cells among the different groups ($\text{No} - \text{FS} = 79 \pm 5$, $\text{FS} = 56 \pm 7$; $p = 0.047$ Figure 5(d)). However, the analysis of CldU/Arc-labelled cells revealed that mice exposed to forced-swim stress had more activated cells at six weeks post-CldU labelling in the DG ($\text{No} - \text{FS} = 43 \pm 9$, $\text{FS} = 75 \pm 5$; $p = 0.031$; Figure 5(e)).

4. Discussion

This study showed that newborn neurons of the DG exhibit differential activation after three or six weeks postlabelling

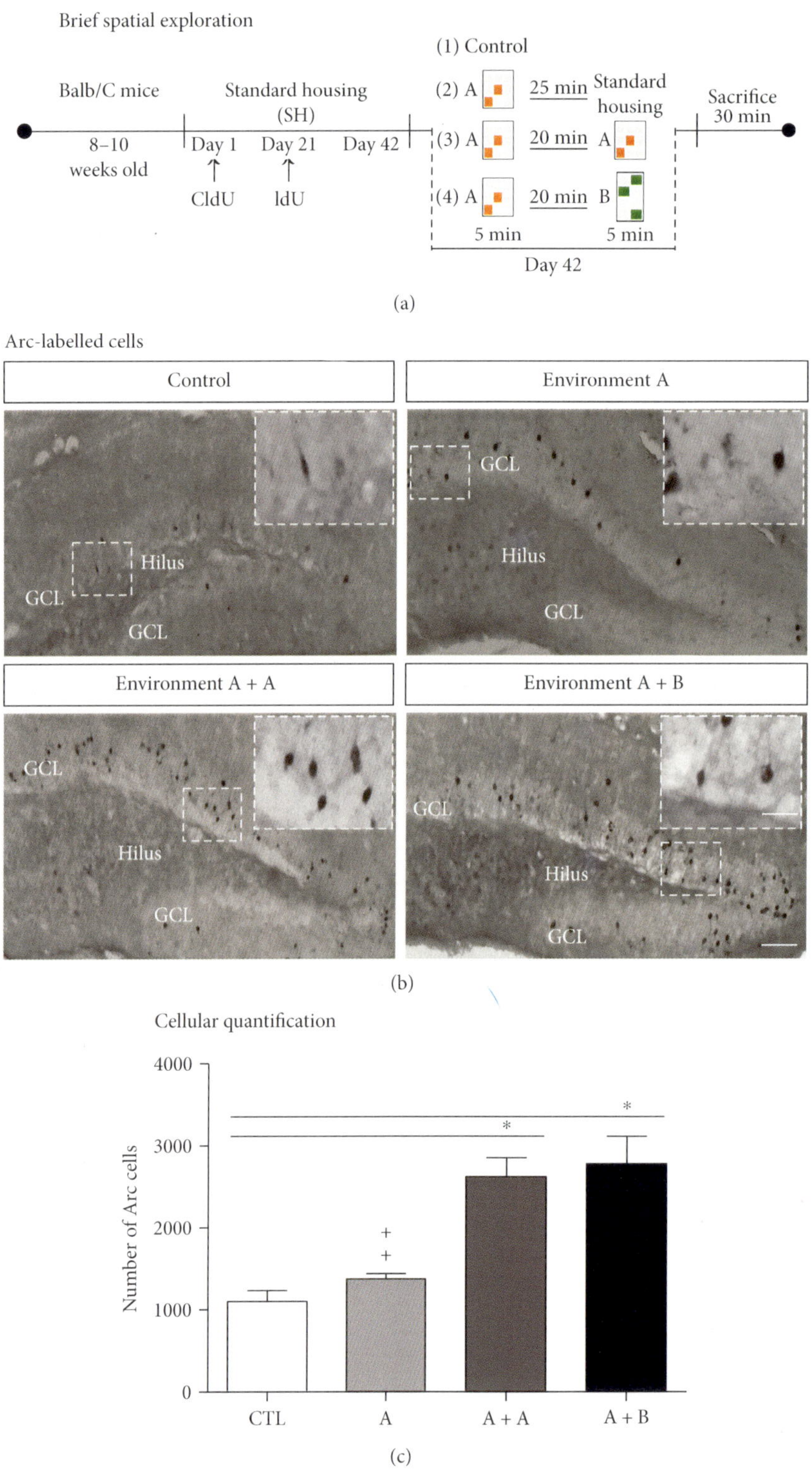

Figure 3: Neuronal activation in the dentate gyrus of adult mice after brief spatial exploration. (a) Experimental design. Female Balb/C mice kept under standard housing conditions were exposed to environment A, A + A, or A + B for 5 minutes as is described in Materials and Methods. (b) Representative micrographs of Arc-labelled cells in mice exposed to the different environments are shown. Scale bar in B is equal to 100 μm. Insets correspond to high-power images of Arc-positive cells. The scale bar in the inserts is equal to 40 μm. (c) Quantification of Arc-labelled cells showed more in the A + A and A + B groups than in the control (CTL) group. Asterisks indicate $p = 0.001$. Crosses indicate a significant difference between A and A + A ($p = 0.006$) or A and A + B ($p = 0.002$). Data are expressed as the mean ± SEM of the absolute number of Arc-cells, and comparisons in (c) were performed with a one-way ANOVA followed by Student-Newman-Keuls post hoc test. $n = 4 - 5$ per group.

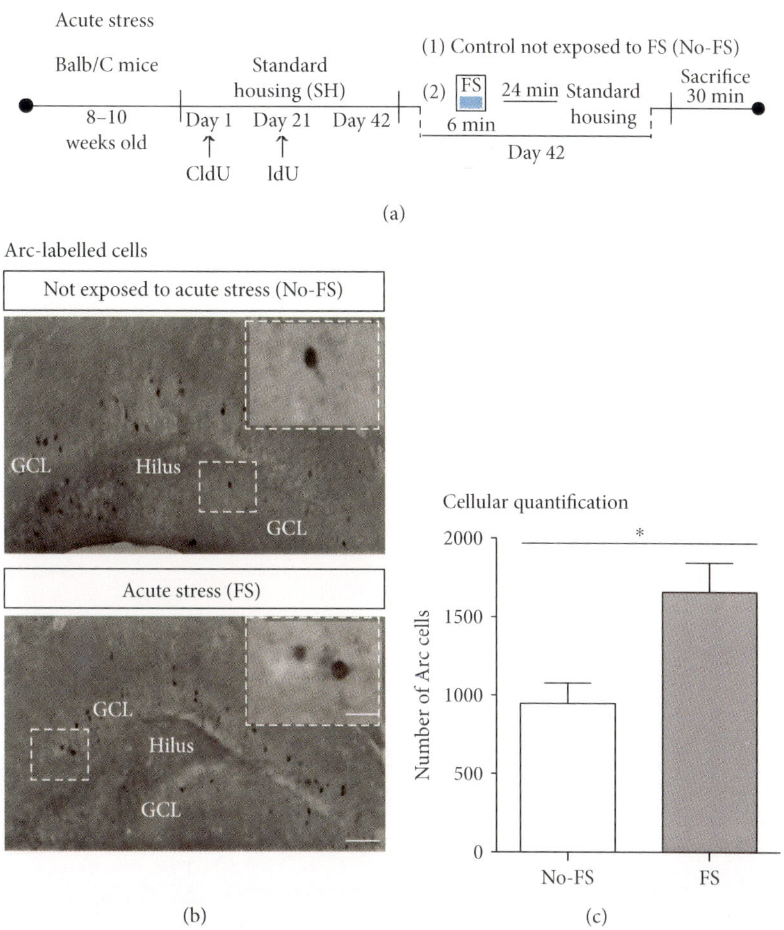

FIGURE 4: Neuronal activation in the dentate gyrus of adult mice after forced-swim exposure. (a) Experimental design. Female Balb/C mice kept under standard housing conditions were exposed to forced-swim stress (FS) for 5 minutes as described in Materials and Methods. (b) Representative micrographs of Arc-labelled cells in mice exposed to forced-swim are shown. The scale bar in B is equal to 100 μm. Insets correspond to high-power images of Arc-positive cells. The scale bar in the insets is equal to 20 μm. (c) Quantification of Arc-labelled cells showed more in the FS group than in the No-FS group. Asterisk indicate $p = 0.035$. Data are expressed as the mean ± SEM of the absolute number of Arc-cells, and comparisons in (c) were performed with unpaired Student's t-test. $n = 4 - 5$ per group.

in adult female Balb/C mice housed in standard conditions further exposed to a spatial exploration paradigm or to forced-swim stress (Figure 6).

4.1. Expression of Arc in the Dentate Gyrus of Adult Mice. Newborn hippocampal neurons are key elements that process information related to spatial exploration (i.e., [8]). In this regard, several studies have explored activation of newborn hippocampal neurons and have shown evidence of the enrolment of these cells in the processing of several types of information (i.e., [11–19]). Here, we exposed mice housed in standard conditions to a paradigm of spatial exploration that has been used mainly in rats and that assures standardization of the amount of space explored by each rodent (i.e., [11, 21]). In this sense, during spatial exploration, rodents are known to create a representation of the environment by activating neuronal circuits in the hippocampus (i.e., [11]). Thus, neuronal activation in the granular cell layer of the dentate gyrus has been studied by the expression of IEGs including Arc, c-Fos, or zif268 (i.e., [11–19]).

In this sense, Arc is distributed in the nucleus, dendrites, and synapses of activated neurons [31, 32]. Interestingly, neuronal activation is observed in granular cells distributed in the inner, middle, or outer layers of the granular cell layer of the dentate gyrus (i.e., [13]). Previous studies have reported that a "small population of granular neurons in the dentate gyrus expressed Arc after exploration suggesting a sparse dentate gyrus code for spatial information" (i.e., [11, 13]).

In this sense, our mice exposed to the spatial exploration paradigm showed different levels of neuronal activation measured with the expression of Arc.

Contrary to what was previously reported in rats (i.e., [11, 13]), we did not find an increase in activation in mice exposed to a new environment once. This result is similar to previous data showing neuronal activation evaluated with zif268 expression in male mice exposed to the Morris water maze after 42 days of standard housing conditions [12]. Moreover, the exposure of adult female Balb/C mice to two identical or different environments

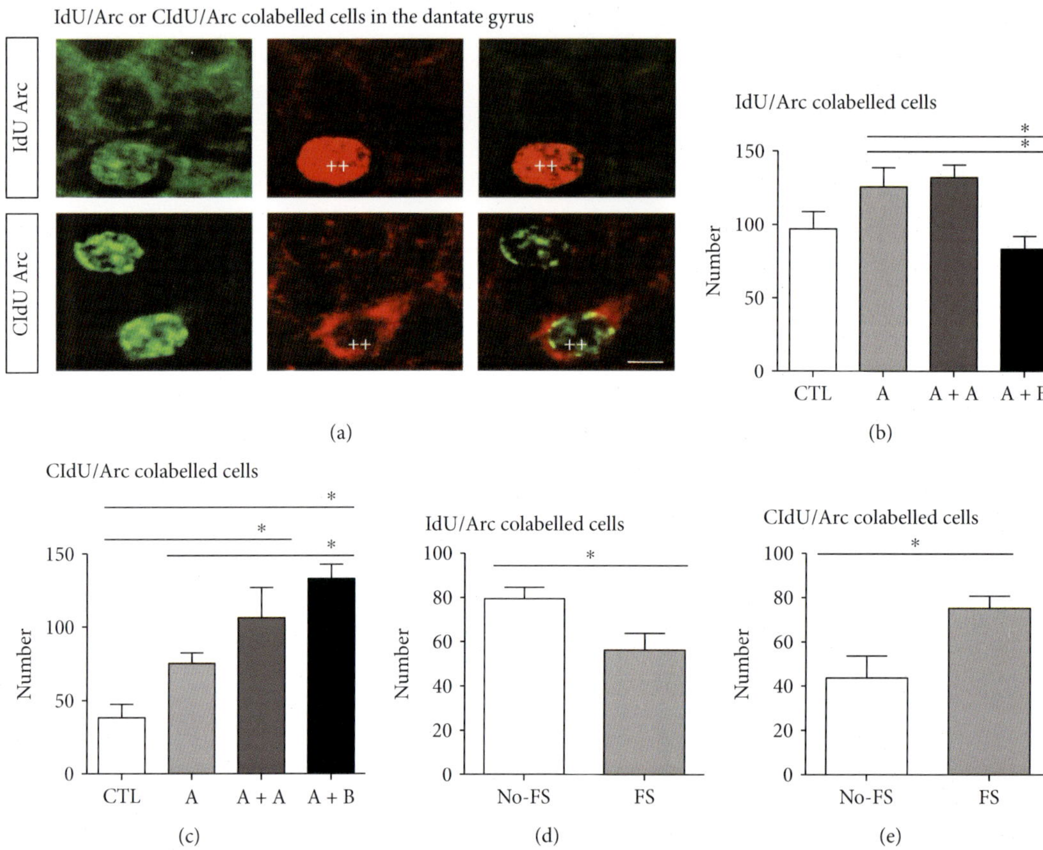

Figure 5: Activation of newborn cells in the dentate gyrus of adult mice. (a) Representative micrographs of IdU/Arc- and CldU/Arc-labelled cells are shown. IdU or CldU (green), Arc (red), and the merged micrographs are shown. The scale bar is equal to 10 μm. (b–c) Quantification of IdU- and CldU-activated (Arc) cells in mice exposed to brief spatial exploration is shown. The number of newborn activated (Arc) cells was calculated by multiplying the ratio of newborn activated IdU or CldU cells with the absolute number of IdU- or CldU-labelled cells, respectively. (b) The number of IdU/Arc-labelled cells increased in mice exposed to environment A once or twice in comparison to that in mice subsequently exposed to environments A and B. Asterisks indicate $p < 0.05$. However, an increase in the number of CldU/Arc-labelled cells was found in mice exposed to environment A twice or in mice subsequently exposed to environment (a and b) in comparison to that in mice exposed to environment A or the control group (c). Asterisks indicate $p = 0.03$ and $p = 0.001$, respectively. Data are expressed as the mean ± SEM, and comparisons were performed with a one-way ANOVA followed by Student-Newman-Keuls post hoc test. $n = 4 - 5$ per group. (d, e) The number of IdU/Arc-labelled cells was significantly lower compared to mice exposed to forced swim (FS) than that found in mice not exposed to forced swim (No-FS). However, CldU/Arc-labelled cells were significantly higher in mice exposed to forced swim (FS). The asterisk in (d) indicates $p = 0.047$. The asterisk in (e) indicates $p = 0.031$. $n = 4 - 5$ per group. Data are expressed as the mean ± SEM, and comparisons were performed with unpaired Student's t-test.

similarly increased neuronal activation, which is different than what has been shown in rats (i.e., [11, 33]). Those reports have indicated different levels of neuronal activation determined with the expression of the messengers coding for Arc and zif268. Additionally, reexposure of rats to the same environment resulted in activation of the same neural ensemble for each exposure, but the exposure of rats to two different environments resulted in activation of a newborn population of neurons in response to the exposure to the second environment [11, 33], an effect that we did not find in our study. Our data indicate that mice exposed to the same environment twice or to two different environments showed an increase in neuronal activation compared to mice with or without a single exposure. These data suggest that, independently of the configuration of the second environment, there is a neuronal population with the capability to respond to the stimuli provided by the second environment. Similar to the neuronal activation presented in spatial exploration paradigms [11, 33], exposure to a stressful situation has also been described to involve the codification of information allowing the animal to exhibit a better coping strategy in the second exposure [34]. Here, mice exposed to the forced-swim stress, which is a stressful situation for rodents [28], after normal housing showed increased levels of neuronal activation. Our results are in line to a previous study in which male C57Bl6 mice exposed to forced swim show increase neuronal activation in the dentate gyrus [17].

4.2. Expression of Arc in Newborn Cells in the Dentate Gyrus of Adult Mice after Spatial Exploration. Newly generated hippocampal neurons are able to functionally integrate into neuronal circuits, which can be analysed by the expression

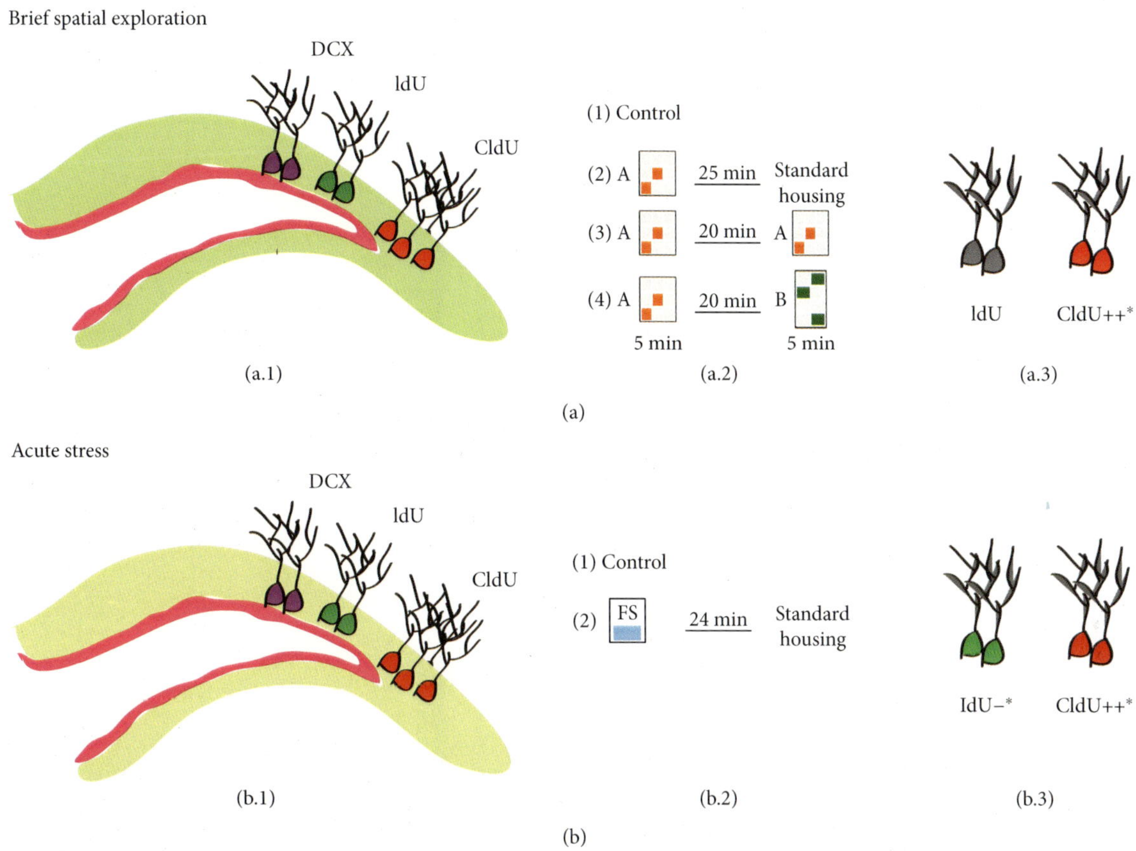

FIGURE 6: Representation of the results derived from the present study. (a) Brief spatial exploration. (a.1) Illustration representing the newly generated cells analysed in our study that corresponds to IdU (green)- and CldU (red)- labelled cells. (a.2) Illustration representing the experimental design indicating the three groups tested with a brief spatial exploration and the control group. The illustration also indicates the duration of the explorations and the amount of time between both environment configurations. (a.3) The representative drawings indicate that newborn cells (CldU, 42 days postlabelling) mainly respond to brief spatial exploration. (b) Forced-swim stress (acute stress). (b.1) Illustration representing the newly generated cells analysed in our study that corresponds to IdU (green)- and CldU (red)- labelled cells. (b.2) The illustration represents the experimental design showing the two groups tested in experiment 2. The illustration also indicates the duration of the test and the time until the mice were sacrificed. (b.3) The representative drawings indicate that newborn cells (CldU, 42 days postlabelling) mainly respond to forced-swim exposure whereas IdU-labelled cells (21 days postlabelling) decrease activation in mice housed in standard conditions but exposed to forced swim.

of IEGs, which are related to plasticity and memory. Thus, several studies have reported expression of c-Fos, zif268, or Arc in response to behavioural stimuli in newborn hippocampal neurons (i.e., [14, 21, 35, 36]). Here, we found a trend towards a decrease in activation of granule cells after 3 weeks post-IdU labelling in mice exposed to two different environments; however, an increase in activation was evident in newborn cells analysed after 6 weeks post-CldU labelling in mice exposed to the environments once or twice, with a higher increase in mice exposed to different environments. The analysis of CldU/Arc-colabelled cells reflected similar results to those found in rats (i.e., [11]), suggesting that, in the mouse hippocampus, there are different ensembles of newborn cells with the capability of being activated in response to the exposure to different environments. Additionally, our data are in line with previous studies performed in rats that indicated that the response to exposure to spatial exploration paradigms involved activation of new hippocampal neurons analysed 30 and 45 days after BrdU-labelling (i.e., [13, 35, 36]).

4.3. Expression of Arc in Newborn Cells in the Dentate Gyrus of Adult Mice after Forced-Swim Stress. Newborn hippocampal neurons are involved in the adaptation to complex and stressful environments, particularly because newborn neurons can help buffer against the effects of stress (i.e., [9, 10]). Interestingly, we found that mice exposed to forced-swim stress showed significant increase activation of newborn cells analysed six weeks post-CldU labelling (CldU/Arc) concomitantly to a significant decrease in the activation of newborn cells analysed three weeks post-IdU labelling (IdU/Arc). These results strongly suggest that the swimming performed by mice during the forced-swim task may include the activation of a neuronal ensemble that involves cells of long survival here identified with CldU labelling. Interestingly, our results are in line to what was previously reported for mice that were exposed to cold forced-swim stress [17]. In that study, the authors found a decrease in the activation of newborn cells in mice housed in voluntary physical activity conditions but not in mice housed without the physical activity stimuli. Here, it is important to note that among the differences found between that study and ours is an important aspect related to the age of the cells analysed. In our study, the newborn cells were analysed three (IdU) or six (CldU) weeks postlabelling, whereas in the previous study, the newborn cells analysed may correspond to cells ranging between 28 and 42 days postcumulative BrdU labelling [17]. Also, we found that cells analysed three weeks post-IdU labelling show decreased activation in mice exposed to forced-swim stress and similar results were recently reported with restrained stress that reduces levels of zif268, another IEG, in immature neurons but not in mature neurons. The newborn cells analysed in that study may correspond to cells ranging between 18 and 30 days postcumulative BrdU labelling [37].

5. Conclusion

Finally, it is important to note that we did not perform the identification of a third population of newborn neurons (CldU/IdU-cells); however, it has been reported that the number of these cells is very low [38], and it remains to be determined in the context of the paradigms used in our study. However, our data confirmed that long-survival newborn neurons in the DG, here cells analysed 42 days postlabelling, mainly respond to a paradigm including spatial exploration, as in the brief spatial exploration paradigm, in adult female Balb/C mice [11]. In addition, our study showed that cells analysed 42 days postlabelling also respond to forced-swim stress. Interestingly, previous studies suggest the possibility that newborn neurons of four or more weeks postlabelling may be preferentially recruited into circuits in the adult brain that are involved in spatial exploration and memory formation events [7–15, 36] but also after acute stress [17]. Moreover, a decrease in the activation of cells analysed 21 days postlabelling was also observed in adult female Balb/C mice (Figure 6). Thus, our study adds information related to the enrolment of newborn neurons of the DG into the neural representation of different environmental stimuli, enrolment that *may be* dependent on the age of the newborn neurons and the type of environment.

Conflicts of Interest

The authors have no conflicts of interest to declare.

Authors' Contributions

Gerardo Bernabé Ramírez-Rodríguez and María del Ángel Ocaña-Fernández designed the study and collaborated in experimental performance and/or in data collection with the respective analysis. Leonardo Ortiz-López performed the phenotype analysis by confocal microscopy. Gerardo Bernabé Ramírez-Rodríguez analysed the findings based on the present hypothesis, wrote the manuscript, and prepared the final figures.

Acknowledgments

This work was financially supported through the budget of INPRFM (SIC-2000) to Gerardo Bernabé Ramírez-Rodríguez. María del Ángel Ocaña-Fernández was a fellowship recipient from Consejo Nacional de Ciencia y Tecnología (Ciencia Básica 2008; Grant 101316 to Gerardo Bernabé Ramírez-Rodríguez). Some of the equipment used in the present study was kindly financed by CONACYT (Grant Infraestructura 2015; 254773 to Gerardo Bernabé Ramírez-Rodríguez). This manuscript was edited for proper English language.

References

[1] G. Kempermann, H. G. Kuhn, and F. H. Gage, "More hippocampal neurons in adult mice living in an enriched environment," *Nature*, vol. 386, no. 6624, pp. 493–495, 1997.

[2] H. van Praag, G. Kempermann, and F. H. Gage, "Running increases cell proliferation and neurogenesis in the adult mouse dentate gyrus," *Nature Neuroscience*, vol. 2, no. 3, pp. 266–270, 1999.

[3] H. van Praag, G. Kempermann, and F. H. Gage, "Neural consequences of environmental enrichment," *Nature Reviews Neuroscience*, vol. 1, no. 3, pp. 191–198, 2000.

[4] M. V. Llorens-Martin, N. Rueda, C. Martinez-Cue, I. Torres-Aleman, J. Florez, and J. L. Trejo, "Both increases in immature dentate neuron number and decreases of immobility time in the forced swim test occurred in parallel after environmental enrichment of mice," *Neuroscience*, vol. 147, no. 3, pp. 631–638, 2007.

[5] N. M. Vega-Rivera, L. Ortiz-Lopez, A. Gomez-Sanchez, J. Oikawa-Sala, E. M. Estrada-Camarena, and G. B. Ramirez-Rodriguez, "The neurogenic effects of an enriched environment and its protection against the behavioral consequences of chronic mild stress persistent after enrichment cessation in six-month-old female Balb/C mice," *Behavioural Brain Research*, vol. 301, pp. 72–83, 2016.

[6] V. Lemaire, M. Koehl, M. Le Moal, and D. N. Abrous, "Prenatal stress produces learning deficits associated with an inhibition of neurogenesis in the hippocampus," *Proceedings of the National Academy of Sciences*, vol. 97, no. 20, pp. 11032–11037, 2000.

[7] A. Garthe and G. Kempermann, "An old test for new neurons: refining the Morris water maze to study the functional relevance of adult hippocampal neurogenesis," *Frontiers in Neuroscience*, vol. 7, 2013.

[8] A. Garthe, I. Roeder, and G. Kempermann, "Mice in an enriched environment learn more flexibly because of adult hippocampal neurogenesis," *Hippocampus*, vol. 26, no. 2, pp. 261–271, 2016.

[9] A. Sahay, K. N. Scobie, A. S. Hill et al., "Increasing adult hippocampal neurogenesis is sufficient to improve pattern separation," *Nature*, vol. 472, no. 7344, pp. 466–470, 2011.

[10] A. S. Hill, A. Sahay, and R. Hen, "Increasing adult hippocampal neurogenesis is sufficient to reduce anxiety and depression-like behaviors," *Neuropsychopharmacology*, vol. 40, no. 10, pp. 2368–2378, 2015.

[11] M. K. Chawla, J. F. Guzowski, V. Ramirez-Amaya et al., "Sparse, environmentally selective expression of Arc RNA in the upper blade of the rodent fascia dentata by brief spatial experience," *Hippocampus*, vol. 15, no. 5, pp. 579–586, 2005.

[12] J. S. Snyder, L. R. Glover, K. M. Sanzone, J. F. Kamhi, and H. A. Cameron, "The effects of exercise and stress on the survival and maturation of adult-generated granule cells," *Hippocampus*, vol. 19, no. 10, pp. 898–906, 2009.

[13] C. J. Sandoval, M. Martinez-Claros, P. C. Bello-Medina, O. Perez, and V. Ramirez-Amaya, "When are new hippocampal neurons, born in the adult brain, integrated into the network that processes spatial information?," *PLoS One*, vol. 6, no. 3, article e17689, 2011.

[14] P. J. Clark, T. K. Bhattacharya, D. S. Miller, R. A. Kohman, E. K. DeYoung, and J. S. Rhodes, "New neurons generated from running are broadly recruited into neuronal activation associated with three different hippocampus-involved tasks," *Hippocampus*, vol. 22, no. 9, pp. 1860–1867, 2012.

[15] C. A. Denny, N. S. Burghardt, D. M. Schachter, R. Hen, and M. R. Drew, "4- to 6-week-old adult-born hippocampal neurons influence novelty-evoked exploration and contextual fear conditioning," *Hippocampus*, vol. 22, no. 5, pp. 1188–1201, 2012.

[16] E. D. Kirby, S. E. Muroy, W. G. Sun et al., "Acute stress enhances adult rat hippocampal neurogenesis and activation of newborn neurons via secreted astrocytic FGF2," *eLife*, vol. 2, article e00362, 2013.

[17] T. J. Schoenfeld, P. Rada, P. R. Pieruzzini, B. Hsueh, and E. Gould, "Physical exercise prevents stress-induced activation of granule neurons and enhances local inhibitory mechanisms in the dentate gyrus," *Journal of Neuroscience*, vol. 33, no. 18, pp. 7770–7777, 2013.

[18] J. Vukovic, G. G. Borlikova, M. J. Ruitenberg et al., "Immature doublecortin-positive hippocampal neurons are important for learning but not for remembering," *Journal of Neuroscience*, vol. 33, no. 15, pp. 6603–6613, 2013.

[19] J. L. Workman, M. Y. T. Chan, and L. A. M. Galea, "Prior high corticosterone exposure reduces activation of immature neurons in the ventral hippocampus in response to spatial and nonspatial memory," *Hippocampus*, vol. 25, no. 3, pp. 329–344, 2015.

[20] B. Perez-Cadahia, B. Drobic, and J. R. Davie, "Activation and function of immediate-early genes in the nervous system," *Biochemistry and Cell Biology*, vol. 89, no. 1, pp. 61–73, 2011.

[21] V. Ramirez-Amaya, D. F. Marrone, F. H. Gage, P. F. Worley, and C. A. Barnes, "Integration of new neurons into functional neural networks," *Journal of Neuroscience*, vol. 26, no. 47, pp. 12237–12241, 2006.

[22] M. Llorens-Martin, G. S. Tejeda, and J. L. Trejo, "Antidepressant and proneurogenic influence of environmental enrichment in mice: protective effects vs recovery," *Neuropsychopharmacology*, vol. 36, no. 12, pp. 2460–2468, 2011.

[23] G. Kempermann, H. G. Kuhn, and F. H. Gage, "Genetic influence on neurogenesis in the dentate gyrus of adult mice," *Proceedings of the National Academy of Sciences*, vol. 94, no. 19, pp. 10409–10414, 1997.

[24] G. Ramirez-Rodriguez, H. Babu, F. Klempin et al., "The α crystallin domain of small heat shock protein b8 (Hspb8) acts as survival and differentiation factor in adult hippocampal neurogenesis," *Journal of Neuroscience*, vol. 33, no. 13, pp. 5785–5796, 2013.

[25] L. Ortiz-Lopez, C. Perez-Beltran, and G. Ramirez-Rodriguez, "Chronic administration of a melatonin membrane receptor antagonist, luzindole, affects hippocampal neurogenesis without changes in hopelessness-like behavior in adult mice," *Neuropharmacology*, vol. 103, pp. 211–221, 2016.

[26] G. Ramirez-Rodriguez, M. A. Ocana-Fernandez, N. M. Vega-Rivera et al., "Environmental enrichment induces neuroplastic changes in middle age female Balb/c mice and increases the hippocampal levels of BDNF, p-Akt and p-MAPK1/2," *Neuroscience*, vol. 260, pp. 158–170, 2014.

[27] M. D. Brandt, E. Ellwardt, and A. Storch, "Short- and long-term treatment with modafinil differentially affects adult hippocampal neurogenesis," *Neuroscience*, vol. 278, pp. 267–275, 2014.

[28] R. D. Porsolt, G. Anton, N. Blavet, and M. Jalfre, "Behavioural despair in rats: a new model sensitive to antidepressant treatments," *European Journal of Pharmacology*, vol. 47, no. 4, pp. 379–391, 1978.

[29] G. Ramirez-Rodriguez, F. Klempin, H. Babu, G. Benitez-King, and G. Kempermann, "Melatonin modulates cell survival of new neurons in the hippocampus of adult mice," *Neuropsychopharmacology*, vol. 34, no. 9, pp. 2180–2191, 2009.

[30] G. Kempermann, D. Gast, G. Kronenberg, M. Yamaguchi, and F. H. Gage, "Early determination and long-term persistence of adult-generated new neurons in the hippocampus of mice," *Development*, vol. 130, no. 2, pp. 391–399, 2003.

[31] S. Farris, G. Lewandowski, C. D. Cox, and O. Steward, "Selective localization of arc mRNA in dendrites involves activity- and translation-dependent mRNA degradation," *Journal of Neuroscience*, vol. 34, no. 13, pp. 4481–4493, 2014.

[32] O. Steward, S. Farris, P. S. Pirbhoy, J. Darnell, and S. J. Van Driesche, "Localization and local translation of Arc/Arg3.1 mRNA at synapses: some observations and paradoxes," *Frontiers in Molecular Neuroscience*, vol. 7, 2015.

[33] D. F. Marrone, V. Ramirez-Amaya, and C. A. Barnes, "Neurons generated in senescence maintain capacity for functional integration," *Hippocampus*, vol. 22, no. 5, pp. 1134–1142, 2012.

[34] S. Ons, O. Marti, and A. Armario, "Stress-induced activation of the immediate early gene Arc (activity-regulated cytoskeleton-associated protein) is restricted to telencephalic areas in the rat brain: relationship to c-fos mRNA," *Journal of Neurochemistry*, vol. 89, no. 5, pp. 1111–1118, 2004.

[35] N. Kee, C. M. Teixeira, A. H. Wang, and P. W. Frankland, "Imaging activation of adult-generated granule cells in spatial memory," *Nature Protocols*, vol. 2, no. 12, pp. 3033–3044, 2007.

[36] N. Kee, C. M. Teixeira, A. H. Wang, and P. W. Frankland, "Preferential incorporation of adult-generated granule cells into spatial memory networks in the dentate gyrus," *Nature Neuroscience*, vol. 10, no. 3, pp. 355–362, 2007.

[37] E. Todorova, S. Cahill, T. O'Leary, and J. Snyder, "Stressful experiences differentially regulate immediate-early genes and stress hormone receptors in immature and mature dentate gyrus neurons," *Matters Select*, 2017.

[38] M. A. Bonaguidi, C. Y. Peng, T. McGuire et al., "Noggin expands neural stem cells in the adult hippocampus," *Journal of Neuroscience*, vol. 28, no. 37, pp. 9194–9204, 2008.

16

Knock-In Mice with Myo3a Y137C Mutation Displayed Progressive Hearing Loss and Hair Cell Degeneration in the Inner Ear

Peipei Li, Zongzhuang Wen, Guangkai Zhang, Aizhen Zhang, Xiaolong Fu, and Jiangang Gao

School of Life Science, Shandong University, Jinan 250100, China

Correspondence should be addressed to Jiangang Gao; jggao@sdu.edu.cn

Academic Editor: Renjie Chai

Myo3a is expressed in cochlear hair cells and retinal cells and is responsible for human recessive hereditary nonsyndromic deafness (DFNB30). To investigate the mechanism of DFNB30-type deafness, we established a mouse model of Myo3a kinase domain Y137C mutation by using CRISPR/Cas9 system. No difference in hearing between 2-month-old Myo3a mutant mice and wild-type mice was observed. The hearing threshold of the ≥6-month-old mutant mice was significantly elevated compared with that of the wild-type mice. We observed degeneration in the inner ear hair cells of 6-month-old Myo3a mutant mice, and the degeneration became more severe at the age of 12 months. We also found structural abnormality in the cochlear hair cell stereocilia. Our results showed that Myo3a is essential for normal hearing by maintaining the intact structure of hair cell stereocilia, and the kinase domain plays a critical role in the normal functions of Myo3a. This mouse line is an excellent model for studying DFNB30-type deafness in humans.

1. Introduction

Deafness presents the highest incidence among sensory defects. One-third of the global population suffer from hearing impairment. Approximately 300 million people currently possess hearing disabilities [1–3]. Presbyacusis, also known as age-related hearing loss (ARHL), refers to the gradual onset of sensorineural hearing loss with age. According to WHO statistics, over one-third of the >65-year-old population are currently affected by senile deafness. The contribution of hearing loss to the general health of individuals during that extended lifespan is of considerable clinical and economic significance [4]. ARHL inevitably causes communication difficulties and is associated with social isolation and depression and decreases physical and cognitive function [5, 6]. Therefore, determining ways to prevent presbyacusis and identifying its pathogenesis have become crucial. Senile deafness is related to environmental factors, such as disease, ear-toxic drugs, noise, and mental trauma, and genetic factors play an important role in this process. Nearly 50% of age-related deafness is determined by genetic factors [7]. Senile deafness is a complex disease that can be affected by a variety of environmental factors, and differences in the genetic background of different populations can interfere with research. Therefore, the use of gene knock-out/knock-in mouse model can strictly control environmental conditions and reduce the influence of genetic background, thereby providing important tools for the validation of age- and deafness-related genes. Therefore, the establishment of presbyacusis animal model has become an important method in studying presbyacusis.

Our hearing depends on hair cells in the inner ear, which can convert the vibrations of sound into electrical signals. At the apical surface of each hair cell, three rows of stereocilium are arranged in high and low orders [8, 9]. When sound is introduced into the inner ear, sound waves cause a slight vibration of the cochlear basilar membrane. The basilar membrane vibration is transduced into an electric signal by a mechanoelectro transduction (MET) protein, which can open the ion channel at the top of the stereocilium and generate a membrane potential. The mechanical signal transduction that occurs at the top of the hair cell stereocilium may comprise a complex of proteins called MET protein complex [10, 11]. In mammals, Myo3a is mainly expressed in the retina [12] and cochlea [13, 14]. In inner ear hair cells, Myo3a is specifically expressed near the tips of the stereocilium, where the MET protein is located [13]. Myo3a protein localization implies its importance in hearing. Myo3a mutations in humans can cause nonsyndrome-type deafness (DFNB30) [14], where patients experience progressive bilateral hearing loss. Hearing loss usually begins at the second decade and becomes severe by the age of 50. In addition, Myo3a is a candidate gene for the disease Bardet-Biedl syndrome, an important human retinal disease [15].

Based on different C-terminal cargo-binding domains, myosin superfamily members are classified into conventional myosins (class II) and unconventional myosins (classes I and III–XV) [16–18]. Myo3a is a class III myosin. The Myo3a protein contains a kinase domain at the N-terminal, followed by a highly conserved motor region and three IQ motifs. Two of the IQ motifs are located at the conserved neck region, and the third motif is located at the center of the tail domain [19]. Myo3a is special because it is autophosphorylated by a kinase domain [20]. In 2010, Walsh et al. generated the Myo3a knock-out mouse model, which showed the characteristics of senile deafness [21]. The knock-out mouse model converts the 1041th codon of Myo3a into a termination codon, which is located at the 28th exon, allowing the knock-out of the protein after the 27th exon. However, the head kinase domain, motor domain, and the regulatory neck domain still remain. The mutation site of Myo3a in humans frequently appears in the head domain of the protein. Our collaborators and our team found that a Myo3a Y129C mutation within the kinase domain can cause ARHL in humans (data not shown). Mimicking this point mutation, we established knock-in mice by changing the tyrosine (Y137) to cysteine in Myo3a. A series of experiments was conducted on these mutant mice to determine the function of Myo3a in the cochlea. The mutant mice displayed progressive hearing loss and inner ear hair cell degeneration. The mouse we generated is a good model for studying DFNB30-type deafness in human and provides valuable material for the study of ARHL.

2. Materials and Methods

2.1. Ethics Statement. All animal experimental procedures were approved by the Ethics Committee of Shandong University. Animal management was performed strictly in accordance with the standards of the Animal Ethics of Shandong University.

2.2. Generation of Myo3a Y137C Mouse. Myo3a mutant mice were generated using the CRISPR-Cas9 genome-editing technology and maintained on the CBA/CaJ background. pX330 plasmid was obtained from Addgene (plasmid ID number 42230). The CRISPR-Cas9 genome-editing technology in mice was used as previously described [22–26]. In brief, a pair of oligonucleotides for the target sequence (5′-CACCGTGTAAAATATATGCAATTAC-3′ and 5′-AAACGTAATTGCATATATTTTACAC-3′) was annealed and ligated to pX330 that was previously digested with BbsI. The pX330 plasmid containing sgRNA and Cas9 was purified and eluted in RNase-free water. The following repair template, which contained the target mutation and two synonymous mutations, was commercially synthesized as follows: ggatttctgaagaggggagaaagaatgagcgagcctgtaatCgcCtGtattttacacgaagcactaatggtaaggctatttgaactctt.

CBA/CaJ female mice were superovulated and mated with CBA/CaJ male mice. The fertilized eggs were removed from the oviducts on the next day. pX330 plasmid (5 ng/μL) mixed with 10 ng/μL repair template was microinjected into the pronucleus of fertilized eggs. After injection, eggs were incubated for 10 min. The eggs were then transferred into the oviducts of pseudopregnant CD1 female mice.

Genomic DNA was extracted from the tails of newborn pups. The genomic DNA fragment around the gRNA target site was amplified by PCR using the Myo3a forward primer 5′-AGCTGTGACCTTTTTGAAGATAGC-3′ and the Myo3a reverse primer 5′-ATCAACAAACACCAAGCTGCC-3′. The total reaction volume of 40 μL contains Taq DNA polymerase, PCR buffer, 2 μL 10 mM forward primers, 2 μL 10 mM reverse primer, and 1 μL DNA fragment. Amplification was performed for 3 min at 95°C, followed by 33 cycles, with each consisting of 30 S at 95°C, 30 S at 60°C, and 30 S at 72°C, with a final extension step of 10 min at 72°C. The obtained PCR products were directly sequenced or cloned using the T/A cloning method and then sequenced to identify the mutation.

2.3. Measurement of Hearing Thresholds. ABR was measured to determine the hearing thresholds of mice in a sound-isolated room as previously described [27, 28]. Mice were anesthetized with 0.007 g/mL pentobarbital sodium by intraperitoneal injection (50 mg/kg body weight). Three needle electrodes were placed subcutaneously in the anesthetized mice. Ground, active, and reference electrodes were placed at the back near the tail, above the vertex between the eyes, and underneath the ear, respectively. Hearing thresholds were measured using a Tucker-Davis Technologies System (TDT, USA) workstation that runs the SigGen32 software (TDT, USA). Mice were presented with click and tone burst stimuli at frequencies of 4, 8, 16, and 32 kHz. Auditory thresholds (dB SPL) were determined by decreasing the sound intensities from 90 dB to 10 dB until the lowest sound intensity at which waveforms lose their reproducible morphology is reached. Myo3a mutant mice were compared with their wild-type littermates at each age. More than five animals were used in each experiment.

2.4. Paraffin Sectioning and Hematoxylin and Eosin (H&E) Staining. The cochleae from Myo3a mutant and wild-type mice were removed, fixed with 4% formaldehyde in 10 mM phosphate buffer at 4°C overnight, decalcified in 10% EDTA in 10 mM phosphate-buffered saline (PBS) at room temperature for 2 d, dehydrated with 30% to 100% ethanol series, and treated with xylene for transparency. The cochlea was embedded in paraffin, and the specimen was sectioned at 7 mm thickness using a thin semiautomatic microtome.

Sections were deparaffinized using xylene and 100% to 30% ethanol series, stained with H&E, and viewed under a light microscope (Nikon YS100).

2.5. Whole-Mount Staining. Wild-type and Myo3a mutant mice were anesthetized with 0.007 g/mL pentobarbital sodium. The cochleae were removed from anesthetized mice, fixed in 4% formaldehyde in 10 mM PBS at 4°C overnight, and decalcified in 10% EDTA at room temperature for 2 days [24, 26]. We isolated the basilar membrane from the cochlea under the Nikon TE2000 fluorescence microscope. The basilar membrane was washed with 10 mM PBS and blocked in 5% goat serum for 30 min at 37°C. Primary antibodies were diluted in 10 mM PBS and incubated with the basilar membrane at 4°C overnight. After being washed with 10 mM PBS, the basilar membrane was incubated at 37°C for 1 h in anti-rabbit TRITC-conjugated secondary antibody diluted in PBS [29, 30]. The basilar membrane was washed again with PBS, and Alexa Fluor 488-conjugated phalloidin (2 μg/mL, Sigma) was applied to the samples for 30 min and 4,6-diamidino-2-phenylindole (DAPI) for 15 min. Finally, the basilar membrane was washed thrice with 10 mM PBS. Morphologic changes in hair cells and stereocilia were observed in the basilar membrane-stretched preparation, and images were acquired using a Leica LSM 700 laser scanning microscope.

2.6. Scanning Electron Microcopy (SEM). Myo3a mutant mice and wild-type mice were anesthetized using pentobarbital sodium and perfused with 4% PFA. The cochleae from Myo3a mutant and wild-type mice were removed, fixed with 2.5% glutaraldehyde in 0.1 M PBS at 4°C overnight, and decalcified in 10% EDTA [31]. The cochleae were dissected out from the temporal bone, and the stria vascularis, Reissner's membrane, and tectorial membrane were removed [32]. The organ of Corti was exposed and postfixed in 1% osmium tetroxide in 0.1 M phosphate buffer [33] for 2 h before dehydration in an ethanol series and critical drying point in an Autosamdri-815A (Tousimis) [32]. Samples were mounted with carbon tape, coated with gold, and imaged with a JEOL 7000 field emission gun scanning electron microscope.

2.7. FM1-43 Staining Experiments. FM1-43 staining experiments were performed as previously reported [34]. First, the Myo3a mutant and wild-type mice were anesthetized, and their cochleae were removed. Cochlear samples were bathed with 3 mM FM1-43 solution for 20 s. The cochlear samples were treated with 4% PFA at 4°C overnight. On the next day, the cochlear samples were washed with 10 mM PBS for 10 min for several times. The cochleae were then observed under an LSM 780 confocal microscope.

2.8. Noise Exposure. Nine 4.5-month-old Myo3a mutant mice and seven wild-type mice were anesthetized with 0.007 g/mL pentobarbital sodium by intraperitoneal injection (50 mg/kg body weight) and placed in a 24 cm × 24 cm × 18 cm stainless steel cage for full white noise handling. The loudspeaker was located just in front of the cage. Sound intensity was calibrated using a standard sound level meter prior to exposure to noise. The mice were continuously treated with 98 ± 2 dB SPL for 2 h to produce a temporary change in auditory threshold shifts.

2.9. Statistical Analysis. All data were expressed as mean ± SD, and all experiments were repeated at least thrice to ensure the data accuracy and repeatability. Statistical analyses were implemented using Microsoft Excel, and charts were constructed using GraphPad Prism 5 software. Two-tailed, unpaired Student's t-tests were used to determine statistical significance when comparing two groups. $P < 0.05$ was considered statistically significant [35].

3. Results

3.1. Generation of Myo3a Y137C Mice Using CRISPR/Cas9. To mimic Myo3a Y129C mutation in human, we introduced the A410G (Y137C) mutation in mice by using CRISPR/Cas9 technology (Figure 1). To introduce the A410G mutation, we first induced a double-strand break (DSB) near the A410 and then repaired the DSB using the repair template with the point mutation of interest.

The sgRNA containing the 20 bp target sequence complexed with Cas9 protease can introduce DSB into the target sequence near a protospacer-adjacent motif (PAM) sequence. On the basis of this principle, we designed a specific sgRNA targeting the sequence near the A410 and cloned the sgRNA into the Px330 plasmid containing the Cas9 gene sequence. Thereafter, we designed a repair template with the mutation of interest based on the location of the DSB. The two synonymous mutations on the repair template aim to prevent a secondary targeting of sgRNA. The Px330 plasmid (5 ng/μL) and the repair template (10 ng/μL) were injected into the pronucleus of the fertilized mouse eggs. Exactly 113 fertilized eggs with clear pronucleus were injected, and 58 fertilized eggs with normal morphology after injection were transferred to the fallopian tubes of three pseudopregnant CD1 female mice. A total of 17 mice were born at 19 days after the transplantation. According to the PCR analysis results of the 17 mice, the mutation of interest was observed in 2 mice—a homozygous mouse and a heterozygous mouse (Figure 1(c)). We also performed sequencing at easy-off sites and found no off-targets. To obtain homozygous Myo3a KI/KI mice, we mated F0 mice with wild-type CBA/CaJ mice to generate F1 heterozygous mice, which were self-crossed to obtain homozygous Myo3a mutant mice. The Myo3a mutant mice were found to harbor cysteine in 137 rather than tyrosine in WT mice, similar to the mutation observed in humans.

Myo3a mutant mice were viable and fertile with no apparent abnormalities in their gross morphology (Figure 1(d)). We then examined the presence of an abnormal structure in the Myo3a mutant mice cochlea by paraffin sectioning and H&E staining. Structural abnormality was not observed in the Myo3a mutant mouse cochlea (Figure 1(e)).

3.2. Progressive Hearing Loss in Myo3a Mutant Mice. In humans, Myo3a mutation can cause nonsyndrome-type deafness. Thus, we wanted to test whether Myo3a mutant mice show the same symptoms. To determine whether

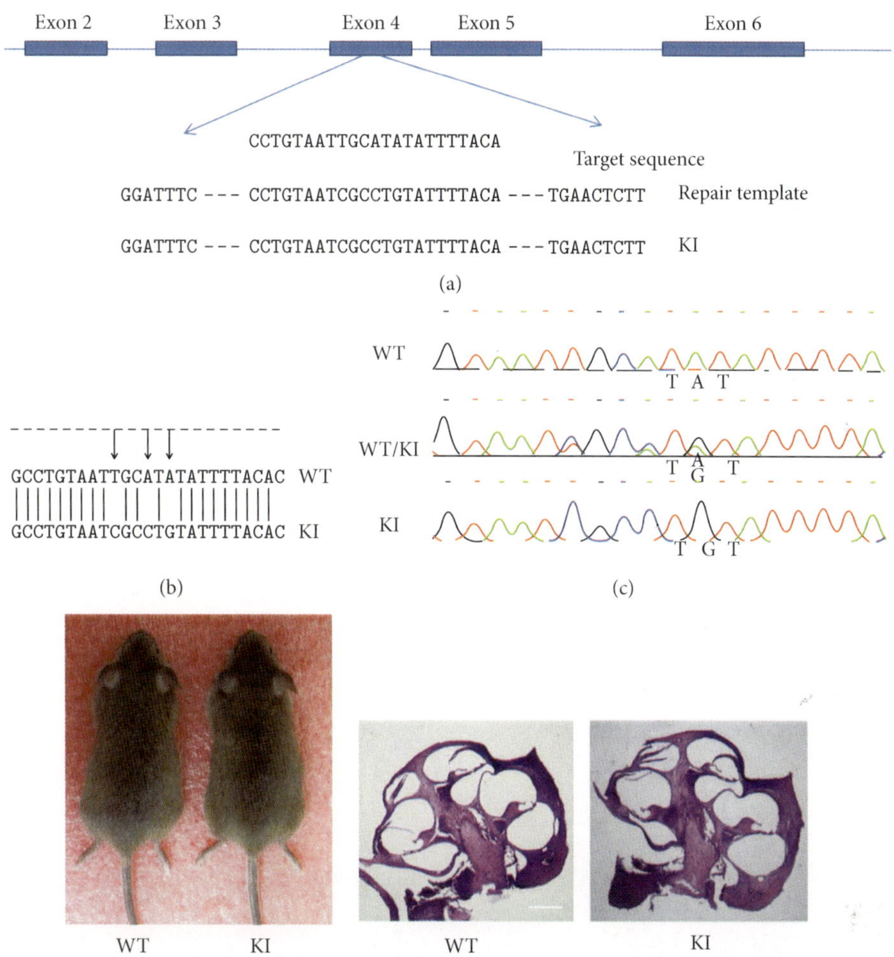

Figure 1: The generation of Myo3a mutant mice using CRISPR/Cas9. (a) Schematic diagram of targeting the mouse myosin IIIA gene. sgRNA was at exon 4 (indicated by the blue rectangles). The point mutation is in red. (b) The comparison of DNA sequences between Myo3a mutant mice (now referred to as Myo3a KI/KI mice) and wild-type mice. (c) Sequence of wild-type mice, heterozygous mice, and homozygous Myo3a KI/KI mutant mice. TAT was changed to TGT, demonstrating the missense mutation at mouse Y137C. (d) Gross morphology of Myo3a KI/KI and wild-type mice at the age of two months. There was no obvious difference. (e) Cochlea morphology is normal in Myo3a mutant mice. Hematoxylin and eosin (HE) staining showed no prominent difference between Myo3a mutant and wide-type mice cochlear at the age of two months. Scale bar = 20 μm.

Myo3a mutant mice demonstrate age-related deafness, we tested the hearing threshold of 2-, 6-, and 12-month-old Myo3a mutant and wild-type mice by ABR measurement. There results indicated no significant difference in the hearing threshold between 2-month-old wild-type ($n = 6$) and Myo3a mutant mice ($n = 7$) (Figure 2(b)). However, by the age of 6 months, Myo3a mutant mice ($n = 7$) exhibited a significantly higher hearing threshold than the wild-type mice ($n = 6$) ($P < 0.05$, Student's t-test) in both the click stimuli and at different frequencies (4, 16, and 32 kHz, Figures 2(a) and 2(c)). Hearing differences between the wild-type and Myo3a mutant mice were increasingly pronounced ($P < 0.01$) at 12 months in the broadband click and tone burst stimuli at frequencies of 4, 8, 16, and 32 kHz (Figures 2(a) and 2(d)). Therefore, we can conclude that Myo3a mutant mice exhibited a gradual hearing loss, which is similar to the characteristics of presbyacusis in humans.

3.3. Progressive Stereocilium Degeneration and Hair Cell Loss in Myo3a Mutant Mice. We investigated the mechanism of senile deafness in Myo3a mutant mice and examined cochlear changes. We dissected the cochleae of 2-, 6-, and 12-month-old wild-type and mutant mice and used phalloidin, DAPI, and Myo7a to stain hair cell stereocilia, hair cell nucleus, and hair cells, respectively. Confocal images of the basilar membrane showed that the stereocilia and hair cells of the wild-type and Myo3a mutant mice were intact at the age of 2 months; by contrast, the stereocilia of the Myo3a mutant mice started to degenerate, and the hair cells began to disappear at 6 months. By the age of 12 months, stereocilium degeneration and hair cell loss became incrementally serious (Figure 3). The confocal image showed that stereocilium degeneration was consistent with hair cell loss.

To further verify the accuracy and reliability of the above result, we used SEM to observe the hair cells of mutant and

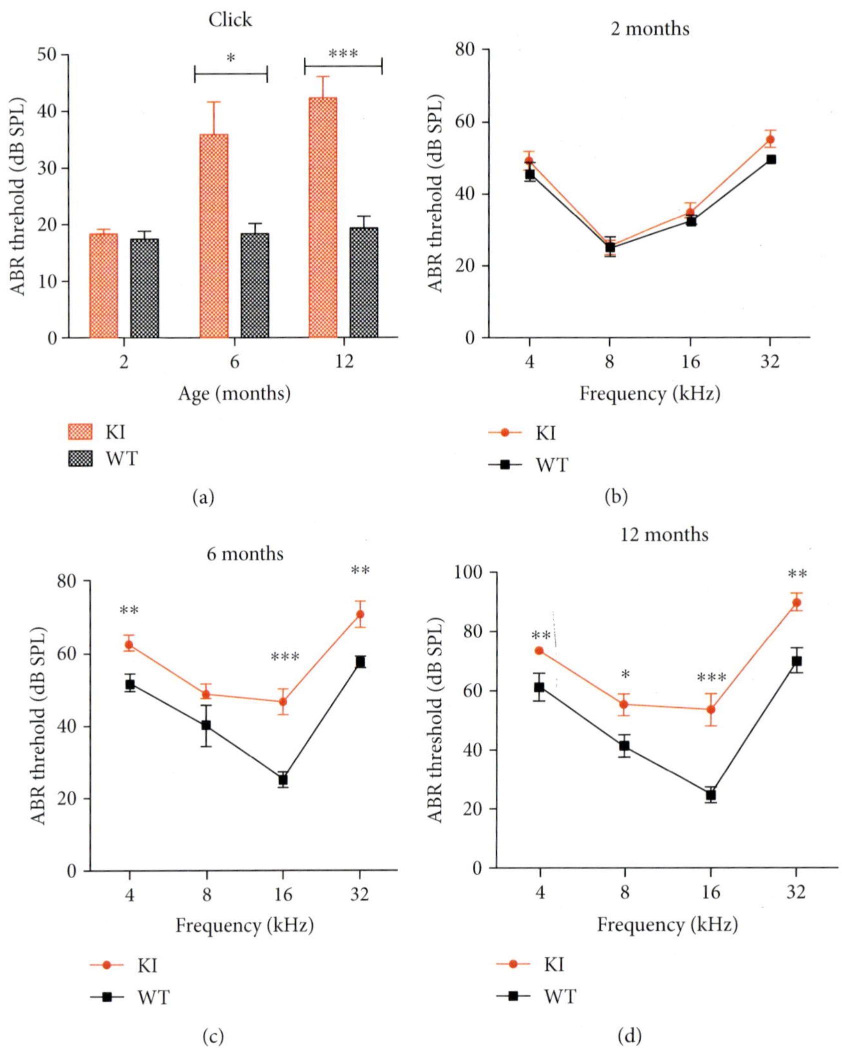

FIGURE 2: ABR analysis in Myo3a mutant mice (red) and wild-type mice (black) at two months, six months, and twelve months. (a) ABR measurements for broadband click. (b) Frequency-specific pure tone stimulation of Myo3a KI/KI mice and wild-type mice at two months old (b), six months old (c), and twelve months old (d). In contrast to wild-type mice, Myo3a KI/KI mutant mice showed progressive hearing loss. Compared with WT threshold at the corresponding frequency as determined by Student's *t*-test. $^{*}P < 0.05$; $^{**}P < 0.01$; $^{***}P < 0.001$. Error bars indicate SEM. $n > 5$ for control and mutant mice for each experiment.

wild-type mice in detail. Consistent with the above results, stereocilium degeneration and hair cell loss occurred in 6-month-old Myo3a mutant mice, especially in the stereocilia of inner hair cells (Figure 4(e)), whereas relatively complete hair cells and stereocilia were observed in wild-type mice (Figure 4(b)). By the age of 12 months, Myo3a mutant mice exhibited intensive stereocilium loss (Figure 4(f)), and this finding agreed with the ABR measurement. Through SEM, we also found structural abnormality in the remaining stereocilia in Myo3a mutant mice, in which the stereocilia of certain outer hair cells began to shorten and degenerate from the innermost line of stereocilia (Figure 5(c)). Fusion phenomenon was also noted in certain stereocilia (Figure 5(b)). The results were consistent with the expression location of Myo3a, in which morphological changes were also observed at the tips of the stereocilia in Myo3a mutant mice (Figure 5(d)). Most of the inner hair cells possess cuspidal stereocilia.

During hearing formation, transformation from mechanical energy to electric energy is crucial, and ion channel plays a critical role in this process. The ion channel is located at the tip of the stereocilia where Myo3a is expressed. Thus, we investigated whether the function of the MET activity was affected in Myo3a mutant mice. We used the FM1-43 dye to stain the hair cells of wild-type and Myo3a mutant mice to determine whether the function of the MET activity was affected. The results are shown in Figure 6. Both the wild-type and Myo3a mutant mice showed positive FM1-43 staining in hair cells. This finding indicated that the MET activity of Myo3a mutant mice remained intact and that Myo3a is not a direct component of MET channels.

3.4. No Difference in Noise Resistance between Myo3a Mutant and Wild-Type Mice. Presbyacusis is highly similar to noise-induced deafness in clinical pathology. Numerous senile deaf individuals are extremely sensitive to noise. To verify

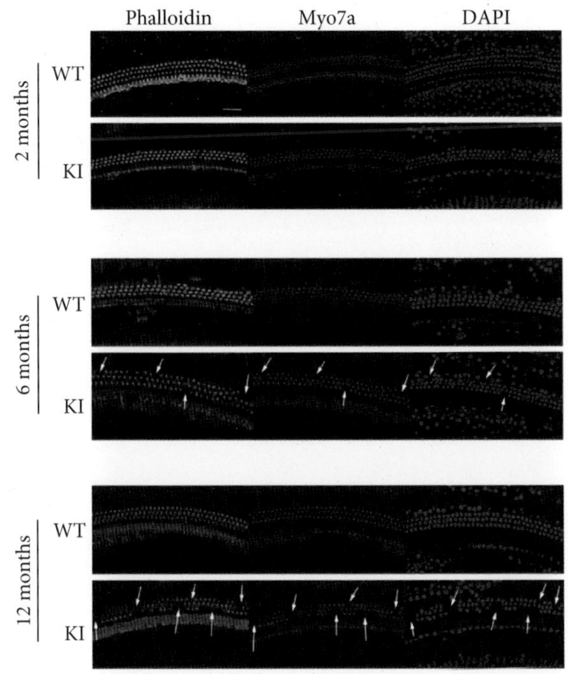

FIGURE 3: The degeneration of stereocilia and the hair cell loss in the Myo3a mutant mice showed by confocal images. Confocal images of the stereocilia, hair cells, and nucleus in Myo3a mutant and WT mice at two months old, six months old, and 12 months old. Images were taken from the middle turn of the cochlea. Scale bar = 20 μm. The stereocilium degeneration and the loss of hair cells can be seen in the Myo3a mutant mice from 6 months old, and this phenomenon becomes more serious in 12-month-old Myo3a mutant mice.

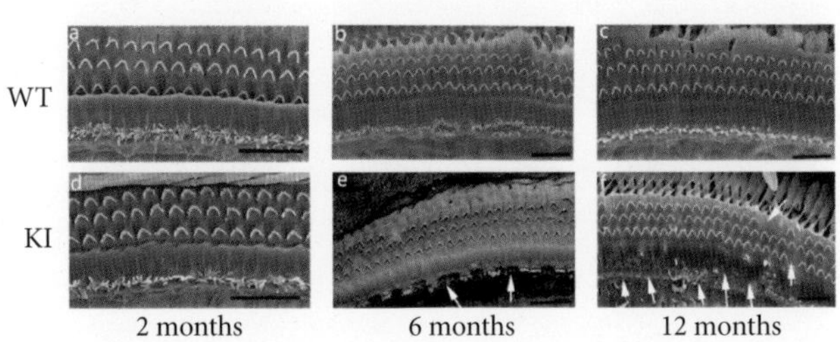

FIGURE 4: The degeneration of stereocilia in the Myo3a mutant mice showed by SEM. SEM images of the hair cells in Myo3a mutant and WT mice at two months old (a, d), six months old (b, e), and 12 months old (c, f). The inner hair cell stereocilium loss was found in 6-month-old Myo3a mutant mice (e), and this phenomenon becomes more serious in 12-month-old Myo3a mutant mice (f). Scale bar = 20 μm.

whether the noise resistance in the Myo3a mutant mice was affected, we performed continuous white-noise experiment for 2 h in 4.5-month-old wild-type and Myo3a mutant mice. Hearing test was conducted in wild-type and mutant mice before, at 4 h after, and at 1 week after noise treatment. The experimental results are shown in Figure 7; here, the line graph depicts no difference in noise resistance between Myo3a mutant and wild-type mice. The hearing threshold of the wild-type and Myo3a mutant mice significantly increased at 4 h after the white-noise experiment. Statistical analysis showed no difference in hearing between mutant and wild-type mice after the noise treatment. However, no difference in hearing was observed between the wild-type and Myo3a mutant mice. We repeated the noise experiment twice to verify the results. No difference in hearing was determined between the wild-type and Myo3a mutant mice after the noise treatment. Therefore, we conclude that the noise resistance of Myo3a mutant and wild-type mice was similar. However, there remains unanswered question. In our experiments, noise exposure seems to "erase" the initial difference in ABR thresholds between WT and KI, but the mechanism of this phenomenon is still unknown. We will perform further investigation in our future experiments.

4. Discussion

Using CRISPR/Cas9 technology, we generated a model of Myo3a Y137C mice consisting of a mutation in the kinase domain similar to that observed in the human Myo3a Y129C mutation. Through ABR hearing detection in mutant mice and wild-type mice, we found that the mutant mice exhibited progressive hearing loss. In 6 months, the hearing threshold of the mutant mice increased relative to that of the wild-type mice, whereas the hair cells of the 6-month-old mice started to degenerate. At 12 months of age, mutant mice exhibited significantly different hearing threshold and a more severe hair cell degeneration in the inner ear compared with that in the wild-type mice. The increased hearing threshold coincided with the loss of hair cells. This finding shows that kinase activity is crucial for the function of Myo3a and inner hair cells. Progressive hearing loss in Myo3a mutant mice was similar to that observed in human Myo3a mutants. Thus, the Myo3a mutant mouse model that we constructed was not only a good model for presbyacusis but also a satisfactory human disease model.

4.1. Kinase Domain Is Important to Myo3a. As a member of the myosin family, Myo3a transports cargo Espin1 to the top of the stereocilia [36]. In contrast to a previous mouse model that contains a stop codon at 1041 but maintains kinase activity, the mouse model in the current study involves mutation at the kinase domain of Myo3a. Our study has proved that kinase domain is important to the function of Myo3a.

Myo3a retains its motility by using the motor domain and the C-terminal THDII domain in combination with actin. In the wild-type mice, the THDI domain specifically binds to cargo Espin1, ensuring that Myo3a can transport Espin1 to the tip of the stereocilia to stabilize its structure [37]. The phosphorylation-dephosphorylation mechanism plays an essential role in normal Myo3a function [38]. Myo3a concentrates at the tip of the stereocilia, and the kinase domain interacts with and phosphorylates the motor domain because of high Myo3a concentration in the stereocilia; furthermore, motor activity is decreased by phosphorylation, and the phosphorylated motor domain loses its affinity with actin and tends to be transported back to the cell body to bind Espin1 again [39]. In the cell line, wild-type Myo3a localizes along the length of the filopodia, and

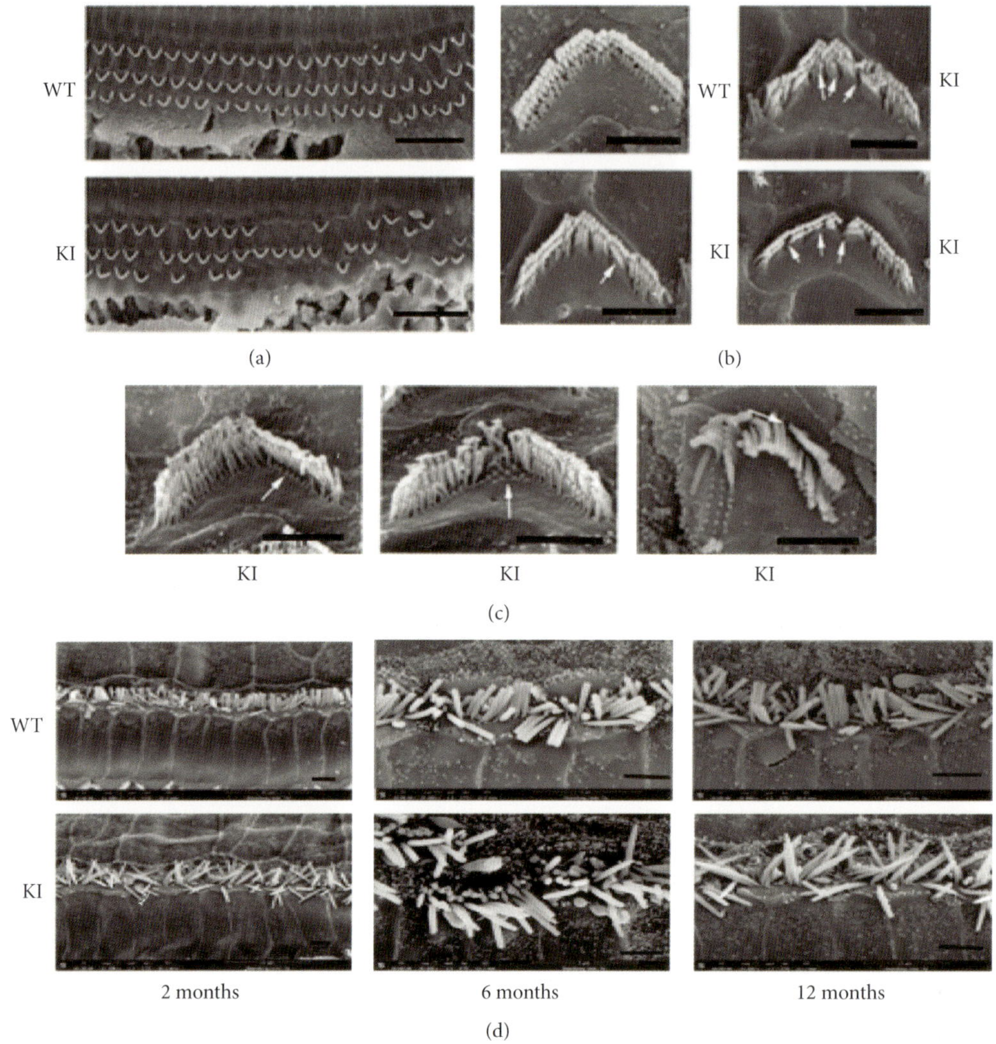

FIGURE 5: SEM images showed the abnormal structure of the stereocilia in Myo3a mutant mice. (a) The outer hair cell stereocilium loss was serious in 6-month-old Myo3a mutant mice. (b) Fusion phenomenon was observed in some stereocilia of mutant mice. (c) The stereocilia of some outer hair cells were found to be shorter, and the degeneration started from the innermost line of the stereocilia. (d) The stereocilia of inner hair cells become sharp in Myo3a mutant mice at the age of 2 months, 6 months, and 12 months. Scale bar = 10 μm for (a) and 2 μm for (b, c, and d).

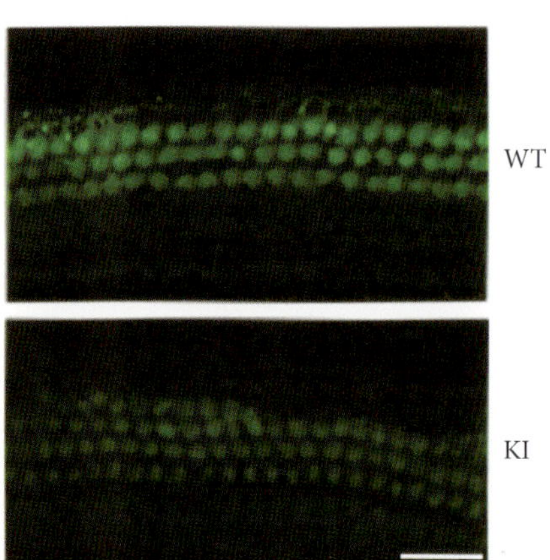

FIGURE 6: MET activity is not affected in Myo3a mutant mice. FM1-43 staining showed that the MET activity is normal in Myo3a mutant mice. Scale bar = 20 μm.

the kinase-deleted construct present increases tip localization [13]; thus, Myo3a, which does not exhibit kinase activity, may demonstrate difficulty in returning to the cytoplasm to bind with Espin1 again.

Myo3a kinase activity may be disrupted in our mutant mouse model. Myo3a autophosphorylation cannot occur even at high Myo3a concentration at the top of the stereocilia so that the motor domain cannot be phosphorylated. The active motor domain tightly binds with actin and cannot be detached from actin. Thus, Myo3a that is located at the tip of the stereocilia cannot return to the cytoplasm and continue to transport Espin1. Thus, the structure of the top of the stereocilia is abnormal, thereby affecting the normal stereocilia functioning and causing progressive hearing loss.

4.2. Myo3b May Compensate for the Function of Myo3a. We observed normal hearing threshold and normal inner ear hair cell development in the 2-month-old Myo3a mutant

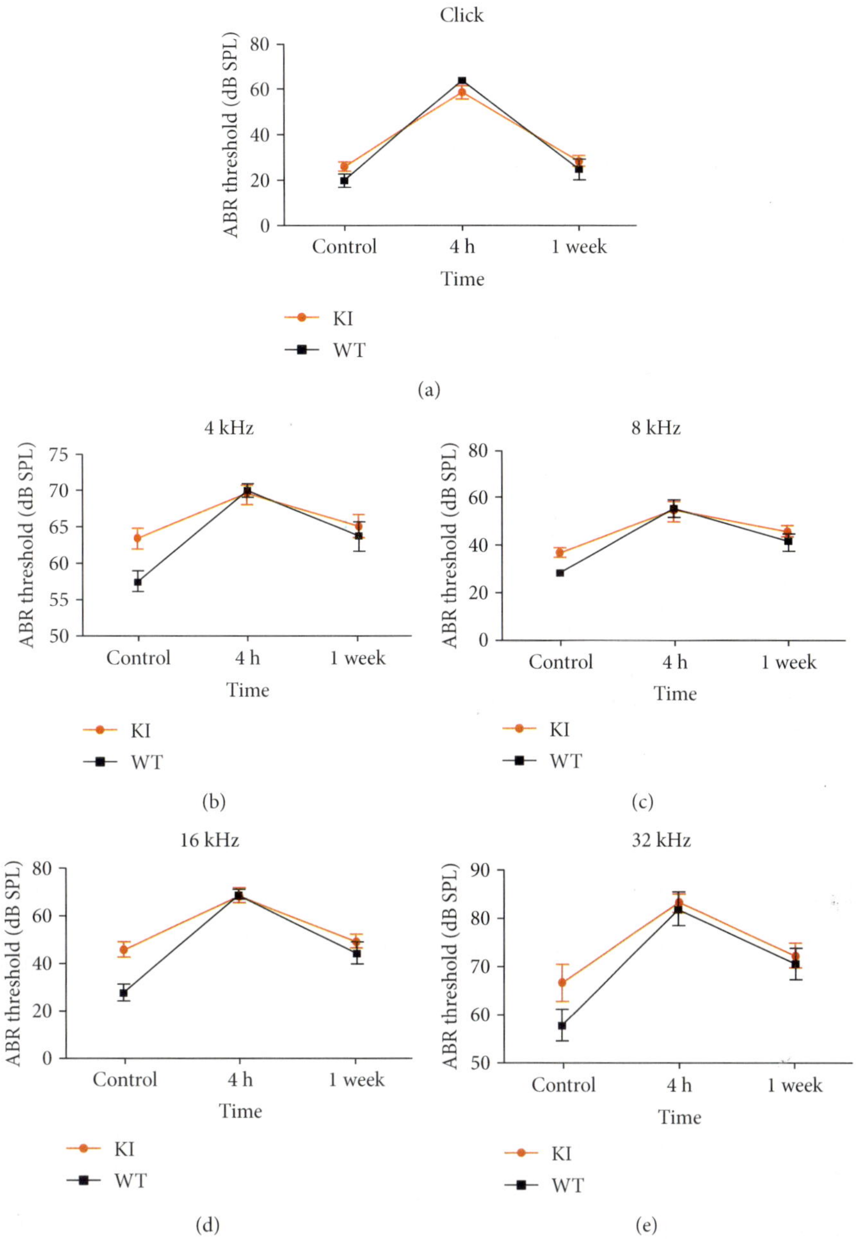

FIGURE 7: ABR analysis in Myo3a mutant and wide-type mice after noise exposure. ABR threshold was tested for broadband click (a) and frequency-specific pure tone (b, c, d, e) on Myo3a mutant and wide-type mice before (control), 4 h after, and 1 week after noise exposure ($n \geqq 7$); error bars indicate SEM.

mice. The elevated hearing threshold and hair cell degeneration of mutant mice presented at ≥6 months of age. The explanation why mutant mice exhibit progressive rather than profound hearing loss at a young age is unknown. We speculate that Myo3b compensates for the loss of Myo3a.

Compensatory effects in higher organisms are highly common. Myo3b localizes at cochlear hair cell stereocilium tips, similar with the localization of Espin1 and Myo3a [37]. Myo3b contains the motor domain and the THDI domain but lacks the THDII domain, which is contrary to Myo3a, which lacks the ability to "walk along" actin [37]. In COS7 cell line, Myo3a that lacks THDII-actin-binding domain does not localize to filopodial tips but moves toward the tip and promotes filopodial elongation when coexpressed with Espin1 Myo3a. This finding suggests that when lacking the THDII-actin-binding domain, Myo3a can bind to the cargo Espin1 with its THDI domain and then use its motor domain and the Espin1 ABM domain to travel along actin [36]. Similarly, when using the THDI domain combined with Espin1, Myo3b can obtain its capability to "walk along" actin by using its motor domain and the Espin1 ABM domain and perform the function of transporting Espin1 to the tip of stereocilia [37]. In an Espin1 knock-out mouse model, Myo3b is not detectable at the stereocilium tips of extrastriolar hair cells [40], demonstrating that Myo3b can transport Espin1 to the tip of stereocilia only when combined with Espin1. Nevertheless, Myo3b compensates for Myo3a for Espin1 shipping.

In Myo3a mutant mice, Myo3b can compensate for the loss of function of Myo3a because Myo3b is located at the stereocilium tip of the inner ear hair cells. Thus, we observed normal development of the inner ear hair cells. Myo3a and Myo3b double knock-out mice are profoundly deaf, demonstrating that class III myosins play redundant roles in hearing function [41].

Unlike a previous Myo3a knock-out mouse model [21, 41], the Myo3a mutant mice in the current study were maintained on the CBA/CaJ background. Our mouse model is suitable for studying DFNB30-type deafness in human because the B6 mice exhibit the characteristic of senile deafness.

5. Conclusion

The knock-in mice with Myo3a kinase domain mutation displayed progressive hearing loss and stereocilium degeneration in inner ear hair cells. Our mouse model of Myo3a point mutation made by CRISPR/Cas9 technology can simulate human diseases well and provide a good mouse model for the study of senile deafness.

Conflicts of Interest

The authors declare no conflict of interests regarding the publication of this paper.

Authors' Contributions

Jiangang Gao and Peipei Li conceived and designed the experiments. Peipei Li and Zongzhuang Wen performed the experiments. Peipei Li analyzed the data. Jiangang Gao contributed reagents/materials/analysis tools. Peipei Li, Zongzhuang Wen, and Jiangang Gao wrote the paper.

Acknowledgments

This work was supported by grants from the Natural Science Foundation of China (31171194), the National 973 Basic Research Program of China (2014CB541703), and Shandong Provincial Science and Technology Key Program (2009GG10002039).

References

[1] T. B. Friedman and A. J. Griffith, "Human nonsyndromic sensorineural deafness," *Annual Review of Genomics and Human Genetics*, vol. 4, no. 1, pp. 341–402, 2003.

[2] C. C. Morton and W. E. Nance, "Newborn hearing screening–a silent revolution," *The New England Journal of Medicine*, vol. 354, no. 20, pp. 2151–2164, 2006.

[3] D. Raviv, A. A. Dror, and K. B. Avraham, "Hearing loss: a common disorder caused by many rare alleles," *Annals of the New York Academy of Sciences*, vol. 1214, no. 1, pp. 168–179, 2010.

[4] G. Stevens, S. Flaxman, E. Brunskill et al., "Global and regional hearing impairment prevalence: an analysis of 42 studies in 29 countries," *European Journal of Public Health*, vol. 23, no. 1, pp. 146–152, 2013.

[5] R. K. Gurgel, P. D. Ward, S. Schwartz, M. C. Norton, N. L. Foster, and J. A. T. Tschanz, "Relationship of hearing loss and dementia: a prospective, population-based study," *Otology & Neurotology*, vol. 35, no. 5, pp. 775–781, 2014.

[6] C. M. Li, X. Zhang, H. J. Hoffman, M. F. Cotch, C. L. Themann, and M. R. Wilson, "Hearing impairment associated with depression in us adults, National Health and Nutrition Examination Survey 2005-2010," *JAMA Otolaryngology. Head & Neck Surgery*, vol. 140, no. 4, pp. 293–302, 2014.

[7] R. J. H. Smith, J. F. Bale Jr, and K. R. White, *Sensorineural Hearing Loss in Children*, Elsevier, 2005.

[8] C. Petit and G. P. Richardson, "Linking genes underlying deafness to hair-bundle development and function," *Nature Neuroscience*, vol. 12, no. 6, pp. 703–710, 2009.

[9] M. Schwander, B. Kachar, and U. Müller, "Review series: the cell biology of hearing," *The Journal of Cell Biology*, vol. 190, no. 1, pp. 9–20, 2010.

[10] P. Kazmierczak, H. Sakaguchi, J. Tokita et al., "Cadherin 23 and protocadherin 15 interact to form tip-link filaments in sensory hair cells," *Nature*, vol. 449, no. 7158, pp. 87–91, 2007.

[11] Z. Xu, A. W. Peng, K. Oshima, and S. Heller, "Magi-1, a candidate stereociliary scaffolding protein, associates with the tip-link component cadherin 23," *Journal of Neuroscience*, vol. 28, no. 44, pp. 11269–11276, 2008.

[12] A. C. Dosé and B. Burnside, "Cloning and chromosomal localization of a human class III myosin," *Genomics*, vol. 67, no. 3, pp. 333–342, 2000.

[13] M. E. Schneider, A. C. Dose, F. T. Salles et al., "A new compartment at stereocilia tips defined by spatial and temporal patterns of myosin IIIa expression," *Journal of Neuroscience*, vol. 26, no. 40, pp. 10243–10252, 2006.

[14] T. Walsh, V. Walsh, S. Vreugde et al., "From flies' eyes to our ears: mutations in a human class III myosin cause progressive nonsyndromic hearing loss DFNB30," *Proceedings of the National Academy of Sciences of the United States of America*, vol. 99, no. 11, pp. 7518–7523, 2002.

[15] A. C. Dose and B. Burnside, "A class III myosin expressed in the retina is a potential candidate for Bardet-Biedl syndrome," *Genomics*, vol. 79, no. 5, pp. 621–624, 2002.

[16] M. J. T. Cope, J. Whisstock, I. Rayment, and J. Kendrick-Jones, "Conservation within the myosin motor domain: implications for structure and function," *Structure*, vol. 4, no. 8, pp. 969–987, 1996.

[17] A. Wang, Y. Liang, R. A. Fridell et al., "Association of unconventional myosin *MYO15* mutations with human nonsyndromic deafness *DFNB3*," *Science*, vol. 280, no. 5368, pp. 1447–1451, 1998.

[18] C. Montell and G. M. Rubin, "The drosophila *ninaC* locus encodes two photoreceptor cell specific proteins with domains homologous to protein kinases and the myosin heavy chain head," *Cell*, vol. 52, no. 5, pp. 757–772, 1988.

[19] T. B. Friedman, J. R. Sellers, and K. B. Avraham, "Unconventional myosins and the genetics of hearing loss," *American Journal of Medical Genetics*, vol. 89, no. 3, pp. 147–157, 1999.

[20] K. P. Ng, T. Kambara, M. Matsuura, M. Burke, and M. Ikebe, "Identification of myosin III as a protein kinase," *Biochemistry*, vol. 35, no. 29, pp. 9392–9399, 1996.

[21] V. L. Walsh, D. Raviv, A. A. Dror et al., "A mouse model for human hearing loss DFNB30 due to loss of function of myosin IIIA," *Mammalian Genome*, vol. 22, no. 3-4, pp. 170–177, 2011.

[22] H. Yang, H. Wang, and R. Jaenisch, "Generating genetically modified mice using CRISPR/CAS-mediated genome engineering," *Nature Protocols*, vol. 9, no. 8, pp. 1956–1968, 2014.

[23] Y. Fujihara and M. Ikawa, "CRISPR/Cas9-based genome editing in mice by single plasmid injection," *Methods in Enzymology*, vol. 546, pp. 319–336, 2014.

[24] K. A. Steigelman, A. Lelli, X. Wu et al., "Polycystin-1 is required for stereocilia structure but not for mechanotransduction in inner ear hair cells," *Journal of Neuroscience*, vol. 31, no. 34, pp. 12241–12250, 2011.

[25] J. Gong, X. Wang, C. Zhu et al., "Insm1a regulates motor neuron development in zebrafish," *Frontiers in Molecular Neuroscience*, vol. 10, p. 274, 2017.

[26] Y. He, X. Lu, F. Qian, D. Liu, R. Chai, and H. Li, "*Insm1a* is required for zebrafish posterior lateral line development," *Frontiers in Molecular Neuroscience*, vol. 10, p. 241, 2017.

[27] X. Fu, L. Zhang, Y. Jin et al., "Loss of myh14 increases susceptibility to noise-induced hearing loss in CBA/CaJ mice," *Neural Plasticity*, vol. 2016, Article ID 6720420, 16 pages, 2016.

[28] Y. Wang, J. Li, X. Yao et al., "Loss of CIB2 causes profound hearing loss and abolishes mechanoelectrical transduction in mice," *Frontiers in Molecular Neuroscience*, vol. 10, p. 401, 2017.

[29] X. Lu, S. Sun, J. Qi et al., "Bmi1 regulates the proliferation of cochlear supporting cells via the canonical Wnt signaling pathway," *Molecular Neurobiology*, vol. 54, no. 2, pp. 1326–1339, 2016.

[30] C. Cheng, L. Guo, L. Lu et al., "Characterization of the transcriptomes of Lgr5+ hair cell progenitors and Lgr5− supporting cells in the mouse cochlea," *Frontiers in Molecular Neuroscience*, vol. 10, p. 122, 2017.

[31] R. Hertzano, E. Shalit, A. K. Rzadzinska et al., "A *Myo6* mutation destroys coordination between the myosin heads, revealing new functions of myosin VI in the stereocilia of mammalian inner ear hair cells," *PLoS Genetics*, vol. 4, no. 10, article e1000207, 2008.

[32] T. Self, M. Mahony, J. Fleming, J. Walsh, S. D. Brown, and K. P. Steel, "Shaker-1 mutations reveal roles for myosin VIIA in both development and function of cochlear hair cells," *Development*, vol. 125, no. 4, pp. 557–566, 1998.

[33] Z. He, L. Guo, Y. Shu et al., "Autophagy protects auditory hair cells against neomycin-induced damage," *Autophagy*, vol. 13, no. 11, pp. 1884–1904, 2017.

[34] A. Lelli, Y. Asai, A. Forge, J. R. Holt, and G. S. G. Géléoc, "Tonotopic gradient in the developmental acquisition of sensory transduction in outer hair cells of the mouse cochlea," *Journal of Neurophysiology*, vol. 101, no. 6, pp. 2961–2973, 2009.

[35] Y. Chen, L. Liu, Y. Zhang, R. Chai, and H. Li, "Wnt activation protects against neomycin-induced hair cell damage in the mouse cochlea," *The Journal of Laryngology & Otology*, vol. 130, no. S3, pp. S105–S105, 2016.

[36] F. T. Salles, R. C. Merritt, U. Manor et al., "Myosin IIIa boosts elongation of stereocilia by transporting espin 1 to the plus ends of actin filaments," *Nature Cell Biology*, vol. 11, no. 4, pp. 443–450, 2009.

[37] R. C. Merritt, U. Manor, F. T. Salles et al., "Myosin IIIB uses an actin-binding motif in its espin-1 cargo to reach the tips of actin protrusions," *Current Biology*, vol. 22, no. 4, pp. 320–325, 2012.

[38] B. C. An, T. Sakai, S. Komaba et al., "Phosphorylation of the kinase domain regulates autophosphorylation of myosin IIIA and its translocation in microvilli," *Biochemistry*, vol. 53, no. 49, pp. 7835–7845, 2014.

[39] O. A. Quintero, W. C. Unrath, S. M. Stevens Jr, U. Manor, B. Kachar, and C. M. Yengo, "Myosin 3A kinase activity is regulated by phosphorylation of the kinase domain activation loop," *Journal of Biological Chemistry*, vol. 288, no. 52, pp. 37126–37137, 2013.

[40] S. Ebrahim, M. R. Avenarius, M.'. Grati et al., "Corrigendum: stereocilia-staircase spacing is influenced by myosin III motors and their cargos espin-1 and espin-like," *Nature Communications*, vol. 8, p. 16133, 2017.

[41] A. Lelli, V. Michel, J. Boutet de Monvel et al., "Class III myosins shape the auditory hair bundles by limiting microvilli and stereocilia growth," *Journal of Cell Biology*, vol. 212, no. 2, pp. 231–244, 2016.

17

Role of Adiponectin in Central Nervous System Disorders

Jenna Bloemer,[1] **Priyanka D. Pinky**,[1] **Manoj Govindarajulu**,[1] **Hao Hong**,[2] **Robert Judd**,[3] **Rajesh H. Amin**,[1,4] **Timothy Moore**,[1,4] **Muralikrishnan Dhanasekaran**,[1,4] **Miranda N. Reed**,[1,4] **and Vishnu Suppiramaniam**[1,4]

[1]*Department of Drug Discovery and Development, Auburn University, Auburn, AL, USA*
[2]*Department of Pharmacology, Key Laboratory of Neuropsychiatric Diseases, China Pharmaceutical University, Nanjing, China*
[3]*Department of Anatomy, Physiology and Pharmacology, College of Veterinary Medicine, Auburn University, Auburn, AL, USA*
[4]*Center for Neuroscience, Auburn University, Auburn, AL, USA*

Correspondence should be addressed to Miranda N. Reed; reedmir@auburn.edu and Vishnu Suppiramaniam; suppivd@auburn.edu

Academic Editor: Massimo Grilli

Adiponectin, the most abundant plasma adipokine, plays an important role in the regulation of glucose and lipid metabolism. Adiponectin also possesses insulin-sensitizing, anti-inflammatory, angiogenic, and vasodilatory properties which may influence central nervous system (CNS) disorders. Although initially not thought to cross the blood-brain barrier, adiponectin enters the brain through peripheral circulation. In the brain, adiponectin signaling through its receptors, AdipoR1 and AdipoR2, directly influences important brain functions such as energy homeostasis, hippocampal neurogenesis, and synaptic plasticity. Overall, based on its central and peripheral actions, recent evidence indicates that adiponectin has neuroprotective, antiatherogenic, and antidepressant effects. However, these findings are not without controversy as human observational studies report differing correlations between plasma adiponectin levels and incidence of CNS disorders. Despite these controversies, adiponectin is gaining attention as a potential therapeutic target for diverse CNS disorders, such as stroke, Alzheimer's disease, anxiety, and depression. Evidence regarding the emerging role for adiponectin in these disorders is discussed in the current review.

1. Introduction

Adiponectin, a hormone produced by adipocytes, regulates metabolic processes and improves insulin sensitivity. Adiponectin signaling has been widely studied in multisystem diseases, for example, obesity, diabetes, dyslipidemia, atherosclerosis, and comorbid metabolic dysfunction in the setting of cardiovascular disease such as hypertension. Serum adiponectin levels appear to be inversely correlated with the presence and severity of metabolic dysfunction, that is, lower serum adiponectin is seen in patients with disease [1–5]. Serum adiponectin levels also appear to be altered in various neurological disorders in which the etiologies of these conditions involve both metabolic and inflammatory components. Furthermore, adiponectin receptors are highly expressed in a number of brain regions, and adiponectin exerts neuroprotective and antidepressant properties, likely through specific adiponectin receptors expressed in the central nervous system (CNS). Therefore, this review provides an overview of adiponectin and discusses recent evidence supporting adiponectin's role in stroke, Alzheimer's disease (AD), anxiety, and depression.

2. Overview of Adiponectin

2.1. Structure and Production of Adiponectin. Adiponectin is a 244-amino acid polypeptide protein which belongs to the complement 1q family [6]. Adiponectin is produced in adipocytes, and its transcription is regulated by sirtuin 1/forkhead box O-1 and peroxisome proliferator-activated receptors (PPARs) [7]. It forms a characteristic homomultimer composed of an NH_2-terminal collagenous region and a COOH-terminal globular domain [8]. Usually, adiponectin exists as a full-length protein of 30 kDa (fAd) that circulates in trimeric, hexameric, and higher order complexes [9]. Adiponectin is further identified based on the molecular weight of these multimers as low (trimer), middle (hexameric), and high (higher order complexes) [10]. In the circulation, adiponectin is present as either these full-length forms or a smaller, globular fragment. Full-length adiponectin is cleaved by leukocyte esterase to form globular adiponectin (gAd). Both gAd and fAd mediate tissue-specific effects, as well as regulate distinct signaling pathways in the same tissue. Studies report that a sexual dimorphism exists in serum adiponectin levels. Adiponectin serum levels are approximately 2.5-fold higher in female than in male mice [11], and this sexual dimorphism is also confirmed in humans [12]. Furthermore, the associations between adiponectin and certain disease states appear to be sex specific [13–15]. Because adiponectin may have sex-specific effects, differentiating the effects of altered adiponectin levels in both males and females is important, although the vast majority of rodent studies have only been performed in males.

It was initially thought that adiponectin does not cross the blood-brain barrier (BBB) [16]. However, adiponectin is observed in human cerebral spinal fluid (CSF) [17, 18], with evidence that the adiponectin trimer is the predominate form [17]. In addition, studies in mice show that peripheral intravenous application of adiponectin leads to a concurrent rise in CSF adiponectin [19]. Therefore, adiponectin does cross the BBB, although concentrations in the CSF are approximately 1000-fold lower than that in serum [17].

2.2. Adiponectin Receptors. Adiponectin is known to bind 3 receptors: adiponectin receptor 1 (AdipoR1), adiponectin receptor 2 (AdipoR2), and T-cadherin. AdipoR1 and AdipoR2 were isolated from a human skeletal muscle cDNA library with AdipoR2 showing >60% homology to AdipoR1 [20]. Though AdipoR1 and AdipoR2 are surface membrane proteins containing seven transmembrane domains, they differ from other G protein-coupled receptors, because the amino terminal of the receptor is located intracellularly while the carboxyl terminal is located extracellularly [21]. AdipoR1 and AdipoR2 are expressed abundantly in the liver, muscle, brain, and adipose tissue in humans. These receptors have differing affinities for specific forms of adiponectin. While AdipoR1 is a high-affinity receptor for gAd, it acts as a low-affinity receptor for fAd in skeletal muscle. In contrast, AdipoR2 is an intermediate-affinity receptor for both gAd and fAd in the liver [22]. Mouse studies indicate that AdipoR1 and AdipoR2 mediate metabolic actions of adiponectin in peripheral tissues [23]. These effects are apparent in AdipoR1-AdipoR2 double knockout mice, which are glucose intolerant and hyperinsulinemic under certain conditions. This indicates that AdipoR1 and AdipoR2 are important for regulating basal glucose levels and insulin sensitivity. In the CNS, AdipoR1 and AdipoR2 are expressed in various areas of the brain, including the hypothalamus, brainstem, hippocampus, and cortex [24]. In the hypothalamus and brainstem, adiponectin is thought to regulate food intake and energy expenditure via AdipoR1-mediated AMP-activated protein kinase (AMPK) signaling [25]. This signaling may relate to the association between adiponectin and metabolic disease including atherosclerosis, which is a precipitating factor for stroke. In the hippocampus, adiponectin appears to promote neurogenesis via AdipoR1 [26] and directly affects synaptic function via AdipoR2 [27]. Adiponectin signaling in various areas of the brain, including the cortex, appears to be neuroprotective against damage induced by metabolic insults, such as a high-fat diet, in part through AdipoR1 [28].

High molecular weight forms of adiponectin can bind to T-cadherin, which is traditionally thought of as a receptor that binds low-density lipoprotein (LDL) with signaling cascades related to cell growth, proliferation, and migration. T-cadherin, a glycosylphosphatidylinositol-anchored membrane protein, is abundantly present in the cardiovascular system [29]. Deficiency in T-cadherin leads to exacerbation of cardiac hypertrophy during chronic pressure overload, suggesting a cardioprotective role of T-cadherin [30]. T-cadherin is a unique receptor, because it lacks cytoplasmic and transmembrane domains [30]. Therefore, the mechanism by which T-cadherin influences intracellular signaling is unclear, and it has been suggested that this receptor may require interaction with transmembrane proteins for some physiological actions [31].

Several studies have established a link between the gene that encodes T-cadherin, cadherin 13, and various metabolic diseases [32–34]. Furthermore, in human aortic smooth muscle cells, adiponectin's ability to inhibit inflammation was negated after knockdown of T-cadherin [35]. This evidence suggests that adiponectin interactions with T-cadherin may account for some of adiponectin's metabolic effects. T-cadherin is also present in the brain [36]. However, whether interactions between adiponectin and T-cadherin occur in the brain is unclear. T-cadherin's preference for binding high molecular weight adiponectin isomers over lower molecular weight isoforms [29] may preclude the interaction, as the major adiponectin isoform in the brain is the trimeric form (~80%) with the other 20% predominately being lower molecular weight forms [17]. Because metabolic dysfunction may be a precipitating factor in cognitive dysfunction [37, 38], the mechanistic relationship between peripheral adiponectin signaling through T-cadherin and any downstream effects on cognition should be further explored.

2.3. Peripheral Adiponectin Receptor Signaling. Adiponectin receptor signaling in the periphery regulates insulin sensitivity, reduces oxidative stress, and inhibits inflammation. In the downstream signaling pathways of AdipoR1 and AdipoR2, the adapter protein containing a pleckstrin homology domain, phosphotyrosine binding domain, and leucine zipper motif (APPL1) links the adiponectin receptors to various signaling molecules including AMPK and p38 mitogen-activated protein kinase (p38MAPK), which are important for many metabolic actions of adiponectin [39]. AMPK further mediates important downstream effects of adiponectin, including enhanced insulin sensitivity in part through serine phosphorylation of insulin receptor substrate 1 (IRS-1) [40]. While AdipoR1 regulates insulin sensitivity via activation of the AMPK pathway, AdipoR2 is more involved with activation of the peroxisome proliferator-activated receptor alpha (PPARα) pathway, which stimulates energy dissipation and inhibits inflammation and oxidative stress [23].

Overall, adiponectin appears to reduce inflammation cascades *in vivo* and *in vitro* by several mechanisms, although there is some conflicting data concerning overall effects in immunological diseases [41]. Adiponectin decreases the expression of proinflammatory cytokines such as tumor necrosis factor-α (TNF-α) [42] and increases the expression of anti-inflammatory molecules such as interleukin 10 (IL-10) [43]. In return, some proinflammatory factors, such as TNF-α and IL-6, appear to inhibit the production of adiponectin [44] suggesting bidirectional modulation.

Adiponectin also has a role in the reduction of oxidative stress through AMPK-mediated reduction of reactive oxygen species [45]. Furthermore, disruption of AdipoR1 and AdipoR2 signaling results in significantly increased expression of genes encoding chemokines, such as chemokine C-C motif ligand 2, and decreased expression of genes encoding molecules that reduce oxidative stress [23]. In pancreatic beta cells and cardiomyocytes, overexpression of adiponectin decreases caspase-8-mediated cell death, whereas genetic ablation of adiponectin enhances apoptosis [46, 47]. In summary, the proposed beneficial effects of adiponectin in the periphery include improved insulin sensitivity, reduced inflammation, and reduced oxidative stress.

While the previously mentioned peripheral effects of adiponectin are mainly due to AdipoR1 and AdipoR2 signaling, less is known about adiponectin-T-cadherin-specific signaling. Overall, T-cadherin appears to be important in anti-atherogenesis and cardioprotection. T-cadherin is necessary for adiponectin-mediated phosphorylation of AMPK in some models of ischemia [48]. Interestingly, T-cadherin may not independently mediate signaling, but instead may function to localize circulating adiponectin at target tissues. Following ischemia, T-cadherin appears to localize adiponectin to vascular tissue, where adiponectin promotes revascularization and prevents atherosclerotic plaque formation [31, 35].

2.4. Central Adiponectin Receptor Signaling. In the brain, adiponectin appears to play a role not only in energy homeostasis, but also in neuroprotection in various disease states. In the hypothalamus, adiponectin signaling influences satiety, as well as energy homeostasis. Intracerebroventricular (i.c.v.) delivery of adiponectin improves peripheral insulin sensitivity and glucose homeostasis [49], suggesting that central actions of adiponectin may also influence metabolic diseases. In the hippocampus, adiponectin signaling regulates neurogenesis and synaptic plasticity. *In vitro*, adiponectin increases proliferation in hippocampal progenitor cells and Neuro2a cells through AdipoR1 signaling [26]. In the hippocampal dentate gyrus (DG) of adult male mice, reductions in adiponectin lead to reduced neurogenesis, and adiponectin i.c.v. infusion increases neurogenesis [50]. This effect is mediated by activation of p38MAPK and the resultant inactivation of glycogen synthase kinase 3 beta via phosphorylation of Ser-389 [51]. A reduction in adult neurogenesis may be linked to depression since stressful conditions reduce hippocampal neurogenesis, whereas antidepressant treatment increases neurogenesis [52]. However, a causal relationship for reduced neurogenesis in depression is not well established [53]. Thus, additional research is required to elucidate a possible role for promotion of neurogenesis via adiponectin as a therapeutic option in treatment of depression.

2.5. Summary. Our understanding of adiponectin and its role in maintaining metabolic homeostasis and modulating various systemic disease states has greatly increased over the past decade. The role for adiponectin in CNS disorders is becoming more appreciated, although much remains unknown. The remainder of this review will focus on the role of adiponectin in cerebrovascular disease/stroke, mild cognitive impairment (MCI) and AD, anxiety, and depression (Figure 1). A summary of major studies related to the neuroprotective effects of adiponectin in these CNS disorders is provided in Table 1.

3. Adiponectin in Atherosclerosis/Stroke

3.1. Overview and Adiponectin Levels in Stroke. According to American Heart Association Statistics Committee and Stroke Statistics Subcommittee, approximately 700,000 people experience a new or recurrent stroke every year, and on an average, every 45 seconds someone in the United States suffers from a stroke [54]. Since adiponectin is associated with many cardiovascular risk factors, such as hypertension, type II diabetes, and an altered lipid profile, a link between adiponectin and stroke is expected [55]. However, a meta-analysis of prospective cohort studies determined that plasma adiponectin levels are not a risk factor for the occurrence of the disease [56]. Yet, low plasma adiponectin levels have been observed poststroke, and in fact, decreased adiponectin levels predict increased risk of 5-year mortality after a first-ever ischemic stroke [57]. Thus, the utility of plasma adiponectin levels in management of risk factors for stroke versus management of poststroke sequelae may differ, and this difference may be due to varying mechanisms of action elicited by adiponectin receptor signaling under differing conditions.

3.2. Adiponectin Protective Effects in Stroke. Despite unclear data on the correlations between serum adiponectin levels and stroke risk or recovery from stroke, there are several studies demonstrating adiponectin-mediated mechanistic effects that are protective against atherosclerosis as well as stroke pathogenesis. Circulating adiponectin inhibits monocyte adhesion to endothelial cells [58] and inhibits macrophage transformation to foam cells by reducing oxidized LDL binding and uptake [59]. This process is a crucial step in atherosclerosis as well as stroke pathogenesis. Adiponectin also inhibits induction of vascular cell adhesion molecule-1 (VCAM-1) and intracellular cell adhesion molecule-1 (ICAM-1) [60], which typically bind to leukocytes and initiate formation of atheroma following endothelial cell injury [61]. The mechanism for reduction in adhesion molecules may be through activation of AdipoR2

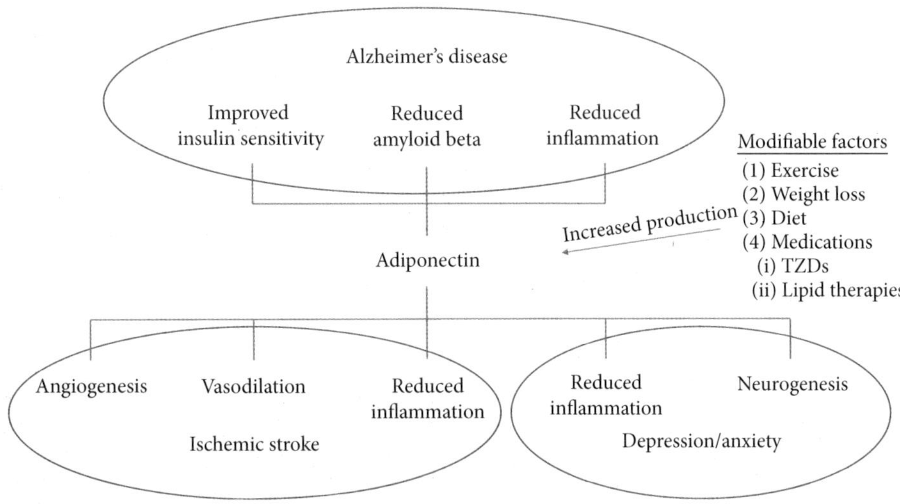

Figure 1: Proposed beneficial effects of adiponectin in central nervous system disorders. Adiponectin receptor signaling is under investigation for central nervous system disorders including Alzheimer's disease (AD), ischemic stroke, and depression. In models of AD, adiponectin receptor activation appears to reduce amyloid beta and improve insulin sensitivity. Adiponectin receptor signaling increases angiogenesis and enhances vasodilation, which may be of benefit in the treatment or prevention of ischemic stroke. Reductions in inflammation related to adiponectin may be beneficial to decrease risk of various diseases, including ischemic stroke, AD, and depression/anxiety. Adult neurogenesis may be reduced in depression, and adiponectin promotes neurogenesis especially in response to exercise. There are a number of modifiable factors that enhance production of adiponectin and may reduce risk of the previously mentioned disorders. In particular, exercise, weight loss, a diet rich in omega-3 polyunsaturated fatty acids, and certain medications such as lipid-lowering therapies and thiazolidinediones (TZDs) all increase circulating adiponectin levels.

which increases PPARα activity [23], since PPARα agonists can also reduce VCAM-1 [62] and ICAM-1 [63]. Interestingly, a clinical trial with the PPARγ agonist rosiglitazone resulted in increased circulating levels of adiponectin and reduced circulating VCAM-1 [64], indicating that PPARγ agonists may confer antiatherogenic properties [65] through an increase in adiponectin.

Other studies show that elevated plasma adiponectin protects endothelial cells from hypercholesterolemia-induced vascular injury and suppresses the uptake of modified LDL into foam cells. In mouse models of atherosclerosis, adiponectin reduces the size of atherosclerotic lesions [66], whereas adiponectin knockout (APN-KO) mice exhibit excessive vascular remodeling in response to acute ischemic insult [67]. While APN-KO mice exhibit increases in breadth of cerebral infarct after ischemia-reperfusion, exogenous adiponectin reduces the infarct size in both APN-KO and wild type mice. Furthermore, adiponectin overexpression increases indices of positive behavioral outcomes as well as stimulates angiogenesis following ischemic injury [68]. Therefore, adiponectin may regulate vascular remodeling, confer antiatherogenic properties within the vasculature, and afford protection against stroke and/or stroke severity.

3.3. Adiponectin Influences Nitric Oxide. Protective actions of adiponectin in stroke may also be due to stimulation of nitric oxide (NO) synthesis from endothelial cells [69], through AdipoR1 signaling [70, 71]. In case of acute stroke, intense vasospasm may occur over the first few weeks which can lead to increased morbidity and mortality. NO plays a significant protective role, since it causes vasodilation and increases blood flow [72]. Adiponectin increases NO production through stimulation endothelial NO synthase (eNOS), and therefore, adiponectin may be neuroprotective following stroke [70]. Usually, plasma NO production is increased in response to hypoxia/ischemia, but this response is absent in APN-KO mice [69]. Adiponectin treatment of bovine aortic endothelial cells increases NO production significantly, an effect mediated by phosphorylation of both Akt at Ser^{473} and eNOS at Ser^{1179} via phosphatidylinositol-4,5-bisphosphate 3-kinase (PI3K) [73]. Akt can also directly phosphorylate eNOS at Ser^{117}, resulting in NO production and the regulation of vasomotor responses [74]. Phosphorylation of Akt is activated by calmodulin-dependent protein kinase kinase (CaMKK), which then concomitantly phosphorylates eNOS in response to increased calcium in the cytoplasm [75]. The calcium-dependent activation of calmodulin stimulates CaMKK and the recruitment of calmodulin to eNOS, causing a "burst-like" release of NO. AMPK, which is also activated by adiponectin signaling, activates cardiac and endothelial cell eNOS by phosphorylation at Ser^{1177} (human sequence) *in vitro* [56]. AMPK signaling is also required for vascular endothelial growth factor -stimulated endothelial cell NO production, migration, and differentiation in response to hypoxic conditions and increased oxidative stress in stroke [76], which also promotes angiogenesis in vivo. Therefore, adiponectin may play a significant protective role in stroke via influence on NO.

3.4. Summary. Because adiponectin reduces cerebrovascular infarct size and improves behavioral outcomes following cerebral ischemia, therapeutic strategies targeting the adiponectin signaling pathways (Figure 2) should be considered for further study. However, achieving beneficial therapeutic

Table 1: Major animal and *in vitro* studies regarding neuroprotective effects of adiponectin in various CNS disorders.

Related pathology	Model	Treatment	Key effect(s) and mechanism(s)	Reference
Stroke	Male apo$E^{-/-}$ mice (12–14 weeks)	Ad-APN (i.v.) 14 days prior to measurements	Effects: Ad-APN treatment reduced atherosclerotic lesion size, reduced the diameter of lipid droplets, and reduced VCAM-1 mRNA	Okamoto [66]
Stroke	Male AdipoKO, eNOS KO, and WT mice (10–12 weeks)	Ad-APN (i.v.) 5 days prior to ischemia (1 hour of middle cerebral artery occlusion followed by 23 hours of reperfusion)	Effects: larger infarct size in AdipoKO mice compared to WT; reduced infarct size in AdipoKO and WT mice when pretreated with Ad-APN Mechanism: adiponectin reduces infarct size through eNOS; there was no alteration in infarct size in eNOS KO mice pretreated with Ad-APN	Nishimura [69]
Stroke	Male CD-1 mice (young: 3 months; age: 22–24 months)	AAV-APN (striatal injection) 7 days prior to transient middle cerebral artery occlusion	Effects: AAV-APN treatment improved motor function (neurological score, beam walk test, rotarod test, and corner test) and increased angiogenesis in young and aged mice	Miao [68]
Alzheimer's disease	SH-SY5Y$_{swAPP}$ cell line	Adiponectin (10 μg/ml) for 2 h followed by hydrogen peroxide (200–800 μM)	Effect: improved neuronal survival with adiponectin incubation prior to insult Mechanisms: adiponectin is neuroprotective against oxidative stress via AdipoR1, AdipoR2, and APPL1; improved neuronal survival was prevented by knockdown of AdipoR1, AdipoR2, or APPL1	Chan [115]
Alzheimer's disease	Male C57BL/6J mice (8–14 weeks)	Osmotin (15 mg/kg, i.p.) at 3 or 40 days following administration of $A\beta_{1-42}$ (i.c.v.)	Effects: osmotin treatment improved Y-maze spontaneous alternations performance, reduced $A\beta_{1-42}$ accumulation, and reduced tau hyperphosphorylation	Ali [118]
Alzheimer's disease	Male AdipoKO and WT mice (9 and 18 months)		Effects: AdipoKO mice had impaired performance on MWM and increased expression of $A\beta_{1-42}$, hyperphosphorylated tau, and pIRS-1^{S616} at 18 months	Ng [103]
Alzheimer's disease	SH-SY5Y$_{swAPP}$ cell line	Adiponectin (10 μg/ml, trimeric)	Effects: adiponectin reduced $A\beta_{1-42}$ expression and increased insulin sensitivity Mechanisms: adiponectin reduces $A\beta_{1-42}$ through AdipoR1 and increases insulin sensitivity through AdipoR1 and AMPK; effects blocked by knockdown of AdipoR1 or inhibition of AMPK	Ng [103]
Alzheimer's disease	Male APP/PS1 mice (5–12 months)	Osmotin (12 mg/kg/day i.p.) for 2 days or osmotin (5 mg/kg/day, i.p.) twice a week for 2–4 weeks	Effects: osmotin treatment increased NMDAR expression, improved hippocampal CA1 LTP, and improved performance on MWM	Shah [119]
Alzheimer's disease	SH-SY5Y$_{swAPP}$ cell line	Osmotin (0.2 μM) for 24 hours	Effects: osmotin reduced expression of $A\beta$ and increased expression of AMPK and SIRT1 Mechanism: osmotin alters expression of these proteins via AdipoR1; knockdown of AdipoR1 prevented these effects	Shah [119]
Alzheimer's disease	Male C57BL/6J mice (5–11 weeks)	AdipoR1 knockdown (shRNA, i.v., weekly injection)	Effects: AdipoR1 knockdown mice displayed impaired performance on MWM, increased body weight, increased $A\beta$, and reduced $pAMPK^{T172}$	Kim [104]

TABLE 1: Continued.

Related pathology	Model	Treatment	Key effect(s) and mechanism(s)	Reference
Depression	Male Adipo$^{+/-}$ and WT mice (9–12 weeks)	Globular (0.3 μg, i.c.v.) or full length (1 μg, i.c.v.) adiponectin	Effects: adiponectin deficient mice displayed increased susceptibility to depressive behaviors (social interaction, sucrose preference test, and learned helplessness following a social defeat paradigm); globular or full length adiponectin had antidepressant effect in WT mice (forced swim test)	Liu [132]
Depression	Male AdipoKO and WT mice (8-9 weeks)		Effects: running enhanced hippocampal neurogenesis and increased hippocampal adiponectin in WT but not AdipoKO mice	Yau [26]
Depression	Neuro2a cell line	Trimeric adiponectin (3 μg/ml)	Effect: adiponectin incubation promoted cell proliferation Mechanism: adiponectin promotes cell proliferation through AdipoR1 in the Neuro2a cell line; siRNA knockdown of AdipoR1 but not AdipoR2 abolished adiponectin induced proliferation	Yau [26]
Anxiety	Male AdipoKO and WT mice (9 and 18 months)		Effect: increased anxiety behavior in 9- and 18-month AdipoKO mice (open-field test)	Ng [103]
PTSD	Male AdipoKO, AdipoR1 conditional KO, AdipoR2 KO, and WT mice (8–2 weeks)	Adiponectin (0.25 μg, intra-DG infusion) daily 3 days prior to fear extinction and 30 min prior to each extinction session	Effects: AdipoKO and AdipoR2 KO mice, but not AdipoR1 conditional KO mice, displayed slower contextual fear extinction learning; adiponectin infusion to DG of hippocampus facilitated extinction learning in WT mice Mechanism: adiponectin facilitations extinction learning via AdipoR2; adiponectin infusion failed to facilitate extinction learning in AdipoR2 KO mice	Zhang [27]
Misc.	Primary hippocampal neurons from Sprague-Dawley rats	Adiponectin (5 or 20 μg/ml) for 48 h followed by kainic acid (100 μM) for 12 h	Effects: adiponectin incubation improved neuronal survival, reduced expression of reactive oxygen species, and reduced caspase-3 activity Mechanism: adiponectin promotes neuronal survival through AMPK; adiponectin enhancement of survival was prevented by an AMPK inhibitor	Qiu [114]
Misc.	Primary neuronal stem cells from ICR mice	Adiponectin (30 μg/ml) for 4 days prior to high glucose (120 mM)	Effects: adiponectin incubation enhanced neurogenesis, increased AdipoR1 expression, and increased TLX expression	Song [28]

Aβ: amyloid beta; AAV-APN: adeno-associated virus expressing adiponectin; Ad-APN: adenovirus expressing adiponectin; AdipoKO: adiponectin knockout; AdipoR1: adiponectin receptor 1; AdipoR2: adiponectin receptor 2; AMPK: 5$'$ AMP-activated protein kinase; apoE: apolipoprotein E; APPL1: adaptor protein, phosphotyrosine interacting with PH domain, and leucine zipper 1; CA1: cornu ammonis 1; DG: dentate gyrus; eNOS: endothelial nitric oxide synthase; i.c.v.: intracerebroventricular; i.p.: intraperitoneal; i.v.: intravenous; IRS-1: insulin receptor substrate 1; KO: knockout; LTP: long-term potentiation; Misc.: miscellaneous; MWM: Morris water maze; NMDAR: N-methyl-D-aspartate receptor; SIRT1: sirtuin 1; TLX: tailless; VCAM-1: vascular cell adhesion molecule 1; WT: wild type.

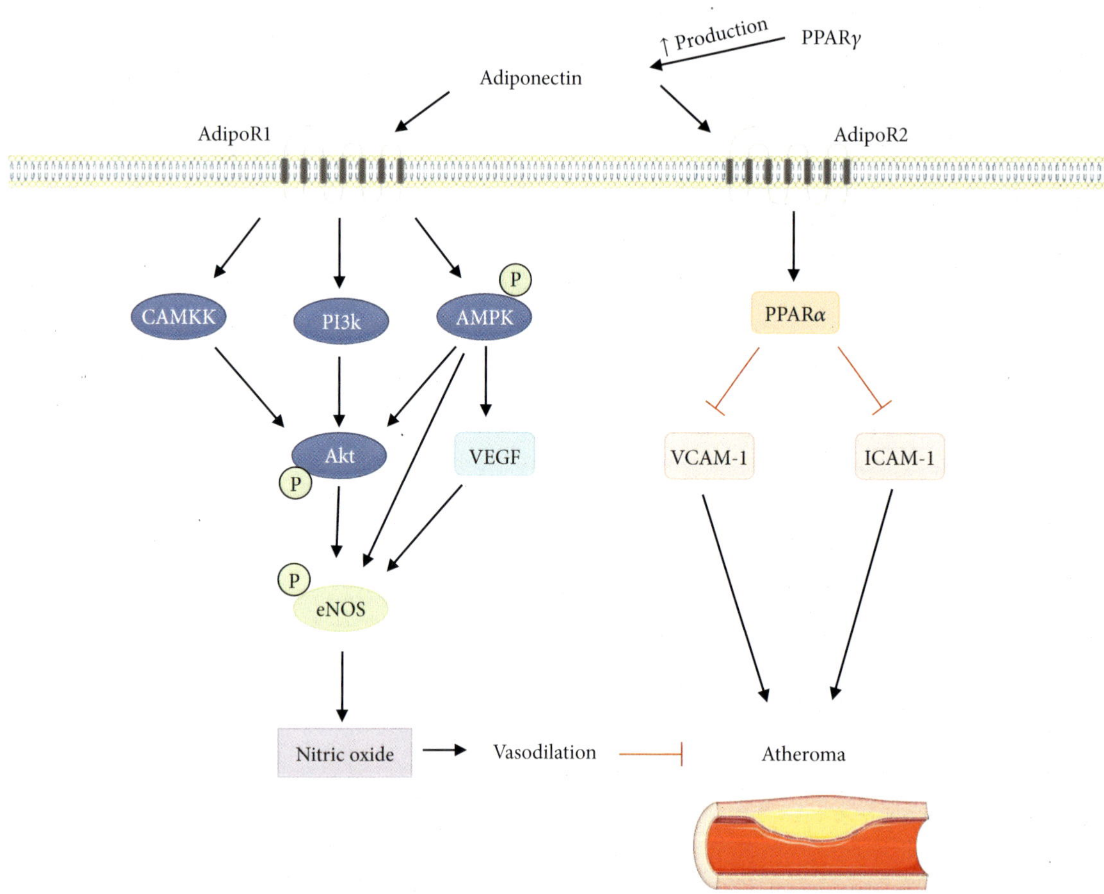

FIGURE 2: Proposed signaling mechanisms of adiponectin in prevention of ischemic stroke. Signaling through AdipoR1 and AdipoR2 can reduce formation of atheroma. AdipoR1 activates the AMP-activated protein kinase (AMPK) pathway resulting in phosphorylation of protein kinase B (Akt) and activation of vascular endothelial growth factor (VEGF). Activation of Akt through calcium calmodulin kinase kinase (CAMKK), phosphatidylinositol-4,5-bisphosphate 3-kinase (PI3K), and AMPK contributes to activation of endothelial nitric oxide synthase (eNOS). Additionally, AMPK and VEGF also increase eNOS activity leading to nitric oxide (NO) production. Increase in production of NO leads to vasodilation, which is beneficial in prevention of atheroma and ischemia. Adiponectin signaling reduces vascular cell adhesion molecule 1 (VCAM-1) and intracellular adhesion molecule 1 (ICAM-1), and these adhesion molecules increase atheroma size. Peroxisome proliferator-activated receptor alpha (PPARα) also reduces VCAM-1 and ICAM-1, and PPARα is activated by AdipoR2 signaling. PPARγ increases production of adiponectin and also leads to reduction of VCAM-1 and ICAM-1. This figure was produced using Servier Medical Art (http://www.servier.com/).

concentrations of adiponectin has been difficult due to its high serum concentrations and multimeric structure. Therefore, research designed to develop novel adiponectin mimetics and/or receptor agonists which mimic physiological functions of adiponectin are currently under development.

4. Adiponectin and Alzheimer's Disease

4.1. Overview and Adiponectin Levels in MCI and AD. Currently, more than 5 million Americans are living with AD, and death rates from AD have increased by 89% since 2000 [77]. AD is associated with brain insulin resistance, leading to the possibility that the insulin-sensitizing properties of adiponectin may confer protection in AD and other cognitive disorders [78–80]. Similar to the studies on correlations between adiponectin levels and stroke risk or stroke recovery, contrasting reports exist on the association between adiponectin levels and MCI and/or AD. In a cohort of participants from the Framingham Heart Study, elevated serum adiponectin levels were associated with increased risk for development of AD and dementia in women, but not in men [81]. Additional studies of serum adiponectin levels in MCI and AD have found an increase [82–84], decrease [85], or no change [86, 87] in adiponectin levels. Several factors may account for these disparate findings. For example, one strong predictor of circulating adiponectin levels is body weight; increased body weight is inversely correlated to adiponectin levels [88]. In MCI and AD patients, weight is reduced, [89] which may explain the increase in serum adiponectin in some studies. However, when the Framingham Heart Study adjusted for age, body mass index (BMI), and weight change, there was still a significant increase in the risk of AD, but not all-cause dementia, in women with elevated adiponectin levels [81]. Diet is another consideration for adiponectin levels, as increased intake of omega-3 polyunsaturated fatty acids increases plasma adiponectin [90]. Another potential confounder is drug therapies that affect adiponectin levels

[91]. Drugs used in AD treatment, such as acetylcholinesterase inhibitors, may increase levels of adiponectin [92]. Of note, most studies examining serum levels of adiponectin in MCI/AD have not adjusted for medication factors. One group reported increased serum adiponectin levels following treatment with donepezil, but BMI was concurrently reduced, which confounds the results [92]. Thiazolidinediones [93, 94], which are PPARγ agonists, and lipid-lowering drugs such as niacin [95, 96], fibrates [97, 98], and certain statins [99–101] can also increase adiponectin levels.

Studies are now also evaluating correlations between CSF adiponectin levels and disease onset or progression. In one study, a reduction in CSF adiponectin in AD patients was reported with a concurrent increase in serum adiponectin [102]. In the CSF of these patients, adiponectin was negatively correlated with hyperphosphorylated tau (p-tau), but in contrast, adiponectin was positively correlated with amyloid beta (Aβ). This is interesting as p-tau containing tangles and Aβ plaques are both hallmarks of AD. Reduced adiponectin CSF levels were correlated with declining scores on the mini-mental status exam, a clinical test for cognitive function in which higher scores indicate better memory. This may indicate that as AD progresses, adiponectin in the CSF decreases. Adiponectin was also colocalized with p-tau in neurofibrillary tangles in AD, suggesting that sequestering may occur, which could explain the reduced CSF adiponectin levels [102]. In a separate study, adiponectin levels were increased in the CSF of patients with MCI, but this correlation was not present in AD [82]. Based on these studies, one hypothesis is that increased adiponectin in the CSF may initially indicate MCI, but declining levels may mark disease progression (from MCI to AD). It remains difficult to make conclusions from correlative data on adiponectin levels alone without mechanistic studies, given that adiponectin levels are affected by multiple intrinsic and extrinsic factors.

4.2. Reduced Adiponectin Signaling and Cognitive Deficits. There is growing interest in the role of adiponectin in memory and synaptic plasticity. APN-KO mice historically used to examine peripheral metabolic disorders are now being used to investigate the role of adiponectin in the brain. In one study, APN-KO mice were utilized as a model of insulin resistance and associated memory pathology [103]. The APN-KO mice displayed a number of behavioral changes indicating memory impairments and increased anxiety at 9 and 18 months. Furthermore, the APN-KO mice had increased protein levels of $A\beta_{42}$ and p-tau, pathological markers of AD, in various areas of the brain by 18 months of age compared to age-matched controls. These knockout mice also displayed cerebral insulin resistance and reduced AMPK activation, which is a potential mechanism for the cognitive deficits and pathological markers observed.

A separate group utilized AdipoR1 knockdown mice via shRNA tail vein injection [104]. These mice exhibited approximately a 50% reduction in AdipoR1 protein expression in the brain, liver, kidney, and spleen with metabolic dysfunctions including increased body weight, increased LDL, and hepatic dysfunction after about 6 weeks of shRNA injections. Interestingly, these animals displayed a similar phenotype to APN-KO mice in terms of central effects, including deficits in hippocampal-dependent Morris water maze performance, hippocampal neuronal loss, and increased Aβ. In fact, these deficits were seen in 11-week-old mice after only about 5-6 weeks of AdipoR1 knockdown. Therefore, it appears that reduction of adiponectin or AdipoR1 signaling negatively affects cognition and leads to increases in pathogenic markers of AD. The role of AdipoR2 is less clear. It is noted that in the periphery, both AdipoR1 signaling and AdipoR2 signaling appear to be beneficial in reducing metabolic dysfunction [105], suggesting that signaling through AdipoR2 may also affect cognition. It is also unclear whether the central effects noted in knockout or knockdown mice are the result of peripheral changes, central changes, or a combination of both. Additional mechanistic studies will be highly useful to determine the role of central versus peripheral adiponectin.

4.3. Adiponectin and Brain Insulin Signaling. As reduced insulin signaling is associated with cognitive impairment and AD [106], adiponectin may influence cognition via reductions in insulin resistance. In human studies, AD patients appear to have reduced insulin activity in the brain as demonstrated by elevated levels of phosphorylated IRS-1 at Ser^{616} and Ser^{636} [79] along with reduced insulin receptor (IR) expression [107]. Based on this, there is an immense interest in the use of insulin-sensitizing agents in animal models of AD [108–110], and there is a phase II/III clinical trial examining intranasal insulin in MCI or mild AD with results from the trial expected to emerge soon. As adiponectin is an insulin-sensitizing hormone, there is interest in adiponectin as a treatment for AD to restore insulin signaling in the brain. As expected, aged APN-KO mice have increased pIRS-1 at Ser^{616} and reduced IR levels in the frontal cortex indicating brain insulin resistance [103]. However, unexpectedly, these aged APN-KO mice have increased IR expression in the hippocampus. This may be due to compensatory mechanisms, and despite the increase in IR, the aged APN-KO animals still displayed neuroinflammation, increased apoptosis, and synaptic loss in the hippocampus. In the human neuroblastoma SH-SY5Y cell line, adiponectin enhances insulin sensitivity via activation of AMPK through AdipoR1 signaling [103]. Therefore, adiponectin receptor signaling and effects on insulin sensitivity in the brain may be an interesting mechanism to target in the treatment of AD.

4.4. Adiponectin Acute Effects at Hippocampal Synapses. Adiponectin may also influence cognition by directly affecting hippocampal synaptic plasticity. Adiponectin injection in the DG of the hippocampus leads to a chemical long-term potentiation (LTP) characterized by a 20% increase in excitatory post-synaptic potential slope [111], indicating that adiponectin may have a beneficial effect on memory. Furthermore, adiponectin applied 10 minutes prior to stimulation protocols potentiates LTP via high-frequency stimulation and prevents induction of long-term depression (LTD) via low-frequency stimulation, suggesting that adiponectin may play a role in both LTP and LTD. In contrast to the

DG, in the cornu ammonis 1 (CA1) region of the hippocampus, the adiponectin receptor agonist AdipoRon reduces LTP [112], suggesting subregional variation in adiponectin responses. In addition, these studies found subregion-specific alterations in paired pulse facilitation, indicating potential presynaptic mechanisms of adiponectin signaling. As both AdipoR1 and AdipoR2 are expressed in the hippocampus, it is unclear which receptor is responsible for the synaptic plasticity effects in these regions of the hippocampus. Interestingly, AdipoR2 deletion, but not AdipoR1 deletion, leads to increased hyperexcitability in DG neurons in acute brain slices [27]. Thus, it appears that adiponectin signaling has direct and acute effects on hippocampal synapses, and further research in this area is needed.

4.5. Neuroprotective Properties of Adiponectin. Despite some controversy in human correlational studies, there is strong evidence for the neuroprotective effects of adiponectin in cell culture and animal models [113]. Many studies in cell culture models have described neuroprotective properties of adiponectin against neurotoxic insults. Adiponectin is protective against kainate-induced excitotoxicity [114], Aβ toxicity during oxidative stress [115], and high glucose concentrations [28]. Many of these effects appear to be due to increased AMPK signaling [114, 115]. Interestingly, adiponectin signaling also can occur in astrocytes where it may actually promote expression of proinflammatory cytokines [116], but relatively little work has been done to delineate the role of adiponectin signaling in these cells. In the periphery, adiponectin promotes anti-inflammatory mediators and inhibits production of TNFα [117]. Therefore, it will be interesting to determine how adiponectin may differentially influence inflammation in the periphery versus the CNS and the role of glia cells in adiponectin-mediated neuroinflammation.

In addition to *in vitro* models, *in vivo* models also support a neuroprotective role of adiponectin against pathological markers of AD. A single intraperitoneal injection of the adiponectin receptor agonist, osmotin, improves performance in the Y-maze task in mice exposed to Aβ_{1-42} peptides [118]. In addition, the osmotin-exposed mice demonstrate attenuated expression of Aβ, beta-secretase 1, and p-tau and increased expression of the presynaptic proteins synaptophysin and synaptosomal-associated protein 25. It is interesting to note that only one dose of osmotin is needed to produce these changes in protein expression. Osmotin also reduces Aβ production in APPswe-transfected SH-SY5Y cells through a pathway dependent on AMPK [119]. Furthermore, in osmotin-treated APP/PS1 mice, Aβ expression is reduced and LTP deficits reversed in the hippocampal CA1 region. Taken together, these results indicate that adiponectin signaling is neuroprotective, especially in models of Aβ neurotoxicity.

4.6. Summary. In summary, adiponectin demonstrates a number of neuroprotective properties and also appears to directly influence hippocampal synapses and synaptic plasticity in a subregion-specific manner. This highlights an important role for adiponectin in modulating development of neurocognitive disorders and influencing severity. Further delineation of the role of adiponectin signaling in the brain, particularly the role of specific receptors, is needed.

5. Adiponectin in Anxiety and Depression

5.1. Overview and Adiponectin Levels in Depression. Statistics from the Anxiety and Depression Association of America state that anxiety disorders are one of the most common mental illnesses, affecting 40 million adults, or around 18% of the population, yearly in the United States. Anxiety disorders and depression often coexist, and nearly half of those diagnosed with depression are also diagnosed with an anxiety disorder. A recent meta-analysis found a significant reduction in adiponectin plasma levels in patients with depression compared to those without the disorder [120]. Although Weber-Hamann et al. reported no changes in plasma adiponectin concentrations of depressed patients during 6 weeks of antidepressant treatment [121], Narita et al. showed that plasma adiponectin levels were higher in depressed patients treated with an antidepressant drug for more than 12 months [122], suggesting time-dependent effects in antidepressant-induced alterations in adiponectin levels. However, variations such as age, BMI, additional medications, and other comorbid factors, like heart disease or diabetes, should be kept in mind while interpreting these data, as all have been demonstrated to affect circulating adiponectin levels. As evidence for a role for adiponectin in anxiety disorders, APN-KO mice demonstrate increased anxiety in an open-field test at ages 9 months and 18 months [103]. Further delineation of a specific role for adiponectin in anxiety and/or depressive disorders is needed, as well as more mechanistic studies to help in designing therapeutic strategies around adiponectin signaling.

5.2. Adiponectin and the HPA Axis. There are many potential mechanisms for adiponectin's role in anxiety and/or depression. One hypothesis involves adiponectin suppression of TNFα, a potent proinflammatory cytokine, which typically activates the hypothalamo-pituitary-adrenocortical (HPA) axis. Overactivity of HPA axis contributes to the pathogenesis of depression, in that activation of the HPA axis leads to activation of neuronal serotonin transporters leading to reduced serotonin availability in the brain [123]. TNF-α is thought to play an important role in the pathogenesis of depression by activating the HPA axis. Adiponectin suppresses the production TNFα and induces production of various anti-inflammatory cytokines [124]. Further supporting this, an inverse correlation between adiponectin and circulating TNF-α concentrations exists [122]. Thus, decreased production of adiponectin can lead to dysregulation of cytokines, which could contribute to depression.

Cortisol, a glucocorticoid, is released with activation of the HPA axis. Interestingly, exogenous glucocorticoid exposure appears to have an inhibitory effect on adiponectin expression [125, 126]. Therefore, in the case of pathological overactivation of the HPA axis, adiponectin expression may be reduced, leading to absence of the inhibitory effect of adiponectin on the HPA axis. However, contradictory to this, patients with higher levels of adiponectin had higher levels of cortisol [127]. In addition, adiponectin levels follow a similar diurnal variation of cortisol, which suggests that adiponectin and cortisol might be influenced by common regulatory factors [128]. Therefore, although cortisol appears to suppress adiponectin expression in case of exogenous administration and adiponectin would be expected to suppress cortisol based on effects on the HPA axis, these effects may either "cancel out" *in vivo* or only become physiologically relevant in the presence of additional factors. In summary, adiponectin appears to reduce activation of the HPA axis by reduction of TNFα, but the relationship between cortisol and adiponectin is less clear.

5.3. Adiponectin and Thyroid Hormone Regulation. Adiponectin may also exhibit a relationship with the thyroid axis. As hypothyroidism can contribute to depression and hyperthyroidism can contribute to anxiety, the effects of adiponectin on the thyroid axis are also of interest. Some conflicting data have been observed between adiponectin levels and the thyroid axis. Subjects in the highest quartile of adiponectin levels also have higher circulating concentrations of free thyroxine in serum [127]. However, another study showed that adiponectin was 2-fold higher in hypothyroid than in healthy patients [129]. Studies in hypothyroid dogs and guinea pigs show elevated levels of serum adiponectin, as well as their reduction after thyroid hormone replacement therapy [130]. These data indicate that both hyperthyroidism and hypothyroidism may be associated with increased adiponectin, but there is currently little known about the effects of thyroid hormones on adiponectin gene expression and vice versa.

5.4. Behavioral Effects of Adiponectin. While i.c.v. injection of an adiponectin neutralizing antibody in a diabetic mouse model produces stress-induced depressive- behavior, exogenous adiponectin administration via i.c.v leads to antidepressant- behavioral effects [131]. Thus, it can be hypothesized that drugs that increase endogenous adiponectin levels may also be beneficial to treat depression. Studies in a mouse model of depression showed that the effects of physical exercise in reducing depression symptoms might be mediated by adiponectin, which in turn promotes hippocampal neurogenesis [26]. Furthermore, the antidepressant activity of the PPARγ agonists may be due to increased expression of adiponectin. The PPARγ agonist rosiglitazone has antidepressant and anxiolytic effects, which are absent in mice lacking adiponectin [132]. In addition, a clinical trial demonstrated improvement in major depressive disorder in patients with comorbid metabolic syndrome following treatment with the PPARγ agonist, pioglitazone [133].

Although the mechanisms responsible for the antidepressant effects of adiponectin are unclear, a recent animal study suggests that adiponectin signaling, specifically through AdipoR2, enhances extinction of fear memories [27]. This effect of adiponectin could be beneficial in treatment of posttraumatic stress disorder (PTSD). In this study, hippocampal infusion of adiponectin facilitated the extinction of contextual fear, but did not affect the acquisition of fear memories. Furthermore, deletion of AdipoR2, but not AdipoR1, reduced fear extinction [27]. Based on these observations, increasing adiponectin production or activating AdipoR2 receptors might be useful for facilitating extinction-based exposure treatments in managing PTSD and other trauma- and stress-related disorders.

5.5. Summary. At present, existing evidence concerning adiponectin and its relationship to depression and anxiety is somewhat controversial. In population-based studies, there appears to be a correlation between adiponectin levels and depression, and adiponectin may indirectly influence anxiety and depression through its actions on the HPA axis and/or thyroid-mediated effects. Additionally, adiponectin's direct effects on neurogenesis and extinction learning support continued research in this area with the goal of developing novel treatments for anxiety and depressive disorders.

6. Conclusion

Accumulating evidence indicates that adiponectin and adiponectin receptors may be important targets for translational studies to find novel treatments and/or prevention strategies for various CNS disorders, such as stroke-induced cerebrovascular dysfunction, AD, and anxiety and/or depressive disorders. Clearly, additional research is needed to more thoroughly examine adiponectin receptor signaling in the brain and roles of specific receptors in treatment of disease. Development of specific adiponectin receptor agonists and antagonists will be highly valuable in differentiation of these roles. We predict that adiponectin receptor signaling will be targeted in future clinical trials as a therapeutic strategy for CNS disorders.

Conflicts of Interest

The authors declare that there is no conflict of interest regarding the publication of this paper.

References

[1] Y. Arita, S. Kihara, N. Ouchi et al., "Paradoxical decrease of an adipose-specific protein, adiponectin, in obesity," *Biochemical and Biophysical Research Communications*, vol. 257, no. 1, pp. 79–83, 1999.

[2] K. Hotta, T. Funahashi, Y. Arita et al., "Plasma concentrations of a novel, adipose-specific protein, adiponectin, in type 2 diabetic patients," *Arteriosclerosis, Thrombosis, and Vascular Biology*, vol. 20, no. 6, pp. 1595–1599, 2000.

[3] V. Mohan, R. Deepa, R. Pradeepa et al., "Association of low adiponectin levels with the metabolic syndrome—the Chennai Urban Rural Epidemiology Study (CURES-4)," *Metabolism*, vol. 54, no. 4, pp. 476–481, 2005.

[4] M. Kumada, S. Kihara, S. Sumitsuji et al., "Association of hypoadiponectinemia with coronary artery disease in men," *Arteriosclerosis, Thrombosis, and Vascular Biology*, vol. 23, no. 1, pp. 85–89, 2003.

[5] M.-C. Chen, C.-J. Lee, C.-F. Yang, Y.-C. Chen, J.-H. Wang, and B.-G. Hsu, "Low serum adiponectin level is associated with metabolic syndrome and is an independent marker of peripheral arterial stiffness in hypertensive patients," *Diabetology and Metabolic Syndrome*, vol. 9, no. 1, p. 49, 2017.

[6] T. Kadowaki and T. Yamauchi, "Adiponectin and adiponectin receptors," *Endocrine Reviews*, vol. 26, no. 3, pp. 439–451, 2005.

[7] M. Liu and F. Liu, "Transcriptional and post-translational regulation of adiponectin," *Biochemical Journal*, vol. 425, no. 1, pp. 41–52, 2010.

[8] Y. Wang, K. S. L. Lam, J. Y. Xu et al., "Adiponectin inhibits cell proliferation by interacting with several growth factors in an oligomerization-dependent manner," *The Journal of Biological Chemistry*, vol. 280, no. 18, pp. 18341–18347, 2005.

[9] R. Palanivel, X. Fang, M. Park et al., "Globular and full-length forms of adiponectin mediate specific changes in glucose and fatty acid uptake and metabolism in cardiomyocytes," *Cardiovascular Research*, vol. 75, no. 1, pp. 148–157, 2007.

[10] H. Waki, T. Yamauchi, J. Kamon et al., "Impaired multimerization of human adiponectin mutants associated with diabetes: molecular structure and multimer formation of adiponectin," *The Journal of Biological Chemistry*, vol. 278, no. 41, pp. 40352–40363, 2003.

[11] U. B. Pajvani, X. Du, T. P. Combs et al., "Structure-function studies of the adipocyte-secreted hormone Acrp30/adiponectin: implications for metabolic regulation and bioactivity," *Journal of Biological Chemistry*, vol. 278, no. 11, pp. 9073–9085, 2003.

[12] W.-S. Yang, W.-J. Lee, T. Funahashi et al., "Weight reduction increases plasma levels of an adipose-derived anti-inflammatory protein, adiponectin," *The Journal of Clinical Endocrinology and Metabolism*, vol. 86, no. 8, pp. 3815–3819, 2001.

[13] A. G. Tabak, M. Carstensen, D. R. Witte et al., "Adiponectin trajectories before type 2 diabetes diagnosis: Whitehall II study," *Diabetes Care*, vol. 35, no. 12, pp. 2540–2547, 2012.

[14] J. L. Durand, A. R. Nawrocki, P. E. Scherer, and L. A. Jelicks, "Gender differences in adiponectin modulation of cardiac remodeling in mice deficient in endothelial nitric oxide synthase," *Journal of Cellular Biochemistry*, vol. 113, no. 10, pp. 3276–3287, 2012.

[15] B. Kollerits, D. Fliser, I. M. Heid, E. Ritz, F. Kronenberg, and for the MMKD Study Group, "Gender-specific association of adiponectin as a predictor of progression of chronic kidney disease: the Mild to Moderate Kidney Disease Study," *Kidney International*, vol. 71, no. 12, pp. 1279–1286, 2007.

[16] J. Spranger, S. Verma, I. Göhring et al., "Adiponectin does not cross the blood-brain barrier but modifies cytokine expression of brain endothelial cells," *Diabetes*, vol. 55, no. 1, pp. 141–147, 2006.

[17] C. M. Kusminski, P. G. McTernan, T. Schraw et al., "Adiponectin complexes in human cerebrospinal fluid: distinct complex distribution from serum," *Diabetologia*, vol. 50, no. 3, pp. 634–642, 2007.

[18] M. Neumeier, J. Weigert, R. Buettner et al., "Detection of adiponectin in cerebrospinal fluid in humans," *American Journal of Physiology-Endocrinology and Metabolism*, vol. 293, no. 4, pp. E965–E969, 2007.

[19] Y. Qi, N. Takahashi, S. M. Hileman et al., "Adiponectin acts in the brain to decrease body weight," *Nature Medicine*, vol. 10, no. 5, pp. 524–529, 2004.

[20] T. Yamauchi, J. Kamon, Y. Ito et al., "Cloning of adiponectin receptors that mediate antidiabetic metabolic effects," *Nature*, vol. 423, no. 6941, pp. 762–769, 2003.

[21] X. Mao, C. K. Kikani, R. A. Riojas et al., "APPL1 binds to adiponectin receptors and mediates adiponectin signalling and function," *Nature Cell Biology*, vol. 8, no. 5, pp. 516–523, 2006.

[22] T. Kadowaki, T. Yamauchi, N. Kubota, K. Hara, K. Ueki, and K. Tobe, "Adiponectin and adiponectin receptors in insulin resistance, diabetes, and the metabolic syndrome," *The Journal of Clinical Investigation*, vol. 116, no. 7, pp. 1784–1792, 2006.

[23] T. Yamauchi, Y. Nio, T. Maki et al., "Targeted disruption of AdipoR1 and AdipoR2 causes abrogation of adiponectin binding and metabolic actions," *Nature Medicine*, vol. 13, no. 3, pp. 332–339, 2007.

[24] J. Thundyil, D. Pavlovski, C. G. Sobey, and T. V. Arumugam, "Adiponectin receptor signalling in the brain," *British Journal of Pharmacology*, vol. 165, no. 2, pp. 313–327, 2012.

[25] N. Kubota, W. Yano, T. Kubota et al., "Adiponectin stimulates AMP-activated protein kinase in the hypothalamus and increases food intake," *Cell Metabolism*, vol. 6, no. 1, pp. 55–68, 2007.

[26] S. Y. Yau, A. Li, R. L. C. Hoo et al., "Physical exercise-induced hippocampal neurogenesis and antidepressant effects are mediated by the adipocyte hormone adiponectin," *Proceedings of the National Academy of Sciences of the United States of America*, vol. 111, no. 44, pp. 15810–15815, 2014.

[27] D. Zhang, X. Wang, B. Wang et al., "Adiponectin regulates contextual fear extinction and intrinsic excitability of dentate gyrus granule neurons through AdipoR2 receptors," *Molecular Psychiatry*, vol. 22, no. 7, pp. 1044–1055, 2017.

[28] J. Song, S. M. Kang, E. Kim, C.-H. Kim, H.-T. Song, and J. E. Lee, "Adiponectin receptor-mediated signaling ameliorates cerebral cell damage and regulates the neurogenesis of neural stem cells at high glucose concentrations: an *in vivo* and *in vitro* study," *Cell Death & Disease*, vol. 6, no. 8, p. e1844, 2015.

[29] C. Hug, J. Wang, N. S. Ahmad, J. S. Bogan, T.-S. Tsao, and H. F. Lodish, "T-cadherin is a receptor for hexameric and high-molecular-weight forms of Acrp30/adiponectin," *Proceedings of the National Academy of Sciences of the United States of America*, vol. 101, no. 28, pp. 10308–10313, 2004.

[30] T. Takeuchi, Y. Adachi, Y. Ohtsuki, and M. Furihata, "Adiponectin receptors, with special focus on the role of the third receptor, T-cadherin, in vascular disease," *Medical Molecular Morphology*, vol. 40, no. 3, pp. 115–120, 2007.

[31] J. L. Parker-Duffen, K. Nakamura, M. Silver et al., "T-cadherin is essential for adiponectin-mediated revascularization," *Journal of Biological Chemistry*, vol. 288, no. 34, pp. 24886–24897, 2013.

[32] C.-M. Chung, T.-H. Lin, J.-W. Chen et al., "A genome-wide association study reveals a quantitative trait locus of adiponectin on *CDH13* that predicts cardiometabolic outcomes," *Diabetes*, vol. 60, no. 9, pp. 2417–2423, 2011.

[33] C. Fava, E. Danese, M. Montagnana et al., "A variant upstream of the *CDH13* adiponectin receptor gene and metabolic syndrome in Swedes," *The American Journal of Cardiology*, vol. 108, no. 10, pp. 1432–1437, 2011.

[34] E. Org, S. Eyheramendy, P. Juhanson et al., "Genome-wide scan identifies *CDH13* as a novel susceptibility locus contributing to blood pressure determination in two European populations," *Human Molecular Genetics*, vol. 18, no. 12, pp. 2288–2296, 2009.

[35] Y. Fujishima, N. Maeda, K. Matsuda et al., "Adiponectin association with T-cadherin protects against neointima proliferation and atherosclerosis," *The FASEB Journal*, vol. 31, no. 4, pp. 1571–1583, 2017.

[36] T. Takeuchi, A. Misaki, S.-B. Liang et al., "Expression of T-cadherin (CDH13, H-cadherin) in human brain and its characteristics as a negative growth regulator of epidermal growth factor in neuroblastoma cells," *Journal of Neurochemistry*, vol. 74, no. 4, pp. 1489–1497, 2000.

[37] V. H. Taylor and G. M. MacQueen, "Cognitive dysfunction associated with metabolic syndrome," *Obesity Reviews*, vol. 8, no. 5, pp. 409–418, 2007.

[38] K. F. Yates, V. Sweat, P. L. Yau, M. M. Turchiano, and A. Convit, "Impact of metabolic syndrome on cognition and brain: a selected review of the literature," *Arteriosclerosis, Thrombosis, and Vascular Biology*, vol. 32, no. 9, pp. 2060–2067, 2012.

[39] H. Ruan and L. Q. Dong, "Adiponectin signaling and function in insulin target tissues," *Journal of Molecular Cell Biology*, vol. 8, no. 2, pp. 101–109, 2016.

[40] C. Wang, X. Mao, L. Wang et al., "Adiponectin sensitizes insulin signaling by reducing p70 S6 kinase-mediated serine phosphorylation of IRS-1," *Journal of Biological Chemistry*, vol. 282, no. 11, pp. 7991–7996, 2007.

[41] S. Esmaili, A. Xu, and J. George, "The multifaceted and controversial immunometabolic actions of adiponectin," *Trends in Endocrinology & Metabolism*, vol. 25, no. 9, pp. 444–451, 2014.

[42] P.-H. Park, H. Huang, M. R. McMullen, P. Mandal, L. Sun, and L. E. Nagy, "Suppression of lipopolysaccharide-stimulated tumor necrosis factor-α production by adiponectin is mediated by transcriptional and post-transcriptional mechanisms," *The Journal of Biological Chemistry*, vol. 283, no. 40, pp. 26850–26858, 2008.

[43] M. Kumada, S. Kihara, N. Ouchi et al., "Adiponectin specifically increased tissue inhibitor of metalloproteinase-1 through interleukin-10 expression in human macrophages," *Circulation*, vol. 109, no. 17, pp. 2046–2049, 2004.

[44] J. Hector, B. Schwarzloh, J. Goehring et al., "TNF-α alters visfatin and adiponectin levels in human fat," *Hormone and Metabolic Research*, vol. 39, no. 4, pp. 250–255, 2007.

[45] A. Shrestha and P.-H. Park, "Globular adiponectin attenuates LPS-induced reactive oxygen species production in HepG2 cells via FoxO3A and HO-1 signaling," *Life Sciences*, vol. 148, pp. 71–79, 2016.

[46] W. L. Holland, R. A. Miller, Z. V. Wang et al., "Receptor-mediated activation of ceramidase activity initiates the pleiotropic actions of adiponectin," *Nature Medicine*, vol. 17, no. 1, pp. 55–63, 2011.

[47] W. L. Holland, A. C. Adams, J. T. Brozinick et al., "An FGF21-adiponectin-ceramide axis controls energy expenditure and insulin action in mice," *Cell Metabolism*, vol. 17, no. 5, pp. 790–797, 2013.

[48] M. S. Denzel, M.-C. Scimia, P. M. Zumstein, K. Walsh, P. Ruiz-Lozano, and B. Ranscht, "T-cadherin is critical for adiponectin-mediated cardioprotection in mice," *The Journal of Clinical Investigation*, vol. 120, no. 12, pp. 4342–4352, 2010.

[49] S. Park, D. S. Kim, D. Y. Kwon, and H. J. Yang, "Long-term central infusion of adiponectin improves energy and glucose homeostasis by decreasing fat storage and suppressing hepatic gluconeogenesis without changing food intake," *Journal of Neuroendocrinology*, vol. 23, no. 8, pp. 687–698, 2011.

[50] D. Zhang, X. Wang, and X.-Y. Lu, "Adiponectin exerts neurotrophic effects on dendritic arborization, spinogenesis, and neurogenesis of the dentate gyrus of male mice," *Endocrinology*, vol. 157, no. 7, pp. 2853–2869, 2016.

[51] D. Zhang, M. Guo, W. Zhang, and X.-Y. Lu, "Adiponectin stimulates proliferation of adult hippocampal neural stem/progenitor cells through activation of p38 mitogen-activated protein kinase (p38MAPK)/glycogen synthase kinase 3β (GSK-3β)/β-catenin signaling cascade," *Journal of Biological Chemistry*, vol. 286, no. 52, pp. 44913–44920, 2011.

[52] J. E. Malberg, "Implications of adult hippocampal neurogenesis in antidepressant action," *Journal of Psychiatry & Neuroscience*, vol. 29, no. 3, pp. 196–205, 2004.

[53] M. M. Lee, A. Reif, and A. G. Schmitt, "Major depression: a role for hippocampal neurogenesis?," *Current Topics in Behavioral Neurosciences*, vol. 14, pp. 153–179, 2012.

[54] T. Thom, N. Haase, W. Rosamond et al., "Heart disease and stroke statistics–2006 update: a report from the American Heart Association Statistics Committee and Stroke Statistics Subcommittee," *Circulation*, vol. 113, no. 6, pp. e85–e151, 2006.

[55] M. Matsumoto, S. Ishikawa, and E. Kajii, "Association of adiponectin with cerebrovascular disease: a nested case-control study," *Stroke*, vol. 39, no. 2, pp. 323–328, 2008.

[56] Z.-P. Chen, K. I. Mitchelhill, B. J. Michell et al., "AMP-activated protein kinase phosphorylation of endothelial NO synthase," *FEBS Letters*, vol. 443, no. 3, pp. 285–289, 1999.

[57] S. P. Efstathiou, D. I. Tsioulos, A. G. Tsiakou, Y. E. Gratsias, A. V. Pefanis, and T. D. Mountokalakis, "Plasma adiponectin levels and five-year survival after first-ever ischemic stroke," *Stroke*, vol. 36, no. 9, pp. 1915–1919, 2005.

[58] N. Ouchi, S. Kihara, Y. Arita et al., "Novel modulator for endothelial adhesion molecules: adipocyte-derived plasma protein adiponectin," *Circulation*, vol. 100, no. 25, pp. 2473–2476, 1999.

[59] Y. Arita, S. Kihara, N. Ouchi et al., "Adipocyte-derived plasma protein adiponectin acts as a platelet-derived growth factor-BB-binding protein and regulates growth factor-induced common postreceptor signal in vascular smooth muscle cell," *Circulation*, vol. 105, no. 24, pp. 2893–2898, 2002.

[60] D. Kawanami, K. Maemura, N. Takeda et al., "Direct reciprocal effects of resistin and adiponectin on vascular endothelial cells: a new insight into adipocytokine-endothelial cell interactions," *Biochemical and Biophysical Research Communications*, vol. 314, no. 2, pp. 415–419, 2004.

[61] P. Libby, P. M. Ridker, and A. Maseri, "Inflammation and atherosclerosis," *Circulation*, vol. 105, no. 9, pp. 1135–1143, 2002.

[62] Y. Rival, N. Benéteau, T. Taillandier et al., "PPARα and PPARδ activators inhibit cytokine-induced nuclear translocation of NF-κB and expression of VCAM-1 in EAhy926 endothelial cells," *European Journal of Pharmacology*, vol. 435, no. 2-3, pp. 143–151, 2002.

[63] S. Gautier, T. Ouk, M. Pétrault, O. Pétrault, V. Bérézowski, and R. Bordet, "PPAR-alpha agonist used at the acute phase of experimental ischemic stroke reduces occurrence of

thrombolysis-induced hemorrhage in rats," *PPAR Res*, vol. 2015, article 246329, 6 pages, 2015.

[64] R. Dolezalová, M. M. Haluzík, L. Bosanská et al., "Effect of PPAR-γ agonist treatment on markers of endothelial dysfunction in patients with type 2 diabetes mellitus," *Physiological Research*, vol. 56, no. 6, pp. 741–748, 2007.

[65] S. Zhao, C. Zhang, Y. Lin et al., "The effects of rosiglitazone on aortic atherosclerosis of cholesterol-fed rabbits," *Thrombosis Research*, vol. 123, no. 2, pp. 281–287, 2008.

[66] Y. Okamoto, S. Kihara, N. Ouchi et al., "Adiponectin reduces atherosclerosis in apolipoprotein E-deficient mice," *Circulation*, vol. 106, no. 22, pp. 2767–2770, 2002.

[67] M. Matsuda, I. Shimomura, M. Sata et al., "Role of adiponectin in preventing vascular stenosis: the missing link of adipo-vascular axis," *Journal of Biological Chemistry*, vol. 277, no. 40, pp. 37487–37491, 2002.

[68] J. Miao, L.-H. Shen, Y.-H. Tang et al., "Overexpression of adiponectin improves neurobehavioral outcomes after focal cerebral ischemia in aged mice," *CNS Neuroscience & Therapeutics*, vol. 19, no. 12, pp. 969–977, 2013.

[69] M. Nishimura, Y. Izumiya, A. Higuchi et al., "Adiponectin prevents cerebral ischemic injury through endothelial nitric oxide synthase dependent mechanisms," *Circulation*, vol. 117, no. 2, pp. 216–223, 2008.

[70] C.-F. Chen, J. Huang, H. Li et al., "MicroRNA-221 regulates endothelial nitric oxide production and inflammatory response by targeting adiponectin receptor 1," *Gene*, vol. 565, no. 2, pp. 246–251, 2015.

[71] Y. Du, R. Li, W. B. Lau et al., "Adiponectin at physiologically relevant concentrations enhances the vasorelaxative effect of acetylcholine via Cav-1/AdipoR-1 signaling," *PLoS One*, vol. 11, no. 3, p. e0152247, 2016.

[72] Z.-Q. Chen, R.-T. Mou, D.-X. Feng, Z. Wang, and G. Chen, "The role of nitric oxide in stroke," *Medical Gas Research*, vol. 7, no. 3, pp. 194–203, 2017.

[73] H. Chen, M. Montagnani, T. Funahashi, I. Shimomura, and M. J. Quon, "Adiponectin stimulates production of nitric oxide in vascular endothelial cells," *The Journal of Biological Chemistry*, vol. 278, no. 45, pp. 45021–45026, 2003.

[74] D. Fulton, J.-P. Gratton, T. J. McCabe et al., "Regulation of endothelium-derived nitric oxide production by the protein kinase Akt," *Nature*, vol. 399, no. 6736, pp. 597–601, 1999.

[75] S. Yano, H. Tokumitsu, and T. R. Soderling, "Calcium promotes cell survival through CaM-K kinase activation of the protein-kinase-B pathway," *Nature*, vol. 396, no. 6711, pp. 584–587, 1998.

[76] N. Ouchi, H. Kobayashi, S. Kihara et al., "Adiponectin stimulates angiogenesis by promoting cross-talk between AMP-activated protein kinase and Akt signaling in endothelial cells," *The Journal of Biological Chemistry*, vol. 279, no. 2, pp. 1304–1309, 2004.

[77] "Latest facts & figures report | Alzheimer's Association," January 2018, https://www.alz.org/facts/.

[78] Z. Wan and J. P. Little, "Adiponectin and Alzheimer's disease: is there a link?," *Inflammation and Cell Signaling*, vol. 1, no. 2, 2014.

[79] K. Talbot, H.-Y. Wang, H. Kazi et al., "Demonstrated brain insulin resistance in Alzheimer's disease patients is associated with IGF-1 resistance, IRS-1 dysregulation, and cognitive decline," *Journal of Clinical Investigation*, vol. 122, no. 4, pp. 1316–1338, 2012.

[80] R. J. Mullins, T. C. Diehl, C. W. Chia, and D. Kapogiannis, "Insulin resistance as a link between amyloid-beta and tau pathologies in Alzheimer's disease," *Frontiers in Aging Neuroscience*, vol. 9, p. 118, 2017.

[81] T. M. van Himbergen, A. S. Beiser, M. Ai et al., "Biomarkers for insulin resistance and inflammation and the risk for all-cause dementia and Alzheimer disease," *Archives of Neurology*, vol. 69, no. 5, pp. 594–600, 2012.

[82] K. Une, Y. A. Takei, N. Tomita et al., "Adiponectin in plasma and cerebrospinal fluid in MCI and Alzheimer's disease," *European Journal of Neurology*, vol. 18, no. 7, pp. 1006–1009, 2011.

[83] K. Shafique, A. Ishtiaque, and Z. Arain, "Circulating adiponectin levels and its association with Alzheimer's, dementia, and stroke," *Alzheimer's & Dementia*, vol. 10, no. 4, article P260, 2014.

[84] V. K. Khemka, D. Bagchi, K. Bandyopadhyay et al., "Altered serum levels of adipokines and insulin in probable Alzheimer's disease," *Journal of Alzheimer's Disease*, vol. 41, no. 2, pp. 525–533, 2014.

[85] A. L. Teixeira, B. S. Diniz, A. C. Campos et al., "Decreased levels of circulating adiponectin in mild cognitive impairment and Alzheimer's disease," *NeuroMolecular Medicine*, vol. 15, no. 1, pp. 115–121, 2013.

[86] B. Bigalke, B. Schreitmüller, K. Sopova et al., "Adipocytokines and $CD34^+$ progenitor cells in Alzheimer's disease," *PLoS One*, vol. 6, no. 5, article e20286, 2011.

[87] L. Dukic, A.-M. Simundic, I. Martinic-Popovic et al., "The role of human kallikrein 6, clusterin and adiponectin as potential blood biomarkers of dementia," *Clinical Biochemistry*, vol. 49, no. 3, pp. 213–218, 2016.

[88] A. Lubkowska, A. Radecka, I. Bryczkowska, I. Rotter, M. Laszczyńska, and W. Dudzińska, "Serum adiponectin and leptin concentrations in relation to body fat distribution, hematological indices and lipid profile in humans," *International Journal of Environmental Research and Public Health*, vol. 12, no. 9, pp. 11528–11548, 2015.

[89] I. Cova, F. Clerici, A. Rossi et al., "Weight loss predicts progression of mild cognitive impairment to Alzheimer's disease," *PLoS One*, vol. 11, no. 3, article e0151710, 2016.

[90] M. Mostowik, G. Gajos, J. Zalewski, J. Nessler, and A. Undas, "Omega-3 polyunsaturated fatty acids increase plasma adiponectin to leptin ratio in stable coronary artery disease," *Cardiovascular Drugs and Therapy*, vol. 27, no. 4, pp. 289–295, 2013.

[91] D. Wanders, E. P. Plaisance, and R. L. Judd, "Pharmacological effects of lipid-lowering drugs on circulating adipokines," *World Journal of Diabetes*, vol. 1, no. 4, pp. 116–128, 2010.

[92] M. Pákáski, A. Fehér, A. Juhász et al., "Serum adipokine levels modified by donepezil treatment in Alzheimer's disease," *Journal of Alzheimer's Disease*, vol. 38, no. 2, pp. 371–377, 2014.

[93] J. G. Yu, S. Javorschi, A. L. Hevener et al., "The effect of thiazolidinediones on plasma adiponectin levels in normal, obese, and type 2 diabetic subjects," *Diabetes*, vol. 51, no. 10, pp. 2968–2974, 2002.

[94] R. H. Amin, S. T. Mathews, H. S. Camp, L. Ding, and T. Leff, "Selective activation of PPARγ in skeletal muscle induces endogenous production of adiponectin and protects mice from diet-induced insulin resistance," *American Journal of Physiology-Endocrinology and Metabolism*, vol. 298, no. 1, pp. E28–E37, 2010.

[95] E. P. Plaisance, M. Lukasova, S. Offermanns, Y. Zhang, G. Cao, and R. L. Judd, "Niacin stimulates adiponectin secretion through the GPR109A receptor," *American Journal of Physiology-Endocrinology and Metabolism*, vol. 296, no. 3, pp. E549–E558, 2009.

[96] S. Westphal, K. Borucki, E. Taneva, R. Makarova, and C. Luley, "Extended-release niacin raises adiponectin and leptin," *Atherosclerosis*, vol. 193, no. 2, pp. 361–365, 2007.

[97] R. S. Rosenson, "Effect of fenofibrate on adiponectin and inflammatory biomarkers in metabolic syndrome patients," *Obesity*, vol. 17, no. 3, pp. 504–509, 2009.

[98] T. Nakamura, Y. Kodama, H. Takano et al., "Increase in circulating levels of adiponectin after treatment with statin and fibrate in patients with coronary artery disease and hyperlipidemia," *Atherosclerosis*, vol. 193, no. 2, pp. 449–451, 2007.

[99] S. Devaraj, D. Siegel, and I. Jialal, "Simvastatin (40 mg/day), adiponectin levels, and insulin sensitivity in subjects with the metabolic syndrome," *The American Journal of Cardiology*, vol. 100, no. 9, pp. 1397–1399, 2007.

[100] H. Ando, K. Sugimoto, H. Yanagihara et al., "Effects of atorvastatin and pravastatin on glucose tolerance, adipokine levels and inflammatory markers in hypercholesterolaemic patients," *Clinical and Experimental Pharmacology and Physiology*, vol. 35, no. 9, pp. 1012–1017, 2008.

[101] N. Katsiki and C. S. Mantzoros, "Statins in relation to adiponectin: a significant association with clinical implications," *Atherosclerosis*, vol. 253, pp. 270–272, 2016.

[102] M. Waragai, G. Ho, Y. Takamatsu et al., "Importance of adiponectin activity in the pathogenesis of Alzheimer's disease," *Annals of Clinical Translational Neurology*, vol. 4, no. 8, pp. 591–600, 2017.

[103] R. C.-L. Ng, O.-Y. Cheng, M. Jian et al., "Chronic adiponectin deficiency leads to Alzheimer's disease-like cognitive impairments and pathologies through AMPK inactivation and cerebral insulin resistance in aged mice," *Molecular Neurodegeneration*, vol. 11, no. 1, p. 71, 2016.

[104] M. W. Kim, N. B. Abid, M. H. Jo, M. G. Jo, G. H. Yoon, and M. O. Kim, "Suppression of adiponectin receptor 1 promotes memory dysfunction and Alzheimer's disease-like pathologies," *Scientific Reports*, vol. 7, no. 1, article 12435, 2017.

[105] M. Okada-Iwabu, T. Yamauchi, M. Iwabu et al., "A small-molecule AdipoR agonist for type 2 diabetes and short life in obesity," *Nature*, vol. 503, no. 7477, pp. 493–499, 2013.

[106] J. Bloemer, S. Bhattacharya, R. Amin, and V. Suppiramaniam, "Impaired insulin signaling and mechanisms of memory loss," *Progress in Molecular Biology and Translational Science*, vol. 121, pp. 413–449, 2014.

[107] A. M. Moloney, R. J. Griffin, S. Timmons, R. O'Connor, R. Ravid, and C. O'Neill, "Defects in IGF-1 receptor, insulin receptor and IRS-1/2 in Alzheimer's disease indicate possible resistance to IGF-1 and insulin signalling," *Neurobiology of Aging*, vol. 31, no. 2, pp. 224–243, 2010.

[108] P. L. McClean, V. Parthsarathy, E. Faivre, and C. Holscher, "The diabetes drug liraglutide prevents degenerative processes in a mouse model of Alzheimer's disease," *Journal of Neuroscience*, vol. 31, no. 17, pp. 6587–6594, 2011.

[109] N. Nicolakakis, T. Aboulkassim, B. Ongali et al., "Complete rescue of cerebrovascular function in aged Alzheimer's disease transgenic mice by antioxidants and pioglitazone, a peroxisome proliferator-activated receptor agonist," *Journal of Neuroscience*, vol. 28, no. 37, pp. 9287–9296, 2008.

[110] B. L. Adler, M. Yarchoan, H. M. Hwang et al., "Neuroprotective effects of the amylin analogue pramlintide on Alzheimer's disease pathogenesis and cognition," *Neurobiology of Aging*, vol. 35, no. 4, pp. 793–801, 2014.

[111] F. Pousti, R. Ahmadi, F. Mirahmadi, N. Hosseinmardi, and K. Rohampour, "Adiponectin modulates synaptic plasticity in hippocampal dentate gyrus," *Neuroscience Letters*, vol. 662, pp. 227–232, 2018.

[112] F. Weisz, S. Piccinin, D. Mango et al., "The role of adiponectin receptors in the regulation of synaptic transmission in the hippocampus," *Synapse*, vol. 71, no. 5, article e21964, 2017.

[113] L. Letra, T. Rodrigues, P. Matafome, I. Santana, and R. Seiça, "Adiponectin and sporadic Alzheimer's disease: clinical and molecular links," *Frontiers in Neuroendocrinology*, 2017.

[114] G. Qiu, R. Wan, J. Hu et al., "Adiponectin protects rat hippocampal neurons against excitotoxicity," *Age*, vol. 33, no. 2, pp. 155–165, 2011.

[115] K.-H. Chan, K. S.-L. Lam, O.-Y. Cheng et al., "Adiponectin is protective against oxidative stress induced cytotoxicity in amyloid-beta neurotoxicity," *PLoS One*, vol. 7, no. 12, article e52354, 2012.

[116] Z. Wan, D. Mah, S. Simtchouk, A. Klegeris, and J. P. Little, "Globular adiponectin induces a pro-inflammatory response in human astrocytic cells," *Biochemical and Biophysical Research Communications*, vol. 446, no. 1, pp. 37–42, 2014.

[117] A. T. Turer and P. E. Scherer, "Adiponectin: mechanistic insights and clinical implications," *Diabetologia*, vol. 55, no. 9, pp. 2319–2326, 2012.

[118] T. Ali, G. H. Yoon, S. A. Shah, H. Y. Lee, and M. O. Kim, "Osmotin attenuates amyloid beta-induced memory impairment, tau phosphorylation and neurodegeneration in the mouse hippocampus," *Scientific Reports*, vol. 5, article 11708, no. 1, 2015.

[119] S. A. Shah, G. H. Yoon, S. S. Chung et al., "Novel osmotin inhibits SREBP2 via the AdipoR1/AMPK/SIRT1 pathway to improve Alzheimer's disease neuropathological deficits," *Molecular Psychiatry*, vol. 22, no. 3, pp. 407–416, 2017.

[120] Y. Hu, X. Dong, and J. Chen, "Adiponectin and depression: a meta-analysis," *Biomedical Reports*, vol. 3, no. 1, pp. 38–42, 2015.

[121] B. Weber-Hamann, J. Kratzsch, D. Kopf et al., "Resistin and adiponectin in major depression: the association with free cortisol and effects of antidepressant treatment," *Journal of Psychiatric Research*, vol. 41, no. 3-4, pp. 344–350, 2007.

[122] K. Narita, T. Murata, T. Takahashi, H. Kosaka, N. Omata, and Y. Wada, "Plasma levels of adiponectin and tumor necrosis factor-alpha in patients with remitted major depression receiving long-term maintenance antidepressant therapy," *Progress in Neuro-Psychopharmacology and Biological Psychiatry*, vol. 30, no. 6, pp. 1159–1162, 2006.

[123] M. Berthold-Losleben and H. Himmerich, "The TNF-α system: functional aspects in depression, narcolepsy and psychopharmacology," *Current Neuropharmacology*, vol. 6, no. 3, pp. 193–202, 2008.

[124] H. Tilg and A. M. Wolf, "Adiponectin: a key fat-derived molecule regulating inflammation," *Expert Opinion on Therapeutic Targets*, vol. 9, no. 2, pp. 245–251, 2005.

[125] C. de Oliveira, C. Iwanaga-Carvalho, J. F. Mota, L. M. Oyama, E. B. Ribeiro, and C. M. Oller do Nascimento, "Effects of

adrenal hormones on the expression of adiponectin and adiponectin receptors in adipose tissue, muscle and liver," *Steroids*, vol. 76, no. 12, pp. 1260–1267, 2011.

[126] M. Fasshauer, J. Klein, S. Neumann, M. Eszlinger, and R. Paschke, "Hormonal regulation of adiponectin gene expression in 3T3-L1 adipocytes," *Biochemical and Biophysical Research Communications*, vol. 290, no. 3, pp. 1084–1089, 2002.

[127] J. M. Fernández-Real, A. López-Bermejo, R. Casamitjana, and W. Ricart, "Novel interactions of adiponectin with the endocrine system and inflammatory parameters," *The Journal of Clinical Endocrinology and Metabolism*, vol. 88, no. 6, pp. 2714–2718, 2003.

[128] A. Gavrila, C.-K. Peng, J. L. Chan, J. E. Mietus, A. L. Goldberger, and C. S. Mantzoros, "Diurnal and ultradian dynamics of serum adiponectin in healthy men: comparison with leptin, circulating soluble leptin receptor, and cortisol patterns," *The Journal of Clinical Endocrinology and Metabolism*, vol. 88, no. 6, pp. 2838–2843, 2003.

[129] L. Lozanov, D. Gorcheva, B. Lozanov et al., "Role of thyroid deficiency on adiponectin, leptin, and metabolic status in visceral obesity: a cross-sectional study," *Hormone and Metabolic Research*, vol. 49, no. 9, pp. 667–672, 2017.

[130] M. Mazaki-Tovi, S. K. Abood, A. Kol, A. Farkas, and P. A. Schenck, "Increased serum concentrations of adiponectin in canine hypothyroidism," *Veterinary Journal*, vol. 203, no. 2, pp. 253–255, 2015.

[131] J. Liu, M. Guo, D. Zhang et al., "Adiponectin is critical in determining susceptibility to depressive behaviors and has antidepressant-like activity," *Proceedings of the National Academy of Sciences of the United States of America*, vol. 109, no. 30, pp. 12248–12253, 2012.

[132] M. Guo, C. Li, Y. Lei, S. Xu, D. Zhao, and X.-Y. Lu, "Role of the adipose PPARγ-adiponectin axis in susceptibility to stress and depression/anxiety-related behaviors," *Molecular Psychiatry*, vol. 22, no. 7, pp. 1056–1068, 2017.

[133] K. Sepanjnia, A. Modabbernia, M. Ashrafi, M.-J. Modabbernia, and S. Akhondzadeh, "Pioglitazone adjunctive therapy for moderate-to-severe major depressive disorder: randomized double-blind placebo-controlled trial," *Neuropsychopharmacology*, vol. 37, no. 9, pp. 2093–2100, 2012.

18

Aerobic Exercise Intervention Alters Executive Function and White Matter Integrity in Deaf Children: A Randomized Controlled Study

Xuan Xiong,[1] Li-Na Zhu,[1] Xiao-xiao Dong,[1] Wei Wang,[2] Jun Yan,[1] and Ai-Guo Chen[1]

[1]College of Physical Education, Yangzhou University, Yangzhou, Jiangsu 225127, China
[2]Department of Medical Imaging, The Affiliated Hospital of Yangzhou University, Yangzhou University, Yangzhou, Jiangsu 225009, China

Correspondence should be addressed to Ai-Guo Chen; agchen@yzu.edu.cn

Academic Editor: Ping Zheng

This study examined the effects of an 11-week aerobic exercise intervention on executive function (EF) and white matter integrity (WMI). In total, 28 deaf children (aged 9–13 years) were randomly assigned to either an 11-week exercise intervention or the control group. All the children had behavioral assessment and diffusion tensor imaging prior to and following the exercise intervention. The behavioral performance results demonstrated that EF was enhanced by exercise. Relative to the control group, WMI of the exercise intervention group showed (1) lower fractional anisotropy (FA) in the pontine crossing tract (PCT) and right cingulum (hippocampus) (CH), genu of the corpus callosum (gCC), right inferior cerebellar peduncle (ICP), left superior corona radiata (SCR), and left superior frontooccipital fasciculus (SFOF); (2) higher mean diffusivity (MD) in the gCC, right CH, right inferior frontooccipital fasciculus (IFOF), and left anterior limb of the internal capsule (ALIC); and (3) lower MD in the left ICP and left tapetum (TAP). Furthermore, the lower FA in gCC showed a significant negative correlation with improvement in behavioral performance, but the correlation was not significant after FDR correction. These results suggest that exercise can effectively improve deaf children's EF and reshape the WMI in deaf children. The improved EF by exercise is not related to a reshaping of WMI, but more studies on the relationship between EF and WMI by exercise may be needed.

1. Introduction

Executive function (EF), including inhibition, working memory, and shifting, refers to higher and meta-levels of cognitive processes that regulate and organize purposeful and goal-directed behaviors [1, 2] and is at the core of children's cognition, emotion, and social function, playing an important role in the development of children's mental health [3, 4]. Deficits in EF will seriously harm the development of children's physical, mental, and social achievements; conversely, individuals, local communities, and society will benefit from well-developed EF [5–7]. EF is based on the dynamic interaction between the prefrontal cortex and other cortical and subcortical regions [8], and it is flexible and plastic and can therefore be improved through training, especially in high correlation with children's cognitive development [9, 10]. Various fields have paid attention to EF—particularly at the frontier of interdisciplinary research—as the key to effective methods for improving children's EF.

A burgeoning body of literature has emerged on the positive effects of aerobic exercise on the brain and EF. Exercise plays a causal role in improving EF, as exercise training improves performance of EF tasks [11]. A 10-week aerobic exercise program in primary students with Chinese learning difficulties improved EF performance in the exercise group compared to the control group [12]. Another study of deaf children found positive effects on working memory and shifting of executive function in preadolescent deaf children after an 8-week moderate skipping training program [13]. Nevertheless, it remains unclear whether the neural basis of improvement in deaf children's EF is elicited by exercise intervention.

Exercise intervention improved EF and altered brain activation as assessed by functional magnetic resonance imaging (fMRI). Specifically, a 6-month exercise intervention in older adults improved performance and increased prefrontal and posterior parietal activation during a flanker task in the exercise group as compared to the controls [14]. Changes in regions of the brain were also found in studies of children. Our group recently found that 11-week exercise intervention in children aged between 9 years and 13 years improved EF performance compared to the controls. The exercise group also increased frontal lobe, temporal lobe, hippocampus, and cingulate cortex activation during an EF task compared to the control group [15].

With evidence that brain activation is affected by exercise, one issue that warranted investigation was whether exercise alters brain structure. Altered white matter structure may be an underlying cause of functional change, given the evidence that interindividual differences in brain activation reflect white matter integrity (WMI) [16]. WMI reflects axonal membrane structure and myelination and can be assessed by diffusion tensor imaging (DTI), which measures the anisotropy (directional dependence) of water diffusion. Fractional anisotropy (FA) is a frequent measure of interest in DTI and describes the anisotropy of water diffusion. FA values range between 0 and 1, with 1 indicating fully anisotropic diffusion. Higher values are generally interpreted as greater WMI (myelination and axonal membrane structure [17]). Another measure based on the same tensor model is mean diffusivity (MD), which measures water diffusion restricted by water (with higher values indicating less restriction). Taken together, higher FA and lower MD values are often interpreted as primarily reflecting greater myelination.

WMI has been associated with fitness in several cross-sectional studies. Higher aerobic fitness in adults was associated with higher FA in the cingulum and corpus callosum, possibly relating to motor planning and control [18–20]. Fitness was also associated with the integrity of the uncinate fasciculus, which is involved in memory [20]. The longitudinal study also found that the improvement in the WMI of overweight children after an 8-month exercise intervention was related to selective attention [21]. While the literature indicates that exercise affects many cognitive abilities and WMI, this topic has yet to be investigated in relation to EF.

Given the evidence that exercise improved EF and altered associated brain activation in prior studies, we investigated whether an exercise intervention in deaf children improves WMI. Only deaf children were recruited for the current study; the EF of deaf children is retarded, and they are therefore likely to derive greater benefits from exercise [22]. As the brain structure does not completely mature until young adulthood, ongoing development makes it an interesting target for investigation across the ages included in the current study (children aged between 9 years and 13 years). Our hypotheses were generated based on the literature indicating that exercise improves both EF and WMI. Specifically, we hypothesized that a randomized controlled exercise intervention with deaf children would improve their EF behavioral performance and reshape their WMI. Further, improved EF in deaf children may be associated with WMI changes after an exercise intervention, which may help us better understand the biological mechanisms underlying these changes.

Table 1: Participants' demographics and treatment-induced heart rates (M ± SD).

Variables	Control group	Experimental group	P value
N	8	10	—
Sex (male/female)	4/4	3/7	0.52^b
Age (years)	11.50 ± 0.76	10.20 ± 1.23	0.02^a
BMI (height/weight^2)	17.88 ± 1.46	17.90 ± 2.42	0.98^a
n^c	4	4	—
Sex (male/female)	2/2	2/2	—
HR during treatment	89.30 ± 10.30	136.40 ± 0.57	0.03^a

Values are presented as mean ± SD or percentages unless otherwise indicated. $^a t$-test. $^b\chi^2$ test. ^{c}Heart rate value was presented for four participants in each group.

2. Materials and Methods

2.1. Participants. The 28 deaf children recruited from two special education schools who participated in the study had normal or corrected-to-normal vision and were right-handed as assessed by the Edinburgh Test [23]. All participants were free of psychiatric disorders or a history of head trauma. They also completed a set of questions relating to their history of drug abuse or inherited disease and their general intelligence. Exclusions included any medical condition that would limit exercise intervention or affect study results (including neurological or psychiatric disorders). The study was conducted in accordance with the Declaration of Helsinki.

All participants were then randomly assigned to either the control or the exercise intervention group. The exercise group included six females and eight males. The other six females and eight males constituted the control group. Age and gender were well matched between the two groups. MRI was completed with DTI data available for 28 children at baseline and 20 at posttest. Of the 20 children with both baseline and posttest data, one was excluded due to the loss of behavioral performance data and the other was excluded because behavioral performance was an extreme outlier. Thus, the present study included 18 children: 10 in the exercise group and 8 in the control group (Table 1). The study protocol was approved by the Ethics and Human Protection Committee of the Affiliated Hospital of Yangzhou University. Written informed consent was obtained from each participant after the experimental procedures had been fully explained.

2.2. Exercise Intervention. The aerobic exercise program was adapted from Chen et al. [24] and Yin et al. [25]. All subjects in the exercise group were offered an after-school program 4 days per week for 11 weeks. The exercise program consists of three stages, (1) preparation, (2) exercise intervention, and

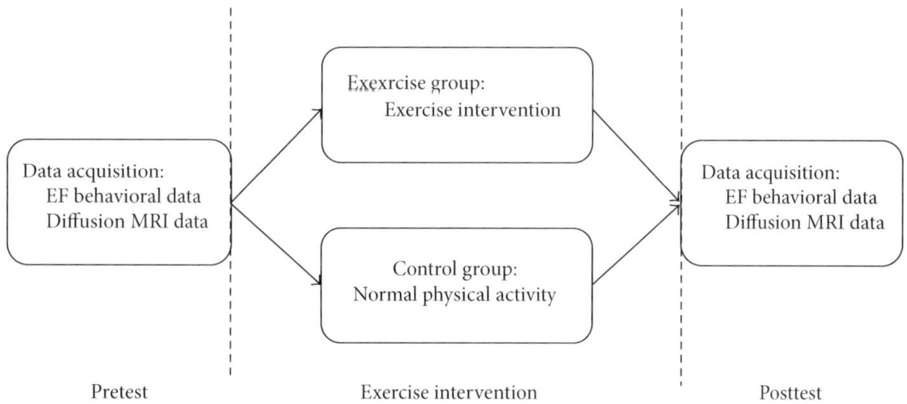

FIGURE 1: Experimental process.

(3) relaxation, all lasting for about 45 minutes. The first stage consisted of warm-up exercises (preparation stage), wherein exercise intensity reached a moderately intense heart rate. This was followed by a 30 min exercise stage that emphasized exercise intensity, enjoyment, safety, repetition, and practice; all activities were selected based on the ease of comprehension, fun, and eliciting of intermittent vigorous movement, including running games, jumping rope, and wushu. The chosen aerobic exercise load was of moderate intensity [60%–69% of maximum heart rate (MHR), wherein MHR = 220—age], based on the aerobic exercise intensity classification defined by the American College of Sports Medicine [26]. Exercise intensity was monitored by heart rate monitors (Polar Electro RS800XSD, Oy, Finland) that were attached throughout the experiment to four subjects (two boys and two girls). The final (relaxation) stage focused on physically relaxing prior to ending the exercise regime.

2.3. Executive Function and Related Assessments. A test-tool designed by Chen et al. [11] was used to assess EF of deaf children. Three computer-based neuropsychological assessments were used to assess inhibition, working memory, and shifting aspects of EF. A modified Eriksen flanker task was used to examine the inhibitory control aspect of EF [27]; the response times (RT) in the congruent and incongruent trials were recorded and used to create an index of inhibition, defined as the RT difference between incongruent and congruent trials. Shorter RT differences reflected better performance. A 2-back task was used to assess the working memory aspect of EF. The RT on correct trials were recorded and averaged as the main behavioral index, wherein shorter RT reflected better performance. A more-odd task adapted from Hillman et al. [28] and Salthouse et al. [29] was employed to investigate the shifting aspect of EF. The shifting index used in the present study was the global switch cost, which was calculated as the RT difference between the heterogeneous (i.e., the average of the c blocks) and homogeneous (i.e., the average of the a and b blocks) blocks. The detail of every test was introduced in our previous paper [11]. The stimulus presentation and response data collection was performed using E-Prime software 1.1 (Psychology Software Tools Inc., Pittsburgh, USA).

2.4. DTI Procedure and Analysis

2.4.1. MRI Acquisition. Images were acquired at the Affiliated Hospital of Yangzhou University on a Siemens Magnetom Tim Verio 3 Tesla scanner. During scanning, head position was stabilized with a vacuum pillow and/or foam padding. Diffusion images were acquired using an echo planar imaging sequence (acquisition matrix = 128 × 128, 60 interleaved slices, voxel size = 1.8 × 1.8 × 4.0 mm, FOV = 230 × 230 mm, TR = 3800 ms, TE = 106 ms, 3 B0 images, 30 diffusion-weighted images, and b = 1000 s/mm^2).

2.4.2. Image Analysis. Diffusion images were processed using a MATLAB toolbox named "Pipeline for Analyzing braiN Diffusion imAges (PANDA) (http://www.nitrc.org/projects/panda/)" [30]. The main procedures included preprocessing and producing diffusion metrics in preparation for statistical analysis: local diffusion homogeneity (LDH) = 7 voxels, smooth: normalizing resolution = 2 mm, and smoothing ker nel = 6 mm. The preprocess steps were executed one by one, including converting DICOM files into Nifti images, estimating the brain mask, cropping raw images, correcting for the eddy-current effects, and calculating diffusion tensor metrics. Then, using the atlas-based analysis, we normalized diffusion metrics (FA and MD) into the MNI space and calculated regional diffusion metrics by averaging the values within each region of the ICBM DTI-81 atlas [31]. All the procedures were fully automated and completed by PANDA.

2.5. Experimental Process. In this longitudinal study, participants were scanned twice with MRI. MRI was performed as follows: a pretest scan performed before exercise intervention (MRI 1) and a posttest scan 11 weeks after completion of the intervention period (MRI 2). The control group, consisting of age- and gender-matched subjects scanned at pretest and posttest, did not participate in any additional aerobic exercise during the 11 weeks (Figure 1).

2.6. Statistical Analyses. All analyses were conducted using SPSS Version 20.0 (IBM, Armonk, N.Y., USA). Demographic variables were compared between the control and exercise groups with independent sample *t*-tests for continuous variables and χ^2 tests for sex proportion. For the performance of executive function tasks, group-by-time repeated-measures

TABLE 2: Performance for three fundamental aspects of executive function (M ± SD).

	Control group		Experimental group	
	Pretest	Posttest	Pretest	Posttest
RT (ms)				
Inhibition	17.80 ± 20.70	29.88 ± 21.55	38.93 ± 16.97	9.80 ± 5.22
Working memory	651.30 ± 104.04	622.51 ± 93.36	724.09 ± 112.13	607.53 ± 71.53
Shifting	277.50 ± 206.72	339.87 ± 160.79	278.43 ± 50.00	225.69 ± 60.81
Accuracy (%)				
Inhibition				
Congruent	88.75 ± 12.08	88.13 ± 14.64	93.50 ± 6.55	95.20 ± 4.13
Incongruent	87.13 ± 11.45	87.13 ± 12.40	87.40 ± 13.60	91.00 ± 7.12
Working memory	64.00 ± 26.79	68.00 ± 19.24	83.80 ± 20.47	90.10 ± 8.48
Shifting				
Homogeneous	80.00 ± 11.46	73.34 ± 24.49	80.20 ± 15.83	84.50 ± 16.22
Heterogeneous	53.25 ± 17.91	46.88 ± 20.32	48.30 ± 30.39	63.30 ± 33.20

analyses of variance (ANOVAs) were conducted separately for inhibition, working memory, and shifting indices, whereas effect size was presented as partial eta-squared (η^2) values. Post hoc analyses were conducted with planned pairwise comparisons when significant interaction effects were revealed. Repeated measures ANOVAs were conducted for both measurements of WMI (FA and MD) on the outcome to examine the effects of group, measurement time, and their interactions. Each model was also controlled for age. Then, we calculated the Pearson correlation coefficient (r) between WMI and EF performance in the exercise group. Results were corrected for multiple comparisons using the false discovery rate (FDR) correction. Probability values < 0.05 were considered statistically significant.

3. Results

3.1. Participants' Characteristics. The participants' demographic details are presented in Table 1. Independent t-tests revealed no significant differences between the control and exercise groups in terms of gender ($\text{chi} - \text{square} = 0.18$, $P > 0.05$) or BMI [$t\,(16) = 0.027$, $P > 0.05$], but because of the reduction in data, the age of the two groups was inhomogeneous; therefore, we used "age" as a covariate in the subsequent statistical analysis to eliminate its influence.

3.2. Exercise Intensity Manipulation. The heart rates for the control and exercise groups were 42.52% and 64.95% of the maximal heart rate, respectively [$t\,(6) = 9.13$, $P < 0.05$]. The different heart rates between the two treatment groups, as well as the percentages of the maximal heart rates, suggested that the consideration of the exercise manipulation of moderate exercise intensity was appropriate.

3.3. Behavioral Performance. The groups did not differ significantly at baseline on any of the characteristics listed in Table 2. Based on a priori hypotheses concerning the effects of physical exercise on cognition, the two groups of deaf children were compared with an ANOVA. A repeated measures ANOVA was conducted to examine group differences in behavioral performance, with time (pretest and posttest) as the within-subject factor and group (exercise intervention and control) as the between-subject factor.

3.3.1. Inhibition. A repeated measures ANOVA revealed the main effects to be time [$F(1, 16) = 1.61$, $P > 0.05$, partial $\eta^2 = 0.09$] and group [$F(1, 16) = 0.04$, $P > 0.05$, partial $\eta^2 = 0.003$]. There was no significant difference between both of them. The interaction between time and group was significant [$F(1, 16) = 9.05$, $P < 0.01$, partial $\eta^2 = 0.38$]. A follow-up analysis deconstructing the interaction revealed significant pretest [$F(1, 16) = 5.68$, $P < 0.05$] and posttest [$F(1, 16) = 8.20$, $P < 0.05$] differences between the exercise and control groups (i.e., the RT of the exercise group were lower than those of the control group after exercise); there was no significant difference between pre- and posttest results in the control group [$F(1, 16) = 2.84$, $P > 0.05$], but there was a significant difference in pre- and posttest condition in the exercise group [$F(1, 16) = 20.66$, $P < 0.001$]; the posttest inhibition RT differences was shorter than the pretest inhibition RT differences in the exercise group.

Regarding accuracy, no significant interaction effect was observed in inhibition effect regarding "congruent" [$F(1, 16) = 0.34$, $P > 0.05$, partial $\eta^2 = 0.02$] and "incongruent" [$F(1, 16) = 0.34$, $P > 0.05$, partial $\eta^2 = 0.02$] behaviors.

3.3.2. Working Memory. A repeated measures ANOVA revealed the main effects for time [$F(1, 16) = 4.38$, $P > 0.05$, partial $\eta^2 = 0.23$] to be not significant, but those for group [$F(1, 16) = 6.51$, $P < 0.05$, partial $\eta^2 = 0.30$] were significant. The interaction of time and group was significant [$F(1, 16) = 18.63$, $P < 0.05$, partial $\eta^2 = 0.55$]. A follow-up analysis deconstructing the interaction effects revealed no significant pretest differences in RT between the exercise and control groups [$F(1, 16) = 1.99$, $P > 0.05$] or in posttest differences [$F(1, 16) = 0.15$, $P > 0.05$]. (However, the RT of the exercise group were longer than those of the control group after exercise.) There was no significant difference between pre- and posttest RT in the control group [$F(1, 16) = 1.68$, $P > 0.05$], but there was a significant difference in the pre-

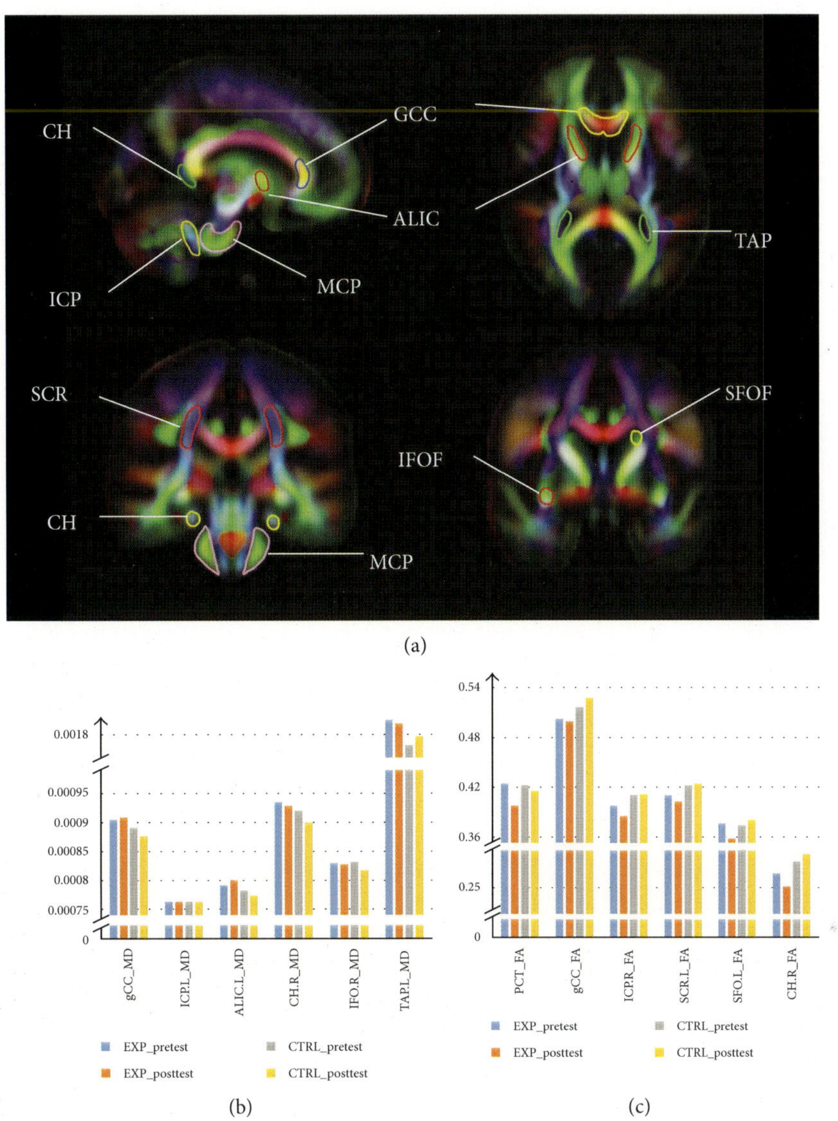

FIGURE 2: (a) nine anatomical regions defined by the ICBM DTI-81 atlas with significant changes after exercise intervention. Difference in MD (b) and FA (c) values for specific fiber tracts in an atlas-based ROI analysis between the experimental group (blue, orange) and the control group (gray, yellow).

and posttest RT in the exercise group [$F(1, 16) = 34.35$, $P < 0.001$] (i.e., in the exercise group, the posttest RT were less than the pretest RT).

Regarding accuracy, no significant interaction effect was observed in working memory [$F(1, 16) = 0.06$, $P > 0.05$, partial $\eta^2 = 0.004$].

3.3.3. Shifting. A repeated measures ANOVA revealed the main effects to be time [$F(1, 16) = 0.01$, $P > 0.05$, partial $\eta^2 = 0.001$] and group [$F(1, 16) = 0.44$, $P > 0.05$, partial $\eta^2 = 0.03$]. There was no significant difference between both of them. The interaction between time and group was significant [$F(1, 16) = 5.07$, $P < 0.05$, partial $\eta^2 = 0.25$]. A follow-up analysis deconstructing the interaction effects revealed no significant differences in pretest [$F(1, 16) = 0.00$, $P > 0.05$] or posttest [$F(1, 16) = 4.33$, $P > 0.05$] conditions between the exercise and control groups (however, the RT of the exercise group were lower than those of the control group after exercise intervention); there was no significant difference in RT between pre- and posttest conditions in the control group [$F(1, 16) = 4.35$, $P > 0.05$] or exercise group [$F(1, 16) = 3.89$, $P > 0.05$]. (However, for the exercise group, the posttest shift in RT was shorter than the pretest shift in RT.)

Regarding accuracy, no significant interaction for shifting was observed in "homogeneous" [$F(1, 16) = 1.01$, $P > 0.05$, partial $\eta^2 = 0.06$] or "heterogeneous" [$F(1, 16) = 3.67$, $P > 0.05$, partial $\eta^2 = 0.19$].

3.4. WM Structure. There was a significant group-by-time interaction between groups in some WMI measures (Figure 2): a decreased FA in the pontine crossing tract (PCT) [$F(1, 16) = 6.83$, $P < 0.05$, partial $\eta^2 = 0.31$] and right cingulum (hippocampus) (CH) [$F(1, 16) = 8.96$, $P < 0.01$, partial $\eta^2 = 0.37$], genu of the corpus callosum (gCC) [$F(1, 16) = 6.20$, $P < 0.05$, partial $\eta^2 = 0.29$] and left superior frontooccipital fasciculus (SFOF) [$F(1, 16) = 5.42$, $P < 0.05$, partial $\eta^2 = 0.27$], right inferior cerebellar peduncle (ICP) [$F(1, 16) = 4.95$, $P < 0.05$, partial $\eta^2 = 0.25$], and left superior corona radiata (SCR) [$F(1, 16) = 6.06$, $P < 0.05$, partial $\eta^2 = 0.29$]; an increased MD in the genu of the corpus callosum (gCC) [$F(1, 16) = 7.37$, $P < 0.05$, partial $\eta^2 = 0.33$] and left anterior limb of the internal capsule (ALIC) [$F(1, 16) = 4.89$, $P < 0.05$, partial $\eta^2 = 0.25$], right inferior frontooccipital fasciculus (IFOF) [$F(1, 16) = 6.80$, $P < 0.05$, partial $\eta^2 = 0.31$], and and right cingulum (hippocampus) (CH) [$F(1, 16) = 8.43$, $P < 0.05$, partial $\eta^2 = 0.36$]; and a lower MD in the left inferior cerebellar peduncle (ICP) [$F(1, 16) = 4.66$, $P < 0.05$, partial $\eta^2 = 0.24$] and left tapetum (TAP) [$F(1, 16) = 4.98$, $P < 0.05$, partial $\eta^2 = 0.25$]. These results indicate that the exercise intervention differentially affected WMI compared to that of the control condition.

3.5. Correlations between WMI and Behavioral Performance. We found a significant negative correlation between WMI and behavioral performance, wherein a decrease in WMI in the gCC (from pretest to posttest) was associated with a lessening in inhibition for deaf children in the exercise intervention group (Flanker task, pretest to posttest) and reaction time ($r = -0.67$, $P = 0.03 < 0.05$); however, there was no significant correlation after correction for multiple comparisons (FDR, $P < 0.05$).

4. Discussion

The current study was designed to explore the effects of aerobic exercise on EF and WMI in deaf children. Children from two similar special education schools were randomly allocated to two groups: an exercise intervention group, receiving an aerobic exercise intervention including running games, jumping rope, and wushu, and a control group that did not attend any additional aerobic exercise. We controlled for all the confounding variables. Consequently, reliable exercise gains emerged, allowing us to observe the neural basis of exercise-improved EF.

4.1. Behavioral Performance. A rapidly growing body of literature indicates that, from both behavioral and neuroelectric perspectives, physical exercise improves EF. As observed here, deaf children's EF performance in the exercise intervention group was better than that in the control group—in agreement with previous studies [11, 32–36]. Accordingly, the present behavioral results have again been verified: physical exercise beneficially impacts children's EF.

4.2. White Matter Integrity. Recently, a number of studies have focused on exploring the effects of exercise on the brain. Some evidence has indicated that exercise intervention can cause microstructural changes in the WM [21, 37, 38]. Our results support existing evidence that exercise intervention causes changes in WMI. Specifically, a decrease in WMI was found in the PCT, right CH, left SFOF, right IFOF, right ICP, left SCR, left ALIC, and gCC, whereas there was an increase in WMI in the left ICP and left TAP.

Previous research shows that, compared with normal-hearing subjects, the microstructural changes of brain white matter in deaf subjects have lower FA in their bilateral auditory [39–41]. Hribar et al. [42] also found lower AD in the left ALIC and left SCR in deaf individuals than in normal-hearing individuals, which are regions important for the transmission of sensory, motor, visual, auditory, and other information between the cerebral cortex, the brainstem, the cerebellum, and the spinal cord. Hribar et al. suggested that the lower anisotropy values found in the large network of projection fibers in deaf people may be due not only to the degradation of their auditory pathways but also to the reorganization of sensory, motor, and visual pathways as a compensation for the absence of auditory input. These WMI changes in brain regions were also observed in our study, wherein the FA declined or MD increased after a prolonged exercise regimen.

Higher MD in deaf children was observed also in the right IFOF. A decreased FA among deaf subjects has been previously reported for the right IFOF [42]. IFOF connects the occipital and frontal lobes [43]. Philippi et al. [44] found that damage associated with the right IFOF impairs recognition of facial expressions and emotions. For deaf subjects, facial expressions are important for interpreting a speaker's emotional state because they cannot hear a speaker's tone of voice; this is also critical for sign language comprehension [42]. Studies have shown that deaf subjects have a keen ability to recognize subtle differences in facial features, which may be related to their experience using sign language [45]. Most studies relate lower anisotropy values to demyelination and degradation of axons, which lead to poorer functioning [46]. However, lower anisotropy values might not always correlate with poorer functional performance, as shown by Hoeft et al., who indicated that increased FA values correlate with poorer visuospatial construction abilities [47]. The increased MD of IFOF of deaf children in our study may have required more recognition of facial expressions and emotional states during exercise, because both attributes are important for comprehending sign language.

Lower FA and higher MD occurred in the gCC in our study, suggesting that the lower FA could be attributable to myelination abnormalities. Previous research found that deaf subjects show lower AD in the gCC relative to normal-hearing subjects, which might be related to impaired motor proficiency and balance problems in people with sensorineural hearing loss [42]. However, in our study, physical exercise seemed to improve motor proficiency and enabled the formation of new connections and reinforcement and degradation of existing connections may also alter FA in the deaf. Because the anterior part of the CC contains fibers projecting into the prefrontal, premotor, and supplementary motor cortical areas [48], we speculate that exercise may promote a compensatory reorganization.

Our results found higher WMI in the left ICP and left TAP after exercising, while WMI was reduced in the PCT, right CH, right ICP, and left SFOF. However, similar results have not been observed in previous relevant studies. It is possible that our results only pertain to our study due to the small sample size of our study. However, even if this is true, our results may provide a basis for future research comprising more test subjects.

The change in diffusion anisotropy of deaf children implies an alteration in WMI, but we cannot draw conclusions from a one-sided index. In our study, we have shown where the changes are, but the interpretation of diffusion indices in deaf children requires further research.

4.3. Correlation between Behavioral Performance and WMI. We found a significant correlation in deaf children (following an imposed exercise regimen) between lower WMI in the gCC and better inhibition behavioral performance (declines in reaction time). Nevertheless, perhaps because our sample size was small or our intervention time was short, the correlation was not significant after FDR correction. The existing theory indicates that exercise improves cognitive functioning by improving brain plasticity (structural components, activation patterns, functional connectivity, etc.) [49, 50]. We had hoped to explore the neural basis of exercise on EF from the perspective of WMI plasticity, but our results did not support our initial hypothesis. In fact, our results did not provide any evidence for a significant correlation between changes in WMI and improvements in EF behavioral performance. Even so, this finding might provide an interesting a priori hypothesis for future studies and so this topic would still be worth exploring in future research.

5. Conclusions

Our results demonstrated that, after establishing an exercise regimen in deaf children, EF improved in three behavioral performance measures and declined for WMI in the PCT, right CH, left SFOF, right IFOF, right ICP, left SCR, left ALIC, and gCC. In addition, WMI increased in left ICP and left TAP after exercise. In summary, our results suggest that exercise intervention may reshape the microstructure of WM in deaf children, which may have some implications for the instruction of alternative sport programs for children with executive dysfunction.

Conflicts of Interest

The authors declare that there is no conflict of interest regarding the publication of this paper.

Acknowledgments

This research was supported by grants from the National Natural Science Foundation of China (31300863 and 31771243) and the Fok Ying Tong Education Foundation (141113) to Ai-Guo Chen.

References

[1] M. D. Lezak, D. B. Howieson, D. W. Loring, H. J. Hannay, and J. S. Fischer, *Neuropsychological Assessment*, Oxford University Press, Oxford, MS, USA, 2004.

[2] A. F. Kramer, S. Hahn, N. J. Cohen et al., "Ageing, fitness and neurocognitive function," *Nature*, vol. 400, no. 6743, pp. 418-419, 1999.

[3] A. Diamond, "Executive functions," *Annual Review of Psychology*, vol. 64, no. 1, pp. 135–168, 2013.

[4] S. Funahashi, "Neuronal mechanisms of executive control by the prefrontal cortex," *Neuroscience Research*, vol. 39, no. 2, pp. 147–165, 2001.

[5] L. S. Siegel and E. B. Ryan, "The development of working memory in normally achieving and subtypes of learning disabled children," *Child Development*, vol. 60, no. 4, pp. 973–980, 1989.

[6] R. Bull, K. A. Espy, and S. A. Wiebe, "Short-term memory, working memory, and executive functioning in preschoolers: longitudinal predictors of mathematical achievement at age 7 years," *Developmental Neuropsychology*, vol. 33, no. 3, pp. 205–228, 2008.

[7] M. C. Passolunghi and L. S. Siegel, "Short-term memory, working memory, and inhibitory control in children with difficulties in arithmetic problem solving," *Journal of Experimental Child Psychology*, vol. 80, no. 1, pp. 44–57, 2001.

[8] M. S. Gazzaniga, R. B. Ivry, G. R. Mangun, and M. S. Steven, "Cognitive neuroscience: the biology of the mind," *Quarterly Review of Biology*, vol. 4, pp. 87–90, 2009.

[9] F. Collette and M. Van der Linden, "Brain imaging of the central executive component of working memory," *Neuroscience & Biobehavioral Reviews*, vol. 26, no. 2, pp. 105–125, 2002.

[10] E. E. Smith and J. Jonides, "Storage and executive processes in the frontal lobes," *Science*, vol. 283, no. 5408, pp. 1657–1661, 1999.

[11] A. G. Chen, J. Yan, H. C. Yin, C. Y. Pan, and Y. K. Chang, "Effects of acute aerobic exercise on multiple aspects of executive function in preadolescent children," *Psychology of Sport and Exercise*, vol. 15, no. 6, pp. 627–636, 2014.

[12] A. G. Chen, L. Cui, and H. C. Yin, "Effect of combined exercise program on the executive function in primary students with chinese learning difficulties," *Chinese Journal of Behavioral Medicine and Brain Science*, vol. 25, pp. 1123–1127, 2016.

[13] A. G. Chen, R. W. Jiang, X. H. Ji, B. Q. Tao, F. S. Zhu, and J. Yan, "Effects of 8-week moderate fancy rope skipping training on executive function in preadolescent deaf children: a school-based experimental study," *Journal of Sports and Science*, vol. 36, pp. 105–109, 2015.

[14] S. J. Colcombe, A. F. Kramer, K. I. Erickson et al., "Cardiovascular fitness, cortical plasticity, and aging," *Proceedings of the National Academy of Sciences of the United States of America*, vol. 101, no. 9, pp. 3316–3321, 2004.

[15] A. G. Chen, L. Jin, L. N. Zhu, X. Xiong, W. Wang, and J. Yan, "Effects of eleven-week aerobic exercise on working memory of deaf children: evidence from behavior and functional mri," *Chinese Journal of Sports Medicine*, vol. 35, pp. 1132–1139, 2016.

[16] E. M. Gordon, P. S. Lee, J. M. Maisog et al., "Strength of default mode resting-state connectivity relates to white matter integrity in children," *Developmental Science*, vol. 14, no. 4, pp. 738–751, 2011.

[17] C. Beaulieu, "The basis of anisotropic water diffusion in the nervous system - a technical review," *NMR in Biomedicine*, vol. 15, no. 7-8, pp. 435–455, 2002.

[18] N. F. Johnson, C. Kim, J. L. Clasey, A. Bailey, and B. T. Gold, "Cardiorespiratory fitness is positively correlated with cerebral white matter integrity in healthy seniors," *NeuroImage*, vol. 59, no. 2, pp. 1514–1523, 2012.

[19] B. L. Marks, L. M. Katz, M. Styner, and J. K. Smith, "Aerobic fitness and obesity: relationship to cerebral white matter integrity in the brain of active and sedentary older adults," *British Journal of Sports Medicine*, vol. 45, no. 15, pp. 1208–1215, 2011.

[20] B. L. Marks, D. J. Madden, B. Bucur et al., "Role of aerobic fitness and aging on cerebral white matter integrity," *Annals of the New York Academy of Sciences*, vol. 1097, no. 1, pp. 171–174, 2007.

[21] C. E. Krafft, D. J. Schaeffer, N. F. Schwarz et al., "Improved frontoparietal white matter integrity in overweight children is associated with attendance at an after-school exercise program," *Developmental Neuroscience*, vol. 36, no. 1, pp. 1–9, 2014.

[22] J. L. Pan, H. C. Yin, A. G. Chen, L. Cui, Y. Wang, and Y. B. Cui, "An experimental study on the effect of exercise intervention on the executive functions of primary students with and without learning difficulties," *China Sport Science*, vol. 36, 2016.

[23] R. C. Oldfield, "The assessment and analysis of handedness: the Edinburgh inventory," *Neuropsychologia*, vol. 9, no. 1, pp. 97–113, 1971.

[24] A. G. Chen, L. N. Zhu, L. Jin, X. Xiong, W. Wang, and J. Yan, "Effect of aerobic exercise on executive control and its brain network in deaf children," *Journal of Sports and Science*, vol. 37, 2016.

[25] H. C. Yin, A. G. Chen, Z. Ma, X. N. Li, and M. Liu, "A follow-up study on two kinds of exercise intervention programs for children's executive functions," *China Sport Science*, vol. 34, pp. 24–28, 2014.

[26] American College of Sports Medicine, *ACSM's Guidelines for Exercise Testing and Prescription*, Lippincott Williams & Wilkins, Philadelphia, PA, USA, 2006.

[27] B. A. Eriksen and C. W. Eriksen, "Effects of noise letters upon the identification of a target letter in a nonsearch task," *Perception & Psychophysics*, vol. 16, no. 1, pp. 143–149, 1974.

[28] C. H. Hillman, A. F. Kramer, A. V. Belopolsky, and D. P. Smith, "A cross-sectional examination of age and physical activity on performance and event-related brain potentials in a task switching paradigm," *International Journal of Psychophysiology*, vol. 59, no. 1, pp. 30–39, 2006.

[29] T. A. Salthouse, N. Fristoe, K. E. McGuthry, and D. Z. Hambrick, "Relation of task switching to speed, age, and fluid intelligence," *Psychology and Aging*, vol. 13, no. 3, pp. 445–461, 1998.

[30] Z. X. Cui, S. Y. Zhong, P. F. Xu, Y. He, and G. L. Gong, "PANDA: a pipeline toolbox for analyzing brain diffusion images," *Frontiers in Human Neuroscience*, vol. 7, p. 42, 2013.

[31] S. Mori, K. Oishi, H. Y. Jiang et al., "Stereotaxic white matter atlas based on diffusion tensor imaging in an ICBM template," *NeuroImage*, vol. 40, no. 2, pp. 570–582, 2008.

[32] C. H. Hillman, K. I. Erickson, and A. F. Kramer, "Be smart, exercise your heart: exercise effects on brain and cognition," *Nature Reviews Neuroscience*, vol. 9, no. 1, pp. 58–65, 2008.

[33] K. I. Erickson and A. F. Kramer, "Aerobic exercise effects on cognitive and neural plasticity in older adults," *British Journal of Sports Medicine*, vol. 43, no. 1, pp. 22–24, 2009.

[34] Y. K. Chang, J. D. Labban, J. I. Gapin, and J. L. Etnier, "The effects of acute exercise on cognitive performance: a meta-analysis," *Brain Research*, vol. 1453, pp. 87–101, 2012.

[35] Y. K. Chang, Y. J. Tsai, T. T. Chen, and T. M. Hung, "The impacts of coordinative exercise on executive function in kindergarten children: an ERP study," *Experimental Brain Research*, vol. 225, no. 2, pp. 187–196, 2013.

[36] E. S. Drollette, M. R. Scudder, L. B. Raine et al., "Acute exercise facilitates brain function and cognition in children who need it most: An ERP study of individual differences in inhibitory control capacity," *Developmental Cognitive Neuroscience*, vol. 7, pp. 53–64, 2014.

[37] D. J. Schaeffer, C. E. Krafft, N. F. Schwarz et al., "The relationship between uncinate fasciculus white matter integrity and verbal memory proficiency in children," *Neuroreport*, vol. 25, no. 12, pp. 921–925, 2014.

[38] D. J. Schaeffer, C. E. Krafft, N. F. Schwarz et al., "An 8-month exercise intervention alters frontotemporal white matter integrity in overweight children," *Psychophysiology*, vol. 51, no. 8, pp. 728–733, 2014.

[39] D. J. Kim, S. Y. Park, J. Kim, D. H. Lee, and H. J. Park, "Alterations of white matter diffusion anisotropy in early deafness," *Neuroreport*, vol. 20, no. 11, pp. 1032–1036, 2009.

[40] Y. Y. Li, G. S. Ding, J. R. Booth et al., "Sensitive period for white-matter connectivity of superior temporal cortex in deaf people," *Human Brain Mapping*, vol. 33, no. 2, pp. 349–359, 2012.

[41] W. Miao, J. Li, M. Tang et al., "Altered white matter integrity in adolescents with prelingual deafness: a high-resolution tract-based spatial statistics imaging study," *American Journal of Neuroradiology*, vol. 34, no. 6, pp. 1264–1270, 2013.

[42] M. Hribar, D. Suput, A. A. Carvalho, S. Battelino, and A. Vovk, "Structural alterations of brain grey and white matter in early deaf adults," *Hearing Research*, vol. 318, pp. 1–10, 2014.

[43] B. J. Jellison, A. S. Field, J. Medow, M. Lazar, M. S. Salamat, and A. L. Alexander, "Diffusion tensor imaging of cerebral white matter: a pictorial review of physics, fiber tract anatomy, and tumor imaging patterns," *American Journal of Neuroradiology*, vol. 25, no. 3, pp. 356–369, 2004.

[44] C. L. Philippi, S. Mehta, T. Grabowski, R. Adolphs, and D. Rudrauf, "Damage to association fiber tracts impairs recognition of the facial expression of emotion," *The Journal of Neuroscience*, vol. 29, no. 48, pp. 15089–15099, 2009.

[45] J. Bettger, K. Emmorey, S. McCullough, and U. Bellugi, "Enhanced facial diserimination: effects of experience with American sign language," *Journal of Deaf Studies and Deaf Education*, vol. 2, no. 4, pp. 223–233, 1997.

[46] S. Chanraud, N. Zahr, E. V. Sullivan, and A. Pfefferbaum, "MR diffusion tensor imaging: a window into white matter integrity of the working brain," *Neuropsychology Review*, vol. 20, no. 2, pp. 209–225, 2010.

[47] F. Hoeft, N. Barneagoraly, B. W. Haas, G. Golarai, D. Ng, and D. Mills, "More is not always better: increased fractional anisotropy of superior longitudinal fasciculus associated with poor visuospatial abilities in williams syndrome," *The Journal of Neuroscience*, vol. 27, no. 44, pp. 11960–11965, 2007.

[48] S. Hofer and J. Frahm, "Topography of the human corpus callosum revisited - comprehensive fiber tractography using diffusion tensor magnetic resonance imaging," *NeuroImage*, vol. 32, no. 3, pp. 989–994, 2006.

[49] A. G. Chen, L. N. Zhu, J. Yan, and H. C. Yin, "Neural basis of working memory enhancement after acute aerobic exercise: fMRI study of preadolescent children," *Frontiers in Psychology*, vol. 7, article 1804, 2016.

[50] A. G. Chen, L. N. Zhu, X. Xiong, and Y. Li, "Acute aerobic exercise alters executive control network in preadolescent children," *Revista de psicología del deporte*, vol. 26, Supplement 4, pp. 132–137, 2017.

19

Noninvasive Brain Stimulations for Unilateral Spatial Neglect after Stroke: A Systematic Review and Meta-Analysis of Randomized and Nonrandomized Controlled Trials

Flávio Taira Kashiwagi,[1] Regina El Dib,[2] Huda Gomaa,[3] Nermeen Gawish,[3] Erica Aranha Suzumura,[4] Taís Regina da Silva,[1] Fernanda Cristina Winckler,[1] Juli Thomaz de Souza,[2] Adriana Bastos Conforto,[5] Gustavo José Luvizutto,[6] and Rodrigo Bazan[1]

[1]*Neurology Department, Botucatu Medical School, Universidade Estadual Paulista (UNESP), Botucatu, SP, Brazil*
[2]*Science and Technology Institute, Universidade Estadual Paulista (UNESP), São José dos Campos, SP, Brazil*
[3]*Department of Pharmacy, Tanta Chest Hospital, Tanta, Egypt*
[4]*Research Institute, Hospital do Coração (HCor), São Paulo, SP, Brazil*
[5]*Neurostimulation Laboratory, University of São Paulo (USP), São Paulo, SP, Brazil*
[6]*Department of Applied Physical Therapy, Federal University of Triângulo Mineiro (UFTM), Uberaba, MG, Brazil*

Correspondence should be addressed to Gustavo José Luvizutto; gluvizutto@fmb.unesp.br

Academic Editor: Michele Fornaro

Background. Unilateral spatial neglect (USN) is the most frequent perceptual disorder after stroke. Noninvasive brain stimulation (NIBS) is a tool that has been used in the rehabilitation process to modify cortical excitability and improve perception and functional capacity. *Objective.* To assess the impact of NIBS on USN after stroke. *Methods.* An extensive search was conducted up to July 2016. Studies were selected if they were controlled and noncontrolled trials examining transcranial direct current stimulation (tDCS), repetitive transcranial magnetic stimulation (rTMS), and theta burst stimulation (TBS) in USN after stroke, with outcomes measured by standardized USN and functional tests. *Results.* Twelve RCTs (273 participants) and 4 non-RCTs (94 participants) proved eligible. We observed a benefit in overall USN measured by the line bisection test with NIBS in comparison to sham (SMD −2.35, 95% CI −3.72, −0.98; $p = 0.0001$); the rTMS yielded results that were consistent with the overall meta-analysis (SMD −2.82, 95% CI −3.66, −1.98; $p = 0.09$). The rTMS compared with sham also suggested a benefit in overall USN measured by Motor-Free Visual Perception Test at both 1 Hz (SMD 1.46, 95% CI 0.73, 2.20; $p < 0.0001$) and 10 Hz (SMD 1.19, 95% CI 0.48, 1.89; $p = 0.54$). There was also a benefit in overall USN measured by Albert's test and the line crossing test with 1 Hz rTMS compared to sham (SMD 2.04, 95% CI 1.14, 2.95; $p < 0.0001$). *Conclusions.* The results suggest a benefit of NIBS on overall USN, and we conclude that rTMS is more efficacious compared to sham for USN after stroke.

1. Background

Stroke is the second leading cause of death worldwide and the primary cause of chronic disability in adults [1]. In the United States, it is the fourth leading cause of death overall [2]. Among people who survive a stroke, unilateral spatial neglect (USN) is the most frequent disorder for right hemisphere lesions [3].

The incidence of USN varies widely from 10% to 82% [4, 5]. USN is characterized by the inability to report or respond to people or objects presented on the side contralateral to the lesioned side of the brain and has been associated with poor functional outcomes and long stays in hospitals and rehabilitation centers [6].

Pharmacological interventions such as dopamine and noradrenergic agonists or procholinergic treatment have been used in people affected by USN after stroke, but the evidence derived from a Cochrane systematic review that included only two available RCTs was very low and inconclusive [7].

Other nonpharmacological rehabilitation techniques have been explored for USN with the aim to facilitate the recovery of perception and behavior, which include right half-field eye-patching [8], mirror therapy [9], prism adaptation [10], left-hand somatosensory stimulation with visual scanning training [11], contralateral transcutaneous electrical nerve stimulation and optokinetic stimulation [12], trunk rotation [13], repetitive transcranial magnetic stimulation [14], galvanic vestibular stimulation [15], and dressing practice [16]. However, their results do not support the use of these techniques in isolation for improvement of secondary outcomes such as performance and sensorimotor functions, activities of daily living (ADLs), or quality of life [9, 14, 17].

Noninvasive brain stimulations (transcranial direct current stimulation (tDCS) and repetitive transcranial magnetic stimulation (rTMS)) have already shown their ability to modify cortical excitability [18]. tDCS is a noninvasive method used to modulate cortical excitability by applying a direct current to the brain that is less expensive than repetitive transcranial magnetic stimulation (rTMS). The latter is an electric current that creates magnetic fields that penetrate the brain and can modulate cortical excitability by decreasing or increasing it and potentially improve perceptual and cognitive abilities [19, 20].

A previous Cochrane systematic review summarized results about the effects of tDCS versus control (sham/any other intervention) on activities of daily living (ADLs) among stroke survivors. The authors included 32 randomized controlled trials (RCTs) and concluded that tDCS might enhance ADLs, but upper and lower limb function, muscle strength, and cognitive abilities should be further explored [21]. Another Cochrane systematic review assessed the efficacy of repetitive transcranial magnetic stimulation (rTMS) compared to sham therapy or no therapy for improving function in people with stroke. The 19 included trials showed that rTMS was not associated with a significant increase in ADLs or in motor function; therefore, the authors do not support the use of rTMS for the treatment of stroke, and they plan to complete further trials to confirm their findings [22].

Previous reviews were, however, limited in that they did not include non-RCT studies nor did they evaluate the newest noninvasive brain stimulation—theta burst. We therefore conducted a systematic review of RCT and non-RCT studies that assessed the impact of tDCS, rTMS, and TBS for unilateral spatial neglect after stroke.

2. Methods

We adhered to methods described in the Cochrane Handbook for Intervention Reviews [23]. Our reporting also adheres to the Preferred Reporting Items for Systematic Reviews and Meta-Analyses (PRISMA) [24] and Meta-Analysis of Observational Studies in Epidemiology (MOOSE) statements [25].

2.1. Eligibility Criteria. The eligibility criteria are as follows:

(1) Study designs: RCTs, quasi-RCTs, and non-RCTs

(2) Participants: adults over 18 years of age, regardless of gender and the duration of illness or severity of the initial impairment, with USN after any type of stroke diagnosis (ischemic or intracranial hemorrhage) measured by clinical examination or radiographically by computed tomography (CT) or magnetic resonance imaging (MRI), regardless of whether they were included after evaluation by standardized USN tests.

(3) Interventions: any noninvasive brain stimulations such as tDCS, rTMS, and including theta burst (continuous TBS (cTBS) or intermittent theta burst (iTBS)) (we considered evaluating both the different types of stimulations (i.e., cathodal tDCS versus anodal tDCS versus dual tDCS) and types of frequency (i.e., high-frequency versus low frequency))

(4) Comparators: interventions were to be compared against sham stimulation or any conventional stroke rehabilitation (e.g., pharmacological therapy or nonpharmacological therapy such as right half-field eye-patching, mirror therapy, prism adaptation, left-hand somatosensory stimulation, and visual scanning training or other conventional treatment)

We also considered noninvasive brain stimulations as an adjunct to any type of conventional stroke rehabilitation.

(5) Outcomes:

(i) Overall USN measured by any paper-and-pencil tests, such as the line cancellation task [26], the line bisection test [27], or the star cancellation test [28], and by any validated specific instrument, such as the Catherine Bergego Scale [29], and the Behavioral Inattention Test [30]

(ii) Disability in neurological and functional abilities as measured by any validated specific instrument, such as the National Institutes of Health Stroke Scale and the Modified Rankin Scale [31], the box and block test [32], or the Fugl-Meyer Assessment [33] after treatment and over the long term

(iii) Daily life functions as measured by any validated measurement scale, such as the Barthel index [31]

(iv) Number of reported falls as measured by diaries of falls, by the Morse Fall Scale [34], or by the Hendrich II Fall Risk Model [35] after treatment and over the long term

(v) Balance as measured by the Berg Balance Scale, the balance subscale of the Fugl-Meyer test, and the Postural Assessment Scale for Stroke Patients [36] after treatment and over the long term

(vi) Depression or anxiety as measured by the Beck Depression Inventory, the Hospital Anxiety and Depression Scale, Symptom Checklist-90 (SCL-90), and the Hamilton Depression Rating Scale [37] after treatment and over the long term

(vii) Evaluation of poststroke fatigue by the Fatigue Severity Scale [38] after treatment and over the long term

(viii) Quality of life (however defined by the study authors) after treatment and over the long term

(ix) Adverse events (e.g., euphoria, hallucinations, orthostatic hypotension, nausea, insomnia, dizziness, and syncope) after treatment and over the long term

(x) Death

2.2. Data Source and Searches. We searched MEDLINE (OvidSP) (1966 to July 2016), EMBASE (OvidSP) (1980 to July 2017), the Cochrane Central Register of Controlled Trials (CENTRAL) (The Cochrane Library, 2017, issue 7), CINAHL (1961 to July 2017), and Latin-American and Caribbean Center on Health Sciences Information (LILACS) (from 1982 to July 2017) without language restrictions. The date of the most recent search was 26 July 2017. All searches were conducted with the assistance of a trained medical librarian. We also searched the reference lists of relevant articles and conference proceedings and contacted the authors of included trials.

The search strategy was: (tDCS OR TDCS OR Cathodal Stimulation Transcranial Direct Current Stimulation OR Cathodal Stimulation tDCSs OR Cathodal Stimulation tDCS OR Transcranial Random Noise Stimulation OR Transcranial Alternating Current Stimulation OR Transcranial Electrical Stimulation OR dual transcranial direct current stimulation OR Transcranial Electrical Stimulations OR Anodal Stimulation Transcranial Direct Current Stimulation OR Anodal Stimulation Tdcs OR Anodal Tdcs OR Anodal Stimulation TDCSs OR Repetitive Transcranial Electrical Stimulation OR repetitive transcranial magnetic stimulation OR RTMS OR rTMS OR High-frequency rTMS OR Trasncranial Magnetic Stimulation OR Transcranial Magnetic Stimulations OR Low-frequency transcranial magnetic stimulation OR Stimulation Transcranial Magnetic OR Stimulations Transcranial Magnetic OR Single Pulse Transcranial Magnetic Stimulation OR Paired Pulse Transcranial Magnetic Stimulation OR Repetitive Transcranial Magnetic Stimulation OR theta burst OR theta burst stimulation OR theta-burst OR theta-burst stimulation OR burst stimulation OR continuous theta burst stimulation OR continuous TBS OR TBS) AND (cerebrovascular disorders OR basal ganglia cerebrovascular disease OR hemispatial neglect OR hemispatial neglect OR spatial attentional asymmetries OR brain ischemia OR carotid artery diseases OR intracranial arterial diseases OR intracranial embolism and thrombosis OR intracranial hemorrhages OR stroke OR brain infarction OR vertebral artery dissection OR post-stroke OR poststroke OR hemineglect OR hemi-neglect OR unilateral visuospatial neglect OR visuospatial neglect OR visual spatial neglect OR spatial neglect OR unilateral neglect of acute stroke patients OR unilateral spatial neglect OR patients with stroke OR stroke patients with spatial neglect OR right hemisphere strokes OR rehabilitation after stroke OR chronic spatial neglect after stroke OR unilateral neglect OR spatial neglect OR hemispatial neglect OR visual neglect OR inattention OR hemi-inattention OR space perception OR visual perception OR perceptual disorders OR perceptual disorder OR extinction OR functional laterality).

2.3. Selection of Studies. Two pairs of reviewers independently screened all titles and abstracts identified by the literature search, obtained full-text articles of all potentially eligible studies, and evaluated them for eligibility. Reviewers resolved disagreement by discussion or, if necessary, with third party adjudication. We also considered studies reported only as conference abstracts.

2.4. Data Extraction. Reviewers underwent calibration exercises and worked in pairs to independently extract data from included studies. They resolved disagreement by discussion or, if necessary, with third party adjudication. They abstracted the following data using a pretested data extraction form: study design, participants, interventions, comparators, outcome assessed, and relevant statistical data.

2.5. Risk of Bias Assessment. Reviewers, working in pairs, independently assessed the risk of bias of included RCTs using a modified version of the Cochrane Collaboration's instrument (http:/distillercer.com/resources/) [39]. That version includes nine domains: adequacy of sequence generation, allocation sequence concealment, blinding of participants and caregivers, blinding of data collectors, blinding for outcome assessment, blinding of data analysts, incomplete outcome data, selective outcome reporting, and the presence of other potential sources of bias not accounted for in the previously cited domains [40]. For incomplete outcome data in individual studies, we stipulated as low risk of bias for loss to follow-up as less than 10% and a difference of less than 5% in missing data between intervention/exposure and control groups.

When information regarding risk of bias or other aspects of methods or results was unavailable, we attempted to contact study authors for additional information.

2.6. Certainty of Evidence. We summarized the evidence and assessed its certainty separately for bodies of evidence from RCT and non-RCT studies. We used the Grading of Recommendations Assessment, Development and Evaluation (GRADE) methodology to rate certainty of the evidence for each outcome as high, moderate, low, or very low [41]. In the GRADE approach, RCTs begin as high certainty and non-RCT studies begin as moderate certainty. Detailed GRADE guidance was used to assess overall risk of bias [42], imprecision [43], inconsistency [44], indirectness [45], and publication bias [46] and to summarize the results in an evidence profile (Table 1).

We planned to assess publication bias through visual inspection of funnel plots for each outcome in which we identified 10 or more eligible studies; however, we were not able to do so because there were an insufficient number of studies to allow for this assessment.

2.7. Data Synthesis and Statistical Analysis. We calculated pooled inverse variance standardized mean difference (SMD) and associated 95% CIs using random-effects models. We addressed variability in results across studies by using I^2 statistic and the P value obtained from the Cochran chi square test. Our primary analyses were based on eligible patients who had reported outcomes for each study (complete case analysis). We used Review Manager (RevMan) (version 5.3; Nordic Cochrane Centre, Cochrane) for all analyses [47].

2.8. Subgroup and Sensitivity Analyses. We planned possible subgroup analyses according to the following characteristics:

(i) Participants (stroke type: ischemic stroke versus intracranial hemorrhage)

(ii) Interventions (type of stimulation: cathodal versus anodal and position of electrodes; type of frequency: high frequency versus low frequency)

(iii) Comparator (type of control intervention: pharmacological therapy versus nonpharmacological therapy)

(iv) Different tests for overall USN (star cancellation test versus line bisection test)

We planned to conduct subgroup analyses only when five or more studies were available, with at least two in each subgroup. We planned to synthesize the evidence separately for bodies of evidence from RCT and non-RCT studies by a sensitivity analysis.

3. Results

3.1. Study Selection. We identified a total of 4129 citations through database searches and a further four studies from the reference lists of the Cochrane reviews [22, 48, 49] (see Figure 1 for search results). After screening by title and then by abstract, we obtained full-paper copies for 30 citations that were potentially eligible for inclusion in the review. We excluded 15 studies for the following reasons: case report, case series, self-controlled study, review, and off-topic. The remaining 12 RCTs [14, 50–60] with a total of 273 participants and four non-RCTs [61–64] with a total of 94 participants met the minimum requirements, and we included them in this review.

3.2. Study Characteristics. Table 2 describes study characteristics related to design of study, setting, number of participants, mean age, gender, inclusion and exclusion criteria, and follow-up. Eight studies [14, 54, 56, 59, 61–64] were conducted largely in Europe and eight in Asia [50–53, 55, 57, 58, 60]. Randomized trials' sample sizes ranged from 10 [56] to 38 [55], and non-RCT studies ranged from 12 [63] to 36 [62]. Typical participants were males in their 40s, 50s, and 60s. Studies followed participants immediately after treatment [50, 57, 58, 62] to one month [51, 52, 54–56].

Table 3 describes study characteristics related to intervention and comparators and assessed outcomes. Of the 16 included studies, nine trials [14, 50, 52, 54, 55, 59–62] evaluated TBS:

(1) Eight trials compared cTBS versus

  (i) sham cTBS (both groups received conventional rehabilitation training [52, 60]);

  (ii) 1 Hz rTMS, 10 Hz rTMS, and sham rTMS (all groups with addition of routine rehabilitation [55]);

  (iii) sham TBS [14];

  (iv) sham cTBS [54, 59, 61, 62].

(2) One trial compared iTBS with 80% resting motor threshold (RMT) versus iTBS 40% RMT [50].

Of the remaining seven studies, four trials [56–58, 64] evaluated tDCS:

(1) Two trials compared tDCS over the left (cathodal) and right (anodal) posterior parietal cortex, one versus placebo at an intensity of 2 mA [56] and the other versus sham tDCS [64].

(2) One trial [57] compared tDCS dual versus either tDCS single or tDCS sham.

(3) One trial [58] compared tDCS versus sham tDCS.

Three further trials [51, 53, 63] evaluated rTMS:

(1) One trial [51] compared rTMS with sham rTMS, both plus conventional rehabilitation therapy (neurodevelopmental facilitation techniques).

(2) Two trials compared 1 Hz rTMS, one versus 10 Hz rTMS and sham rTMS [53] (both groups received conventional rehabilitation), and the other trial compared 1 Hz rTMS versus sham rTMS [63].

None of the included studies evaluated noninvasive brain stimulations as an adjunct to any type of conventional stroke rehabilitation.

3.3. Risk of Bias. Figure 2 describes the risk of bias assessment for the RCTs and non-RCTs, respectively. The major issue

Table 1: GRADE evidence profile for RCTs: noninvasive brain stimulations for unilateral spatial neglect after stroke.

Quality assessment Number of participants (studies) Range follow-up Time in weeks	Risk of bias	Inconsistency	Indirectness	Imprecision	Publication bias	Illustrative comparative risks (95% CI) Assumed risk Sham	Corresponding risk Noninvasive brain stimulations	Certainty in estimates or quality of evidence
Overall USN measured by star cancellation test								
116 (6) Immediately postintervention 4 weeks	Serious limitation[1]	Serious limitation[2]	No serious limitation[3]	Serious limitation[4]	Undetectable	The mean in change in USN measured by star cancellation test was 45.29 (SD 5.94)*	The std. mean in changes in USN measured by star cancellation test in the intervention group was on average 0.51 fewer (1.89 fewer to 0.88 more)	Very low
Overall USN measured by line bisection test								
107 (5) Immediately postintervention 1 month	Serious limitation[1]	Serious limitation[2]	No serious limitation[3]	No serious limitation	Undetectable	The mean in change in USN measured by line bisection test was 35.79 (SD 18.65)*	The std. mean in changes in USN measured by line bisection test in the intervention group was on average 2.33 fewer (3.54 fewer to 1.12 fewer)	Low
Overall USN measured by Motor-Free Visual Perception Test								
38 (2) 2–4 weeks	Serious limitation[1]	No serious limitation	No serious limitation	No serious limitation	Undetectable	The mean in change in USN measured by Motor-Free Visual Perception Test was 16.9 (SD 2.1)**	The std. mean in changes in USN measured by Motor-Free Visual Perception Test in the intervention group was on average 1.46 more (0.73 more to 2.20 more)	Moderate
Overall USN measured by Albert test and line crossing test								
50 (2) 4 weeks	Serious limitation[1]	Serious limitation[2]	No serious limitation	No serious limitation	Undetectable	The mean in change in USN measured by Albert test and line crossing test was 27.33 (SD 4.55)**	The std. mean in changes in USN measured by Albert test and line crossing test in the intervention group was on average 1.01 more (1 fewer to 3.02 more)	Low

SD = standard error; std. = standardized. *Baseline risk estimates for overall USN come from control arm of Fu et al.'s [52] study (lowest risk of bias trial in the meta-analysis). **Baseline risk estimates for overall USN come from control arm of Cha et al.'s [51] study (newest trial in the meta-analysis). [1]The majority of the studies were ranked as high risk of bias for both allocation sequence and allocation concealment. [2]There was a substantial heterogeneity ($I^2 > 70\%$). [3]There was no substantial difference related to the mean age and eligibility criteria throughout the six included studies. [4]95% CI for absolute effects includes clinically important benefit and no benefit.

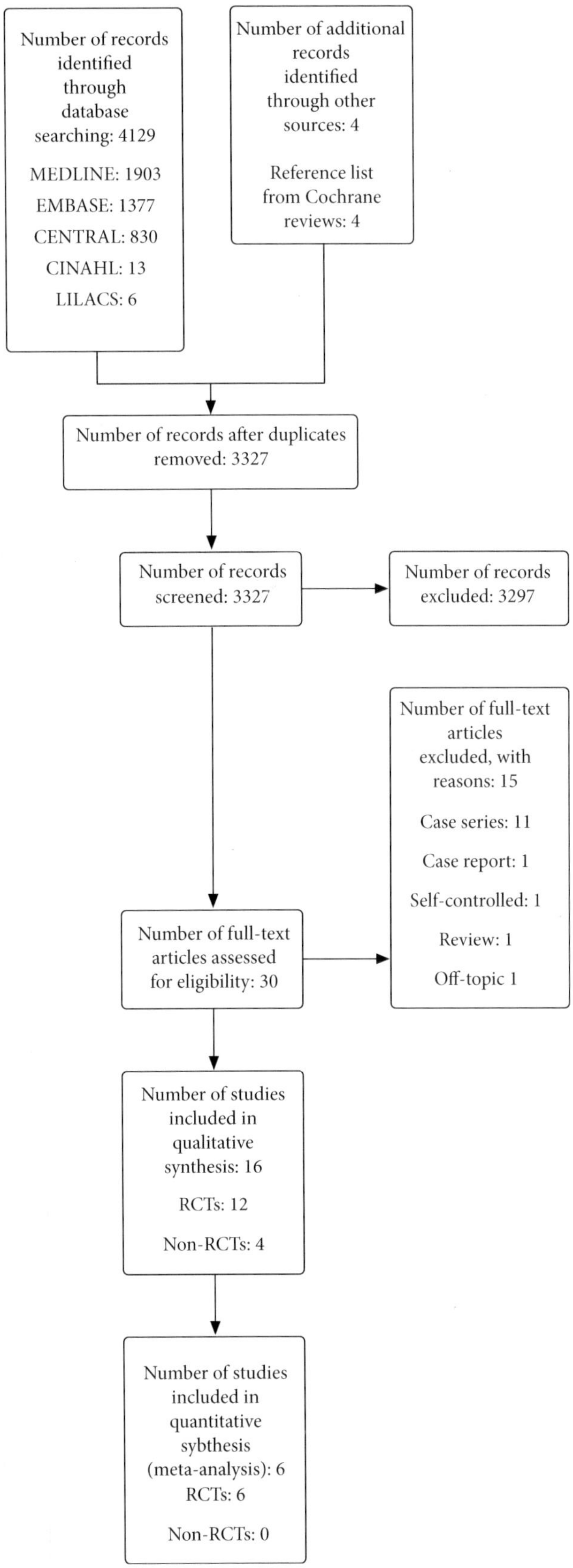

FIGURE 1: Flow diagram of the systematic review.

regarding risk of bias in the RCTs and non-RCTs was problems of random sequence generation [14, 50, 51, 54–59, 61–64] and concealment of randomization [14, 50, 53–59, 61–64]. An additional problem was blinding of the statistician in all included studies.

3.4. Outcomes

3.4.1. Synthesized Results from Randomized Controlled Trials

(1) Overall USN Measured by the Star Cancellation Test. The results from six RCTs [51–55, 57] comparing noninvasive brain stimulations with sham failed to show a benefit in overall USN measured by the star cancellation test (SMD −0.51, 95% CI −1.87, 0.85; $p = 0.46$; $I^2 = 90\%$) (Figure 3). The results were consistent regardless of the type of noninvasive brain stimulations (TBS in three RCTs [52, 54, 55] (SMD −1.61, 95% CI −4.28, 1.06; $p = 0.24$; $I^2 = 93\%$); dual-tDCS in one RCT [57] (SMD −0.12, 95% CI −0.99, 0.76; $p = 0.79$; I^2 = not applicable); and 1 Hz rTMS in two RCTs [51, 53] (SMD 0.57, 95% CI −2.95, 4.10; $p = 0.75$; $I^2 = 95\%$)) (Figure 3). Certainty in evidence was rated as very low because of imprecision, inconsistency, and risk of bias due to the studies that were ranked as high risk of bias for both allocation sequence and allocation concealment (Figure 2).

A sensitivity analysis from the same RCTs using TBS [52, 54, 55], single-tDCS [57], and 10 Hz rTMS [51, 53] yielded results that were also consistent with the primary analysis and failed to show a difference in the effects of noninvasive brain stimulations compared to sham (SMD −0.62, 95% CI −1.89, 0.65; $p = 0.34$; $I^2 = 88\%$) (Figure 4).

(2) Overall USN Measured by the Line Bisection Test. Results from five RCTs [51–53, 55, 57] comparing noninvasive brain stimulations with sham suggested a benefit in overall USN measured by the line bisection test (SMD −2.33, 95% CI −3.54, −1.12; $p = 0.0002$; $I^2 = 81\%$) (Figure 5). The results were inconsistent when the data were analyzed by type of noninvasive brain stimulations: TBS in two RCTs [52, 55] (SMD −3.08, 95% CI −6.54, 0.38; $p = 0.08$; $I^2 = 90\%$) and dual-tDCS in one RCT [57] (SMD −0.66, 95% CI −1.56, 0.25; $p = 0.15$; I^2 = not applicable) except by 1 Hz rTMS in two RCTs [51, 53] that yielded results that were consistent with the overall meta-analysis (SMD −2.33, 95% CI −3.54, −1.12; $p < 0.0002$; $I^2 = 81\%$) (Figure 5). Certainty in evidence was rated as low because of inconsistency and risk of bias due to the studies that were ranked as high risk of bias for both allocation sequence and allocation concealment (Figure 2).

A sensitivity analysis from the same RCTs using TBS [52, 55], tDCS [57], and 10 Hz rTMS [53] yielded results that were also consistent with the primary analysis and suggested a difference in the effects of noninvasive brain stimulations compared to sham (SMD −2.35, 95% CI −3.72, −0.98; $p = 0.002$; $I^2 = 85\%$) (Figure 6).

(3) Overall USN Measured by Motor-Free Visual Perception Test. The results from two RCTs [51, 53] comparing noninvasive brain stimulations with sham suggested a benefit

TABLE 2: Study characteristics related to design of study, setting, number of participants, mean age, gender, and inclusion and exclusion criteria.

Author, year	Design of study	Status of publication	Location	No.* of participants	Mean age	No. of males (%)	Inclusion criteria	Exclusion criteria
Randomized controlled trials								
Cao et al., 2016 [50]	Parallel RCT	Full text	Asia	I: 7 C: 6	I: 55.0 C: 62.0	I: 85.7 C: 83.3	Right-handed patients who had a first-ever stroke in the right hemisphere and visuospatial neglect with normal or corrected-to-normal vision	NR
Cha and Kim, 2016 [51]	Parallel RCT	Full text	Asia	I: 15 C: 15	I: 64.07 C: 63.33	I: 64 C: 60.0	Had a first right hemisphere stroke (cerebral infarction or hemorrhage) more than 2 weeks before the study, which had been confirmed by computed tomography or magnetic resonance imaging (MRI); had VSN determined by line bisection tests (rightward bias > 12%) or star cancelation test (omission of any number of stars); had a Glasgow coma scale score < 15; 18–80 years old; right-handed; normal vision or normal corrected vision; and had the ability to understand the study and signed an informed consent form	All patients did not have brain tumors or other brain pathology. Excluded were patients with hemianopia; subarachnoid hemorrhage, venous sinus thrombosis, transient ischemic attack, reversible ischemia, or a condition exacerbated by a new infarction or hemorrhage site; a medical history or family history of seizure; or with metal devices or claustrophobia preventing MRI
Fu et al., 2015 [52]	Parallel RCT	Full text	Asia	I: 11 C: 11	I: 55.1^{β} C: 59.5^{β}	I: 80.0 C: 80.0	Right-handed patients with right hemisphere stroke (hemorrhagic or ischemic lesion) confirmed by computed tomography or magnetic resonance imaging > 2 weeks before the beginning of the study and diagnosis of visuospatial neglect based on clinician judgement and on deficits in at least one out of two paper-pencil tests	Age < 30 years or > 80 years, history of epilepsy, previous head trauma, drug and alcohol abuse and psychiatric disorders, recurrent stroke, obvious aphasia and communication obstacles, family history of seizures, ever use of tricyclic antidepressants or antipsychotic drugs, diamagnetic metal implants such as cardiac pacemakers, and visual field defects

Table 2: Continued.

Author, year	Design of study	Status of publication	Location	No.* of participants	Mean age	No. of males (%)	Inclusion criteria	Exclusion criteria
Fu et al., 2017 [60]	Parallel RCT	Full text	Asia	I: 6 C: 6	I: 60.17 C: 62	I: 75 C: 75	Had a first right hemisphere stroke (cerebral infarction or hemorrhage) more than 2 weeks before the study, which had been confirmed by computed tomography or magnetic resonance imaging (MRI); had VSN determined by line bisection tests (rightward bias > 12%) or star cancelation test (omission of any number of stars); had a Glasgow coma scale score < 15; 18–80 years old; right-handed; normal vision or normal corrected vision; and had the ability to understand the study and sign an informed consent form; all patients did not have brain tumors or other brain pathology	Patients with hemianopia; subarachnoid hemorrhage, venous sinus thrombosis, transient ischemic attack, reversible ischemia, or a condition exacerbated by a new infarction or hemorrhage site; a medical history or family history of seizure; or with metal devices or claustrophobia preventing MRI
Smit et al., 2015 [56]	RCT cross-over study	Full text	Europe	I: $5^{\text{€}}$ C: $5^{\text{€}}$	I: $64.8^{\text{€}}$ C: $64.8^{\text{€}}$	I: $60.0^{\text{€}}$ C: $60.0^{\text{€}}$	Patients with left hemispatial neglect after right-hemispheric lesion, right-handed, older than the age of 18, more than four months after stroke	Patients with severe language and communication disorders, bilateral cortical damage, psychiatric disorders, alcohol and/or drug addiction, epilepsy, eczema or damages on the scalp, metal or other foreign parts in the head
Yang et al., 2015 [55]	Parallel RCT	Full text	Asia	I: 9 I2: 10 I3: 9 C: 10	I: 46.7 I2: 48.0 I3: 49.4 C: 47.7	I: 66.6 I2: 40.0 I3: 55.6 C: 30.0	Age between 18 and 80; first stroke patients (cerebral infarction or hemorrhage) and in recovery time within 60–180 days; USN confirmed by line bisection test, star cancellation test, or clinical examination; no metallic implant of diamagnetic substance; signed the informed consent	Subarachnoid hemorrhage, venous sinus thrombosis, and reversible or transient ischemic attacks; worsening condition and new-onset infarction or hemorrhage; GCS score < 15; obvious aphasia and severe cognitive-communication disorders; family history of epilepsy; impaired organ function or failure in the heart, lung, liver, kidney, or

Table 2: Continued.

Author, year	Design of study	Status of publication	Location	No.* of participants	Mean age	No. of males (%)	Inclusion criteria	Exclusion criteria
								other vital organs and life expectancy < 6 months; history of claustrophobia and uncooperative during examination; and hemianopsia
Kim et al. [53]	Parallel RCT	Full text	Asia	I: 9 I2: 9 C: 9	I: 68.6 I2: 64.1 C: 68.3	I: 55.6 I2: 44.4 C: 66.7	Patients with right cerebral ischemic or hemorrhagic with visuospatial neglect (confirmed using the line bisection test); all patients were right-handed	Severe cognitive impairment making them unable to understand the instructions; contraindications for TMS, such as a history of epileptic seizure, major head trauma, and presence of metal in the skull or pacemaker; or unstable medical or neurologic conditions
Sunwoo et al., 2013 [57]	RCT cross-over study	Full text	Asia	I: 10 I2: 10 C: 10	62.6[¢]	40.0[β]	Stroke patients with lesion in the right hemisphere involving the parietal cortex, and left USN diagnosed by clinical observation and confirmed by a line bisection test; all patients were previously right-handed	Patients who had metallic implants in the cranial cavity, a skull defect, history of seizure, uncontrolled medical problems, and severe cognitive impairment
Cazzoli et al., 2012 [14]	Parallel RCT	Full text	Europe	24[£]	58.0[¢]	70.8[¢]	Ischemic or hemorrhagic lesion to the right hemisphere and left-sided spatial neglect determined on the basis of deficits in at least two out of three classes of paper-pencil tests and on clinical judgement; all patients had to have normal or corrected-to-normal visual acuity	History of epilepsy, prior head trauma, drug and alcohol abuse, and major psychiatric disorders
Ko et al., 2008 [58]	RCT cross-over study	Full text	Asia	I: 15[€] C: 15[€]	I: 62.1[€] C: 62.1[€]	I: 66.6[€] C: 66.6[€]	Patients with subacute stroke with neglect	Patients who had metal in the cranial cavity or calvarium, skin lesions in the area of electrode, uncontrolled medical conditions, and severe cognitive impairments

Table 2: Continued.

Author, year	Design of study	Status of publication	Location	No.* of participants	Mean age	No. of males (%)	Inclusion criteria	Exclusion criteria
Koch et al., 2012 [54]	Parallel RCT	Full text	Europe	I: 10 C: 10	I: 61.4# C: 71.9#	I: 55.5# C: 55.5#	Right-handed patients, with right hemisphere subacute ischemic stroke affected by hemispatial neglect, confirmed by radiologic (CT or MRI) and clinical examination	NR
Bonnì et al., 2011 [59]	Parallel RCT	Conference abstract	Europe	NR	NR	NR	Subacute stroke patients with neglect	NR
Non-RCTs								
Cazzoli et al., 2015 [61]	Non-RCT cross-over study$	Full text	Europe	I: 8¥ C: 8¥	I: 52.6 and 54.2α C: 53.0	NR	Patients with left-sided, hemispatial neglect after a subacute right-hemispheric stroke; all patients had normal or corrected-to-normal visual acuity	Not clearly reported, however, authors have assessed patients by means of internationally accepted safety guidelines for the application of TMS, which included screening for a history of epilepsy, prior head trauma, drug and alcohol abuse, and major psychiatric disorders
Hopfner et al., 2015 [62]	Non-RCT cross-over	Full text	Europe	I: 18€ C: 18€	I: 64.5€ C: 64.5€	I: 50.0€ C: 50.0€	Left-sided neglect, based on clinical judgement and neuropsychological testing, after subacute right-hemispheric stroke; all subjects had normal or corrected-to-normal visual acuity	NR
Làdavas et al., 2015 [64]	Quasi-RCT	Full text	Europe	I: 8 I2: 11 C: 11	I: 72.0 I2: 66.0 C: 67.0	I: 50.0 I2: 54.5 C: 54.5	Patients with right hemisphere stroke with hemispatial neglect and performance on the Behavioral Inattention Test battery with scores ≤ 129	Presence of widespread mental deterioration (Mini-Mental State Examination score < 20), psychiatric disorders, a history of prior stroke or hemorrhage, any severe internal medical disease, epilepsy, and additional factors influencing the risk of epilepsy

Table 2: Continued.

Author, year	Design of study	Status of publication	Location	No.* of participants	Mean age	No. of males (%)	Inclusion criteria	Exclusion criteria
Agosta et al., 2014 [63]	Non-RCT cross-over study	Full text	Europe	I: 6[€] C: 6[€]	I: 67.83[€] C: 67.83[€]	I: 66.6[€] C: 66.6[€]	Patients with right hemisphere unilateral lesions due to a cerebrovascular stroke, confirmed by radiological examination (CT or MR), in their chronic stage after the stroke (at least six months post onset); besides, participants were right-handed, native Italian speakers, and had normal or corrected-to-normal visual acuity	History or evidence of degenerative disease or psychiatric disorder

C: control group; CT: computed tomography; GCS: Glasgow coma scale; I: intervention; MR: magnetic resonance imaging; No.: number; RCT: randomized controlled trial; TMS: transcranial magnetic stimulation; USN: unilateral spatial neglect. [€]Participants of the experimental group also served as controls. [¥]Five patients were randomized in parallel design, and three further patients included in both groups. [£]The authors did not specify the sample size per studied group. [α]Data comprises three patients that received both experimental and control interventions. [β]Data was calculated from 10 patients (one patient was excluded after randomization). [¢]Data are from the whole sample, as the authors did not specify it per studied group. [#]Data are from 9 patients in each group. [$]The study was a cross-over for only three patients, for the remaining ten patients the study was a RCT.

TABLE 3: Study characteristics related to intervention and control groups, assessed outcomes, and follow-up.

Author, year	Description of interventions	Description of control groups	Measured outcomes	Follow-up
Randomized controlled trials				
Cao et al., 2016 [50]	**iTBS** 80% RMT in the rTMS group: stimulation was applied using an 87 mm butterfly coil connected to a Magstim Rapid2 (Magstim Co., Whitland, UK), with peak intensity of 2.0 T and a maximum pulse length of 250 μs. Pulses (theta burst type) were delivered to the left dorsal lateral prefrontal cortex, the F5 label of the left hemisphere, which is between the F3 and F7, at 80% of resting motor threshold. Two sessions were applied with a 15 min interval on each day. Each session included 20 stimulation trains consisting of three pulses delivered at a frequency of 50 Hz in every 200 ms for 2 s (total 10 bursts, 30 pulses) with an interval of 8 s.	Same as intervention group; however, pulses were delivered at 40% of RMT	Line bisection and star cancellation tests	After intervention
Cha and Kim, 2016 [51]	**Repetitive rTMS** + conventional rehabilitation therapy (neurodevelopmental facilitation techniques) for a total of 40 minutes (rTMS: 10 min; rehabilitation: 30 min) per day, with a 10-minute rest period halfway through the session, for 4 weeks, 5 days per week: stimulation was delivered using figure-of-eight coil with a diameter of 80 mm connected to Magstim Rapid2 (Magstim Co. Ltd., Wales, UK). Stimulation was applied in the right posterior parietal (P3 and P4 areas) based on the electroencephalogram 10/20 system at a frequency of 1 Hz for 5 minutes with 90% of the motor threshold during rest.	Sham rTMS and conventional rehabilitation therapy using the same protocol than the experimental group	Motor-Free Visual Perception Test; line bisection test; Albert test; star cancellation test	4 weeks
Fu et al., 2015 [52]	Left posterior parietal cortex **cTBS** + conventional rehabilitation training: cTBS was set over P5, three-pulse burst was delivered at 30 Hz and repeated every 200 ms for 40 s with intensity was 80% of the resting motor threshold. cTBS was delivered using a Super Rapid 2 magnetic stimulator (Magstim, Whitland, UK) with 2.0-Tesla maximum field strength, connected with a figure-of-eight coil (diameter of outside loop, 87 mm). Patients received 4 trains daily, with an interval of 15 min, for 14 consecutive days.	Sham cTBS + conventional rehabilitation training	Star cancellation test; line bisection test	4 weeks

Table 3: Continued.

Author, year	Description of interventions	Description of control groups	Measured outcomes	Follow-up
Fu et al., 2017 [60]	The cTBS group received continuous TBS with the coil placed tangentially to the scalp at P3 over the left posterior parietal cortex (according to the 10–20 electrode position system of the American Electroencephalographic Association28). The magnitude of the pulses was maintained at 80% resting motor threshold. On each day for 10 consecutive days, 4 sessions of stimulation were delivered, with an interval of 15 min between every 2 sessions. Each session lasted 40 s and contained 600 pulses delivered in 200 bursts at 5 Hz (theta rhythm). Each burst included 3 pulses delivered at 30 Hz.	The active control group received stimulations with the same features at the same position as the cTBS group, but with the coil placed perpendicular to the scalp surface and the amplitude of the stimulation pulses reduced to 40% resting motor threshold	Star cancellation test; line bisection test	1(days
Smit et al., 2015 [56]	**tDCS** was applied for 20 minutes over the left (cathodal) and right (anodal) posterior parietal cortex on five consecutive days with a battery-driven direct current stimulator (NeuroConnDC-Stimulator; serialnumber 0096). Stimulation parameters were set at a current of 2000 mA, and a resistance of <10 kOhm, applied for 1200s with ramping up in 30 s and ramping down in 30 s. Electrodes were located over the posterior parietal lobe, corresponding with P3 (cathodal electrode) and P4 (anodal electrode). Treatment conditions were separated by a four-week washout period.	Placebo was applied for 20 minutes over the left (cathodal) and right (anodal) posterior parietal cortex at an intensity of 2 mA on five consecutive days; treatment conditions were separated by a four-week washout period	Cancellation tests; line bisection tests; drawing tests	1 month
Yang et al., 2015 [55]	Group I: 1 Hz **rTMS** two times a day for 2 weeks + routine rehabilitation: stimulation was administered using a rapid magnetic stimulator (Magstim Company) with a figure-of-eight coil, peak intensity of stimulation at 2 T, and pulse duration of 250 s, at the contralateral hemisphere (P3), intensity 80% of RMT, and frequency of 1 Hz, and stimulus duration for each sequence was 8 s, repeated 82 sequences with a total of 656 pulse numbers. Group I2: 10 Hz **rTMS** two times a day for 2 weeks + routine rehabilitation: stimulation was administered using a rapid magnetic stimulator (Magstim Company) with a figure-of-eight coil, peak intensity of stimulation at 2 T, and pulse duration of 250 s, at the contralateral hemisphere (P3), intensity 80% of RMT, frequency 10 Hz, with a total pulse number of 1000 and stimulation interval of 55 s.	Sham rTMS two times a day for 2 weeks + routine rehabilitation	Star cancellation test; line bisection test	1 month

Table 3: Continued.

Author, year	Description of interventions	Description of control groups	Measured outcomes	Follow-up
	Group I3: **cTBS** two times a day for 2 weeks + routine rehabilitation: stimulation was administered using a rapid magnetic stimulator (Magstim Company) with a figure-of-eight coil, peak intensity of stimulation at 2 T, and pulse duration of 250 s, at the contralateral hemisphere (P3), intensity 80% of RMT, 801 pulses, in bursts of 3 pulses at 30 Hz, repeated every 100 ms.			
Kim et al., 2013 [53]	Group A: 10 sessions of low-frequency (**1 Hz**) **rTMS** over the nonlesioned left posterior parietal cortex (P3) at a 90% motor threshold in 4 trains of 5-minute duration, each separated by 1 minute (resulting in a total stimulation period of 20 minutes). rTMS was delivered using a Magstim Super Rapid Magnetic Stimulator with a 70-millimeter, air-cooled 8-shaped coil. rTMS was performed 5 times per week for 2 weeks. Patients also received conventional rehabilitation treatment (including physical, occupational, and cognitive therapies). Group B: 10 sessions of high-frequency (**10 Hz**) **rTMS** over the lesioned right posterior parietal cortex (P4) at a 90% motor threshold in 4 trains of 5-minute duration, each separated by 55 seconds (resulting in a total stimulation period of 20 minutes). The remaining of the protocol followed the same instructions as group A.	Sham rTMS + conventional rehabilitation	Motor-Free Visual Perception Test; line bisection test; cancellation test; Catherine Bergego scale; Korean-modified Barthel index	2 weeks
Sunwoo et al., 2013 [57]	Group A: dual-mode (**tDCS dual**) direct current was delivered by two sets of battery-powered devices (Phoresor II Auto Mod-elPM850, IOMED, USA) using two pairs of surface saline-soaked sponge electrodes (5 cm × 5 cm). Anodal tDCS of the first circuit over the right PPC (P4) was accompanied by cathodal tDCS of the second circuit over the left PPC (P3). Therefore, in the first tDCS circuit, the anode was placed over P4 and the cathode was placed over the left supraorbital area. In the second tDCS circuit, the anode was placed over the right supraorbital area and the cathode was placed over the P3. A constant current of 1 mA was delivered for 20 min.	Sham mode (tDCS sham) in the first and second tDCS circuits. The stimulator was turned on and the current intensity was gradually increased for 5 s, and was then tapered off over 5 s	Line bisection test; star cancelation test	Immediately after treatment

Table 3: Continued.

Author, year	Description of interventions	Description of control groups	Measured outcomes	Follow-up
	Group B: Single-mode (**tDCS single**) direct current was delivered by two sets of battery-powered devices (Phoresor II Auto Mod-elPM850, IOMED, USA) using two pairs of surface saline-soaked sponge electrodes (5 cm × 5 cm). The anode was placed over P4 and the cathode over the left supraorbital area (the first tDCS circuit), and real stimulation was provided, whereas the second tDCS circuit received sham stimulation. For the real stimulation, a constant current of 1 mA was delivered for 20 min. For the sham stimulation, the stimulator was turned on and the current intensity was gradually increased for 5 s, and was then tapered off over 5 s.			
Cazzoli et al., 2012 [14]	**cTBS** for 2 days on week 1 and sham TBS for 2 days on week 2. cTBS was applied by means of a MagPro X100 stimulator (Medtronic Functional Diagnostics) connected to a round coil with 60 mm outer radius (Magnetic Coil Transducer MC-125). cTBS protocol comprised 801 pulses, delivered in a continuous train and consisting of 267 bursts, each one contained three pulses at 30 Hz, repeated at 6 Hz (total duration of one single, cTBS train was 44 s), and eight cTBS trains were applied over 2 days. cTBS was applied over P3. Besides, patients received neurorehabilitation therapy including 1 h neuropsychological training, 1 h of occupational therapy, and 1 h of physiotherapy per day.	Control A: sham TBS for 2 days on week 1 and cTBS for 2 days on week 2. cTBS protocol was the same described for intervention A. Besides, patients received neurorehabilitation therapy including 1 h neuropsychological training, 1 h of occupational therapy, and 1 h of physiotherapy per day Control B: sham TBS for 2 days on week 1 and sham TBS for 2 days on week 2. Besides, patients received neurorehabilitation therapy including 1 h neuropsychological training, 1 h of occupational therapy, and 1 h of physiotherapy per day	Catherine Bergego scale; Vienna Test System; random shape cancelation test	2 weeks
Ko et al., 2008 [58]	**tDCS** to the right posterior parietal cortex for 20 min (2 mA anodal DC brain polarization) delivery by a battery-powered device (Phoresor II Auto model PM850, IOMED, USA), using a pair of saline-soaked surface sponge electrodes (5 cm × 5 cm). The anode was placed over P4, and cathode was placed over left supraorbital area.	Sham tDCS (current was delivered for 10 s and then turned off)	Line bisection test; shape-unstructured cancellation test; letter-structured cancellation test	Immediately post intervention

Table 3: Continued.

Author, year	Description of interventions	Description of control groups	Measured outcomes	Follow-up
Koch et al., 2012 [54]	**cTBS** was delivered using a MagStim Super Rapid magnetic stimulator (Magstim Company, Whitland, Wales, UK), connected with a figure-of-eight coil with a diameter of 70 mm. In each session, 3-pulse bursts at 50 Hz repeated every 200 ms for 40 s were delivered at 80% of the active motor threshold over the left PPC (600 pulses). Every day, 2 sessions of left PPC cTBS were applied with an interval of 15 minutes and lasted for 10 days (5 days per week, Monday to Friday). Patients also received rehabilitation program consisted of 20 sessions of 45 minutes each, held 5 days per week (based on computerized visuospatial scanning training) and motor rehabilitation when necessary.	Sham cTBS was delivered with the coil angled at 90°, with only the edge of the coil resting on the scalp Stimulus intensity, expressed as a percentage of the maximum stimulator output, was set at 80% of the active motor threshold inducing the same acoustic sensation as for real TBS Patients also received rehabilitation program	Line crossing test; letter cancellation test; star cancellation test; figure and shape copying test; representative drawing test	1 month
Bonnì et al., 2011 [59]	**cTBS** over the left PPC, for two weeks.	Sham cTBS	Standardized behavioural inattention test; excitability of the parieto-frontal functional connections	NR
		Non-RCTs		
Cazzoli et al., 2015 [61]	**cTBS** over the left, contralesional PPC (P3), was applied using a MagPro X100 stimulator, connected to either a round coil (MC-125 Medtronic Functional Diagnostics). The cTBS protocol consisted of 801 pulses delivered in a continuous train. The train was comprised of 267 bursts, where each contained three single pulses at 30 Hz, repeated at 6 Hz, and had a total duration of 44 s. Application consisted on two trains separated by a 15 min interval.	Sham cTBS over the left, contralesional PPC, was applied using a sham coil (MC-P-B70 Medtronic Functional Diagnostics)	Computerised balloon test with eye movement recording; paper-pencil cancellation tasks	8 hours
Hopfner et al., 2015 [62]	**cTBS** comprised 801 pulses, delivered in a continuous train of 267 bursts (each including 3 pulses at 30 Hz, repeated at 6 Hz). The total duration of a single cTBS train was 44 s. Two cTBS trains were applied overP3, with an intertrain interval of 15 min. A MagPro X100 stimulator (Medtronic Functional Diagnostics, Farum, Denmark), connected to around coil (Magnetic Coil Transducer MC-125) was used to deliver biphasic, repetitive magnetic pulses. Besides, 12 (from 18) patients also received smooth pursuit eye movement training.	Sham cTBS connected to a placebo coil (Magnetic Coil Transducer MC-P-B70) Besides, 12 (from 18) patients also received Smooth pursuit eye movement training	Center of cancellation score; x-position of leftmost cancelled target; number of cancelled targets	Right after treatment

Table 3: Continued.

Author, year	Description of interventions	Description of control groups	Measured outcomes	Follow-up
Làdavas et al., 2015 [64]	Group A: 2-week rehabilitation program consisted of 10 sessions of **cathodal tDCS** lasting 30 minutes each and held 5 days per week. tDCS was applied using a battery-driven Eldith (neuroConn GmbH, Ilmenau, Germany) Programmable Direct Current Stimulator with a pair of surface saline-soaked sponge electrodes. In each session, a constant current of 2 mA intensity (current density: 0.57 mA/cm2) was delivered lasting 20 minutes of cathodal tDCS of the left, intact PPC (over P5). Group B: 2-week rehabilitation program consisted of 10 sessions of **anodal tDCS** lasting 30 minutes each and held 5 days per week. The anodal tDCS was placed over the PPC of the damaged hemisphere (P6). The remaining protocol was the same used in group A.	Sham tDCS (montage used in the sham group mimicked that used in the two active groups)	Behavioral Inattention Test	Final follow-up within the first week after the last session
Agosta et al., 2014 [63]	A 10-minute train of repetitive low-frequency (**1** Hz) **rTMS** over the left parietal lobe (P3 site) identified using the 10/20 EEG measurement system. The stimulus was delivered using a 70 mm figure-of-eight coil connected to a Magstim Rapid2 (Magstim Co., UK). Stimulation strength was set to 90% of the threshold to evoke motor responses at rest.	Sham rTMS over the intact left parietal cortex	Visual tracking task; unilateral and bilateral tasks	30 minutes

C: control group; cTBS: continuous theta burst stimulation; I: intervention; iTBS: intermittent theta burst; PPC: posterior parietal cortex; RMT: resting motor threshold; rTMS: repetitive transcranial magnetic stimulation; tDCS: transcranial direct current stimulation; TBS: theta burst stimulation; USN: unilateral spatial neglect.

	Random sequence generation (selection bias)	Allocation concealment (selection bias)	Blinding of patients	Blinding of caregivers	Blinding of data collectors	Blinding of statistician	Blinding of outcome assessors	Incomplete outcome data (attrition bias)	Selective reporting (reporting bias)	Other bias
Agosta 2014	−	−	+	−	+	−	+	+	−	+
Bonní 2011	−	−	+	−	−	−	−	−	−	−
Cao 2016	−	−	+	−	−	−	−	−	−	−
Cazzoli 2012	−	−	+	+	+	−	+	−	−	−
Cazzoli 2015	−	−	+	−	−	−	−	−	−	−
Cha 2016	−	+	+	+	+	−	+	+	+	+
Fu 2015	+	+	+	+	+	−	+	+	+	+
Fu 2017	+	+	+	−	−	−	−	+	+	+
Hopfner 2015	−	−	+	−	−	−	−	+	+	+
Kim 2013	+	−	+	+	+	+	+	−	−	−
Ko 2008	−	−	+	+	+	−	+	+	+	+
Koch 2012	−	−	+	+	−	−	−	−	+	+
Làdavas 2015	−	−	+	+	+	−	+	+	−	−
Smit 2015	−	−	+	−	−	−	−	−	−	−
Sunwoo 2013	−	−	+	+	+	−	+	+	−	−
Yang 2015	−	−	+	−	+	−	+	+	+	+

FIGURE 2: Risk of bias assessment for RCTs and non-RCTs.

in overall USN measured by the Motor-Free Visual Perception Test at 1 Hz (SMD 1.46, 95% CI 0.73, 2.20; $p < 0.0001$; $I^2 = 0\%$), and the difference was not observed using 10 Hz (SMD 0.97, 95% CI −0.02, 1.96; $p = 0.06$; I^2 = not applicable) (Figure 7). Certainty in evidence was rated as moderate because of risk of bias due to the studies that were ranked as high risk of bias for both allocation sequence and allocation concealment (Figure 2).

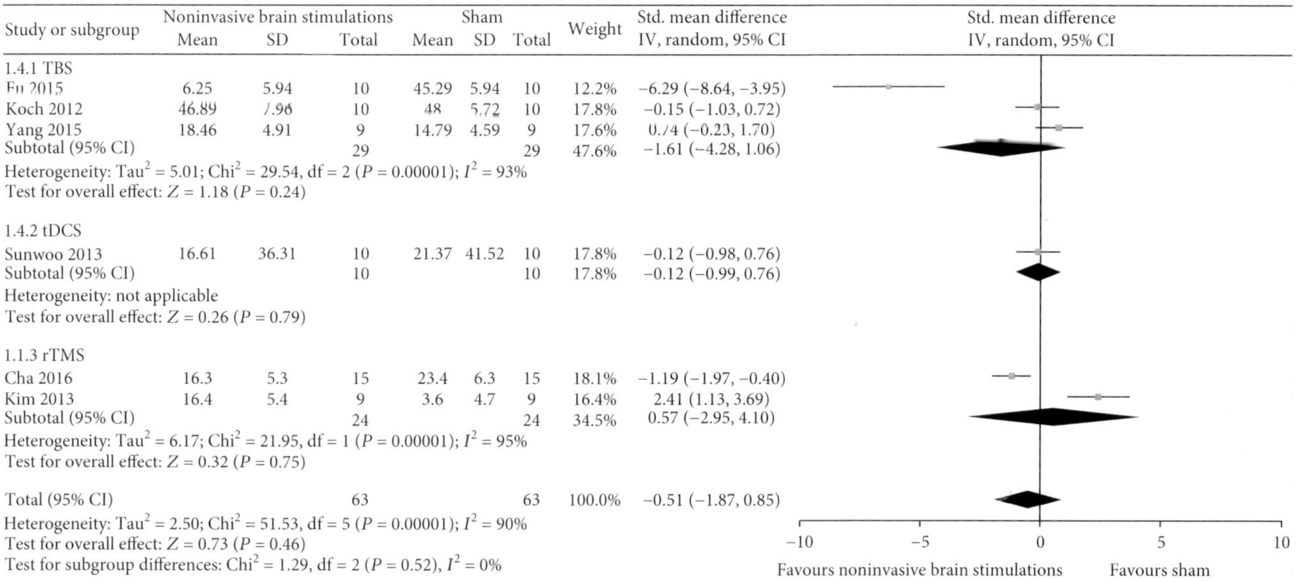

FIGURE 3: Meta-analysis of overall USN measured by the star cancellation test.

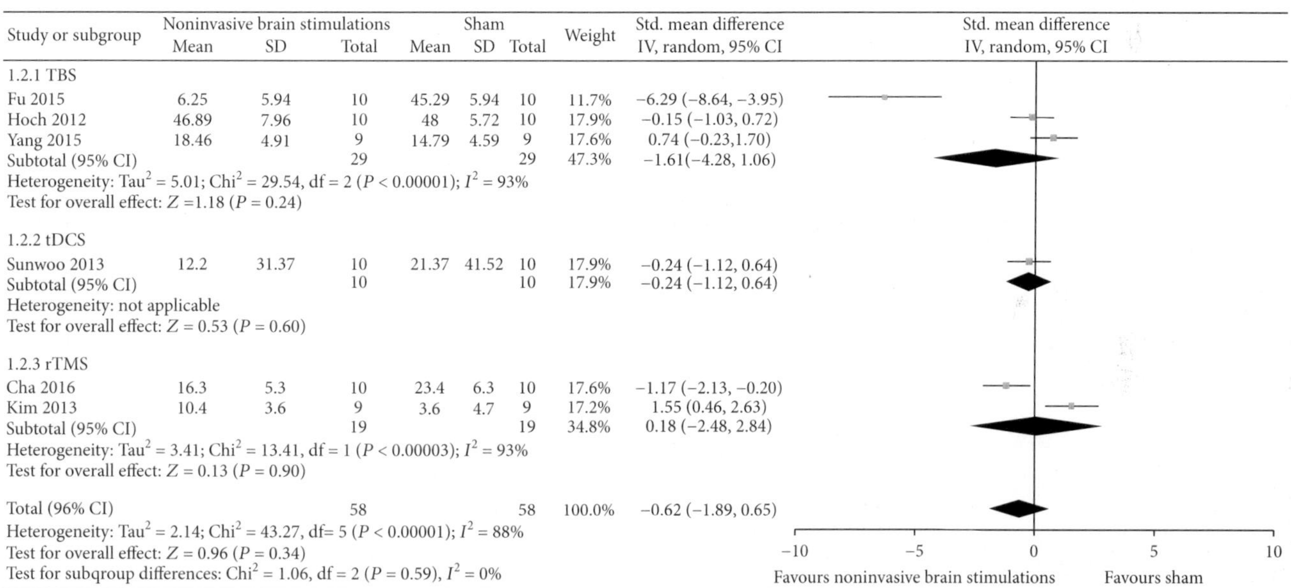

FIGURE 4: Sensitivity analysis of overall USN measured by the star cancellation test using TBS, single-mode tDCS, and 10 Hz rTMS.

(4) Overall USN Measured by Albert's Test and the Line Crossing Test. The results from two RCTs [51, 54] comparing noninvasive brain stimulations with sham failed to show a benefit in overall USN measured by Albert's test and the line crossing test (SMD 1.01, 95% CI −1.0, 3.02; $p = 0.32$; $I^2 = 90.2\%$) (Figure 8). However, in the subgroup analysis with the use of 1 Hz rTMS, we found a statistically significant difference compared to sham (SMD 2.04, 95% CI 1.14, 2.95; $p < 0.00001$; $I^2 =$ not applicable). Regarding the use of TBS, there was no benefit compared to sham (SMD −0.01, 95% CI −0.89, 0.87; $p = 0.98$; $I^2 =$ not applicable). Certainty in evidence was rated as low because of inconsistency and risk of bias due to the studies that were ranked as high risk of bias for both allocation sequence and allocation concealment (Figure 2).

(5) Other Outcomes: Daily Life Functions and Adverse Events. Only Kim et al. [53] reported on daily life functions with a higher mean in the 10 Hz rTMS group than in the sham and 1 Hz rMTS groups; however, there was only a statistically significant difference favoring the 10 Hz rTMS group compared to the sham group (SMD 1.83, 95% CI 0.68, 2.97; $p = 0.002$; $I^2 =$ not applicable). Làdavas et al.'s study [64] was the only study that reported on adverse events; no significant adverse effect of tDCS was reported, except only a few cases of minimal irritation of the skin beneath the electrodes.

None of the included studies reported on the following outcomes: neurological and functional disabilities, loss of balance, depression or anxiety and evaluation of poststroke fatigue, quality of life, and death.

Study or subgroup	Noninvasive brain stimulations Mean	SD	Total	Sham Mean	SD	Total	Weight	Std. mean difference IV, random, 95% CI
1.4.1 TBS								
Fu 2015	11.17	14.27	10	35.79	18.65	10	21.8%	−1.42 (−2.42, −0.42)
Yang 2015	22.36	5.31	9	54.12	6.76	10	15.2%	−4.96 (−6.94, −2.97)
Subtotal (95% CI)			19			20	36.9%	−3.08 (−6.54, 0.38)
Heterogeneity: $Tau^2 = 5.61$; $Chi^2 = 9.70$, df = 1 ($P = 0.002$); $I^2 = 90\%$								
Test for overall effect: $Z = 1.75$ ($P = 0.08$)								
1.3.2 tDCS								
Sunwoo 2013	7.05	7.45	10	14.27	12.85	10	22.4%	−0.66 (−1.56, 0.25)
Subtotal (95% CI)			10			10	22.4%	−0.66 (−1.56, 0.25)
Heterogeneity: not applicable								
Test for overall effect: $Z = 1.42$ ($P = 0.15$)								
1.3.3 rTMS								
Cha 2016	19.33	6.87	15	34.6	4	15	21.7%	−2.64 (−3.66, −1.63)
Kim 2013	−30	9.2	9	−8.3	4.2	9	19.0%	−2.89 (−4.30, −1.48)
Subtotal (95% CI)			24			24	40.7%	−2.73 (−3.55, −1.90)
Heterogeneity: $Tau^2 = 0.00$; $Chi^2 = 0.08$, df = 1 ($P = 0.78$); $I^2 = 0\%$								
Test for overall effect: $Z = 6.49$ ($P < 0.00001$)								
Total (95% CI)			53			54	100.0%	−2.33 (−3.54, −1.12)
Heterogeneity: $Tau^2 = 1.49$; $Chi^2 = 21.15$, df = 4 ($P = 0.0003$); $I^2 = 81\%$								
Test for overall effect: $Z = 3.77$ ($P = 0.0002$)								
Test for subgroup differences: $Chi^2 = 11.49$, df = 2 ($P = 0.003$), $I^2 = 82.6\%$								

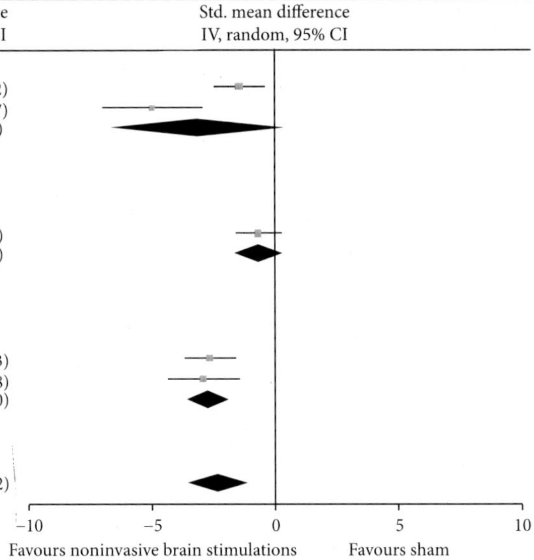

Figure 5: Meta-analysis of overall USN measured by the line bisection test.

Study or subgroup	Noninvasive brain stimulations Mean	SD	Total	Sham Mean	SD	Total	Weight	Std. mean difference IV, random, 95% CI
1.4.1 TBS								
Fu 2015	11.17	14.27	10	35.79	18.65	10	21.5%	−1.42 (−2.42, −0.42)
Yang 2015	22.36	5.31	9	54.12	6.76	10	16.1%	−4.96 (−6.94, −2.97)
Subtotal (95% CI)			19			20	37,6%	−3.08 (−6.54, 0.38)
Heterogeneity: $Tau^2 = 5.61$; $Chi^2 = 9.70$, df = 1 ($P = 0.002$); $I^2 = 90\%$								
Test for overall effect: $Z = 1.75$ ($P = 0.08$)								
1.4.2 tDCS								
Sunwoo 2013	10.4	9.64	10	14.27	12.85	10	22.1%	−0.33 (−1.21, 0.56)
Subtotal (95% CI)			10			10	22.1%	−0.33 (−1.21, 0.56)
Heterogeneity: not applicable								
Test for overall effect: $Z = 0.72$ ($P = 0.47$)								
1.4.3 rTMS								
Cha 2016	19.33	6.87	15	34.6	4	15	21.5%	−2.64 (−3.66, −1.63)
Kim 2013	−36,9	112	9	−8.3	4.2	9	18.8%	−3.22 (−4.73, −1.71)
Subtotal (95% CI)			24			24	40.3%	−2.82 (−3.66, −1.98)
Heterogeneity: $Tau^2 = 0.00$; $Chi^2 = 0.39$, df = 1 ($P = 0.53$); $I^2 = 0\%$								
Test for overall effect: $Z = 6{,}58$ ($P < 0.00001$)								
Total (95% CI)			58			58	100.0%	−2.35 (−3.72, −0.98)
Heterogeneity: $Tau^2 = 2.02$; $Chi^2 = 27.01$, df = 4 ($P < 0.0001$); $I^2 = 85\%$								
Test for overall effect: $Z = 3.35$ ($P < 0.0008$)								
Test for subqroup differences: $Chi^2 = 16.74$, df = 2 ($P = 0.0002$), $I^2 = 88.1\%$								

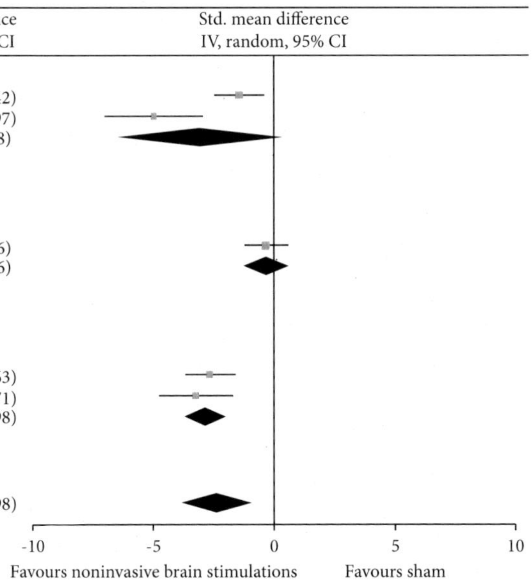

Figure 6: Sensitivity analysis of overall USN measured by the line bisection test using TBS, single-mode tDCS, and 10 Hz rTMS.

3.4.2. Synthesized Results from Non-RCTs. The non-RCTs did not report data in a usable way to allow for any statistical analysis.

4. Discussion

4.1. Main Findings. Based on pooled data from six randomized trials with 116 participants, we found evidence for a benefit in overall USN with noninvasive brain stimulation, especially with the use of rTMS in comparison to the sham (Figures 5, 7, and 8). The evidence is from moderate-quality evidence because of risk of bias due to the studies that were ranked as high risk of bias for both allocation sequence and allocation concealment (Figure 2). Non-RCT studies provided no evidence, suggesting that future trials should adhere to CONSORT guidelines to ensure clarity and reproducibility in the reporting of methods.

We presented the results of overall USN in a forest plot, which showed a statistically significant difference between the noninvasive brain stimulations and sham in the following tests: line bisection test, Motor-Free Visual Perception Test, and Albert's test and line crossing test. Nevertheless, the study also showed a nonsignificant difference between the noninvasive brain stimulations and sham on the star cancellation test.

Several noninvasive brain stimulations have been explored to determine whether some of these techniques might be useful in promoting recovery from USN after stroke. The lesion of the right parietal cortex after stroke causes disinhibition of the left hemisphere and thus a

Study or subgroup	Noninvasive brain stimulations Mean	SD	Total	Sham Mean	SD	Total	Weight	Std. mean difference IV, random, 95% CI
1.5.1 1Hz rTMS								
Cha 2016	21.6	4	10	16.9	2.1	10	53.8%	1.41 (0.41, 2.41)
Kim 2013	6.6	1.8	9	3.3	2.3	9	46.2%	1.52 (0.44, 2.60)
Subtotal (95% CI)			19			19	100.0%	1.46 (0.73, 2.20)
Heterogeneity: Tau^2 = 0.00; Chi^2 = 0.02, df = 1 (P = 0.88); I^2 = 0%								
Test for overall effect: Z = 3.89 (P = 0.0001)								
1.52 10Hz rTMS								
Cha 2016	21.6	4	10	16.9	2.1	10	49.4%	1.41 (0.41, 2.41)
Kim 2013	5.4	1.8	9	3.3	2.3	9	50.6%	0.97 (−0.02, 1.96)
Subtotal (95% CI)			19			19	100.0%	1.19 (0.48, 1.89)
Heterogeneity: Tau^2 = 0.00; Chi^2 = 0.38, df = 1 (P = 0.54); I^2 = 0%								
Test for overall effect: Z = 3.30 (P = 0.0010)								
Test for subgroup differences: Chi^2 = 0.28, df = 1 (P = 0.60), I^2 = 0%								

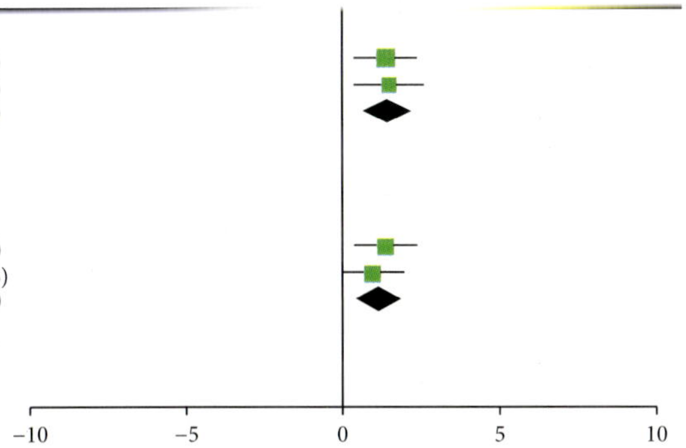

FIGURE 7: Meta-analysis of overall USN measured by the Motor-Free Visual Perception Test.

Study or subgroup	Noninvasive brain stimulations Mean	SD	Total	Sham Mean	SD	Total	Weight	Std. mean difference IV, random, 95% CI
1.6.1 TBS								
Koch 2012	35.44	1.01	10	35.45	0.65	10	50.2%	−0.01 (−0.89, 0.87)
Subtotal (95% CI)			10			10	50.2%	−0.01 (−0.89, 0.87)
Heterogeneity: not applicable								
Test for overall effect: Z = 0.03 (P = 0.98)								
1.6.2 rTMS								
Cha 2016	35.33	2.9	15	27.33	4.55	15	49.8%	2.04 (1.14, 2.95)
Subtotal (95% CI)			15			15	49.8%	2.04 (1.14, 2.95)
Heterogeneity: not applicable								
Test for overall effect: Z = 4.42 (P < 0.00001)								
Total (95% CI)			25			25	100.0%	1.01 (−1.00, 3.02)
Heterogeneity: Tau^2 = 1.90; Chi^2 = 10.19, df = 1 (P = 0.001); I^2 = 90%								
Test for overall effect: Z = 0.99 (P = 0.32)								
Test for subgroup differences: Chi^2 = 10.19, df = 1 (P = 0.001), I^2 = 90.2%								

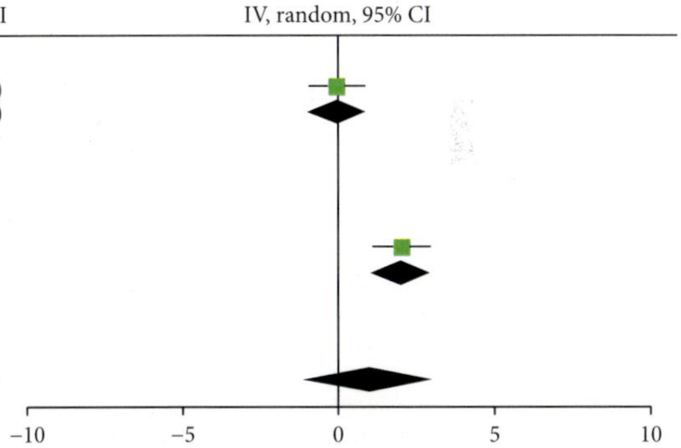

FIGURE 8: Meta-analysis of overall USN measured by Albert's test and the line crossing test.

pathological overactivation of the latter. This overactivation in the left depresses the neural activity by an increased inhibition on the right hemisphere, aggravating the perception. The rTMS can generate currents capable of depolarizing cortical neurons, and tDCS changes cortical activity by means of small electric currents and does not evoke action potentials. The tDCS has the advantage that the device is inexpensive, portable, and easy to use, but rTMS presented more activation of the neural network and induced a neuroplastic response for a long-term potentiation [65].

In three of four meta-analyses, rTMS was responsible for the improvement of overall USN, revealing that an electric current is an effective strategy for generating lasting promising effects in the brain. Unfortunately, we did not find any significant TBS or tDCS effects compared to sham procedures.

4.2. Strengths and Limitation. Strengths of our review include a comprehensive search; assessment of eligibility, risk of bias, and data abstraction independently and in duplicate; assessment of risk of bias that included a sensitivity analysis addressing loss to follow-up; and use of the GRADE approach for rating the certainty of evidence for each outcome (Table 3). Furthermore, there were no language restrictions, and translations of non-English trials were obtained whenever possible.

The primary limitation of our review is the low certainty consequent to study limitations. We identified a small number of RCTs with a modest number of participants resulting in wide confidence intervals. The total number of participants was relatively very low (RCTs $n = 278$, non-RCTs $n = 94$) due to the small sample sizes of individual trials, which led to downgrading the quality of evidence in some instances because underpowered trials are likely to have a greater degree of imprecision.

Moreover, selection bias and unblinding were substantial. Another limitation of this review was having an insufficient number of included studies to allow for the complete statistical analysis that we had planned. We were not able to assess publication bias because there were fewer than 10 eligible studies addressing the same outcome in a meta-analysis. We also planned to perform subgroup analyses according to the characteristics of stroke type, type of stimulation, type of frequency, and comparators (type of control intervention, i.e., pharmacological therapy versus nonpharmacological). However, we also were not able to conduct these analyses because they did not meet our minimal criteria, which was at least five studies available with at least two in each subgroup.

Although this review presents several limitations, the issue is whether one should dismiss these results entirely or consider them bearing in mind the limitations. The latter represents our view of the matter.

4.3. Relation to Prior Work. The research question we investigated in our review has been addressed before from different perspectives using our population of interest but with a different intervention (i.e., pharmacological intervention) [7] or investigating either the intervention or the control arms explored in this review but with a different population (e.g., idiopathic Parkinson's disease (IPD) [48], panic disorder in adults [66], or amyotrophic lateral sclerosis or motor neuron disease) [13].

Two Cochrane reviews [21, 49] evaluated the effect of tDCS in people after stroke but not in comparison with rTMS; instead, the authors compared tDCS with placebo, sham tDCS, no intervention, or conventional motor rehabilitation. The first review's [49] authors found evidence of effect regarding activities of daily living performance at the end of the intervention period and at the end of follow-up. However, the results did not persist in a sensitivity analysis including only trials of good methodological quality. In the second review [21], the authors found that there were no studies examining the effect of tDCS on cognition in stroke patients with aphasia.

Another Cochrane review [22] that addressed the use of rTMS compared to sham treatment or other conventional treatment for improving function after stroke revealed that rTMS treatment was not associated with improved activities of daily living, nor did it have a statistically significant effect on motor function.

Three additional Cochrane reviews also discussed the effects of both tDCS [48] and rTMS [13, 66] but in different populations—in Parkinsonism [48], in patients with amyotrophic lateral sclerosis or motor neuron disease [13], and in adults with panic disorder [66]. All reviews suffered from poor methodological quality, imprecision, and hence low confidence in the estimate of the true effect to draw a consistent conclusion on the effects of noninvasive brain stimulations.

4.4. Implications. Moderate-quality evidence shows that rTMS, at 1 Hz, is more efficacious than sham for unilateral spatial neglect after stroke measured by Motor-Free Visual Perception Test. Furthermore, low-quality evidence also suggests a benefit of noninvasive brain stimulation, particularly with the use of rTMS, for overall USN measured by the line bisection test, Albert's test, and the line crossing test. Future trials should adhere to CONSORT guidelines to ensure clarity and reproducibility in the reporting of methods [67].

Disclosure

The funding agencies played no role in conducting the research or preparing the manuscript.

Conflicts of Interest

The authors have no conflicts of interest.

Authors' Contributions

Flávio Taira Kashiwagi, Regina El Dib, Adriana Bastos Conforto, Gustavo José Luvizutto, and Rodrigo Bazan conceived the review. Erica Aranha Suzumura, Taís Regina da Silva, and Fernanda Cristina Winckler undertake searches. Huda Gomaa, Juli Thomaz de Souza, and Nermeen Gawish screened search results. Flávio Taira Kashiwagi, Regina El Dib, and Gustavo José Luvizutto organized the retrieval of papers. Flávio Taira Kashiwagi, Huda Gomaa, Nermeen Gawish, Erica Aranha Suzumura, Taís Regina da Silva, and Rodrigo Bazan helped in screening retrieved papers against inclusion criteria. Flávio Taira Kashiwagi, Huda Gomaa, Nermeen Gawish, Erica Aranha Suzumura, Taís Regina da Silva, Fernanda Cristina Winckler, Juli Thomaz de Souza, and Rodrigo Bazan appraised the quality of papers. Flávio Taira Kashiwagi, Erica Aranha Suzumura, Taís Regina da Silva, and Fernanda Cristina Winckler extracted data from the papers. Flávio Taira Kashiwagi, Huda Gomaa, Nermeen Gawish, and Erica Aranha Suzumura helped in writing to the authors of papers for additional information. Flávio Taira Kashiwagi, Gustavo José Luvizutto, Juli Thomaz de Souza, and Nermeen Gawish provided additional data about the papers. Flávio Taira Kashiwagi, Erica Aranha Suzumura, Taís Regina da Silva, Nermeen Gawish, and Huda Gomaa obtained and screened the data of unpublished studies. Flávio Taira Kashiwagi, Regina El Dib, Gustavo José Luvizutto, and Rodrigo Bazan managed the data for the review. Flávio Taira Kashiwagi, Regina El Dib, Erica Aranha Suzumura, Gustavo José Luvizutto, and Rodrigo Bazan entered the data into Review Manager (RevMan). Regina El Dib, Gustavo José Luvizutto, Adriana Bastos Conforto, and Rodrigo Bazan analyzed the RevMan statistical data. Flávio Taira Kashiwagi, Huda Gomaa, Nermeen Gawish, Erica Aranha Suzumura, Adriana Bastos Conforto, Gustavo José Luvizutto, Regina El Dib, and Rodrigo Bazan interpreted the data. Flávio Taira Kashiwagi, Regina El Dib, Huda Gomaa, Nermeen Gawish, Erica Aranha Suzumura, Gustavo José Luvizutto, and Rodrigo Bazan made statistical inferences. Flávio Taira Kashiwagi, Gustavo José Luvizutto, Regina El Dib, Erica Aranha Suzumura, and Rodrigo Bazan wrote the review. Flávio Taira Kashiwagi, Huda Gomaa, Nermeen Gawish, Erica Aranha Suzumura, Gustavo José Luvizutto, Adriana Bastos Conforto, and Rodrigo Bazan take the responsibility for reading and checking the review before submission.

Acknowledgments

The authors would like to acknowledge São Paulo Research Foundation (FAPESP) (2015/14231-0) and National Council for Scientific and Technological Development (CNPq) (423924/2016-8) for the grants and financial support.

References

[1] R. Bonita, "Epidemiology of stroke," *Lancet*, vol. 339, no. 8789, pp. 342–344, 1992.

[2] E. C. Jauch, J. L. Saver, Adams HP Jr et al., "Guidelines for the early management of patients with acute ischemic stroke: a

guideline for healthcare professionals from the American Heart Association/American Stroke Association," *Stroke*, vol. 44, no. 3, pp. 870–947, 2013.

[3] N. Gorgoraptis, Y. H. Mah, B. Machner et al., "The effects of the dopamine agonist rotigotine on hemispatial neglect following stroke," *Brain*, vol. 135, no. 8, pp. 2478–2491, 2012.

[4] P. Chen, K. Hreha, P. Fortis, K. M. Goedert, and A. M. Barrett, "Functional assessment of spatial neglect: a review of the Catherine Bergego scale and an introduction of the Kessler Foundation neglect assessment process," *Topics in Stroke Rehabilitation*, vol. 19, no. 5, pp. 423–435, 2012.

[5] S. P. Stone, P. W. Halligan, and R. J. Greenwood, "The incidence of neglect phenomena and related disorders in patients with an acute right or left hemisphere stroke," *Age and Ageing*, vol. 22, no. 1, pp. 46–52, 1993.

[6] M. Vanier, L. Gauthier, J. Lambert et al., "Evaluation of left visuospatial neglect: norms and discrimination power of two tests," *Neuropsychology*, vol. 4, no. 2, pp. 87–96, 1990.

[7] G. J. Luvizutto, R. Bazan, G. P. Braga et al., "Pharmacological interventions for unilateral spatial neglect after stroke," *Cochrane Database of Systematic Reviews*, vol. 1, no. 11, article CD010882, 2015.

[8] M. H. M. Tsang, K. H. Sze, and K. N. K. Fong, "Occupational therapy treatment with right half-field eye-patching for patients with subacute stroke and unilateral neglect: a randomised controlled trial," *Disability and Rehabilitation*, vol. 31, no. 8, pp. 630–637, 2009.

[9] H. Thieme, M. Bayn, M. Wurg, C. Zange, M. Pohl, and J. Behrens, "Mirror therapy for patients with severe arm paresis after stroke: a randomized controlled trial," *Clinical Rehabilitation*, vol. 27, no. 4, pp. 314–324, 2013.

[10] K. Mizuno, T. Tsuji, T. Takebayashi, T. Fujiwara, K. Hase, and M. Liu, "Prism adaptation therapy enhances rehabilitation of stroke patients with unilateral spatial neglect: a randomized, controlled trial," *Neurorehabilitation and Neural Repair*, vol. 25, no. 8, pp. 711–720, 2011.

[11] K. Polanowska, J. Seniów, E. Paprot, M. Leśniak, and A. Członkowska, "Left-hand somatosensory stimulation combined with visual scanning training in rehabilitation for post-stroke hemineglect: a randomised, double-blind study," *Neuropsychological Rehabilitation*, vol. 19, no. 3, pp. 364–382, 2009.

[12] A. Schröder, E. R. Wist, and V. Hömberg, "TENS and optokinetic stimulation in neglect therapy after cerebrovascular accident: a randomized controlled study," *European Journal of Neurology*, vol. 15, no. 9, pp. 922–927, 2008.

[13] J. Fang, M. Zhou, M. Yang, C. Zhu, L. He, and Cochrane Neuromuscular Group, "Repetitive transcranial magnetic stimulation for the treatment of amyotrophic lateral sclerosis or motor neuron disease," *Cochrane Database of Systematic Reviews*, vol. 1, no. 5, article CD008554, 2013.

[14] D. Cazzoli, R. M. Muri, R. Schumacher et al., "Theta burst stimulation reduces disability during the activities of daily living in spatial neglect," *Brain*, vol. 135, no. 11, pp. 3426–3439, 2012.

[15] J. Nakamura, Y. Kita, K. Ikuno, K. Kojima, Y. Okada, and K. Shomoto, "Influence of the stimulus parameters of galvanic vestibular stimulation on unilateral spatial neglect," *Neuroreport*, vol. 26, no. 8, pp. 462–466, 2015.

[16] M. F. Walker, A. Sunderland, J. Fletcher-Smith et al., "The DRESS trial: a feasibility randomized controlled trial of a neuropsychological approach to dressing therapy for stroke inpatients," *Clinical Rehabilitation*, vol. 26, no. 8, pp. 675–685, 2012.

[17] A. J. Turton, K. O'Leary, J. Gabb, R. Woodward, and I. D. Gilchrist, "A single blinded randomised controlled pilot trial of prism adaptation for improving self-care in stroke patients with neglect," *Neuropsychological Rehabilitation*, vol. 20, no. 2, pp. 180–196, 2010.

[18] M. A. Nitsche and W. Paulus, "Excitability changes induced in the human motor cortex by weak transcranial direct current stimulation," *The Journal of Physiology*, vol. 527, no. 3, pp. 633–639, 2000.

[19] L. J. Bindman, O. C. J. Lippold, and J. W. T. Redfearn, "The action of brief polarizing currents on the cerebral cortex of the rat (1) during current flow and (2) in the production of long-lasting after-effects," *The Journal of Physiology*, vol. 172, no. 3, pp. 369–382, 1964.

[20] D. A. Nowak, C. Grefkes, M. Ameli, and G. R. Fink, "Interhemispheric competition after stroke: brain stimulation to enhance recovery of function of the affected hand," *Neurorehabilitation and Neural Repair*, vol. 23, no. 7, pp. 641–656, 2009.

[21] B. Elsner, J. Kugler, M. Pohl, J. Mehrholz, and Cochrane Stroke Group, "Transcranial direct current stimulation (tDCS) for improving aphasia in patients with aphasia after stroke," *Cochrane Database of Systematic Reviews*, vol. 1, no. 5, article CD009760, 2015.

[22] Z. Hao, D. Wang, Y. Zeng, and M. Liu, "Repetitive transcranial magnetic stimulation for improving function after stroke," *Cochrane Database of Systematic Reviews*, vol. 1, no. 5, article CD008862, 2013.

[23] H. JPT, "Cochrane handbook for systematic reviews of interventions," *Version 5.1.0 The Cochrane Collaboration*2011, http://handbook-5-1.cochrane.org/.

[24] D. Moher, A. Liberati, J. Tetzlaff, D. G. Altman, and for the PRISMA Group, "Preferred reporting items for systematic reviews and meta-analyses: the PRISMA statement," *BMJ*, vol. 339, article b2535, 2009.

[25] D. F. Stroup, J. A. Berlin, S. C. Morton et al., "Meta-analysis of observational studies in epidemiology: a proposal for reporting. Meta-analysis of Observational Studies in Epidemiology (MOOSE) group," *Journal of the American Medical Association*, vol. 283, no. 15, pp. 2008–2012, 2000.

[26] M. L. Albert, "A simple test of visual neglect," *Neurology*, vol. 23, no. 6, pp. 658–664, 1973.

[27] T. Schenkenberg, D. C. Bradford, and E. T. Ajax, "Line bisection and unilateral visual neglect in patients with neurologic impairment," *Neurology*, vol. 30, no. 5, pp. 509–517, 1980.

[28] P. W. Halligan, J. P. Burn, J. C. Marshall, and D. T. Wade, "Visuo-spatial neglect: qualitative differences and laterality of cerebral lesion," *Journal of Neurology, Neurosurgery, and Psychiatry*, vol. 55, no. 11, pp. 1060–1068, 1992.

[29] P. Azouvi, S. Olivier, G. de Montety, C. Samuel, A. Louis-Dreyfus, and L. Tesio, "Behavioral assessment of unilateral neglect: study of the psychometric properties of the Catherine Bergego scale," *Archives of Physical Medicine and Rehabilitation*, vol. 84, no. 1, pp. 51–57, 2003.

[30] B. Wilson, J. Cockburn, and P. Halligan, "Development of a behavioral test of visuospatial neglect," *Archives of Physical Medicine and Rehabilitation*, vol. 68, no. 2, pp. 98–102, 1987.

[31] C. Cincura, O. M. Pontes-Neto, I. S. Neville et al., "Validation of the National Institutes of Health stroke scale, modified rankin scale and Barthel index in Brazil: the role of cultural adaptation and structured interviewing," *Cerebrovascular Diseases*, vol. 27, no. 2, pp. 119–122, 2009.

[32] V. Mathiowetz, G. Volland, N. Kashman, and K. Weber, "Adult norms for the box and block test of manual dexterity," *American Journal of Occupational Therapy*, vol. 39, no. 6, pp. 386–391, 1985.

[33] J. Sanford, J. Moreland, L. R. Swanson, P. W. Stratford, and C. Gowland, "Reliability of the Fugl-Meyer assessment for testing motor performance in patients following stroke," *Physical Therapy*, vol. 73, no. 7, pp. 447–454, 1993.

[34] J. M. Morse, C. Black, K. Oberle, and P. Donahue, "A prospective study to identify the fall-prone patient," *Social Science & Medicine*, vol. 28, no. 1, pp. 81–86, 1989.

[35] A. L. Hendrich, P. S. Bender, and A. Nyhuis, "Validation of the Hendrich II fall risk model: a large concurrent case/control study of hospitalized patients," *Applied Nursing Research*, vol. 16, no. 1, pp. 9–21, 2003.

[36] H. F. Mao, I. P. Hsueh, P. F. Tang, C. F. Sheu, and C. L. Hsieh, "Analysis and comparison of the psychometric properties of three balance measures for stroke patients," *Stroke*, vol. 33, no. 4, pp. 1022–1027, 2002.

[37] I. Aben, F. Verhey, R. Lousberg, J. Lodder, and A. Honig, "Validity of the Beck depression inventory, hospital anxiety and depression scale, SCL-90, and Hamilton depression rating scale as screening instruments for depression in stroke patients," *Psychosomatics*, vol. 43, no. 5, pp. 386–393, 2002.

[38] A. Lerdal and A. Kottorp, "Psychometric properties of the fatigue severity scale-Rasch analyses of individual responses in a Norwegian stroke cohort," *International Journal of Nursing Studies*, vol. 48, no. 10, pp. 1258–1265, 2011.

[39] J. P. T. Higgins, D. G. Altman, P. C. Gotzsche et al., "The Cochrane collaboration's tool for assessing risk of bias in randomised trials," *BMJ*, vol. 343, no. oct18 2, p. d5928, 2011.

[40] G. H. Guyatt and J. W. Busse, "Modification of Cochrane tool to assess risk of bias in randomized trials," http://distillercer.com/resources/.

[41] G. H. Guyatt, A. D. Oxman, G. Vist et al., "GRADE guidelines: 4. Rating the quality of evidence—study limitations (risk of bias)," *Journal of Clinical Epidemiology*, vol. 64, no. 4, pp. 407–415, 2011.

[42] G. H. Guyatt, A. D. Oxman, G. Vist et al., "GRADE guidelines: 5. Rating the quality of evidence—study limitations (risk of bias)," *Journal of Clinical Epidemiology*, vol. 64, no. 4, pp. 407–415, 2011.

[43] G. H. Guyatt, A. D. Oxman, R. Kunz et al., "GRADE guidelines 6. Rating the quality of evidence—imprecision," *Journal of Clinical Epidemiology*, vol. 64, no. 12, pp. 1283–1293, 2011.

[44] G. H. Guyatt, A. D. Oxman, R. Kunz et al., "GRADE guidelines: 7. Rating the quality of evidence—inconsistency," *Journal of Clinical Epidemiology*, vol. 64, no. 12, pp. 1294–1302, 2011.

[45] G. H. Guyatt, A. D. Oxman, R. Kunz et al., "GRADE guidelines: 8. Rating the quality of evidence—indirectness," *Journal of Clinical Epidemiology*, vol. 64, no. 12, pp. 1303–1310, 2011.

[46] G. H. Guyatt, A. D. Oxman, V. Montori et al., "GRADE guidelines: 5. Rating the quality of evidence—publication bias," *Journal of Clinical Epidemiology*, vol. 64, no. 12, pp. 1277–1282, 2011.

[47] The Cochrane Collaboration, *Review Manager (RevMan). 5.3.*, The Nordic Cochrane Centre, The Cochrane Collaboration, Copenhagen, Denmark, 2011.

[48] B. Elsner, J. Kugler, M. Pohl, and J. Mehrholz, "Transcranial direct current stimulation (tDCS) for idiopathic Parkinson's disease," *Cochrane Database of Systematic Reviews*, vol. 1, no. 7, article CD010916, 2016.

[49] B. Elsner, J. Kugler, M. Pohl, and J. Mehrholz, "Transcranial direct current stimulation (tDCS) for improving activities of daily living, and physical and cognitive functioning, in people after stroke," *Cochrane Database of Systematic Reviews*, vol. 1, no. 3, article CD009645, 2016.

[50] L. Cao, W. Fu, Y. Zhang et al., "Intermittent θ burst stimulation modulates resting-state functional connectivity in the attention network and promotes behavioral recovery in patients with visual spatial neglect," *Neuroreport*, vol. 27, no. 17, pp. 1261–1265, 2016.

[51] H. G. Cha and M. K. Kim, "Effects of repetitive transcranial magnetic stimulation on arm function and decreasing unilateral spatial neglect in subacute stroke: a randomized controlled trial," *Clinical Rehabilitation*, vol. 30, no. 7, pp. 649–656, 2016.

[52] W. Fu, W. Song, Y. Zhang et al., "Long-term effects of continuous theta-burst stimulation in visuospatial neglect," *The Journal of International Medical Research*, vol. 43, no. 2, pp. 196–203, 2015.

[53] B. R. Kim, M. H. Chun, D. Y. Kim, and S. J. Lee, "Effect of high- and low-frequency repetitive transcranial magnetic stimulation on visuospatial neglect in patients with acute stroke: a double-blind, sham-controlled trial," *Archives of Physical Medicine and Rehabilitation*, vol. 94, no. 5, pp. 803–807, 2013.

[54] G. Koch, S. Bonni, V. Giacobbe et al., "Theta-burst stimulation of the left hemisphere accelerates recovery of hemispatial neglect," *Neurology*, vol. 78, no. 1, pp. 24–30, 2012.

[55] W. Yang, T. T. Liu, X. B. Song et al., "Comparison of different stimulation parameters of repetitive transcranial magnetic stimulation for unilateral spatial neglect in stroke patients," *Journal of the Neurological Sciences*, vol. 359, no. 1-2, pp. 219–225, 2015.

[56] M. Smit, D. J. L. G. Schutter, T. C. W. Nijboer et al., "Transcranial direct current stimulation to the parietal cortex in hemispatial neglect: a feasibility study," *Neuropsychologia*, vol. 74, pp. 152–161, 2015.

[57] H. Sunwoo, Y. H. Kim, W. H. Chang, S. Noh, E. J. Kim, and M. H. Ko, "Effects of dual transcranial direct current stimulation on post-stroke unilateral visuospatial neglect," *Neuroscience Letters*, vol. 554, pp. 94–98, 2013.

[58] M. H. Ko, S. H. Han, S. H. Park, J. H. Seo, and Y. H. Kim, "Improvement of visual scanning after DC brain polarization of parietal cortex in stroke patients with spatial neglect," *Neuroscience Letters*, vol. 448, no. 2, pp. 171–174, 2008.

[59] G. Koch, S. Bonnì, V. Giacobbe et al., "Theta-burst stimulation of the left hemisphere accelerates recovery of hemispatial neglect," *Neurology*, vol. 78, no. 1, pp. 24–30, 2012.

[60] W. Fu, L. Cao, Y. Zhang et al., "Continuous theta-burst stimulation may improve visuospatial neglect via modulating the attention network: a randomized controlled study," *Topics in Stroke Rehabilitation*, vol. 24, no. 4, pp. 236–241, 2017.

[61] D. Cazzoli, C. R. Rosenthal, C. Kennard et al., "Theta burst stimulation improves overt visual search in spatial neglect

independently of attentional load," *Cortex*, vol. 73, pp. 317–329, 2015.

[62] S. Hopfner, D. Cazzoli, R. M. Müri et al., "Enhancing treatment effects by combining continuous theta burst stimulation with smooth pursuit training," *Neuropsychologia*, vol. 74, pp. 145–151, 2015.

[63] S. Agosta, F. Herpich, G. Miceli, F. Ferraro, and L. Battelli, "Contralesional rTMS relieves visual extinction in chronic stroke," *Neuropsychologia*, vol. 62, pp. 269–276, 2014.

[64] E. Làdavas, S. Giulietti, A. Avenanti et al., "A-tDCS on the ipsilesional parietal cortex boosts the effects of prism adaptation treatment in neglect," *Restorative Neurology and Neuroscience*, vol. 33, no. 5, pp. 647–662, 2015.

[65] R. M. Müri, D. Cazzoli, T. Nef, U. P. Mosimann, S. Hopfner, and T. Nyffeler, "Non-invasive brain stimulation in neglect rehabilitation: an update," *Frontiers in Human Neuroscience*, vol. 7, p. 248, 2013.

[66] H. Li, J. Wang, C. Li, and Z. Xiao, "Repetitive transcranial magnetic stimulation (rTMS) for panic disorder in adults," *Cochrane Database of Systematic Reviews*, vol. 1, no. 9, article CD009083, 2014.

[67] F. T. Kashiwagi, *Neon-invasive brain stimulations for unilateral spatial neglect after Strokestroke: a systematic review and meta-analysis of randomized and non-randomized controlled Trials. Dissertation [M.S. thesis]*, Botucatu Medical School, UNESP, 2003.

Permissions

All chapters in this book were first published in NP, by Hindawi Publishing Corporation; hereby published with permission under the Creative Commons Attribution License or equivalent. Every chapter published in this book has been scrutinized by our experts. Their significance has been extensively debated. The topics covered herein carry significant findings which will fuel the growth of the discipline. They may even be implemented as practical applications or may be referred to as a beginning point for another development.

The contributors of this book come from diverse backgrounds, making this book a truly international effort. This book will bring forth new frontiers with its revolutionizing research information and detailed analysis of the nascent developments around the world.

We would like to thank all the contributing authors for lending their expertise to make the book truly unique. They have played a crucial role in the development of this book. Without their invaluable contributions this book wouldn't have been possible. They have made vital efforts to compile up to date information on the varied aspects of this subject to make this book a valuable addition to the collection of many professionals and students.

This book was conceptualized with the vision of imparting up-to-date information and advanced data in this field. To ensure the same, a matchless editorial board was set up. Every individual on the board went through rigorous rounds of assessment to prove their worth. After which they invested a large part of their time researching and compiling the most relevant data for our readers.

The editorial board has been involved in producing this book since its inception. They have spent rigorous hours researching and exploring the diverse topics which have resulted in the successful publishing of this book. They have passed on their knowledge of decades through this book. To expedite this challenging task, the publisher supported the team at every step. A small team of assistant editors was also appointed to further simplify the editing procedure and attain best results for the readers.

Apart from the editorial board, the designing team has also invested a significant amount of their time in understanding the subject and creating the most relevant covers. They scrutinized every image to scout for the most suitable representation of the subject and create an appropriate cover for the book.

The publishing team has been an ardent support to the editorial, designing and production team. Their endless efforts to recruit the best for this project, has resulted in the accomplishment of this book. They are a veteran in the field of academics and their pool of knowledge is as vast as their experience in printing. Their expertise and guidance has proved useful at every step. Their uncompromising quality standards have made this book an exceptional effort. Their encouragement from time to time has been an inspiration for everyone.

The publisher and the editorial board hope that this book will prove to be a valuable piece of knowledge for researchers, students, practitioners and scholars across the globe.

List of Contributors

Najah Alhajri
Graduate Program in Rehabilitation Sciences, University of British Columbia, Vancouver, BC, Canada

Nicola J. Hodges
School of Kinesiology, Faculty of Education, University of British Columbia, Vancouver, BC, Canada

Jill G. Zwicker
Department of Occupational Science and Occupational Therapy, University of British Columbia, Vancouver, BC, Canada
BC Children's Hospital Research Institute, Vancouver, BC, Canada

Naznin Virji-Babul
Department of Physical Therapy, University of British Columbia, Vancouver, BC, Canada
Djavad Mowafaghian Centre for Brain Health, University of British Columbia, Vancouver, BC, Canada

Juan Du, Jingze Hu, Ling Liu, Minmin Ma, Gelin Xu, Xinfeng Liu and Fang Yang
Department of Neurology, Jinling Hospital, Nanjing University School of Medicine, Nanjing 210002, China

Qiang Xu, Qirui Zhang and Jianping Hu
Department of Medical Imaging, Jinling Hospital, Nanjing University School of Medicine, Nanjing 210002, China

Guangming Lu and Zhiqiang Zhang
Department of Medical Imaging, Jinling Hospital, Nanjing University School of Medicine, Nanjing 210002, China
State Key Laboratory of Analytical Chemistry for Life Science, Nanjing University, Nanjing 210002, China

Yong Zhang
MR Research, GE Healthcare, Shanghai 201203, China

Guangfei Li, Dan You, Jiaoyao Ma, Wen Li and Shan Sun
Key Laboratory of Hearing Medicine of NHFPC, ENT Institute and Otorhinolaryngology Department, Shanghai Engineering Research Centre of Cochlear Implant, Affiliated Eye and ENT Hospital, State Key Laboratory of Medical Neurobiology, Fudan University, Shanghai 200031, China

Huawei Li
Key Laboratory of Hearing Medicine of NHFPC, ENT Institute and Otorhinolaryngology Department, Shanghai Engineering Research Centre of Cochlear Implant, Affiliated Eye and ENT Hospital, State Key Laboratory of Medical Neurobiology, Fudan University, Shanghai 200031, China
Institutes of Biomedical Sciences and The Institutes of Brain Science and the Collaborative Innovation Center for Brain Science, Fudan University, Shanghai 200032, China

D. E. Johnson and A. Hudmon
Biochemistry and Molecular Biology, Stark Neuroscience Research Institute, Indiana University School of Medicine, Indianapolis, IN 46202, USA

Kateryna Pysanenko, Jiří Lindovský and Josef Syka
Department of Auditory Neuroscience, Institute of Experimental Medicine, Czech Academy of Sciences, Vídeňská 1083, 14220 Prague 4, Czech Republic

Zbyněk Bureš
Department of Auditory Neuroscience, Institute of Experimental Medicine, Czech Academy of Sciences, Vídeňská 1083, 14220 Prague 4, Czech Republic
Department of Technical Studies, College of Polytechnics, Tolstého 16, 58601 Jihlava, Czech Republic

Andrew Osborne
John van Geest Centre for Brain Repair, Department of Clinical Neurosciences, University of Cambridge, Cambridge, UK

Sara E. Ratican
John van Geest Centre for Brain Repair, Department of Clinical Neurosciences, University of Cambridge, Cambridge, UK
Geisel School of Medicine, Dartmouth College, Hanover, NH, USA

Keith R. Martin
John van Geest Centre for Brain Repair, Department of Clinical Neurosciences, University of Cambridge, Cambridge, UK
Eye Department, Addenbrooke's Hospital, Cambridge, UK
Cambridge NIHR Biomedical Research Centre, Cambridge, UK

Wellcome Trust-MRC Cambridge Stem Cell Institute, University of Cambridge, Cambridge, UK

Louise P. Kirsch
Social Brain in Action Laboratory, Wales Institute for Cognitive Neuroscience, School of Psychology, Bangor University, Bangor, UK
Research Department of Clinical, Educational, and Health Psychology, Division of Psychology and Language Sciences, Faculty of Brain Sciences, University College London, London, UK

Dilini K. Sumanapala
Social Brain in Action Laboratory, Wales Institute for Cognitive Neuroscience, School of Psychology, Bangor University, Bangor, UK
Centre for Brain and Cognitive Development, Birkbeck College, University of London, London, UK

Emily S. Cross
Social Brain in Action Laboratory, Wales Institute for Cognitive Neuroscience, School of Psychology, Bangor University, Bangor, UK
Institute of Neuroscience and Psychology and School of Psychology, University of Glasgow, Glasgow, UK

Nadine Diersch
Aging and Cognition Research Group, German Center for Neurodegenerative Diseases (DZNE), Magdeburg, Germany

Giuseppina Sgandurra, Elisa Sicola, Andrea Guzzetta and Giovanni Cioni
Department of Developmental Neuroscience, IRCCS Fondazione Stella Maris, Calambrone, Pisa, Italy
Department of Clinical and Experimental Medicine, University of Pisa, Pisa, Italy

Laura Biagi and Michela Tosetti
Laboratory of Medical Physics and Biotechnologies for Magnetic Resonance, IRCCS Fondazione Stella Maris, Calambrone, Pisa, Italy

Leonardo Fogassi
Department of Neuroscience, University of Parma and Istituto Italiano di Tecnologia (RTM), Parma, Italy

Adriano Ferrari
IRCCS S. Maria Nuova Hospital, Reggio Emilia, Italy
University of Modena and Reggio Emilia, Modena, Italy

Lauren M. DePoy
Department of Psychiatry, University of Pittsburgh School of Medicine, Pittsburgh, PA, USA

Colleen A. McClung and Ryan W. Logan
Department of Psychiatry, University of Pittsburgh School of Medicine, Pittsburgh, PA, USA
Translational Neuroscience Program, Department of Psychiatry, University of Pittsburgh School of Medicine, Pittsburgh, PA, USA
Center for Neuroscience, University of Pittsburgh, Pittsburgh, PA, USA
The Jackson Laboratory, Bar Harbor, ME, USA

Nicolás Meza-Concha, Marcelo Arancibia and Claudio Córdova
Laboratorio de Estructura y Función Celular, Escuela de Medicina, Facultad de Medicina, Universidad de Valparaíso, Hontaneda 2664, 2341386 Valparaíso, Chile

Ivanny Marchant and Pablo Olivero
Laboratorio de Estructura y Función Celular, Escuela de Medicina, Facultad de Medicina, Universidad de Valparaíso, Hontaneda 2664, 2341386 Valparaíso, Chile
Centro Interoperativo en Ciencias Odontológicas y Médicas, Universidad de Valparaíso, Valparaíso, Chile

Carlo Lozano
Laboratorio de Estructura y Función Celular, Escuela de Medicina, Facultad de Medicina, Universidad de Valparaíso, Hontaneda 2664, 2341386 Valparaíso, Chile
Centro Interoperativo en Ciencias Odontológicas y Médicas, Universidad de Valparaíso, Valparaíso, Chile
Servicio de Anatomía Patológica, Hospital Carlos van Buren, San Ignacio 725, Valparaíso, Chile

Wilfredo González-Arriagada
Centro Interoperativo en Ciencias Odontológicas y Médicas, Universidad de Valparaíso, Valparaíso, Chile
Patología y Diagnóstico Oral, Facultad de Odontología, Universidad de Valparaíso, Valparaíso, Chile

Ramón Sotomayor-Zárate,
Laboratorio de Neuroquímica y Neurofarmacología, Centro de Neurobiología y Fisiopatología Integrativa, Instituto de Fisiología, Facultad de Ciencias, Universidad de Valparaíso, Valparaíso, Chile

Ricardo Ramírez-Barrantes
Escuela de Tecnologia Medica, Universidad Andres Bello, Quillota 980, 2531015 Viña del Mar, Chile

Aiko K. Thompson
Department of Health Sciences and Research, College of Health Professions, Medical University of South Carolina, Charleston, SC 29425, USA

Briana M. Favale, Jacqueline Velez and Patricia Falivena
Helen Hayes Hospital, New York State Department of Health, West Haverstraw, New York City, NY 10993, USA

Efrat Shavit Stein and Avital Artan Furman
Department of Neurology, The Chaim Sheba Medical Center at Tel HaShomer, 52621 Ramat Gan, Israel

Valery Golderman, Joab Chapman and Marina Ben Shimon
Department of Neurology, The Chaim Sheba Medical Center at Tel HaShomer, 52621 Ramat Gan, Israel
Department of Neurology and Neurosurgery, Sackler Faculty of Medicine, Tel Aviv University, 6997801 Tel Aviv, Israel

Nicola Maggio
Department of Neurology, The Chaim Sheba Medical Center at Tel HaShomer, 52621 Ramat Gan, Israel
Department of Neurology and Neurosurgery, Sackler Faculty of Medicine, Tel Aviv University, 6997801 Tel Aviv, Israel
Talpiot Medical Leadership Program, The Chaim Sheba Medical Center at Tel HaShomer, 52621 Ramat Gan, Israel
Sagol School of Neuroscience, Tel Aviv University, 6997801 Tel Aviv, Israel

Krzysztof Miazga, Hanna Fabczak, Ewa Joachimiak, Małgorzata Zawadzka, Łucja Krzemień-Ojak, Marek Bekisz, Anna Bejrowska and Urszula Sławińska
Nencki Institute of Experimental Biology, Polish Academy of Sciences, Warsaw, Poland

Larry M. Jordan
Department of Physiology and Phatophysiology, University of Manitoba, Winnipeg, MB, Canada

Jack J. Q. Zhang and Kenneth N. K. Fong
Department of Rehabilitation Sciences, The Hong Kong Polytechnic University, Kowloon, Hong Kong

Nandana Welage and Karen P. Y. Liu
School of Science and Health, Western Sydney University, Penrith, NSW, Australia

Gerardo Bernabé Ramírez-Rodríguez, María del Ángel Ocaña-Fernández and Leonardo Ortiz-López
Laboratory of Neurogenesis, Division of Clinical Research, National Institute of Psychiatry "Ramón de la Fuente Muñiz", Calzada México-Xochimilco 101, 14370 Mexico City, Mexico

Peipei Li, Zongzhuang Wen, Guangkai Zhang, Aizhen Zhang, Xiaolong Fu and Jiangang Gao
School of Life Science, Shandong University, Jinan 250100, China

Jenna Bloemer, Priyanka D. Pinky and Manoj Govindarajulu
Department of Drug Discovery and Development, Auburn University, Auburn, AL, USA

Rajesh H. Amin, Timothy Moore, Muralikrishnan Dhanasekaran, Miranda N. Reed and Vishnu Suppiramaniam
Department of Drug Discovery and Development, Auburn University, Auburn, AL, USA
Center for Neuroscience, Auburn University, Auburn, AL, USA

Hao Hong
Department of Pharmacology, Key Laboratory of Neuropsychiatric Diseases, China Pharmaceutical University, Nanjing, China

Robert Judd
Department of Anatomy, Physiology and Pharmacology, College of Veterinary Medicine, Auburn University, Auburn, AL, USA

Xuan Xiong, Li-Na Zhu, Xiao-xiao Dong, Jun Yan and Ai-Guo Chen
College of Physical Education, Yangzhou University, Yangzhou, Jiangsu 225127, China

Wei Wang
Department of Medical Imaging, The Affiliated Hospital of Yangzhou University, Yangzhou University, Yangzhou, Jiangsu 225009, China

Flávio Taira Kashiwagi, Taís Regina da Silva, Fernanda Cristina Winckler and Rodrigo Bazan
Neurology Department, Botucatu Medical School, Universidade Estadual Paulista (UNESP), Botucatu, SP, Brazil

Regina El Dib and Juli Thomaz de Souza
Science and Technology Institute, Universidade Estadual Paulista (UNESP), São José dos Campos, SP, Brazil

Huda Gomaa and Nermeen Gawish
Department of Pharmacy, Tanta Chest Hospital, Tanta, Egypt

Erica Aranha Suzumura
Research Institute, Hospital do Coração (HCor), São Paulo, SP, Brazil

Adriana Bastos Conforto
Neurostimulation Laboratory, University of São Paulo (USP), São Paulo, SP, Brazil

Gustavo José Luvizutto
Department of Applied Physical Therapy, Federal University of Triângulo Mineiro (UFTM), Uberaba, MG, Brazil

Index